Psychiatry
in General
Medical Practice

Psychiatry in General Medical Practice

Gene Usdin, M.D.
Clinical Professor of Psychiatry
Louisiana State University
School of Medicine
President, American College of Psychiatrists

Jerry M. Lewis, M.D.
Psychiatrist-in-Chief
Timberlawn Psychiatric Hospital
Clinical Professor of Psychiatry
and Clinical Professor of Family
Practice and Community Medicine
University of Texas
Southwestern Medical School at Dallas

McGraw-Hill Book Company

New York St. Louis San Francisco Auckland Bogotá Düsseldorf
Johannesburg London Madrid Mexico Montreal New Delhi
Panama Paris São Paulo Singapore Sydney Tokyo Toronto

NOTICE

Medicine is an ever-changing science. As new research and clinical experience broaden our knowledge, changes in treatment and drug therapy are required. The editors and the publisher of this work have made every effort to ensure that the drug dosage schedules herein are accurate and in accord with the standards accepted at the time of publication. Readers are advised, however, to check the product information sheet included in the package of each drug they plan to administer to be certain that changes have not been made in the recommended dose or in the contraindications for administration. This recommendation is of particular importance in regard to new or infrequently used drugs.

PSYCHIATRY IN GENERAL MEDICAL PRACTICE

Copyright © 1979 by McGraw-Hill, Inc. All rights reserved. Printed in the United States of America. No part of this publication may be reproduced, stored in a retrieval system, or transmitted, in any form or by any means, electronic, mechanical, photocopying, recording, or otherwise, without the prior written permission of the publisher.

1 2 3 4 5 6 7 8 9 0 F G R F G R 7 8 3 2 1 0 9

Library of Congress Cataloging in Publication Data
Main entry under title:

Psychiatry in general medical practice.

    Includes bibliographical references and index.
    1. Psychiatry. 2. Sick—Psychology. 3. Family
medicine. I. Usdin, Gene L. II. Lewis, Jerry M.,
date   [DNLM: 1. Mental disorders. 2. Family
practice. WM100.3 P976]
RC454.P7825   616.8'9   78-24071
ISBN 0-07-066670-9

This book was set in English Times by Allen Wayne Technical Corp.
The editor was J. Dereck Jeffers;
the cover was designed by A Good Thing, Inc.;
the production supervisor was Milton J. Heiberg.
Fairfield Graphics was printer and binder.

To Cecile and Pat
We dedicate this effort
with and for love

6694

Contents

1

THE EVALUATION OF PATIENTS

2

CHILDREN AND ADOLESCENTS

3

PSYCHIATRIC SYNDROMES OF ADULTS

4

SPECIAL AREAS

5

TREATMENT

List of Contributors

RANSOM J. ARTHUR, M.D.
Professor and Associate Chairman, Department of Psychiatry and Director, Neuropsychiatric Hospital and Clinics, University of California at Los Angeles

JO ANN BROCKWAY, Ph.D.
Instructor (Psychology), Department of Rehabilitative Medicine, University of Washington School of Medicine, Seattle

ROBERT N. BUTLER, M.D.
Director, National Institute on Aging of the National Institutes of Health

DOYLE I. CARSON, M.D.
Medical Director, Timberlawn Psychiatric Hospital; Clinical Assistant Professor, Department of Psychiatry, University of Texas Southwestern Medical School at Dallas

ERIC J. CASSELL, M.D.
Clinical Professor of Public Health, Cornell University Medical College

WILLIAM C. DEMENT, M.D.
Professor of Psychiatry and Behavioral Sciences, Stanford University; Director, Stanford University Sleep Disorders Center; President, Association of Sleep Disorders Centers

JOHN DONNELLY, M.D.
Psychiatrist-in-Chief, Institute of Living, Hartford, Connecticut; Professor of Psychiatry, University of Connecticut School of Medicine; Past President, National Association of Private Psychiatric Hospitals

EVERETT P. DULIT, M.D.
Associate Clinical Professor, Cornell Medical College; Director, Adolescent Psychiatry, New York Hospital—Westchester Division

WILBERT E. FORDYCE, Ph.D.
Professor of Psychology, Department of Rehabilitative Medicine, University of Washington School of Medicine, Seattle; First Vice-President, American Congress of Rehabilitative Medicine

STEVEN R. FORNESS, Ed.D.
Professor in Residence and Special Education Director, Mental Retardation and Child Psychiatry Division, Neuropsychiatric Institute of the University of California at Los Angeles

SHERVERT H. FRAZIER, M.D.
Professor of Psychiatry, Harvard Medical School; Psychiatrist-in-Chief, McLean Hospital; Vice-President, World Psychiatric Association; Vice-President, American College of Psychiatrists; Past President, American Board of Psychiatry and Neurology

KENNETH O. JOBSON, M.D.
Clinical Assistant Professor of Psychiatry, University of Tennessee; Co-Director, Tennessee Psychiatric and Psychopharmacology Clinic

HELEN SINGER KAPLAN, M.D.
Associate Clinical Professor of Psychiatry, Cornell University Medical College; Director of the Human Sexuality Program at Payne-Whitney Clinic, New York Hospital

EDWARD KAUFMAN, M.D.
Associate Clinical Professor, Department of Psychiatry and Human Behavior, University of California, Irvine; Editor, American Journal of Alcohol and Drug Abuse

DONALD G. LANGSLEY, M.D.
Professor and Chairman, Department of Psychiatry, University of Cincinnati College of Medicine; Vice-President, American Psychiatric Association

JERRY M. LEWIS, M.D.
Psychiatrist-in-Chief, Timberlawn Psychiatric Hospital; Director of Research, Timberlawn Psychiatric Research Foundation; Clinical Professor of Psychiatry and Family Practice and Community Medicine, University of Texas Southwestern Medical School at Dallas

MORRIS A. LIPTON, M.D.
Professor of Biochemistry and Kenan Professor of Psychiatry, University of North Carolina School of Medicine, Chapel Hill; Director, Biological Sciences Research Center, Child Development Institute, University of North Carolina; Past President, American College of Neuropsychopharmacology

JUDD MARMOR, M.D.
Franz Alexander Professor of Psychiatry, University of Southern California School of Medicine; Past President, American Psychiatric Association; Past President, Group for the Advancement of Psychiatry

M. J. MARTIN, M.D.
Professor and Chairman, Department of Psychiatry and Psychology, Mayo Clinic and Mayo Medical School; Past President, American Academy of Psychosomatic Medicine

PETER A. MARTIN, M.D.
Clinical Professor of Psychiatry, University of Michigan and Wayne State University Medical Schools; Past President, American College of Psychiatrists

ROBERT MICHELS, M.D.
Barklie McKee Henry Professor of Psychiatry and Chairman of the Department of Psychiatry, Cornell University Medical College; Psychiatrist-in-Chief, The New York Hospital, Payne-Whitney Clinic and Westchester Division

CAROL C. NADELSON, M.D.
Associate Professor of Psychiatry, Harvard Medical School; Director of Medical Student Education in Psychiatry, Beth Israel Hospital

MALKAH T. NOTMAN, M.D.
Associate Clinical Professor of Psychiatry, Harvard Medical School; Liaison Psychiatrist with Obstetrics and Gynecology, Beth Israel Hospital

B. PERRY OTTENBERG, M.D.
Professor of Clinical Psychiatry, University of Pennsylvania Medical School; Senior Attending Psychiatrist, Institute of the Pennsylvania Hospital; Chairperson, Council on Emerging Issues of the American Psychiatric Association

E. MANSELL PATTISON, M.D.
Professor of Psychiatry and Human Behavior, Social Science, and Social Ecology; Acting Chairman, Department of Psychiatry and Human Behavior, University of California, Irvine

MICHAEL A. PERELMAN, Ph.D.
Director of Research, Human Sexuality Program, Payne-Whitney Clinic, The New York Hospital; Instructor in Psychiatry, Cornell University College of Medicine; Director of Training, Institute for Behavior Therapy, New York

CHESTER M. PIERCE, M.D.
Professor of Education and Psychiatry in the Faculty of Medicine and at the Graduate School of Education, Harvard University; President, American Board of Psychiatry and Neurology

JOHN J. SCHWAB, M.D.
Professor and Chairman, Department of Psychiatry, University of Louisville School of Medicine; Past President, American Academy of Psychosomatic Medicine; Past President, American Association for Social Psychiatry

A. C. ROBIN SKYNNER, F.R.C. Psych.
Chairman, Institute of Family Therapy (London); Senior Tutor in Psychotherapy, Institute of Psychiatry; Honorary Associate Consultant, the Bethlem Royal Hospital and the Maudsley Hospital, London

JOHN S. STRAUSS, M.D.
Professor of Psychiatry, Yale University School of Medicine; Director, Yale Psychiatric Institute

GEORGE TARJAN, M.D.
Professor of Psychiatry and Director, Mental Retardation and Child Psychiatry Division, University of California at Los Angeles Neuropsychiatric Institute; President, American Academy of Child Psychiatry; Past President, Group for the Advancement of Psychiatry

GENE USDIN, M.D.
Clinical Professor of Psychiatry, Louisiana State University School of Medicine, New Orleans; President, American College of Psychiatrists

HENRY H. WORK, M.D.
Clinical Professor of Psychiatry, George Washington University and Georgetown University Schools of Medicine; Deputy Medical Director, American Psychiatric Association

Foreword

This textbook attempts to reach the mainstream of general medical practitioners by avoiding exclusively humanistic or exclusively biomedical approaches. Usdin and Lewis have succeeded admirably in putting together a clinical approach that is both scientific and humanistic. Each chapter begins with an editors' introduction portraying dilemmas facing both the patient and the physician in the area covered in that chapter. These vignettes are poignant and empathic in conveying a painful dilemma or a disturbing feeling tone. Each author has gone beyond this humanistic approach in summarizing the relevant data.

　　Several chapters demonstrate the authors' extraordinary personal integration of psychiatry and medicine in such topics as "Reactions to Physical Illness and Hospitalization," "Physical Disease Manifesting as Psychiatric Disorders," "Chronic Pain and Its Management," and "Consultation from the Psychiatrist." Other chapters present a cogent summary of topics directly at the interface of medicine and general psychiatry including "Psychopharmacology," "The Response to Life Stress," "Alcohol and Drug Dependence," "The Geriatric Patient," "Diseases and Illnesses Specific to Women," "The Physician and the Treatment of Sexual Dysfunctions," "Disturbances of Intellectual Functioning," and "Psychosomatic Disturbances." Almost all the remaining chapters focus on problems for which psychiatrists assume significant clinical responsibility but in which general practitioners have a vital interest.

Observations repeated too frequently are often relegated to the soporific department of dusty archives. Occasionally, however, they are rescued by a sudden burst of clarity induced by a shift in understanding, attitudes, or behavior. In my judgment, such a burst of clarification is occurring with regard to observations on psychiatry's relationship to general medical practice.

It has often been stated that:

1 Patients with psychiatric problems constitute a major portion of the work load of those who are primarily engaged in general medical practice.

2 More patients with mental illness are treated by health professionals than by mental health professionals and it is highly likely that the health professionals will continue to retain this therapeutic responsibility.

While these words have been reiterated on many previous occasions, there are indications that the barriers to comprehension of their actual implications are being penetrated. This penetration is beginning to make an impact on the behavior of large numbers of general medical practitioners. Psychiatrists are also demonstrating behavioral changes that give evidence of their perception of these messages. The climate seems most suitable for renewed effort to improve the collaboration between psychiatrists and their colleagues in general medical practice. In helping to achieve this aim, this new textbook by Usdin and Lewis is most timely and pertinent.

Whether one prefers a term like the "remedicalization of psychiatry" or an appropriate analogue, a vigorous effort is now under way to help psychiatrists maintain and enrich their identification with the mainstream of medicine. Simultaneously there are new efforts being made to help general medical practitioners to realize how much of their work pertains to the care of patients with varying degrees and levels of psychiatric problems. In attempting to accomplish these goals, psychiatrists have utilized multiple approaches and perspectives. One commonly used technique in educational practice is to equate psychiatry with the humanistic approach to medical practice. The general medical practitioner is perceived from this perspective as being overly involved with instrumental tasks and thus losing sight of the patient as a human being. In this context, psychiatric education is aimed at broadening physicians' awareness and helping them to deal with patients' emotional problems in a more empathetic and helpful fashion. Conversely, other psychiatrist educators and authors have underemphasized or even eschewed the humanistic aspects of their skills and have stressed a fundamentally biological approach to psychiatry. Since physicians are perceived in this context to be receptive primarily to a biomedical model, it is argued that they will accept only organic theories of diseases and essentially somatic approaches to therapy.

There are serious flaws in both of these approaches. The exclusively humanistic approach denigrates the genuine scientific advances that have been accomplished within psychiatry. It often becomes exhortative, moralistic, and insensitive to the real world of the practitioner. Implicitly, it also tends to define the psychiatrist as an outsider who cannot empathize with the scientific flow of medical practice. The strong partisans of biological approaches also demonstrate several problems in dealing with colleagues in general medical practice. Equating science with that part of psychiatry dealing with somatic explanations and therapies can lead to a significant depreciation of psychosocial theory and practice. Furthermore, this approach underestimates the strong currents of humanistic concerns that permeate all aspects of medicine.

In addition to further integrating psychiatry into general medicine, Usdin and Lewis's textbook serves as an excellent update of recent data and practice. By recognizing the need for renewed efforts in the current context the authors have performed an important service for all physicians. Their particular blending of clinical humanism and scientific medicine points future practice in a direction that will do much to improve patient care.

Melvin Sabshin, M.D.

Preface

This textbook is written for medical students, residents in psychiatry, other physicians, and professionals from a variety of health care disciplines. To many in these groups, psychiatry may seem a confusing hinterland. This book is aimed at clarifying that which psychiatry may contribute to the treatment of patients who turn to physicians with a wide variety of symptoms, illnesses, and diseases. The emphasis is upon the expansion of the physician's knowledge of the role of emotional factors in those processes. It is through such knowledge that new skills may be acquired. The physician's increased capacity for helpfulness may, in turn, lead to greater satisfaction in the practice of medicine.

The experiential aspects of illness are a particular focus of this book. Each chapter is preceded by an "Editors' Introduction" that relates experiential factors to the particular topic of the chapter. What is it like to be delirious, housebound by phobias, severely compulsive, or acutely psychotic? If these syndromes seem rare in the practice of medicine, what about "everyday" events? To be 7 years of age and admitted to a general hospital? To have fever of unknown origin, a lump in the breast, or blood in the stool? To develop a variety of "physical" symptoms in the context of a dissolving marriage, a failing business, or a dying parent? This "What is it like to be sick?" emphasis is of increasing importance as medicine becomes more and more an applied technology. Psychiatry itself has witnessed an increasing emphasis on the neurosciences and, despite the importance and excitement of newer biologic research findings, the patient's experiencing of his or her illness must remain a pivotal point on which sensitive treatment is planned and effected.

We are convinced that such a psychiatric model of medical illness is appropriate because it places the patient and the patient's experiences at the core of medical practice. The emphasis is on viewing each patient as a person with unique feelings, thoughts, life experiences, developmental tasks, family support and strife, and personality strengths and weaknesses. Such an emphasis does not minimize the need to understand the physiochemical processes that have characterized advances in scientific medicine. It does mandate, however, that the physician be comfortable with biological, psychological, and sociological variables which, in concert, produce symptoms, illness, and disease. It stresses the commitment to explore and understand all these areas in the effort to be helpful. No single system of variables is assumed to be always primary, although for some patients treatment may be entirely biological, psychological, or sociological. For most patients, however, illness can best be understood and treated when seen as reflecting the interplay of all three systems of variables.

Readers will be challenged to use their personal feelings in dealing with patients suffering from both emotional and physical illnesses. Sensitive clinicians will recognize much of themselves in the thoughts, fears, hopes, and experiences of patients. In so doing, they may come to understand that what they feel is valuable data to be used in understanding the patient. This use of subjective data is counterbalanced by the traditional skills of detachment: the ability to step back from the patient and observe, hypothesize, and formulate a diagnosis and treatment plan. Both subjective and detached skills are necessary to a practice of medicine that is both scientific and humanistic.

Rather than narrowly prescribe a single model, we encouraged contributors to use their own style of teaching. This approach was made possible by the selection of contributors who are recognized authorities in their respective fields. Some of the contributors focused mainly on their own knowledge, skills, and publications, while others were more encyclopedic, referring to the work of others.

The book is divided into five parts. The first involves the evaluation of the patient and includes material regarding the family, reactions to illness and hospitalization, and the social issues that color and change the practice of medicine.

The second part focuses on children and adolescents and relates the common psychiatric syndromes of those age groups to the developmental tasks particular to each group.

The third part presents material that is useful for the recognition of the common psychiatric syndromes of adulthood.

Ten special areas comprise the fourth part, including chapters on problems faced by all physicians—pain, sleep disorders, psychosomatic conditions, alcoholism and the abuse of drugs, psychiatric emergencies, to name several.

These areas have been selected because of our belief that knowledge about them is crucial for the perceptive clinician.

The final part details the wide range of psychiatric treatments available to the physician.

We have tried, in particular, to be sensitive to the ways in which stereotyping can dehumanize, and have made a singular effort to avoid sexism. The use of trade names for the various drugs mentioned in the text has been avoided. Instead, an appendix lists the generic and trade names of drugs commonly used in psychiatry.

It is our hope that readers will find this book useful and that it will help them develop that balance of empathic compassion and detached scientific objectivity which both supports and heals. Patients are people, and their hopes, fears, families, and experiences are central to the process of both illness and recovery.

Gene Usdin
Jerry M. Lewis

Acknowledgments

Many individuals assist in the preparation of a textbook. Some read manuscripts, others track down obscure references, and still others offer encouragement when the going gets tough. To acknowledge each person who helped this volume come to life is impossible. Three persons, however, have made contributions that merit special mention: Our secretaries, Mrs. Cathy Culmone and Mrs. Nannette Bruchey, spent hundreds of hours typing, proofreading, telephoning, and doing all that was necessary to breathe life into the book—all the while maintaining grace and warmth, and Mrs. Virginia Austin Phillips, Senior Research Associate at the Timberlawn Psychiatric Research Foundation, offered both support and invaluable editorial advice.

In addition, we are grateful to Mr. J. Dereck Jeffers, Health Professions Division, McGraw-Hill Book Company, who invited us to develop this volume and who continued to encourage us in so many ways.

To these, and those not mentioned, we are truly grateful. Without you there might have been a book, but certainly not this one.

Gene Usdin
Jerry M. Lewis

Psychiatry in General Medical Practice

Part One

The Evaluation of Patients

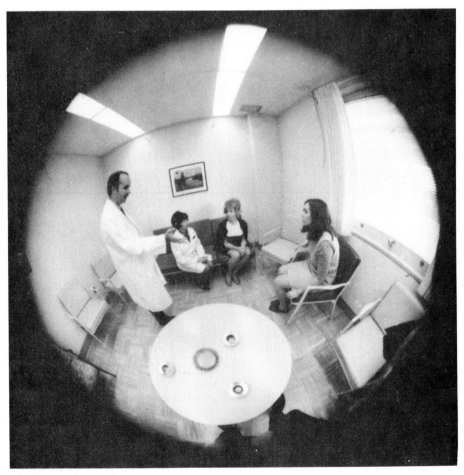

Courtesy of Van Bucher/Photo Researchers, Inc., NYC.

Chapter 1

Disease, Illness, and the Interview

Jerry M. Lewis, M.D.
Gene Usdin, M.D.

EDITORS' INTRODUCTION

An interview, unless rigidly structured, is for both participants an adventure whose outcome is unpredictable. Some interviews move quickly to a smoothly flowing, collaborative tempo; others fail to result in even a trace of human encounter. It is the encounter aspect of an interview that presents both soaring promise and frightening danger. The physician and patient come together primarily to deal with the patient's illness, but in the process the two individuals may achieve moments of closeness, empathy, and sharing. It is this possibility that can provide satisfaction or anxiety for both.

Consider for a moment the tremendous number of two-person interactions each carries as memories into the interview. Patient and physician bring with them bits and pieces of every important "interview" from the past. Being held by a loving mother, soft reprimands from a concerned father, frightening criticisms from a third-grade teacher, gentle suggestions from a loved clergyman, hostile beratings from a tough drill sergeant—all these and many more distant memory traces impinge upon the physician and patient as they face each other in the office or hospital. No wonder their dialogue may seem at first cautious, wary, formal, stilted—strangers from the past are there in the room.

Some data suggest that much of what is unspoken in our interviews involves each participant's concerns about how oneself is being perceived

3

and regarded by the other. No matter how secure or famous one may be it appears that face-to-face interchanges provoke many concerns about acceptability and worth.

It is easy for the physician to rely on a role—the "standard" inquiry that disregards, rather than searches for, the uniqueness of the other. He or she brings much from a personal past into the interview and is then confronted by a specific other, the patient, who has a distinct stimulus value. The aging woman who might be the physician's deceased mother, the sparkling 13-year-old who deeply underscores the physician's childless marriage—each patient brings something that has a personal impact on the physician. Somehow, through all of these currents beneath the surface, the wish to help, to heal, to use science to cure is a dominant force.

On the other side of the desk the patient reaches out for help, but so often the message is subtle, hidden, distorted. The physician may be seen as faithful friend, ultimate authority, censuring judge, scientific wizard, and more. Often the patient is very frightened of the lump, pain, blood, or whatever, and the physician may hardly be seen through this wall of fear.

Learning how to interview is no easy task. It is a very personal process to find the proper balance of detachment and empathy. It is, however, at the core of being a physician and is therefore best not left to the office secretary, nurse, or physician's assistant.

Physicians trained in the twentieth-century scientific tradition are apt to emphasize special examinations and laboratory procedures as the major approach to diagnosis and subsequent treatment of disease. This may lead a physician to treat only disease processes in organ systems rather than focusing on the specific patient's illness. The patient may, therefore, come to feel that the physician is more interested in disease than in people.

What a patient feels about the physician—what trust is put in the doctor's judgment—is determined by the relationship established between them. Crucial in determining the quality of the doctor-patient relationship is the initial interview, and particularly its structure. This chapter presents two decidedly different, but salient, forms of interviewing, and points out what indications there are for one or the other or perhaps both. This is not to minimize the importance of the physician's scientific knowledge of disease processes. Such knowledge alone, however, does not, by itself, make one a physician. To *be* a physician means much, much more.

Unfortunately, many medical schools pay scant attention to the teaching of interviewing skills. If a course in such skills is offered, it is usually taught in the psychiatric division, implying that the skills of interviewing are needed only in dealing with emotionally ill persons and are not germane to the diagnosis, treatment, and outcome of medical and surgical illnesses. An almost exclusive focus on disease, coupled with a teaching hospital's tendency to deal with unusual diseases, often leaves the student and house officer ill prepared to deal with more or less typical patients, their illnesses, their families, and their need for continuity of care over extended periods.

THE PATIENT, THE ILLNESS, AND THE DISEASE

Interviewing techniques or style must consider the obvious: one interviews patients according to a personal model of what a patient is and what illness is about. The rapid growth of scientific knowledge has led to the definition of disease in chemical and cellular terms, as if only symptoms that can be observed or related directly to underlying physiochemical processes are "real." Too often all else is considered either irrelevant or of minimal importance. It appears that medicine, in its focus on disease, has forgotten that patients are first and foremost people, who happen to be be experiencing illness. This is an oversight with many unfortunate consequences. Cassell defines the problem with eloquence: "The doctor sees his role as the curer of disease and 'forgets' his role as a healer of the sick, and patients wander disabled but without a culturally acceptable mantle of disease with which to clothe the nakedness of their pain."[1]

This distinction between disease and illness is at the root of much that is ailing medicine today in the sense that physicians often treat only the disease, thereby neglecting both the patient and the individual illness. A basic premise of this chapter is that treating only the disease, i.e., the underlying physiochemical processes, is inadequate for most patients. Such treatment can succeed only to the extent that the disease *is* the illness, and this situation is represented in only a relatively small fraction of the patients seen by physicians. What is needed is greater emphasis on a holistic approach to patients, without diminishing our attention to specific disease processes.

Mounting evidence suggests that illness must be understood from two broad perspectives: the adaptive consequences of the illness, and the illness behavior itself. For the most part, illness is not a random phenomenon. A large percentage of illness is concentrated in a small percentage of individuals. For many, illnesses tend to cluster in time. Difficult or stressful life disturbances, significant changes in one's life situation, and the loss of a loved one appear to render many individuals more vulnerable to all illness.[2,3,4,5,6] There may be ways of "being" a family—of communicating, loving, fighting, and meeting stress—that result in family members' being more or less vulnerable to illness. It appears, therefore, that the physician must focus on multiple factors in order to understand a given patient's illness, and must use this understanding in planning effective treatment.

Fabrega has pointed out the differences in illness models among various cultures.[7] In Western medicine, we tend to minimize the role of life circumstances, feelings, relationship patterns, and other experiential factors, and think narrowly of disease processes. Some cultures, however, accept life experiences as a usual, everyday part of their illness models. It is no surprise that cultures differ in their models of illness or that participants in a particular culture come to feel that their model is the "real," the "right," or the "true" one. Such participants attend only to data that fit into their model. Their way of interviewing and relating to patients searches specifically for the data that are congruent with their culture's model of illness and disregards the data that are not. To cite an example:

A 39-year-old executive was seen by a physician after he had complained of chest pain. The quality of the pain, plus changes in the electrocardiogram, led to the patient's hospitalization. The pain subsided shortly after his admission. There was no evidence of tissue damage, but coronary arteriography revealed evidence of significant multiple-vessel coronary atherosclerosis. The patient was given a low cholesterol diet, advised about a graduated exercise program, given a prescription for a vasodilator, and discharged from the hospital, to be seen in a few weeks as an outpatient.

No specific effort was made by the patient's physician to deal with anything other than the underlying coronary artery disease. If such an effort had been made, the following data might have been elicited: the patient was tense, hard-driving, and overly perfectionist. Three weeks prior to his episode of chest pain, he had received word that his mother had developed a recurrence of a malignancy. Recent confrontations with his teenage daughter about "the company she kept" and her drug use had led to almost total estrangement. Two weeks before the chest pain, he had been offered a major promotion entailing new responsibilities which would involve a greatly increased travel schedule. His wife, who was obese and was taking mild tranquilizers, was upset by the possibility of his traveling more. She had urged him to consider his responsibilities to her and to their children, and decline the promotion. Worried about his mother, concerned about his relationships with his wife and daughter, the patient found himself increasingly tense, insomniac, and conflicted. In this setting, chest pain developed.

The patient's disease was clearly coronary atherosclerosis, but what was his illness? Did it involve his relationship with his mother and the threat of her death, his sense of responsibility to and conflicts with his wife and children, his ambition, his drive for success, his hopes and fears?

Our basic contention is that these factors were very much a part of the man's illness. They would not, however, be present as clinical data unless the physician-patient relationship had encouraged their exploration. Although some physicians are beginning to understand the profound and unique significance of such factors to the individual patient, many are not. The reasons for the failure are multiple, but the narrow Western model of disease is a principal consideration. Our increasing concern with physiochemical processes and their measurement influences the way we relate to, and communicate with, patients. Too frequently, the way we interview a patient may exclude data crucial to a broader understanding of the illness involved.

A second issue is that of illness behavior. Cassell has written about the more or less inevitable consequences of becoming ill, and suggests that illness precipitates four responses that in turn become part of the illness.[1] These include (1) a feeling of disconnectedness which may range from a modest sense of alienation from one's usual supportive interpersonal networks to a profound sense of loss of connection and hopelessness; (2) loss of a sense of indestructibility, the importance of which is reflected in how far many patients go to deny, in the face of overwhelming symptomatology, that they are ill; (3) a disturbance in the patient's capacity to think rationally about his or her illness; and (4) the patient's feeling of having lost control of one's own world, perhaps the most distressing consequence of all. These four responses vary with the severity of the illness, the patient's personality, the idiosyncratic "meaning" of the illness, and the setting in which the illness occurs. The sensitive physician is, intuitively or otherwise, aware of the presence of these disturbances and uses this awareness in whatever ways seem helpful to a particular patient. From the standpoint of interviewing techniques, the physician must realize that certain approaches to interviewing encourage the patient to share and explore these crucial experiential aspects of illness with the doctor, and other approaches discourage such explorations.

In short, unless the physician understands that life experiences may play a precipitating role in all illnesses, and that there are significant disturbances in feelings and thoughts associated with most episodes of illness, he or she will not consider it important to explore these areas with patients. This may lead to less than adequate treatment for the patient and a corresponding feeling that the doctor is not interested. Indeed, "my doctor doesn't listen to me" is one of the most frequent complaints patients have.

Even if the physician's model of illness does include the roles of life experiences, feelings, and interpersonal relationships as important parts of illness, the interviewing techniques learned in training often are not adequate to help the patient express and explore these feelings and relationships. Most learning about interviewing is influenced by the question book medical students receive, which presents the numerous areas in which the student must seek specific information. "Have you ever fainted?" "Has any member of your family had diabetes?" "Do you have chest pain?" This review of body systems and family history is an indispensable part of a thorough patient evaluation. It is, and should be, a part of the physician's basic approach to data collection. Unfortunately, however, it is not designed to encourage the patient's sharing with the doctor the fears, hopes, and experiences that are so much a part of illness. To rely solely on the traditional form of interviewing, which is primarily *directive,* may prevent those underlying features of illness from surfacing. For this reason, this chapter will emphasize a less directive form of interviewing, *collaborative exploration.* Both styles of interviewing are useful and have a place in a physician's approach to patients. Before they are discussed, however, there are some more general considerations that merit attention.

GENERAL PRINCIPLES OF INTERVIEWING

A patient needs to feel that the doctor is interested and concerned. This important aspect of the doctor-patient relationship is so fundamental that it is taken for granted, but it may be useful to ask how interest and concern are communicated in any interpersonal relationship. First, there is the matter of the quality of the time spent together. The *quantity* of time may vary from several minutes to much longer, but the *quality* of time must be unhurried. One does not feel another's interest and concern if the other appears anxious to leave. "From the moment I enter the office, my doctor seems to be in a hurry to get rid of me," one patient indicated. Another expressed the same feeling by saying, "My doctor's always looking at the time; she seems to be bored with me." Most physicians are busy and have limits on the amount of time they can spend with each patient. Yet some are able to communicate an unhurried sense of being with the patient, even though the actual duration of the visit may be no longer than a visit with a hurried-appearing physician.

A second characteristic of caring involves the level of the physician's attention. Does he or she maintain eye contact, listen carefully, and acknowledge, by word or gesture, hearing what the patient says? How often a patient says that the doctor never looks at him or her, seems preoccupied with the chart, and rarely acts as if what the patient is saying has been heard or understood.

Then there is the matter of the doctor's warmth. This, too, engenders a cared-about feeling in the patient. Many physicians have grave reservations about expressing their warmth, and strive to maintain a cool, remote, or detached demeanor. The assumption is that professionalism involves maintaining great distance from the patient. Such physicians voice the fear that not maintaining great interpersonal distance will end their capacity for detached objectivity. There is a need, of course, for a detached and analytic appraisal of the patient's illness, but this does not mean that a physician should eliminate warmth and caring in relating to patients. Actually, these two aspects of relating to patients, the empathic and the objective, are central qualities of a good interview and vary from moment to moment. Perhaps they can best be thought of as attitudes the physician has toward the patient. The patient needs to experience both capacities of the physician: the warm and caring human being as well as the skilled expert able to decipher and give meaning to illness.

The physician may need to maintain or increase interpersonal distance from the patient when something about the patient precipitates the physician's anxiety. Perhaps an elderly, dying patient evokes memories of the death of the physician's parent; the childlike behavior of a particularly helpless patient may cause discomfort; an attractive patient of the opposite sex may stimulate sexual fantasies. Each physician is vulnerable to anxiety, and for some the response to anxiety is to become increasingly distant. This may be interpreted by the patient as a lack of caring.

None of what has been said about the physician's capacity to relate to the patient with warmth and caring is meant to suggest being artificial. Personalities and styles vary, and each physician will have a personal way of communicating. What is important is to recognize the patient's worries, fears, and confusion about the illness, and the consequent need to feel protected. The physician should not deliberately adopt a distant, remote, "professional" role unless there are clear signals that the patient is more comfortable with such distance. Most patients need evidence of the doctor's caring, and most doctors come to care about patients once they get to know them.

Another factor is the physician's capacity for tenderness. Tenderness involves not only the minimizing of physical pain, but also the sensitivity to emotional distress. Tenderness is usually thought of purely in relation to the physical examination, but it is also an essential factor in the interview. In both situations, it is the way in which the physician communicates an intent to minimize hurt for the patient. Just as the palpatation of the abdomen can be painful, certain feelings and experiences can be painful for patients to discuss. Just as there are varied approaches to examining a physically painful area, there are varied approaches to helping a patient discuss the death of a family member or a painful event of any kind. The responsible physician recognizes these areas and, if it seems important to explore them, proceeds with gentleness. Likewise, there are symptoms, signs, or indications that a particular area (physical or emotional) cannot yet be explored without doing harm.

These factors do not exhaust the list of interview variables that determine the style of the interview. Whether a directive or exploratory approach is being used, the physician is obligated to accept the patient compassionately and humanely. The physician's scientific knowledge about disease processes does not lessen this obligation, but rather increases it.

The study of interpersonal communication patterns provides a mechanism for comparing and contrasting different interviewing styles. Several patterns are helpful to the reader in distinguishing between directive interviewing and collaborative exploration: (1) the source of the interview's flow, which is a reflection of who controls the interview; (2) the techniques the physician uses to accomplish the type of interview felt appropriate for a given patient with a given illness; (3) the objective goal of the interview; and (4) the physician's model of illness that is stated implicitly in the style of the interview.

Let us now turn to directive interviewing because most physicians are more familiar with this approach, and it is the only way many of them interview patients.

Directive Interviewing

The term *directive* is used for interviews in which the physician controls the direction through asking direct questions, thus dominating the interaction between doctor and patient. This happens despite the fact that the patient's answer to a given question influences, to some degree, the nature of the physician's next question. Major changes in the direction of the interview most often come from the physician.

In directive interviewing, the physician clearly assumes the role of expert and, in this sense, is the more powerful. The inferred statement is, "I know what questions to ask, and if you will only answer my questions to the best of your ability I will arrive at the correct diagnosis." A patient's attempt to share something felt to be important may be treated by the doctor as irrelevant. The questions of the physician tend to become more and more focused as the interview proceeds. "Do you have pain in the chest?" may soon be followed by "Is it burning or pressing?", a move in the direction of a more narrow focus.

As a consequence of this basic pattern, the physician talks a great deal, and this is reflected in the cadence of the interview: *Dr.* _____, *Patient*_____, *Dr.* _____, *Patient*_____ is a frequent style of verbal activity. Even when the physician's level of warmth is high, this type of interview is not conducive to a particularly close relationship; interpersonal distance is great, in part because the balance of power between doctor and patient is so unequal.

The object of this type of interviewing is to clarify the nature of the patient's symptoms. By clearly defining the qualities of a given symptom ("pressing or burning?" "dull or sharp?" "seconds or minutes?"), and its correlates ("before or after meals?" "with exertion or at rest?" "when recumbent or standing?"), the physician is accumulating data for a hypothesis about a specific underlying disease. These data, along with the results of the physical examination, special examinations, and laboratory studies, lead to understanding the pathology on which specific treatment will be based. Nonresponsive remarks are considered extraneous and the physician may feel annoyed that the cadence is interrupted, yet the nonresponsive remarks may signal a crucial area warranting exploration.

The physician's model of the patient and illness in this type of interview would appear to be one of pure disease in the sense that minimal effort is exerted to elicit information about the patient as a specific person, a unique human being with fears and hopes, with both past and present life circumstances.

The structure and techniques of directive interviewing are well known. This type of interview is not only characteristic of the practice of medicine, but also of many other professional relationships (i.e., teacher-student, lawyer-client). It is a central part of the doctor's approach to the patient. The point to be emphasized, however, is that if the directive approach is the doctor's *only* interviewing technique, many crucial features of the individual and the illness will not be detected and consequently not understood.

Collaborative Exploration

With collaborative exploration the approach is much less directive in that the physician simply attempts to facilitate the patient's spontaneous flow of conversation. The physician's major responsibility is to listen intently to what the patient says. The flow of the interview should come from the patient's thoughts and feelings, which then determine the direction of the interview. The physician shares with the patient the responsibility of directing the flow; hence, their interaction is seen as collaborative. The physician asks few direct and focused questions, but attempts instead to encourage the patient's continued communication through reflections, general requests for more information, empathic statements, and brief summaries. In this type of interview, it is the patient who talks a lot: *Dr.*_____, *Patient* _____, *Dr.*_____, *Patient*_____.

Reflections are restatements of what the patient has said, often in question form: "You say it was after your husband's death that the pain began?" "The fatigue is often worse in the morning?" Frequently the physician merely paraphrases the patient's statements. Essentially the patient is encouraged to elaborate.

General requests for more information take many forms: "Tell me more." "Help me to understand that better." "Do you have any idea why?" "Please go on.'' The important aspect of this form of facilitation is that the physician does not direct the patient to a very narrow and focused area of the physician's own interest, but encourages the data to evolve from the patient.

At times the patient grows quiet, and during such pauses the physician may summarize briefly what the patient has said. ''Well, let's see, you said that several months ago the pain in your joint became worse. About that time your husband got a promotion and your youngest child left for college?'' Often, the patient will continue or, at times, move off in another direction.

Empathy can be defined in different ways, but for our purposes can be thought of as a sensitivity to what the patient is feeling (along with some type of communication that lets the patient know that one is aware of those feelings). ''You seem sad.'' ''I sense that you're feeling pretty overwhelmed by all of this.'' ''At times like that you feel both hopeless and angry.'' Empathy also can be communicated by a look, a shrug, or a movement. It is not only the foundation of most helping relationships, but for many it is the strongest invitation to further self-exploration. It leads to a deep sense that another person is really with you, understands, and may provide you with the support to reveal previously hidden feelings. It is the essence of most helpful relationships.

Unless physicians are taught specifically about empathy, they may come away from medical training with the feeling that they must always communicate a sense of ''objectivity'' that disregards the patient's feelings. While some physicians grow up in families with high empathy levels and seem to be very empathic naturally, others do not have this natural ability, and there may be little in their medical education to help them develop or even be aware of the importance of such skills.

In talking about empathy, physicians often emphasize that one must not lose objectivity. That is, of course, true, and in certain situations we can overidentify and become overinvolved with patients. A skill central to the physician as interviewer, however, is to combine both empathy and objectivity, to be able to shift from one to the other many times in the course of a single interview. It is this capacity for switching back and forth that is both a challenge to, and the hallmark of, the skillful physician interviewer.

The physician involved in this type of interviewing listens very intently. What is he or she listening for? Primarily, the physician notes the flow of the patient's feelings and thoughts, and the ways in which these seem to be associated or connected. The physician particularly attends to the verbal or nonverbal communication of feelings, but notes even more; e.g., when the patient grows silent, and what thoughts precede the silence. The physician observes changes in the intensity and rate of the patient's speech, notes the patient's posture and bodily movements, and is sensitive to unusual word choices and other presumptive evidence of conflict and anxiety.

A major difference between collaborative and directive approaches to interviewing is the focus of the physician's attention. In directive interviewing, the physician concentrates almost entirely on the patient's answers to questions. In collaborative exploration, the physician notes not only the verbal and nonverbal behavior of the patient, but also clues from within the physician (difficulty with attention, feelings, thoughts unrelated to the patient), and the nature of the interaction between the patient and the physician. By allowing and encouraging awareness of his or her own personal feelings the physician may become a responsive instrument. If, for example, the patient describes a particular event and does not appear to express associated feelings, the physician may relate to it through some inner personal feeling such as anger, sadness, or fear. Such personal feelings can be used to understand what the patient is feeling or may be struggling to avoid. The astute physician may realize that the patient is depressed, for example, when the physician feels brief melancholy.

The physician should always be aware of his or her impact on the patient's behavior in both directive interviewing and collaborative exploration. Perhaps it is more important in the latter technique because the physician will attach more significance to the patient's flow of associations and feelings. If, for example, the physician has a formal office with only straight-back chairs and sits behind the desk in a stiff way, speaking precise English, a distinct tone may be set as to acceptable feelings and behavior. For the physician to then note that the patient seems unable to relax and is tense or rigid is to label as pathological the very behavior that the physician has invited.

What to do with all these observations? Very little in an overt or expressive way. Certainly one does not make deep interpretations of what is wrong. However, the physician lets the patient know that he or she has been heard and, to some degree, understood. Of great importance is the fact that the physician has accumulated valuable data about the patient's feelings and life circumstances, data which offer crucial insights about the individual and the illness. The patient, in turn, is more apt to feel that the physician is interested in him or her as a person.

In addition to the influences of the narrow Western model of disease, other factors may cause many physicians to rely on directive interviewing only. One concern is what to do with the data elicited during collaborative exploration. Many physicians feel that once they have heard about the patient's fears, hopes, feelings, and life circumstances, they somehow become responsible for them and must find a solution, a cure of sorts. Nothing could be farther from the truth. First, most patients only need to be heard. The relief that can result from simply venting feelings is often surprising. Patients struggling with complex life situations can be helped to explore their options. Decision making, except in rare situations, must be left in the patient's hands. It is important for physicians to understand that collaborative exploration may lead to a patient-physician relationship in which responsibility is shared rather than assumed entirely by the physician.

Another factor involves the tendency of faculty members in medical schools and training programs to discourage students from reporting the experiential aspects of their patients' illnesses. How many medical students, for example, have been told that the type of understanding discussed here is irrevelant "for the management of the disease?"

Some physicians have developed a natural ability for collaborative interviewing. Others, even when they have been exposed to both styles, feel more comfortable with the more controlled directive interviewing. This can happen even in cases where physicians understand the advantage of having both styles as part of their approach to patients; they, too, are products of their own past life experiences, and are unable or unwilling to change.

SELECTING THE RIGHT APPROACH

Both directive and collaborative styles are useful in interviewing most patients. If patients are seen by a number of specialists, one needs to be clearly designated as the primary physician. Usually, this will be the family doctor, the internist, or the pediatrician. Each patient deserves to have one physician who knows him or her as a person, and who will direct all treatment in a way that is influenced by such knowledge.

How does the physician use these two different interviewing styles? The answer is that *context* determines the sequence and emphasis placed upon these two different approaches. Clearly, the patient's condition demands a symptom-oriented directive interviewing approach in some situations. This is so particularly when the complaint presented necessitates urgent treatment. The physician's primary responsibility is to move quickly and directly if the presenting complaint suggests a medical emergency.

A second but less urgent indication for a directive interviewing approach is illustrated by the patient who presents an isolated symptom, such as a sore throat or pain in one joint. Here a series of focused questions aimed at clarification of the symptom and its correlates is the most reasonable approach. In such instances, the physician should consider following the directive interview with a period of collaborative exploration. This should occur either at the end of the initial visit or, if the patient's condition is too precarious, at a later time. It is often appropriate to bridge the two different interviewing approaches with a statement such as, "Well, that is what I needed to know about your shoulder. In general, how have you been feeling?" A great many patients will respond in a tentative way as if they are not certain the doctor is interested.

"Well, pretty good."

"Just *pretty* good?"

"Maybe a little down."

"You do look sort of sad, would you care to tell me about it?"

Such active listening and interest on the part of the physician greatly facilitates the patient's capacity to share what may be crucial aspects of the illness.

Many patients come to their physician with diffuse complaints of considerable duration. "I just don't feel right." "There's something wrong, I'm just not certain exactly what it is." Others bring multiple and seemingly unrelated symptoms. "I have a pain in my arm; I'm tired all the time; I've lost my zest." Others come to the physician with symptoms that may sound "psychiatric."

They complain openly of depression, anxiety, fearfulness, or other feeling states. For these three groups of patients, it is preferable to approach the interview as a collaborative exploration. This communicates to the patient that you are concerned with the person as a whole. A very general question helps the patient to be open. "You look and sound as if you're having a tough time. Tell me how you feel." After a period of collaborative exploration, one can move to a more directive style and ask specific, symptom-oriented questions. Again, a bridging summary is helpful. "You've told me a great deal about how depressed you've been. Let's switch now to some specific questions about your symptoms."

The doctor cannot use both interviewing styles simultaneously. Because, as we have noted, each requires a different kind of "being with" another person. Moment-to-moment variation in style would confuse the patient. By separating the two explicit goals of interviewing, knowledge of the person and knowledge of the symptoms, this confusion may be minimized.

The following brief vignettes of both interviewing styles may be helpful:

A Brief Directive Interview

Hello, Mrs. Overby, I'm Doctor Stewart.
Pt.: Hello.
Dr.: Tell me what the trouble is.
Pt.: I have a pain in my chest.
Dr.: Show me where it is.
Pt.: Here. (pointing to substernal area)
Dr.: What kind of pain is it?
Pt.: Kind of dull.
Dr.: Not sharp?
Pt.: No—dull and pressing.
Dr.: Does the pain go anywhere else?
Pt.: No—just in my chest.
Dr.: When did you first notice it?
Pt.: Last night after dinner.
Dr.: Has it been with you constantly since then?
Pt.: Yes.
Dr.: Were you able to sleep?
Pt.: I dozed a little.
Dr.: Have you ever had this type of pain before?
Pt.: No—but I think it's indigestion.
Dr.: Have you noticed any shortness of breath?
Pt.: A little—but I think I'm just upset.
Dr.: Is it worse when you walk to the bathroom or car?
Pt.: Yes.
Dr.: Have you felt weak?
Pt.: Kind of tired all over.
Dr.: I want to examine you, get some laboratory studies, and then the nurse will take an ECG.

A Brief Collaborative Exploration

Dr.: Hell, Mr. Holt, I'm Doctor Stewart.

Pt.: Hello.

Dr.: Tell me what the trouble is.

Pt.: I just don't feel well.

Dr.: Can you tell me more about how you feel?

Pt.: Tired all the time.

Dr.: It's a tired feeling?

Pt.: Well, mostly that. I don't seem to have any energy—nothing interests me.

Dr.: Go ahead—help me to understand more about it.

Pt.: Well, I don't understand it—three or four months ago things just gradually changed. Lost my pep, work isn't fun anymore; I lost interest in sex.

Dr.: What else have you noticed?

Pt.: I'm irritable with my family and find myself taking a very negative outlook about everything. Even food doesn't taste good.

Dr.: You look sort of sad or down.

Pt.: (sighs) I really am. I feel blue—kind of teary some of the time. I don't understand what's happening to me. What do you think is wrong?

Dr.: Let's try to find out. What kind of thoughts have you had about what's happening to you?

Pt.: Well, at first I thought I had some infection—or, this is really crazy—cancer or something. More recently, though, I've wondered if I'm losing my mind.

Dr.: In addition to feeling down, you've been very afraid of cancer or losing your mind?

Pt.: I really am scared, but I haven't told anyone. People are beginning to notice, though, particularly since I've lost so much weight.

Dr.: What other feelings or thoughts have you had?

Pt.: Well, it kind of shocks me—but I've—Doctor, I've begun to feel that I'd be better off dead. It just isn't worth it to feel this way.

Dr.: You've been able to share a lot of it with me and . . .

Pt.: I didn't think I could talk about it, but it hasn't been hard to tell you.

Dr.: Good. For a moment let me switch to something different and ask you some specific questions. (Now, the physician goes into a directive phase of the interview.)

Although these examples are brief, the differences in the structures of the two interviewing styles are apparent. In both interviews, the physician took the nature of the patient's presenting complaint as the cue. In the directive interview, the appropriate concern about the etiology of the patient's chest pain led to a more directive approach and a series of specific questions regarding the most serious hypothesis, that the pain reflected underlying coronary artery disease.

The diffusiveness of the second patient's complaint led the physician to initiate the second interview with a general inquiry. In this collaborative exploration, the physician offered the patient a series of invitations to share what was being experienced, and the patient responded at increasingly intimate levels. As a consequence, the flow of interview came more clearly from the patient. In addition, the physician's role can be seen as a facilitative one of being "with" the patient as a total person rather than primarily being concerned with the opening symptom.

Doing a simple word count will reveal that in 9 of the 13 directive interview exchanges, the physician's question was longer than the patient's answer. In the collaborative interview, the cadence was different. Following the 3 opening exchanges, the remaining 8 statements by the patient were much longer. This observation suggests that the physician successfully involved the patient in collaborative exploration.

These two interviewing styles do not conflict with each other, nor is one inherently better than the other. The directive interview is symptom-oriented; the collaborative exploration is person-oriented. It encourages patients to express their feelings and life circumstances, and assumes that everything the patient has experienced may be involved directly or indirectly in the illness. It is important, however, for physicians to recognize that the approach which is indicated for one patient may not be appropriate for another. Both approaches have their indications and contraindications, and both should be part of the sensitive physician's repertoire. In some situations, the physician must take charge and, insofar as possible, firmly direct the course of events. But in many other situations, the role is one of collaboration with the patient. They work together, and each accepts part of the responsibility. When patients resist this responsibility, the road is apt to be rough and rocky for both patient and physician. It is important to realize that the physician's interviewing technique communicates to the patient the nature of their relationship. To imply to a patient that the disease requires extensive doctor-patient collaboration and then to direct rather than collaborate is to present the patient with a difficult and conflicting message.

THE PHYSICIAN AND THE DIFFICULT PATIENT

Most physicians find some of their patients difficult to treat. Perceptive and introspective physicians develop an awareness of the types of patients or patient behavior that bother them personally. There is considerable variation in this regard. Some physicians, for example, find passive, compliant patients difficult, while others experience difficulty with aggressive patients. Awareness and honesty with oneself regarding the type of behavior that is most disturbing is the first step in dealing constructively with the problem.

At times, however, the difficult patient is difficult only in the sense of making the physician anxious. Something about the patient impinges upon a vulnerability of the physician and rather than exploring the discomfort within oneself, the physician labels the patient as difficult.

A physician may also invite certain types of doctor-patient relationships, and if the patient does not respond positively to the invitation, reacts by thinking of the patient as difficult. For example, a physician may be so authoritarian as to invite passive, compliant behavior. A patient who merely insists on a modest degree of personal autonomy regarding decisions about treatment may be seen by the authoritarian physician as difficult.

There are, therefore, many ways in which patients come to be seen as difficult or bothersome. Despite the complexity, it is well to focus on some patient behaviors that pose problems for many physicians.

The Hostile Patient

Physicians who are sincere in their wish to be helpful are often perplexed, offended, or made defensive by the hostile patient. Under all but rare circumstances, it is best to comment openly about the patient's hostility. As with most confrontations, this should be done with respect and gentleness. "Somehow you seem angry" or "I have the feeling you're angry with me today" may be followed by a helpful exploration. The patient may report some real circumstances involving physician or staff for which the physician may wish to apologize or explain. Often, however, the patient's hostility may be a response to underlying fear. The frightened patient may be able to explore these fears once the defensive hostility has been dealt with in the interview. On some occasions, however, the hostility is a part of all the patient's relationships and may be denied by the patient. The knowledge that the patient's hostility is characteristic of all relationships can help make the patient seem less difficult for the physician. In essence, the physician should understand the hostility as a pattern and not take it personally.

The Uncooperative Patient

Patients may be uncooperative in different ways. Failure to follow instructions, missing appointments, and forgetting to take prescribed medications are all common forms. Once a pattern of such behavior has been noted, it is best to consider a respectful confrontation. "I notice how often you forget your appointments and wonder what that is about?" "I get the feeling that there is something about not taking your medicine that I don't understand. Do you have any idea about the reason? Can you help me understand it better?" This type of nonjudgmental approach clearly communicates the physician's interest and concern. It increases the possibility that the behavior can be understood and, hopefully, modified. Not to deal openly with the uncooperative behavior may result in increasing frustration on the part of the physician and, in some instances, behavior that is clearly retaliatory. Uncooperative patients may be threatening to the physician, particularly since all physicians wish to be successful with as many of their patients as possible. The physician may ask, what right does this patient have not to take the medication that I prescribed to improve the condition? Then, too, the physician must bear in mind the complexities of personality adjustment cause many people to be self-destructive, even in the area of their own medical care. The physician may become riled at the diabetic patient who continues to eat candy.

The physician should be aware of the orality of some patients who secure their dependency gratification by eating. What right does a patient have to disobey the physician's orders regarding alcohol when cirrhosis of the liver is already present? Why won't the alcoholic patient recognize the gravity of the condition and cooperate with the physician? After all, the unsuccessful patient is a poor advertisement for the physician. Appreciation of the patient as an individual with certain drives and needs which may conflict with compliance and with staying or getting well, and appreciation of other unconscious factors, can decrease the physician's irritation and probably increase the physician's effectiveness.

The Seductive Patient

Patients who are openly seductive with the physician may be communicating a variety of underlying needs. Often, these needs are truly sexual; the patient is interested in a sexual relationship. On other occasions, however, the patient's apparent seductiveness represents an attempt to gain nonsexual attention or control of the relationship. The seductive patient presents a difficulty for many physicians who may be capable of being attracted sexually to specific patients. This in itself cannot be considered abnormal. It is when the physician either acts upon the sexual attraction, or becomes so uncomfortable that it interferes with medical responsibilities, that difficulty is encountered. For many physicians, the recognition that a mildly seductive patient is relating in a way characteristic to all of his or her relationships is sufficiently reassuring for the physician to enjoy the interchange. Patients who are aggressively seductive, however, require such confrontations as "At times you make me feel that you are interested in something more than my being a doctor" or "Somehow I sense that you want something more from me than being your doctor, and I am uncomfortable with that feeling." These confrontations may offer the patient an opportunity to explore with the physician the underlying needs, conflicts, or life circumstances that are involved in the behavior. If, however, the patient is unwilling or unable to explore the subject, and continues aggressive seductiveness, the possibility of referral to a colleague should be considered. Above all, the physician has to be aware of the transference potential inherent in the healer's profession. Patients may confuse respect for and dependence on the physician with sexuality. The need to be taken care of may transform itself into what the patient considers the most intimate of all relationships, namely, sexuality. Thus the patient may have gratitude or a need to express and receive gratitude that becomes equated with sexual intimacy.

The Incompetent Patient

Patients who are mentally incompetent pose special problems to the physician. The incompetence may be due to diseases of aging, functional mental illnesses, space-occupying brain lesions, toxic deleria, and other conditions. Patients may be apathetic, agitated, or inappropriate in their actions. The etiology may vary, but dealing with such patients poses additional specific problems to which the physician should be alert. Friends and relatives may be valuable historians, and the legal rights of the patient should be kept in mind. Especially with toxic or organic conditions, the etiology should be established as soon as possible, and appropriate therapy initiated. Patience and diligence are necessary to see that such patients do not hurt themselves. Likewise, the physician has the obligation to see that the patient does not get into any legal transactions. The physician should be aware of the patient's inability to cooperate. Appropriate medication may be required, but caution regarding such medication must be kept in mind, depending on the etiology of the condition.

The Patient as "Crock"

Some patients present themselves with multiple and frequently changing complaints. This can be so frustrating to the physician that the patient is often seen as difficult and labeled with a pejorative term. Most such patients are extremely anxious and some are seriously disturbed. If the source and magnitude of the anxiety does not become readily apparent through collaborative interviewing, consideration should be given to confronting the patient. "Have you noticed that when we finish dealing with one symptom, another one seems to come up?" can, if respectfully offered, lead to important exploration. If the behavior persists, a psychiatric consultation should be considered in order to evaluate the underlying psychiatric pathology. Serious depression or paranoid states may underlie this type of hypochondriacal behavior, and treatment aimed at the underlying pathology may alter remarkably the multiple, ever-changing complaints.

THE PHYSICIAN AND THE PSYCHIATRIC PATIENT

The situation is no different for one who is identified as a psychiatric patient. Generally, it is more useful to start the interview in the exploratory mode and later, if necessary, switch to a more directive approach to elicit and clarify specific symptoms. This holistic approach emphasizes the need of all patients, but especially those who are frightened, depressed, or anxious: to perceive the physician as a concerned humanist who will pay serious attention to all that the patient feels and thinks. Another advantage is that by careful listening to a patient's train of thoughts and feelings, noting the nonverbal clues and recognizing and using one's own inner feelings, the physician is often able to learn more about the patient's disturbance than by asking carefully focused questions and noting only the content of the patient's responses. What the patient considers most vital or upsetting may be more pertinent than what the physician feels to be most important initially.

The more directive interview approach also adds much to the understanding of a patient if the physician tactfully probes omissions or matters that are unclear. Correlations in time may be examined, significant family history may be obtained, prior treatment attempts clarified, drug and toxic history obtained, a survey of the patient's physical health reviewed, and other important information clarified.

Several topics that are essential to a thorough history merit special attention: sexuality, aggressive tendencies, and the patient's moral values. These are sensitive areas and are emotionally charged subjects for all of us. Often the physician is reluctant to question the patient about such areas, not because of the patient's discomfort, but because of his or her own. However, it is mandatory that the patient be offered the opportunity to share feelings and concerns about these vital matters. The repeated experience of discussing sensitive areas may decrease the physician's discomfort.

To elaborate on one sensitive area: despite increasing sexual permissiveness, many patients are confused, worried, or guilty about their sexual feelings or behavior. The opportunity to share and perhaps clarify concerns with a trusted doctor can be extremely helpful. The physician who can inquire about such matters with tact and directness can be most helpful. Starting with general questions is often more comfortable for both patient and physician. "How are you feeling about your sexual needs?" "Do you have some concerns about your sexual life?" This type of broad question may allow the patient to discuss material that is producing significant conflicts. As the patient becomes more comfortable, the physician's questions can be more specific. All of this presumes that the physician has an understanding of both the physiology and psychology of sexuality and is personally comfortable with sexual feelings and behavior.

The physician is also consulted by patients who are having great difficulty controlling anger and aggressive impulses. Most of these patients desperately need to talk with someone about their feelings. Not infrequently there is a risk to others. Behind the subtle "I seem to be overreacting" or "I find myself losing control with my children" may lie behavior which ranges from overconcern about everyday frustration and anger, to serious assaultive acts. The physician must be aware of these possibilities and gently help the patient to clarify the situation. To discount such comments automatically as exaggerations may lead to tragedy. A series of increasingly specific questions is often illuminating and may be greeted with obvious relief by the patient.

The patient's transcendent values may seem to be an issue to be discussed with a clergyman, yet increasingly patients are turning to their physicians for answers to moral and ethical issues that impinge upon their health. Contraception, abortion, and euthanasia are current examples of such issues. By helping some patients distinguish between the medical and moral aspects of these questions, the physician is offering a very real form of help. If he or she is insensitive to the significance of respecting the patient's personal values, the physician's own moral code may be propagated under the guise of "good health." Perhaps one may not wish to make one's own values known to patients, but at the minimum the physician should know where he or she stands and endeavor not to proselytize patients while promoting "health."

THE PHYSICIAN AS HELPER

Overall, the physician is primarily a helper. The assistance offered is determined by the nature of the patient's illness. In both medical and emotional emergencies the doctor may have to take over for the patient temporarily, and function with all the power which medical and personal expertise provides. Most illnesses, however, do not require this type of intervention. Rather, they call for an effective alliance in which physician and patient collaborate about the nature and outcome of treatment. The ultimate success of the doctor-patient relationship—the "healing connection"—is determined by what occurs between them in their interviews. The physician's full awareness of the importance of this enhances greatly the help provided. Our medical education system often fails to emphasize the gratification that nonpsychiatric physicians may derive from treating the patient as a total human being with pains, aches, thoughts, and feelings—a goal that may be most effectively accomplished not by treating the patient as helpless or incompetent, but rather as a partner in a collaborative treatment alliance.

REFERENCES

1   Cassell, Eric: *The Healer's Art,* Philadelphia: J. B. Lippincott, 1976.
2   Canter, A., J. F. Imboden, and L. E. Cluff: "The Frequency of Physical Illness as a Function of Prior Psychological Vulnerability and Contemporary Stress," *Psychosom. Med.,* **28**:344, 1966.
3   Hinkle, L. E., et al.: "An Investigation Between Life Experiences, Personality Characteristics and General Susceptibility to Illness," *Psychosom. Med.,* **20**(4):278, 1958.
4   Rahe, R. H.: "Life Change Measurement as a Predictor of Illness,"*Proceedings of the Royal Society of Medicine,* **61**:1124, 1968.
5   Engel, G. L.: "A Psychological Setting of Somatic Disease: The 'Giving-Up' Complex," *Proceedings of the Royal Society of Medicine,* **60**:533, 1967.
6   Rahe, R. H., et al.: "Social Stress and Illness Onset," *J. Psychosom. Research,* **8**:35, **1964.**
7   Fabrega, H. and K. Manning: "An Integrated Theory of Disease: Ladino-Mestigo Views of Disease in the Chiapas Highlands," *Psychosom. Med.,* **35**(3):223, 1973.

Chapter 2

The Mental Status Examination

Donald G. Langsley, M.D.

EDITORS' INTRODUCTION

So much goes on in each doctor-patient interview—much of it fleeting and subtle—that the physician often feels a strong need to find a way of organizing the emerging data. The physician needs to know what the condition is, the diagnosis, therapy (if any), the probable course, and the prognosis. How can this best be accomplished? One method is to focus narrowly on but one aspect, such as the content of the patient's responses. Another approach is to control the interview format carefully by asking a series of questions and discouraging the patient from any excursions that are not related directly to the questions. It is surprising, therefore, that the more structured part of the evaluation, the mental status examination, is used so little. It should be a part of most patient examinations. Its format is clear and concise and it is so obviously an examination. The key to its underutilization may well be that the *mind* (long considered sacrosanct), not the *body,* is the focus.

The physician may wish to avoid both appearing inappropriate and embarrassing a depressed accountant by asking him to subtract serial sevens. Asking an executive to remember the names of three cities or requesting an aging pastor to tell the meaning of a common proverb may provoke the same type of discomfort. "How do these questions make me appear to my patient?" "Do I look silly questioning the patient's capacity for these basic thought processes?" "Am I embarrassing this advertising executive by asking such questions—even if I am concerned about his possibly having Alzheimer's disease?" The physician may wish to avoid painful memories of situations in which he or she felt interrogated—oral examinations, courtroom testimony, or any situation in which the physician's competence was questioned.

The mental examination may provoke concern that the physician is questioning what for many patients is central to their sense of personhood, the ability to think, reason, recall. The fear of being seen as wrong, dumb, deficient, incompetent, or "slipping" may impinge on the patient during the struggle to remember the capital of the United States, the number of pints in a quart, or the difference between a lie and a mistake. "What *does* 'people in glass houses shouldn't throw stones' mean? I've heard it all my life . . . what must the doctor think of me? He trades at my store. . . ." More out of fear and/or denial mechanisms, the 53-year-old woman executive recovering from a cardiovascular accident may be irritated when the physician questions her about "how her mind is functioning" and whether or not she is depressed. Concern about the physician's questioning regarding happiness, sadness, and aspects of personality may be most upsetting to some patients when the questioning is done poorly and possibly without an introduction.

Physicians can become more comfortable with the opportunity to assess total patient functioning. The physician is examining the patient and it may be this central feature that is experienced with discomfort. Yet, if the mental status is approached with the same gentle, deliberate, straightforward manner as the physical, it will be accepted more easily by the patient as appropriate and reassuring evidence of thoroughness and concern.

Awareness that the mental exam may provoke strong feelings in both patient and physician makes it easy to omit. The physician, however, must accept the responsibility for accomplishing this examination with great sensitivity and tact. This can be accomplished in a few moments of careful explanation about the examination's importance. The approach to the mental status examination is no different from the sensitive physician's approach to other intrusive examinations, that is the hallmark of the "compleat physician."

Then, too, how does the physician get information about the patient's history, past life experiences, recent stresses, relationships with other individuals, and the situation which brings him or her to the physician? Does the physician have to pursue aggressively—probing, interrogating, and directing to get the necessary material? Most of this has been covered in the chapter on interviewing. Contradictory as it may seem, pertinent information does come forth if the physician settles back, lets the patient relate the history, and directs or interjects only occasionally. But what data are required for an adequate history? In the following chapter, the author details some of the general information that should be helpful. However, the reader should bear in mind that each patient is an individual, and the history will vary because of this individuality. It has been said that physicians, especially psychiatrists, have little need to read fiction. Patients may be their fiction, with the physician having the opportunity to see each chapter as the history unfolds and the condition changes. If things go well, the physician can look forward to a happy ending to the story in which he or she plays such an integral role.

The first chapter suggested interviewing techniques for obtaining information from the patient. In this chapter we will emphasize the content of the interview and highlight the content of past psychiatric history which should be obtained.

The psychiatrist (like other physicians) uses the clinical method. The clinical approach is one which gathers data from patients about their current problems and their past histories. The clinician then performs a physical examination and laboratory tests to complete the workup. Historical information is designed to place the present problem within the context of the patient's prior experiences with health and illness. Certain techniques called the Review of Systems are used to be sure that the physician does not overlook pertinent data. Under the Review of Systems, the physician will go through all the functional and anatomical systems of the body, and ask specific questions about symptoms which the patient may have forgotten to mention. The complete medical workup thus focuses on a clinical process in which the physician attends to the present illness in great detail but tries to explain and understand it in terms of the past medical history. The physical examination and laboratory tests offer further data to enlarge on the conditions which the physician suspects to have caused the present symptoms.

The psychiatrist uses a similar method in focusing on present illness and trying to relate it to past history. The mental status exam may be likened to the physical examination in that it attempts to reveal behavior, thought, or emotion which is characteristic of a given clinical syndrome.

THE PSYCHIATRIC HISTORY

The Psychiatric History (Personal History) is similar in function to the Review of Systems in that it seeks to cover all potential areas of information that may throw light on the present illness. One of the major differences might be that the psychiatric approach pays special attention to family interaction, social setting, and the culture in which the patient has developed. Another special emphasis in the psychiatric history is a developmental point of view that assumes that adult behavior and mental functioning relate to earlier experiences.

The process is not dissimilar to that which occurs when a patient comes into the family physician's office complaining of abdominal pain. The physician will proceed from asking very general questions about the symptoms in an open-ended fashion, to gradually focusing on more specific questions that could be answered by a simple yes or no. The physician will ask for a description of the abdominal pain and events related in time. He or she will ask about similar occurrences in the past, including treatment and result of treatment, before proceeding to a more general examination of the patient's prior past medical history.

Out of the knowledge of pathophysiology and past clinical experience, the physician will ask questions that may finally elicit a history of the recent onset of mid-abdominal pain, which subsequently began to radiate to the right lower quadrant and localize in that region. He may also obtain a history of subsequent nausea and vomiting. The physician notes the information that this young patient had previously enjoyed good health and had not experienced prior serious illnesses or complaints referable to the abdominal region. When the subsequent physical examination demonstrated point tenderness and guarding in the right lower quadrant, and when the laboratory tests showed a granulocytic leukocytosis, he would make a diagnosis of acute appendicitis and plan for surgery.

When the patient complains of fatigue and loss of energy, a further examination of the current illness may reveal subjective depression, psychomotor retardation, weight loss, sleep disturbance, and a feeling of worthlessness. the psychiatrically oriented physician would then seek data about prior mental and physical disorders and would take a careful history, including a review of past events. After doing a mental status which displayed the characteristic symptoms, he or she would come to the diagnosis of depression. This is the clinical process.

The history may be recorded in a number of forms. The write-up may be in the traditionally organized fashion (identifying information; chief complaint; present illness; past history; family history; mental exam) or it may be recorded in other fashions. The Problem-Oriented Medical Record (POMR) organizes similar information but in a different style, starting with a data base, a problem list, and progress notes based on the identified problems. A number of automated formats have been developed for use in computerized techniques or machine methods. These are some of the ways to organize and record the data but the clinical process remains the same.

A note of caution is in order. Many of us forget that medical records are subject to scrutiny by others and may easily be subpoenaed. Physicians must train themselves to be thoughtful about recording information and must walk the tightrope of including sufficient data to make the clinical process understandable, while at the same time guiding others who may depend on the record to treat the patient while maintaining adequate confidentiality—especially about material which may be embarrassing, distressing, or dangerous to the patient. Younger physicians (like sophomore medical students) are inclined to keep overly complete records; some highly experienced physicians tend to abbreviate the process and keep minimal records. At times when malpractice action may be threatened by inadequate records, physicians must consider the need for detail to protect patients and themselves from legal action.

The history and workups should be recorded under the headings of Present Illness, Past Medical History, Family History, and Personal History.

Present Illness

The Present Illness should start with the chief complaint; ask the patient what it is that troubles him or her. Then the doctor asks the patient about the present illness. As outlined in Chapter 1, the doctor should move from general and open-ended questions to more specific questions. Responses such as "Tell me more about that" or "Can you describe that" will help the patient to tell the story. The details of how this problem started and its duration (questions about timing) are often important. The physician will also want to know about precipitating events. It is easier to ask general questions such as "What was happening at that time?" The general questions may then lead to more specific ones about stress at home, trouble at the job, difficulty in interpersonal relationships, or physical illness. One should also ask about similar problems in the past. This is often done because many psychiatric problems are repetitive or even cyclical in nature. The response that there have been similar problems in the past should lead to questions about the prior course of events and about what was helpful or otherwise with prior episodes. The pattern of referral (often called "The Pathway to the Doctor") should be explored. The physician will want to know whether the patient came of his or her own accord, or was urged to do so by a family member, a friend, or some authority (employer or court). In almost every case the physician will want to know about certain dangerous symptoms. The history of depression will automatically lead to questions about suicide. A history of violence or suspiciousness will lead the physician to ask about aggressive outbursts and homicidal thoughts. Suicide is an issue which should be approached gently but directly. A series of questions is often helpful and may start with "Have you ever felt depressed? Have you felt so low that it didn't seem worth going on? Have you had thoughts about ending your life? Have you had specific plans about suicide? Have you ever made a suicide attempt?" Each physician will determine a pattern he or she finds most compatible with personal style, but this series illustrates an approach which generally works.

Past Medical History

The primary physician (to whom this book is directed) will not require a detailed outline of what constitutes a past medical history; nevertheless, for the sake of completeness it is worth suggesting that the Past Medical History include a statement about general health and prior serious illnesses including hospitalizations, operations, and trauma. One would also wish to take a family medical history to learn about illnesses which may be genetic or cultural in origin. The Past Medical History should also include information about childhood illnesses and such general areas as sleep patterns, appetite and diet habits, allergies, the use of drugs and alcohol, and the abuse of these substances. One should specifically seek information about head injuries and other trauma, or illness which may result in disturbance of consciousness. Epilepsy and other types of common neurological disorders which may affect behavior should be part of the inquiry.

Family History

We all need to remember that the patient has a family and that the family grew up in some type of cultural setting. The history should indicate something about the sociocultural context of the family, including information about whether the environment was rural, urban, and whether the family grew up in a particular subculture. A history of the family should also comment on changes in composition and geographic location. The stability of the family is of importance in understanding the development of an individual. In view of the high incidence of divorce, it would be wise to seek information about this type of change in family structure. The divorce issue also raises questions about placement of the children, custody, and what influence this had as the patient grew up. The relationship of parents to one another and to their own families of origin (extended family) is important information and should be part of the data sought in the workup. In addition to questions about the relationship between parents, the physician will wish to inquire more specifically about the relationship of the family to the patient. This information can be sought by asking directly about parents, by inquiring about the patient's relationship with each of the parents, and about ways in which this relationship has changed in the course of a lifetime.

Personal History

The Personal or Developmental History (sometimes called Psychiatric History) is of special importance since it differs somewhat from the general medical history. The areas to be explored include childhood development, social development, dating and sexuality, marriage and children, involvement with various social groups, school, work, and legal problems. Under the development history of childhood one should ask about the usual motor milestones. This will indicate whether or not there was major alteration in the expected developmental pattern. The information to be sought includes data on age of walking and talking, and specific questions about whether there was any delay in development of other motor skills. The issue of intellectual development is implied but this information should be sought sensitively. A history of slowness in speech development may lead to questions about early problems in school and in learning patterns. On the other hand, a diversity in motor development and the attainment of intellectual skills may suggest other types of childhood problems.

It is especially important to understand any patient's history of relationships with other people. This begins with the story of relationships with parents in childhood and the changes in those relationships through the years. The psychiatric history should take into account any changes in the composition of the family, as mentioned above. This will lead to questions about whether the relationship changed as the patient became a teenager, and later an adult. Along with inquiries about parents, there should be questions about relationships with siblings and about the place of the patient within the sibship. Ordinal rank has been known to influence personality development, and although generalization may oversimplify, oldest children do seem to be more responsible and obsessional while youngest children tend to be more relaxed and dependent. The history should include information about relationships with friends at various stages throughout life. This would include information on whether friendships had been long-lasting. Some people tend to maintain relationships for long periods of time in spite of a tendency toward geographic mobility. Others never make close friends, or if they do have close relationships at some stage of life, do not maintain them. Friendships during adolescence are often of special importance and it is worthwhile to inquire about friends both of the same and opposite sexes during the teen years, and to ask whether any of those relationships have persisted. Some psychiatrists find it of interest to ask whether a patient had a special friend or a "best friend" during early adolescence.

The whole area of dating and sexuality is important and has implications for a major area of mental health. The questions should begin in the area of dating and then might lead to inquiries about sexuality. It is always best to assume that sexual behavior *has* occurred rather than asking *whether* it took place. A usual sequence of events might be to ask whether masturbation was a problem during adolescence or later in life (note that this asks whether it was a problem and not whether it occurred). It is also useful to know whether the patient feels that he or she has been active sexually and whether there have been any problems in relation to sexuality. Depending on whether there are any indications of deviant sexuality, one might ask whether homosexual experiences ever took place. Questions about sexual adjustment in marriage are important.

There is more to marriage than sexuality and the history should include information on the quality of the marital relationship. The doctor will want to know about children, the size of the family, and the relationship of the parent to his or her children. In addition to the nuclear family, this includes the relationship to the extended family.

The history should include information about relationships with organizations and groups. Does the patient belong to any organized clubs or social activities? Is he or she active in community affairs? Does he or she belong to a church, and what is the extent of activity within the church? All of these areas will highlight problems in social relationships if they exist. The individual who is socially involved and active in groups or clubs appropriate to age and socioeconomic group is not likely to have the same problems as the social isolate.

School is another area that should be included in the data gathered. How far has the individual gone in school and what type of problems were encountered during education? The quality of the patient's relationship to schooling will point to areas of accomplishment as well as problems. The same is true of work, and a detailed job history will reveal successes and problems in this area. The physician will be interested in accomplishments and problems at work as well as in the frequency with which jobs have been changed. The relationships to supervisors and peers will also need to be explored.

Finally, one should ask about difficulties, both legal and financial. These may require specific inquiry if sufficient information is to be obtained. In a sense the entire Psychiatric History is a Review of Systems, since it explores areas in which the patient may not have reported problems unless specifically asked.

In summary, the Psychiatric History includes attention to the present illness, the past medical history, the family history, and a personal history (sometimes called a psychiatric history). This personal history includes information of a developmental nature, including childhood development, social development, information about dating, marriage, sexuality and children, as well as data about relationships with family, with social groups, accomplishments and problems at school and work.

THE MENTAL EXAM

The mental exam is designed to elicit information about the patient's behavior and to understand the emotional, cognitive, and intellectual functions. Like the physical exam, it is a total part of the workup. Experienced physicians are used to making observations about mental functioning in each contact with the patient. In the initial or follow-up contact, the physician will instinctively observe the patient's emotional state while taking a history or doing a physical examination. These clinical skills are often taught and discussed separately, as the interview and mental exam are in this book. In practice, however, they are generally combined with other skills and the physician usually gathers important data about mental status while eliciting a history or obtaining information about recent changes in symptoms. Just as the experienced physician often obtains data for the Review of Systems while doing a physical examination, the information relevant to mental functioning may be obtained during the interview.

Some physicians feel that a formal mental status exam suggests that the patient may be psychotic. Actually, an examination of mental functioning should be part of the effort to diagnose any functional or organic brain disease. It is part of the physician's work to be aware of psychological reactions to organic disease as well as to primary functional illnesses. Such reactions may throw light on the relevant psychological factors. The mental exam should be concerned with strengths and assets as well as pathology and dysfunction. It is important to know which functions are preserved since they aid recovery.

Like the physical findings, mental functioning changes and must be rechecked with each contact. Yesterday's confusion and disorientation may have improved or worsened. The clinician will not know this unless the findings are checked repeatedly. Just as one follows the patient's blood pressure during treatment for hypertension, the signs of psychiatric illness must be monitored. It is equally important to be sure that the findings are representative (check with the nurse's notes or with a family member) and that they are not altered by cultural determinants. What is "normal" in one culture may be considered delusion in another. Under certain circumstances such as an intensely emotional religious meeting, it may not be pathological to have an isolated hallucinatory experience. It is equally important to perform the mental status examination tactfully. The patient will be reassured by an explanation that certain routine and standardized questions help the physician to elicit information about mental functioning. The college professor who might otherwise be annoyed at proverb interpretation will be more accepting if told first that these are standardized questions. It is equally important to avoid the check-list approach. The form for recording the mental examination (like the forms used for recording the physical exam) is a standardized way of organizing data and not a step-by-step system for collecting it.

The record of the mental examination should include data under each of the following headings:

1 Appearance
2 Motor activity and behavior

   3   Speech and communication
   4   Mood
   5   Organization and content of thought
   6   Perception
   7   Level of awareness, orientation, and concentration
   8   Memory, recall, and fund of knowledge
   9   Abstract thinking and judgment
 10   Patient's understanding of own condition

Appearance

A careful look at the patient usually reveals a great deal. The experienced physician will make a mental sketch. For example, he or she may say "This is a middle-aged woman who moves slowly, displays a sad demeanor and downcast gaze. She is unkempt and lacks makeup. She sits almost motionless, and demonstrates frequent deep sighs." Such a sketch is immediately suggestive of areas in the mental exam to be explored. This requires keen observation of the patient's appearance. Is it consistent with age and position? Does the manner of dress indicate cleanliness? Is it garish, meticulous, or careless? The patient's facial expressions should be observed. They may be alert or perplexed and sad. Physical posture and bearing are other indicators of emotional state. Is the patient tense or relaxed? Does the facial expression indicate anxiety or is the patient phlegmatic rather than animated? The attitude toward the examiner should be another matter of concern. Some patients are hostile while others are submissive. An attitude of cooperativeness is important to note, as well as an attitude which is suspicious or evasive.

It is also important to consider the circumstances of the examination itself. Has the patient been physically ill for some time and yet is being seen for the first time in the hospital or physician's office? Was the contact made voluntarily, or has the patient been brought under some duress by a family member?

It is important to determine this overall view of the patient's appearance during the first contact. Patients experiencing organic brain syndromes or functional psychotic reactions often exhibit deterioration in dress and personal appearance. It is equally necessary to repeat the observations in subsequent contacts. A change in appearance may indicate improvement or regression. It is frequently possible to judge improvement from a depression or an organic brain syndrome simply by observation of the patient's physical appearance. The depressed woman who begins to use makeup and the formerly disheveled man who displays concern about his clothing are giving evidence of improvement.

Motor Activity and Behavior

Emotions and mental activity are often expressed in physical movement. Attention should be paid to the overall movement, including the amount of motion, the type of physical activities, and whether destructive behavior is apparent. Depressed patients frequently demonstrate reduced motor activity, as do myxedematous patients. Manic patients reveal increased motor activity which they are able to sustain for long periods of time. With schizophrenic reactions, the motor activity may be either increased or decreased. The patient's gait when entering the room will reveal something about function of the nervous and motor systems. Even if the gait is not neurologically abnormal, there may be functional reasons for an unusual type of walk or movement. The amount of motion is equally important. Is the patient in constant motion, perhaps agitated, or is the patient retarded, slow in all kinds of physical activity, or even immobile? The movements of the face or around the face should be noted especially. Are there grimaces, tics, or tremors? Are the movements of the face and other parts of the body repetitive and stereotyped? Movements may also be compulsive, such as tapping. Other movements could be described as posturing. Still others may be specific kinds of mannerisms. All motor activity should be observed as being indicative of inner emotional states as well as the integrity (or lack thereof) of the nervous system. In addition to classical motor activity, the physician should be concerned about destructive behavior. This is suggested in the amount of tension and in the degree of control a patient exhibits. Telling a story about anger to the accompaniment of clenching fists and threatening gestures should raise questions about the possibility of loss of control and paranoid states.

Speech and Communication

Speech is one of the most important modalities of communication, and the physician should take careful note of it. The areas to be observed include rate, volume, modulation, flow, and abnormalities of speech pattern, as well as the content itself. One should note whether or not the speech is spontaneous, logical, relevant, and appropriate. In seriously disturbed individuals there may be monosyllabic answers to direct questions, or there may be a highly personalized, illogical, and inappropriate type of speech. The rate of speaking will probably be consistent with other motor activity, and psychomotor retardation will often affect speech. The elated or manic patient may speak rapidly and loudly in contrast to the depressed individual. Modulation is another characteristic of spoken communication. The voice may be vivacious and modulated, or monotonous and dull. All of these factors may be influenced by accent or by a special dialect. The other element of speech is the motor activity (gesticulation) which accompanies it. The clinician will want to note whether it is reasonable in amount and appropriate to the content of speech, or whether there is an inhibition of gesticulation. As with all other conditions, it is frequently more important to note a change in speech or gesticulation than it is to note the baseline which has been characteristic for that individual over a long period of time. Many persons habitually speak softly and in a controlled manner, with little gesticulation or modulation. That type of behavior carried on consistently is not indicative of a special problem. The rapid change from speech and communication styles so described to the opposite would be cause for concern.

Some patients are mute. The physician can write simple questions or instructions on a piece of paper, and some patients who are unresponsive to spoken questions or instructions will respond in this manner. If this does not work, the intervention of a family member may be helpful.

Persistent mutism is contrasted with intermittent stoppages of speech called *blocking.* Blocking is usually due to intrusion of unusual or sudden thought, but may also be an expression of lack of energy or "running-down." The flow of speech should be noted. Is there a pushed or forced quality to it? A *flight of ideas* is noted in those who have a hypomanic or manic episode. A flight of ideas occurs when there is a series of expressions whose connections can be seen logically, but which jump rapidly from one topic to another. The patient is often stimulated by an object or person clearly visible and then jumps associatively (but logically) to a series of other topics. Other abnormalities in the flow of speech include *perseveration* (the same answer to all questions) and *echolalia* (the patient repeats whatever the examiner says). Patients may make up totally new and private words (*neologisms*) or may tell a story in far too much detail (*circumstantiality*). Another item to be noted is *distractability*, because it may indicate either a lack of control or too much attention to internal stimuli.

Disturbances in speech and communication are noted in a wide variety of clinical syndromes. Psychotic patients in particular may demonstrate abnormalities in the rate, flow, and content of speech.

Mood

Emotional state or mood is often expressed in terms of high and low. Those with sadness, hopelessness, or a sense of remorse are frequently depressed. The opposite emotional state would be elation, optimism, and uncritical self-confidence. One might see both ends of the spectrum at different times in the manic-depressive, or to a lesser extent in the cyclothymic personality. These emotional states need to be examined in terms of thought and their relevance to thought. Is the emotional state related to spoken content or is there some marked disparity between them? Another aspect of mood relates to its constancy. Though all of us have certain alterations, marked swings within hours or minutes may indicate a serious mental disturbance. The clinician should also ask whether or not the mood is appropriate, and whether it is expressive or flat and constricted.

Organization and Content of Thought

Throughout the interview, the physician should look for the overall content of thought, the hopes, dreams and aspirations, beliefs, fears, and concerns expressed in the communication of the patient. These might be the themes associated with thought processes. The clinician should consider cognition, especially the speed, organization, and content of thought. In considering speed, slowing or acceleration should be noted. Slowing of thought may progress to frank mutism, while in accelerated thought there may be mental processes which race uncontrollably to a flight of ideas. Under organization of thought, one should consider whether it is controlled and tightly organized (not spontaneous) or whether it is loose to the point of incoherence. Patients may make up neologisms or may demonstrate blocking due to intrusion of thoughts.

The content of thought is always of concern, since this expresses the special concerns and preoccupations of the patient. One might wonder whether there are realistic, serious concerns connected with external events. When there is anxiety, thoughts are accompanied by a subjective feeling of impending disaster. There are somatic accompaniments of dry mouth, muscle tension, flushing, and perspiration. Thought content may demonstrate special fears or phobias. One should ask whether there are unrealistic concerns about height, crowds, closed spaces, or other special fears. Other patients may demonstrate uncontrolled thoughts and fears. These may be intrusive, repetitive thoughts which cannot be kept out of mind. The patient fears that harm will be done to him or her. There are certain compulsive acts which may be reported in response to direct questioning. Examples are the need to check doors many times or to wash hands an unusual number of times during the day.

Unusual thoughts may progress from *ideas of reference* to frank delusions. When patients feel that they are constantly the subject of everyone's concern, these feelings are called ideas of reference. They may progress to such frank *delusional ideas* as the belief that words on the television are special messages directed toward the individual. Delusional ideas (totally false beliefs) are often persecutory. One can look for these in carefully phrased, open-ended questions such as "Do you believe something unusual is happening to you?" or "Is someone trying to keep you from success?" or "Do you have special powers or a special mission?" Delusions or perception and/or grandiosity suggest the possibility of paranoid states.

Perception

Perceptions of self and environment say a great deal about mental activity. The clinician will wish to determine whether there are distorted perceptions of the self. Does the patient feel that he or she has frequently experienced this situation before (déjà vu)? Does he or she experience *depersonalization* (feeling that oneself is unreal)? This sense of depersonalization may go on to frank *derealization* (a sense of estrangement from self or a feeling of being dead). These sensations may be accompanied by somatic delusions or a feeling that parts of the body are missing or grossly altered.

In examining perceptions of the environment, the clinician would ask the patient whether the world seems altered or whether things seem in a fog. Some patients may report that objects are altered in size or shape. Some may experience *illusions* (distortions of actual external stimuli), while others experience *hallucinations.* Hallucinations are perceptions with no external source and are presumed to be projections of internal mental needs onto the outside world. Hallucinations may be visual, auditory, tactile, gustatory, or olfactory. Auditory hallucinations may be experienced as external accusatory voices or voices which demand action. Visual hallucinations are more frequently associated with organic syndromes (delirium or dementia), but this is inconstant. Likewise, auditory hallucinations are far more frequent in schizophrenia and in other functional psychoses. Noting the specific type of hallucination may aid in deciding whether the postoperative patient is experiencing a schizophrenic reaction or a toxic delirium. The examiner must find ways of asking about such alterations of perception in a sensitive manner. It is not helpful to barge in with the direct question, "Do you hear voices?'' It is often more effective to seek this information in a series of questions starting from the more acceptable and moving toward the more pathological. One might approach it with ''Do your ears play tricks on you?'' ''Do you hear sounds you can't explain?'' ''Do you hear your own thoughts out loud?'' or ''Do you hear voices speaking to you when there is no one around?''

Other types of perceptual distortion are experienced at the time of falling asleep (*hypnogogic*) or on waking up (*hypnopompic*). These perceptions are frequently auditory (such as hearing one's name being called), though they may also be visual or associated with another sensation. They are occasionally reported by individuals who do not have a psychiatric illness, and isolated hypnogogic or hypnopompic phenomena are described by otherwise normal individuals.

Level of Awareness, Orientation, and Concentration

The level of awareness is often associated with brain functioning. Chemical, circulatory, or physical trauma may interfere, and the patient may demonstrate an alteration in level of awareness. Frank coma is obvious, but the more subtle signs of drowsiness or somnolence require careful observation. Fluctuations in the level of attention may best be determined from ongoing observations of family members, or from nursing staff if the patient is hospitalized. The other extreme of awareness consists of hyperalert or especially watchful behavior. Unusually suspicious individuals, or those who are experiencing the beginning of a psychotic episode, may demonstrate this state of hyperalertness.

Concentration is also related to effective brain functioning. The clincian will be interested in whether the patient can demonstrate sustained, purposeful thinking, or is either too easily diverted or simply unable to maintain concentration. Clouding of consciousness is a condition usually due to chemical intoxication. It is the classic evidence that there is some process which interferes with cerebral functioning. Concentration can be tested during the interview itself by observing how the patient tells a story, or it can be evaluated by such specific tasks as serial subtraction by sevens or threes from one hundred. That particular task demonstrates ability to concentrate on a sustained task as well as the ability to do mathematical calculations.

Orientations as to time, place, person, and situation should be tested. In asking about such fundamental questions, the examiner will do best to begin cautiously with a series of questions. One example of such a series would go ''Are there times when you get confused about dates? For example, could you give me today's date (day, month, and year)?'' ''Can you tell me what place this is?'' ''Do you understand why you're here?'' ''Can you tell me why we are having this examination?'' ''Do you remember my name?'' The clinician must also be cautious about automatic answers. Some patients may correctly say that this is a hospital or even name it, but they will get confused about the situation and the reason for being in a hospital. It is important to note in examining this function, as in examining all others, that the mental exam is tailored to suit the patient and situation, and does not consist of a series of automatic queries. The physician most often notes disturbances in orientation in organic brain syndromes.

Memory, Recall, and Fund of Knowledge

Tests of memory should consider both recent and remote events. It is important to differentiate the types, since some of the earliest signs of brain disorder are disturbance of recent memory. It can be tested by asking the patient to describe certain events of the past 24 hours. However, the examiner must be in a position to verify the information, since some patients confabulate or make up events. Another way to test recent memory is to list three items or an address and ask the patient to remember the information. The physician then asks for the items or the address 5 or 10 minutes later. Remote memory is tested by asking about important events in the past such as birth dates, marriage anniversaries, and addresses from prior years. Again, the examiner must be in a position to verify the accuracy of the responses. Remote memory that is intact while recent memory is impaired is frequently the earliest indication of organic brain disease.

Recall is tested by the digit span exam. The examiner asks the patient to repeat a series of numbers which are pronounced slowly and distinctly, one at a time. Then the test is made more difficult by asking the patient to say the digits backwards. The average individual should be able to do six or seven digits forward, and four or five digits backward.

Sustained performance in calculations and other mental functioning may be tested by serial subtraction as mentioned above. Asking the patient to serially subtract 7 from 100 (or 3 from 100 as an easier test) is a simple and standardized procedure, but the instructions must be given carefully so that the patient understands what is expected of him or her. One technique is to say "Now, I'd like to give you a test which we often use. How much is 7 from 100? How much is 7 from that answer? Now, subtract 7 from 100, and 7 from each answer so that you go backwards from 100 by sevens." For those who cannot do serial subtraction by sevens or threes, an even simpler task is to ask the patient to count backwards from twenty. It is more important to observe the pattern of sustained concentration in performance than simply to record the accuracy of the mathematical operations.

General fund of knowledge is another indication of mental functioning. It is presumed that the examiner has already made a rough estimate of the patient's general intelligence level, based on such things as vocabulary, topics discussed, and accomplishments in school or work. However, specific tests for fund of knowledge may be carried on by asking for a list of items in a certain category, e.g., colors, animals, vegetables. One might also ask for the past four presidents or for the names of countries or cities in a certain region. General fund of information may also be tested by asking the patient to do simple mathematical calculations such as multiplication or division.

Abstract Thinking and Judgment

Abstract thinking may be tested by proverb interpretation or by object sorting. The easiest approach is to ask for interpretation of proverbs, since object sorting requires that one carry a series of items or cards. In asking patients to interpret proverbs, one must be sure that the patient does understand the nature of the task and that the proverb is not inappropriate to the patient's culture or language. Proverbs should be reasonably simple, although the more intelligent patient might be challenged by an uncommon proverb. The examiner may ask the patient to explain what is meant by the proverb "A rolling stone gathers no moss" or "People who live in glass houses should not throw stones." If the patient does not understand the nature of the task immediately, some explanation may be required. If the initial response is *concretistic* (the literal interpretation), the patient may even be encouraged to interpret how the proverb applies to people. Concrete responses are said to be indicative of organic brain disorder, although they are also seen in psychotic states like schizophrenia. Highly personalized responses are more frequently seen in schizophrenic or paranoid disorders.

Judgment may be tested by asking the patient what to do in certain social situations. The usual questions involve asking a patient what would be done if a stamped, addressed envelope were found, or what one might do if one were in a theater and became aware of a fire. Judgment is often impaired in organic psychoses, schizophrenic reactions, and psychotic depression.

Examination for Suspected Brain Disease

Detre and Kupfer offer a simple 16-question outline for the examination of patients with suspected cerebral disease:*

> The patient is asked to (1) name several objects; (2) point to the objects named by the examiner; (3) recognize four letters in the alphabet; (4) recognize four numbers; (5) copy a square, a triangle, and a Greek cross; (6) produce a schematic drawing of a clock, with the hands showing the time specified by the examiner; (7) follow simple directions (such as to go to the door and open it; come back and sit down; place the ashtray on the floor; and move the chair that is closest to the table); (8) guess the approximate distance between two pairs of objects placed on the table by saying which two objects are close to each other and which two objects are far away from each other; (9) point on command to various parts of his own body; (10) move, on command, parts of the right and left sides of his body; (11) imitate simple movements shown by the examiner; (12) read a simple sentence; (13) repeat a simple sentence after the examiner; (14) write down a simple sentence dictated by the examiner; (15) copy a simple sentence from a book; (16) name the colors of four objects laid on the table.

Patient's Understanding of Condition

It is of special interest whether or not patients realize they are ill, and whether they consider their various conditions organic or functional in their etiology. It is important to determine whether patients see their condition as temporary or permanent, and what future plans they have. The patient should be asked these questions by the examiner.

*Thomas P. Detre and David J. Kupfer, "Psychiatric History and Mental Status Examination," in Freedman et al. (eds.), *Comprehensive Textbook of Psychiatry, II,* Baltimore: Williams and Wilkins, 1975, p. 732.

MENTAL EXAMINATION OF THE PATIENT IN CRISIS

Although all patients complaining of a problem may be considered in crisis, there has been increasing attention paid to the concept of crisis and crisis intervention. A patient is considered in crisis when there is rapid development of acute symptoms in response to some external stress. The patient responding to the loss of a job or a relative, or to a change in the composition of the family, with acute anxiety and mental decompensation may be considered in crisis. The actual coping patterns of that person have not been able to master the external stress.

The history of recent events is more important to understanding a crisis than a detailed past history can be. When psychopathology appears rapidly and suddenly, the diagnostic interview should focus on recent changes. Careful questioning should suggest the traumatic events which precipitated the decompensation. It requires equally diligent questioning to determine the mental state of the patient prior to the decompensation. Relatives or friends should be questioned about the patient's mental state prior to the crisis in order to document recent changes in behavior, speech, mood, thought content, or intellectual functioning.

The symptoms accompanying a crisis most frequently are anxiety or depression, but the clinical picture may demonstrate any disturbance of the mental state. Anxiety, especially the free-floating variety, will suggest that the process is very acute and recent. The patient should be questioned about the usual symptoms of anxiety, but special attention should be paid to dating the onset and development of crisis symptoms. If the presenting problem is a recent onset of depression, the course of the symptoms should be explored. The examiner will want to know about the usual somatic concomitants of depression, including psychomotor retardation, subjective hopelessness, diminution of appetite, sleep disturbance, and remorseful thought content. In addition, the clinician should ask about suicidal thoughts and plans. Those who have had experience in crisis intervention know that prompt treatment, along with the promise of immediate aid and the active techniques of crisis resolution, will help these symptoms subside rapidly. It is especially important to see such patients as soon as possible, to use various psychological and pharmacological techniques to reduce tension, and to aid the patient and family in the solution of the specific problems which precipitated the crisis.

MENTAL EXAMINATION FOR MEDICOLEGAL PURPOSES

Physicians are often involved in examinations of patients for forensic purposes. The exam may be to determine mental competency or to justify the need for involuntary hospitalization. Other examinations are done when there is a plea of not guilty by reason of insanity. The mental examination for medicolegal purposes is done in the same manner as any other mental exam. However, it is especially appropriate to be quite thorough and to be sure that all elements of mental functioning are tested. It is also important to make a thorough record of the results of the examination, since the doctor may be questioned closely about the results of the exam during a court hearing. If the examination is precipitated by an alleged criminal act, and the individual being examined pleaded not guilty by reason of insanity, the interview should focus carefully on events at the time of that crime. The patient's mental state just prior to and during the alleged crime should be closely questioned and recorded. It should be compared with the patient's behavior and mental state at the time of the examination. In such situations, it is of value to seek corroborative data about the behavior during the alleged incident. Such information cannot be used directly in coming to a finding, since physicians must use only information that can be documented or that they themselves have observed. Observations from others, however, may suggest questions or areas of inquiry which will be of value in making one's own examination. The distinction about what the physician has observed or heard from the patient personally, and what is reported by others, should be made in the record.

THE VALUE OF THE MENTAL STATUS

Rather than being an onerous, laborious task, the formal Mental Status Examination can be an adventure for the physician, an adventure which often supplies surprising information. This is not only relevant to functional psychopathology, but may also serve as a clue to discovering physical disease that has its first manifestations in subtly impaired cognitive thinking.

The Mental Status Examination taught in medical school is too often neglected by the physician once the confines of the medical school are left behind. Through its use early senile brain changes or functioning may be detected. The hastening of vascular changes throughout the body of the diabetic patient may be observed. The difference between organic and functioning psychoses may be clarified. Space-occupying lesions may first be considered during the Mental Status Examination.

The physician, although hesitant to embarrass the patient by asking seemingly irrelevant, depreciating questions, may reap a surprising harvest of significant findings from a mental examination. Some conditions can be detected early only by the thorough physician who is comfortable with the Mental Status Examination.

BIBLIOGRAPHY

Morgan, William L., and George L. Engel: *The Clinical Approach to the Patient,* Philadelphia: W. B. Saunders, 1969.
Stevenson, Ian: *The Psychiatric Examination,* Boston: Little, Brown, 1969.
Strub, Richard L., and F. William Black: *The Mental Status Examination in Neurology,* Philadelphia: F. A. Davis, 1977.

Chapter 3

Personality Development, Conflict, and Mechanisms of Defense

Doyle I. Carson, M.D.

EDITORS' INTRODUCTION

What is it like to attempt to combat certain undesirable personality characteristics with the awareness, or lack of, that these characteristics are products of one's past life and were developed largely in the early years? How difficult it is for many to accept the crucial role that unconsious conflicts play in emotional illness as well as in day-to-day life. If behavioral scientists emphasize the early years as being so crucial, what is the purpose of psychotherapy? Why not just feel hopeless? What are the id, ego, and superego? How do they affect each other (or interact)? Can there be too much of one or the other? Understanding this kind of issue can be a useful framework for physicians in dealing with patients.

How difficult is it for a person to consider that the infidelity that is suspected in a spouse is actually one's own impulse projected to a mate in order to avoid feeling guilty?

What is it like to be fastidious, preoccupied with bowel movements, meticulous and well organized, and then to be told that the degree of these traits is pathological and possibly related to childhood conflicts? How can that be?

What is it like to be compelled by some inner drive to wash one's hands several times an hour because of a "feeling" of "bad germs," even though one's hands are inflamed and bleeding, yet to be aware of the tremendous illogicality of the hand-washing and at the same time try to avoid others' knowing about the compulsion?

Patients have difficulty understanding mental mechanisms, especially as they relate to themselves. Many of these mechanisms are normal and healthy. Others, when carried to an extreme, are psychotic.

The physician who recognizes that there are unconscious mechanisms permitting some patients to express forbidden impulses while avoiding responsibility for them may find it easier to understand multiple personalities. The physician who sees a patient with a hysterical paralysis of an upper extremity would recognize that the mental mechanisms of repression and conversion are operative; he or she would do well to search for the patient's conflict and consider psychiatric consultation carefully.

Physicians who deal with death recognize the mental mechanism of denial and often should not disturb it. On the other hand, they should be aware of pathological degrees of denial that impede functioning. One frequent mental mechanism is projection, an example of which may be the extreme hostility of some people toward homosexuals when they themselves are struggling with unconscious homosexual impulses.

These are but examples of the numerous mental mechanisms which may be looked upon as constructive, reparative, or destructive. All physicians can benefit from an understanding of personality development, conflict, and mechanisms of defense, regardless of their medical specialities.

In this chapter a clinician, who is the medical director of a major psychiatric facility, introduces the reader to a conceptual framework with which to understand personality development and functioning. The chapter offers a structure around which physicians may organize their observations and construct clinical hypotheses that are essential for effective, sensitive, and individualized treatment. Such understanding will not only be helpful to the patient, but will make the physician more comfortable in his or her functioning.

INTRODUCTION

Psychiatrists strive to develop rational systems to explain the behavior of patients, by basing their theoretical models upon the best available scientific information. The process of constructing rational explanations for human behavior is fraught with the dangers of contradictory information, uncertainties, and the unknown. However, neglect of the best available information regarding human behavior leads to irrational belief systems that lack sound judgment, and to promotion of practices that are not helpful and may even border on quackery.

How, then, do we develop a logical understanding of human nature? Multiple theoretical approaches have evolved to explain the forces that activate human behavior, that drive us toward action. Theories supporting psychoanalysis, neurobiology, behaviorism, environmental influence, ethology, instinctual forces, and family interaction have all offered information that is useful in understanding the forces that motivate mankind. These divergent approaches may be organized under two main headings:

1 Internal forces that drive people toward action
2 Environmental stimuli to which people respond with action

One approach emphasizes innate, driving forces that push an individual toward action, forces that are genetically predetermined and controlled from within, regardless of environmental influence. The other approach emphasizes the importance of environmental stimuli, and pictures the individual as a neutral organism developing along various pathways in response to different environmental influences. This "nature versus nurture" debate has a long history in the behavioral science field. The essential question becomes "Is the individual motivated from within or from without?" Clinical data offer support to both viewpoints, but neither approach alone can do justice in discerning the motivational forces of man.

This chapter considers both viewpoints as essential to understanding the human personality, and stresses that each individual is motivated from within by innate forces and from without by environmental stimuli. Understanding the integration of these two motivational systems offers the best approach for comprehending behavior. A discussion of both these viewpoints will follow.

DEVELOPMENTAL THEORY

Once the decision is made to study both innate forces and responses to environmental stimuli, the next step to be taken in constructing a rational system for understanding behavior is to decide at what time during a person's lifetime the study should be done. At what point during a life span can the most comprehensive understanding of a person be achieved? Is it possible to examine an adult carefully only in the "here and now" and fully comprehend the complexities of that individual's personality? If one accepts the thesis that the personality is *preformed* (present in the fully organized form from birth on), it matters little when a person is evaluated. The personality organization would be the same at any point during the life span. Such sagittal glimpses of individuals, which rely entirely on data obtained in relation to one's current life situation, have been found to be incomplete, and the notion of a fully organized personality from birth on is inconsistent with valid clinical and common sense observations.

In fact, there is little in the way of personality organization at birth. The best explanation for personality development is that it evolves slowly through a series of successive stages from birth to death.[1] The time period to be studied for comprehending an individual personality is the entire life span, from birth to the present. This longitudinal view of a personality evolving slowly through a series of sequential stages from birth to death is known as *developmental theory*. It finds support in the following observations:

1 Intensive psychotherapy and psychoanalysis of adults. Freud's treatment of adult patients led to the conclusion that childhood development stages are important to the formation of personality. These conclusions were based upon recollections of adult patients about their childhood.[2]

2 Direct observation of children. Direct observations of young children have supported the concept of development stages in personality formation and have added to an understanding of the details involved in these stages.[3,4,5]

3 Extrapolation from developmental theories regarding the central nervous system. The famous neurologist, John Hughlings Jackson, had been influenced by the evolutional theories of Charles Darwin, and applied the concept of evolution to explain the function and development of the central nervous system in health and disease.[6] He postulated that the central nervous system had evolved through a series of developmental stages, with each new level of function being more complex. This created a hierarchical organization of anatomy and function. He accounted for many neurological symptoms as resulting from the loss of a higher-level function, and the reappearance of lower-level functions that had been submerged as growth had evolved. He further postulated that the same evolutionary principles could be applied to the development of mental functioning, thereby supporting a theory regarding progressive personality development through a series of stages of increasingly more complex functions.

4 Common sense observations. The importance of the early years in molding personality has long had support in the general population, as found in commonplace practices and attitudes. Popular phrases have evolved to depict this, including "It is better to build boys than repair men"[7] or "The child is the father of man."[8]

Developmental theory has evolved into a major cornerstone of modern psychiatric thinking. It is best viewed as a dynamic theory in contrast to the static, mechanistic view of man that preceded it. Developmental theory takes into account the importance of innate forces for motivating the individual, responsiveness of the individual to external stimuli, and the gradual maturation of the personality that occurs through a series of sequential stages. It stresses dynamic activity from within, crucial influences from without, and continuous evolution toward progressively higher levels of maturation.

The Epigenetic Principle of Development

An important principle of embryonic development is that which is referred to as *epigenesis*. According to this principle, the embryo develops from a stage of minimal anatomic and functional differentiation to a stage of maximal anatomic and functional complexity. Development proceeds in a fixed, biologically innate sequence and at a genetically determined rate. There are critical times that are genetically determined, when clumps of cells differentiate into special organ systems. Gradually, multiple organ systems develop and are integrated into a coordinated whole.

In this stepwise process, each organ differentiates at a critically appointed time. It must form by genetic mandate at this time—no sooner or later. If a noxious environmental influence prevents the organ formation at the critical time, it will not form later. Its lack of formation will alter the differentiation and the functioning of all subsequent organ systems with which it would ordinarily be integrated. For example, certain viral infections during the first trimester of pregnancy affect certain organ system development adversely. Once the damage is done during the critical period, it cannot be corrected by later development. The damage will affect not only the one organ system primarily altered, but all systems that are integrated with that organ system.

The earlier that a distorting influence occurs during embryonic development, the greater the resulting effect, because the cells are more undifferentiated then, and any abnormal development at that point will affect more of the subsequently developing organ systems.

It is helpful to apply the epigenetic principle to personality development. One proponent of this concept is Erik Erikson, who believes that personality develops by predetermined steps that drive the developing child into certain types of interaction with the surrounding world.[1]

When applying the epigenetic principle to personality development, three important points emerge:

1 The earlier that a developing child is affected adversely by noxious influences, the more serious and pervasive will be the impairment.

2 Each stage of development involves phase-specific "critical periods" for each personality component. Proper environmental conditions are necessary to enhance the healthy development of each component at the proper time. Otherwise, healthy components will not emerge and will remain undeveloped or distorted.

3 Each stage of development is dependent upon successful completion of a preceding stage. Impairment at any stage affects the subsequent ones. Early faults lead to pervasive psychological problems. Early success enhances personality strength.

If the epigenetic principle is accepted as applicable to human personality development, the extreme importance of healthy environmental stimuli during critical developmental periods early in life is self-evident.

PERSONALITY DEVELOPMENT

Definition of Terms

Familiarity with certain key terms frequently used in discussing personality development is essential.

Instinct is an inborn, unlearned pattern of behavior that is triggered by a specific external stimulus. This term emphasizes the importance of the specific stimulus in arousing the innate potential for action. Without the stimulus, there is no action response. The response of the organism is not readily delayed once the stimulus occurs, nor is it modified easily by learning.

Many examples of instinctual responses can be found in nature. Migratory birds respond to the external stimuli of decreased sunlight and temperature with a behavioral response of flight patterns to a warmer climate. This response is fixed and dependent upon specific external stimuli for arousal.

Life-necessary drives is a term that refers to basic human drives that must be satisfied for purposes of survival. This includes drives for water, air, food, regulation of body temperature, elimination of excreta, and avoidance of bodily harm. These drives are inborn, require specific substances for their satisfaction, are not basically altered by learning or experience, and failure to gratify them jeopardizes life.

Ordinarily, a life-necessary drive would not be an important driving force within a person because it would be gratified continuously. However, if a person is lost in the desert, the craving for water becomes the most important driving force in the person's life. Failure to gratify life-necessary drives results in a situation where these drives assume an all-important dominance in the individual's life. Only water will gratify this particular drive. An individual in the desert may hallucinate about a beautiful oasis, but this hallucination will not gratify the thirst. Failure to find water will lead to death.

Instinctual drives is a term that refers to innate needs that are not essential to life, but have a biological basis and "press" or "drive" the individual into various patterns of behavior. The goal of the behavior is to achieve gratification of the needs. Instinctual drives have a biological basis and trigger an inner desire or "need" for certain types of behavior that will achieve a sense of gratification. Freud classified the sexual and aggressive drives as falling within this group. In contrast to the life-necessary drives, the instinctual drives are highly displaceable and can be at least partially satisfied in a number of different ways. If a person needs oxygen, there is no substitute. In contrast to this, an aggressive drive can be directed toward a different person, toward an inanimate object, or channelled into constructive activity. A sexual urge can be forgotten, dealt with in fantasy, gratified in autoerotic activity, or channelled into activity that is seemingly unrelated to sex.

An external stimulus is not required in order to activate instinctual drives. These drives "push" an individual into behavior because of their continuing "force" from within. An individual may be in a highly aroused state because of instinctual drives, and the appropriate external stimulus may spark a sudden escalation of the intensity of the internal drive. In other words, environmental stimuli may increase the intensity of instinctual drives, but they have a continuing, internal "push" of their own, independent of environmental influence. For instance, a female may be in a state of high sexual tension because of internal sexual drives, and may respond to an attractive, appealing male with a sudden marked increase in the sexual drive. Both internal, biological forces and external stimuli increase the intensity of instinctual drive. The words instinctual drives, sexual drives, aggressive drives, sexual urges, and aggressive urges are frequently used interchangeably.

Personality is a term that, in general, refers to the "unique whole" that is formed by the integration of the many different components of the psychobiologic organization. These components include temperament, intelligence, character traits, beliefs, desires, and adaptive tendencies. Together they are the personality. In psychoanalytic theory, personality refers to specific functional components known as the id, ego, and superego. This will be elaborated later in the chapter.

Affect refers to feelings or emotions. Important affects are anxiety, depression, guilt, shame, joy, and love. Since affects are both felt and expressed, some investigators refer to the subjective part as feelings and the behavioral expression part as emotion. Affects serve as signals that alert a person to his or her current situation, both internally and externally. They carry basic orienting information and may be pleasurable or unpleasurable. Affects are psychological states that are concomitant with drives. How the affective components of drives are managed by an individual is important to mental health and illness. Unpleasurable affective states may become so intense as to become unbearable, and require psychological maneuvers to diminish their effect. The maneuvers used by an individual in dealing with intolerable affect has a great deal to do with the degree of health or illness in that individual.

Cognition refers to thinking and is uniquely characteristic of human behavior. Thinking involves the use of signs and symbols and gives humans great adaptive advantages. The great accomplishments of humanity are related to cognitive skills. However, the use of signs and symbols makes thinking vulnerable to error and distortion, and may result in adaptive problems. Thinking is a personality component that depends on innate capacity and learning from the environment for its development.

Innate Characteristics

In the attempt to understand the development and organization of personality, the issue of inborn, innate characteristics must be addressed. With what personality components does the infant begin life? In previous centuries, the prevailing view was that the infant was a homunculus, and at birth had his or her final adult psychological structure. This structure was thought to be in minute but complete form that would come to full expression through the process of development. In this view, the parents could enforce specific modifications of behavior and thinking by discipline and suggestion, but were unable to alter the primary aspects of the personality. This concept represents the extreme form of the hereditary-constitutional point of view, and attributes personality organization entirely to innate characteristics, thus minimizing the role of environmental influence.

During this century, the importance of the hereditary-constitutional viewpoint has been replaced gradually with an ideology that emphasizes environmental influences. Psychoanalytic theory played an important role in focusing attention on the importance of psychological factors in shaping personality during childhood. From the 1920s through the 1950s, the importance of the environment in shaping personality assumed an increasingly dominant role in professional literature, teaching, and practice.[10]

Gradually, important studies that once again support the concept of innate characteristics at birth have begun to emerge. In the 1930s Gesell and Ames[11] and Shirley[12] did pioneering work on significant behavioral differences in infants. These studies stressed that differences appear to be due to innate factors and not environmental influences. These studies have not presumed to show that innate characteristics are the sole determinants of personality, but that innate characteristics do exist at birth and play a role in personality formation. The longitudinal research of Thomas and Chess[13] led to the identification of nine categories of temperament that are present in infancy. They used temperament as a general term describing the "how" of behavior, thus equating the term to behavioral style. These behavioral styles are unique for each newborn infant and appear to be innate, present at birth, and not developed in response to environmental influences, although modified by them. These nine categories of temperament are:

1 Activity level—the degree of motor activity versus inactivity.

2 Rhythmicity (regularity)—the predictability or unpredictability in the time of any function.

3 Approach or withdrawal—the nature of the initial response to a new stimulus. The response may be positive in nature as with approach behavior, involving, for example, smiling, reaching, or swallowing new food; or it may be negative as with withdrawal behavior, involving for example, crying, fussing, spitting out new food, or pushing away new toys.

4 Adaptability—response to new situations. This refers to modification of behavior in a desired direction, not to the initial response.

5 Threshold of responsiveness—the intensity level of stimulation that is necessary for sensory stimuli, environmental objects, and social contacts.

6 Intensity of reaction—the energy level of response, irrespective of its quality or direction.

7 Quality of mood—the amount of pleasant, joyful, friendly behavior, as contrasted with unpleasant, crying, and unfriendly behavior.

8 Distractability—the extent to which extraneous environmental stimuli interfere with the direction of ongoing behavior.

9 Attention span and persistence—these two categories are related. Attention span refers to the length of time a particular activity is pursued by a child, and persistence refers to the continuation of the activity in the face of obstacles.

Thomas and Chess observed that the different categories grouped together in various combinations to form "temperamental constellations." They describe three such constellations:

1 The first is characterized by regular rhythms, positive approach responses to new stimuli, high adaptability to change, and mild to moderately intense moods that are preponderantly positive. Children in this category develop regular sleeping and feeding schedules quickly, smile at strangers, take new food readily, accept most frustration without a fuss, and are a joy to parents. They are fun to show off to neighbors and are classified appropriately as "easy children."

2 The second group of temperamental constellations is a group with irregularity of biological functions, negative withdrawal responses to new stimuli, nonadaptability or slow adaptability to change, and intense mood expressions which are frequently negative. Children in this group are slow to develop regular sleep and feeding schedules, do not adjust readily to new people or situations, and frequently have periods of loud crying. Frustration typically produces a violent tantrum. Mothers find such children difficult to manage, and they are aptly called "difficult children."

3 The third constellation is marked by a combination of negative responses of mild intensity to new stimuli, and slow adaptability after repeated contact. In contrast to difficult children, these youngsters show mild intensity of reactions, whether positive or negative, and show less in the way of irregularity of biological functions. The mildly negative responses to new stimuli can be seen in any of a series of new encounters such as with bathing, eating, strangers, or a new school situation. If given the opportunity to reexperience new situations over time and without pressure, such children gradually come to show quiet and positive interest and involvement. Thomas and Chess referred to this group of children as "slow-to-warm-up."

To repeat, these characteristics and temperamental constellations are innate, present at birth. The presence of these traits produces behavioral patterns that influence important people in the environment positively or negatively. The environmental responses in turn will affect the development of youngsters greatly. Long-term studies show that for many children the temperamental traits persist unchanged. In others they were modified, probably by environmental influences. In essence, these studies of innate temperamental traits show that important building blocks of the personality are present at birth.

Studies show that the newborn infant enters life with a highly developed sensory apparatus, but is relatively helpless in the motor sphere. Right out of the uterus, the infant turns its head to the sound of the human voice, chooses a female vocal pitch over any other, and will follow with its eyes a picture of the human face. Within two weeks, the newborn infant responds very differently to the mother than to anyone else. The sensory system is sufficiently advanced to allow the infant to recognize and respond to the mother as a special person. This leads to an early reciprocal relationship between mother and infant that is important for development. When the mother senses that the infant knows her and responds to her in a special way, this encourages more loving and caring for the infant. This early mother-infant reciprocity occurs because of the innate, highly developed sensory system at birth.[14]

Drives

The next group of important characteristics is referred to as drives, and specific information about them is more difficult to obtain, in contrast to the information from studies of temperament. The temperament studies focused on behavioral styles that could be observed and measured directly. The presence of drives must be inferred, and much remains to be clarified about them. The drive concept is used to explain what makes behavior "go," what drives people toward action. Drives are sometimes labeled as instincts, needs, urges, motivations, or presses. The concept of drive rests upon the observation that a number of fundamental behavioral patterns appear to unfold inexorably because of internal motivations or cues.[15] This array of basic directions in behavior is best explained by drive theory, and, accordingly, the notion of drives should be seen as a conceptual convenience that is useful clinically but lacks solid scientific support.

The concept of drive is used to explain various fundamental states of disequilibrium that may be experienced inwardly as tension, frustration, urgency, or a want. The subjective tension is discharged by certain types of behavior, and the individual then experiences inner gratification, harmony, and restfulness. For instance, hunger increases inner tension until the behavior of obtaining and ingesting food terminates it. Lack of oxygen will produce a subjective feeling of intense urgency, which motivates behavioral action until oxygen is obtained. A drive is a biologically determined psychic constituent that produces a state of excitation or tension.

An outline of the events that are involved in drives can be visualized by using the example of the hunger drive:

1   Internal stimuli: Lack of food and inadequate levels of nutritional substances in the body lead to an increase in internal stimuli that signal the status of affairs to the central nervous system.

2   Central nervous system excitation and drive increases: This link in the chain is not well understood. Complicated biological processes are utilized for perceiving and signaling the central nervous system about the status of nutrition within the organism. This involves the interplay between complicated biochemical, hormonal, intracellular, and other factors. The hunger drive increases in intensity in response to the internal perception of inadequate nutrition, and coincides with subjective tension felt as hunger.

3   Development of need: The hunger drive leads the individual to experience a need for food. In this sense, a drive leads to a subjectively experienced need, though the terms are frequently used interchangeably.

4   Motor activity (behavior): The state of tension that is recognized as a need for food motivates the individual to action behavior for purposes of obtaining and ingesting food.

5   Subjective satisfaction: A decrease in tension follows ingestion of food. The need for food has been gratified. The series of events repeats itself when the level of internal nutrition falls below a critical point that is determined biologically.

During this series of events, the perception of food serves as an external stimulus that adds suddenly to the state of inner tension and motivates behavior to obtain the food quickly. In any form of complicated behavior, external and internal stimuli are usually related.

There is much that can be criticized about the drive concept as outlined, but it conveys the essential points of stimuli, increase in drive intensity, a state of disequilibrium and tension, internal recognition of a need, behavioral activity that gratifies the need, and a decrease in tension. A drive is seen then as an innate, biologically determined urge to action.

Freud tried to base his psychologic theories on a physiologic framework, and firmly believed that someday mental phenomena would be explained entirely in terms of brain functioning. For the most part he abandoned the attempt, but within psychoanalytic theory he did retain the concept of instinctual drives as the bridge between mental phenomena and the biologic substrate.[19] He viewed sexual and aggressive drives as arising biologically and creating a state of tension or excitation. However, sexual and aggressive drives do not necessarily produce immediate motor activity to bring about gratification. Their gratification can be delayed, modified, and influenced by learning and experience. In contrast to the life-necessary drives that require highly specific responses for their gratification, the sexual and aggressive drives can be totally or partially satisfied by a variety of responses. For example, a sexually aroused person may achieve some degree of satisfaction with a fetish.

Freud postulated that the sexual drive was present at birth and exercised an important influence on personality development throughout childhood. He theorized that the infantile sexual drive developed along a maturational continuum through different stages and culminated in full adult sexuality. He coined the term *psychosexual development* and described the developmental stages as oral (first year), anal (second year), phallic or genital (3 to 6 years), latency (6 to 12 years), and adolescence (13 to 18 years or so). His theory proposed that sexual stimuli arose from sensitive body parts that were genetically determined at different stages of development. These included the oral mucosa, the anal region, and the genitals. These infantile sexual stimuli increased the sexual drive and produced a state of inner tension. However, immediate motor discharge did not always occur. Instead, an elaborate personality organization developed as a means of dealing with the sexual drives without allowing immediate, direct gratification. Freud postulated that the more developed forms of civilization were achieved because people developed the ability to postpone, modify, and alter gratification of the instinctual drives. The mechanisms of defense were described as important personality components that had been developed to defend the individual against internal sexual drives, and that formed important building blocks in the personality.

Freud's concept of infantile sexual drives was formulated from data obtained in his psychoanalytic therapy. He encouraged patients to engage in retrospective fantasies about their childhood, and stories tinged with sexuality emerged repeatedly. He became convinced that direct observation of children confirmed his theories. As a concept, infantile sexuality has been controversial, but over the last several decades it assumed a dominant role in formulations about development and personality formation.

Freud pointed out that many of the pleasurable activities of children are used in adult sexuality as foreplay. He noted that at times adults under stress will relinquish adult sexual behavior and "regress" or fall back on earlier modes of infantile pleasurable activity. This supported the theory of a continuum of sexuality from infancy to adulthood, a single thread of an instinctual drive running through life. This singular, continuing instinctual drive undergoes modifications. Therefore, the infantile form was hard to recognize as the precursor of the adult form. By infantile sexuality, Freud did not mean sensual eroticism in the adult sense, but an immature form of pleasure, a life force, which would develop into adult sexuality.

Freud did not emphasize the aggressive drive to the same extent as sexuality. The sexual and aggressive drive concepts were important components of his developmental theory, but they are highly theoretical, not soundly supported by research, and undoubtedly will continue to undergo modifications as pertinent new information emerges.

Other Views of Innate Characteristics

In addition to the concepts of temperamental traits and drives, other variations of innate characteristics are presented from time to time. Thirty-seven years ago, Sheldon and Stevens proposed that physical typology was correlated with personality type and attempted to show that various body builds were invariably associated with certain types of personality.[20] Ten years ago Jensen postulated that intelligence is inherited not only individually but also racially.[21] These views have not been supported by research and are not generally accepted.

Environmental Influences

One extreme position taken in the "nature versus nurture" conflict is the point of view espousing environmental influence as all important in development. The infant is viewed as a *tabula rasa* (clean slate), and the parents may mold the personality into any shape they wish. Sixty-five years ago, the famous behaviorist John Watson said, "Give me a dozen healthy infants, well-formed, and my own specified world to bring them up in, and I'll guarantee to take any one at random and train him to become any type of specialist I might select—doctor, lawyer, artist, merchant, chief, and yes, even, beggar man and thief, regardless of his talents, tensions, abilities, vocations, and the race of his ancestors."[22] This view has continued to be a powerful one.

This attitude has a number of important implications. If a child's personality at birth is a "clean slate," then healthy development is entirely dependent upon universally recognized techniques for good parenting. All children should react identically to a given parent attitude or approach. Mental health professionals would only have to teach good-parenting techniques to prospective parents. They, in turn, if they had the proper interest and attitude toward their children, would use the techniques in molding the personalities of their children into healthy adult constellations. If the children turn out well, then the parents did a good job. If the children turn out poorly, the parents did a bad job. The only variable in developmental outcome would be the parents, since all children would be viewed as starting life from the same "clean slate" point. As a result of this attitude, the problems of children and adults were explained as being caused by faulty parenting techniques.

This extreme environmentalist viewpoint has been questioned by studies that show innate characteristics in infants. Different parenting techniques appear to be needed for different children. It is impossible to teach parents a set of parenting techniques that will apply equally well to all newborn infants. The presence of certain behavioral styles in children cannot be attributed automatically to the aptitude, interest, or love of the father, nor to the ineptitude, disinterest, or hostility of the mother. The styles may be related to inborn characteristics. Even so, clinical experience and research studies show that environmental influences, while not acting alone in shaping personality, play a powerful role.

Stimuli and Development   Studies support the importance of environmental stimulation for normal cellular development of some sensory systems.[23] Animals that are deprived of normal visual stimuli early in life will develop permanent visual impairment. The development of normal, healthy cellular functioning in the visual system requires certain types of external visual stimulation at a specified time early in the animal's life.

Recent reports indicate that some early experiences involved in the mother-infant interaction serve as necessary stimuli for the normal development of certain central nervous system cells. These studies indicate that cuddling, holding, and rocking of the newborn infant serve as stimuli necessary to cellular development and that early-life environmental influences affect the physical, cellular process in certain body systems.[24]

Another study reported that infants show a maturational crisis at about 3 to 4 weeks of age. At this age babies show a marked increase in overall sensitivity to external stimulation. This was assumed to be due to a rapid maturation of the sensory apparatus at that age, with a resultant increase in tension accumulation through external stimulation. Without intervention of a mother figure to help in tension reduction, the infant may become overwhelmed by stimuli, which can result in increased crying and undifferentiated negative affect.[25]

Many studies have reported the onset of smiling at the age of 2 to 2½ months. The smile is elicited by the human face or by a drawing of the human face (in particular, a drawing of the two eyes, a nose, and forehead).[26] The schema of the human face appears to be a stimulus that provokes a specific smiling response in the infant. Perhaps the tension reduction that the infant has come to associate with the mother's face is a factor in bringing this response about.

Various responses that have social value develop in relation to a variety of environmental stimuli. Social smiling is an example of one such response.

Social Contact Experiences and Development   The quality of interpersonal contacts early in life plays an important role in shaping the infant's adaptiveness to the surrounding world. In general, influences early in life tend to have more lasting, pervasive impact and may affect subsequent stages and adult functioning. This is in keeping with the epigenetic principle of development.

The work of ethologists in studying imprinting has caught the attention of behavioral scientists. Ethologists have demonstrated, especially in birds, that there is a critical period shortly after birth in which the newborn becomes "imprinted" on a moving, sound-producing object. In the animal's natural environment, this is the mother. That object will subsequently elicit following behavior in the infant. Objects other than mothers can be imprinted onto newborn birds, and the birds will follow that object as they would ordinarily follow the mother. Although imprinting has not been demonstrated in humans, the concept of critical developmental periods has been applied to early mother-child relationships in terms of the developing attachment between infant and mother.

Numerous studies have substantiated the impact of deprivation on the developing infant. H. E. Harlow studied monkeys while focusing on social deprivation experiences and their long-term effects. Monkeys isolated for long periods in infancy became permanently impaired socially, unable to defend themselves from attack, and showed abnormal sexual behavior as adults.[27] This type of animal deprivation study is used to show the importance of early mother-child interaction, though such conclusions are open to criticism. The direct application of animal research data to human functioning is questionable.

The detrimental effects on human infants when they are deprived of social and cognitive experiences has long been recognized. Bowlby concluded that early separation of infant from mother had persistent and irreversible effects on personality and intelligence.[28] Abandoned children placed in orphanages during the first 3 years of life do not fare nearly so well as those placed in foster homes. When seen at adolescence, the children who have been in institutions during their first 3 years show lower IQ's, inferior school performance, and a higher likelihood of sociopathic traits.[29]

A classic study of maternal neglect and deprivation was reported by Spitz.[30,31] He found that for infants who had been raised in a foundling home where insufficient attention was paid to social and emotional interaction during the first year of life, the result was severe developmental retardation, physical wasting, and a shockingly high death rate. He also described nursery babies who, when deprived of maternal attention, developed severe depression. In general, these studies and similar ones support the concept that maternal deprivation in early childhood has a serious, lasting, deleterious impact on development.

Another early environmental influence reported to lead to a wide range of behavioral disorders is maternal overprotection.[32] Overprotection has been reported to foster dependence on parents, and to interfere with ability to master anxiety, or develop autonomy, confidence, and a sense of identity. Maternal overprotection may impair the normal mother-child emotional separation that occurs during the second and third year of life and may play a causative role in the development of the borderline syndrome (considered to be a problem of separation-individuation).[33]

Another social contact pattern that may cause developmental difficulty is the pattern of inconsistent child rearing. Conditioning experiments and clinical observation offer support for this concept. Many children, however, appear to develop normally despite what would appear to be an inconsistent home environment.

Another category of social contact stress is unreasonable, cruel punishment of children. This tends to produce either extremely aggressive attitudes or the opposite, a capitulation with passive attitudes; both interfere with adult adjustment. Significantly, and seemingly paradoxically, children who are abused tend to become child abusers themselves. The important point is that early environmental influence is carried into adult life as a part of the behavioral style.

Another environmental influence is modeling. Children tend to become like their parents in many ways, even to the point of exhibiting qualities that the child abhorred. The adaptive mechanism of identification will be discussed later in the chapter. The way a parent behaves in the presence of a child will influence the child's personality. A loving, caring parent is more likely to raise a loving, caring child, because of the modeling process.

The list of studies of environmental influences is lengthy. A few of the more pertinent examples have been given. The importance of appropriate environmental stimuli, imprinting, early social deprivation, maternal overprotection, inconsistent parenting, child abuse, and modeling are well established in most developmental theories. In essence, environmental influence is important in personality development. It is difficult to measure the exact impact of these influences, but from all indications they contribute to a major degree in shaping the developing individual.

THE UNCONSCIOUS AND THE CONSCIOUS

A basic concept of personality organization is that of the unconscious part of the mind. It is necessary to conceive of an unconscious in order to explain many aspects of mental functioning and personality formation. Freud became convinced that most functions of the mind were unconscious. He observed many discontinuities in the mental lives of patients that could only be explained by conceiving of an unconscious aspect of mental functioning. For example, a person may find him- or herself having a recurring thought, yet not know why. Someone else might point out that a day earlier the individual had been given important information that would explain the thought. Yet the subject had forgotten the information. This information and its importance in the individual's mind must have continued at some level in order to account for the recurring thought. Where was the information kept? The concept of an unconscious mind explains the storage of the information without the individual's awareness of it.

Other support for the unconscious is found in the productions of patients in psychoanalysis, psychotherapy, hypnotherapy, or narcoanalysis. Important, emotionally laden material about which the patient had no previous awareness may be verbalized in such situations. Where was the information stored previously? The concept of the unconscious explains the storage. The idea of the unconscious is supported further by observations of posthypnotic suggestions. An individual in a hypnotic trance can be given a command to carry out an act after the trance has been terminated. The individual may then carry out the precise act at the exact time commanded, without having any awareness of the previous command.

Some definitions relating to the unconscious are in order. The term *conscious* refers to mental functions of which a person is aware at a given moment. *Unconscious* refers to psychologic processes of which a person is unaware and cannot become aware of by ordinary effort. *Preconscious* is used to describe mental functions of which an individual is unaware at a given moment, but which can be recalled and brought into awareness by effort or by being reminded.

Certain personality components are usually unconscious. The drives (both instinctual and life-necessary) are ordinarily unconscious. Many of the moral dictates of the personality are unconscious (the moral dictates are referred to as superego components). Many of the adaptive functions of the personality operate unconsciously (an example would be defense mechanisms, to be discussed later).

Freud theorized that many of the infantile drives are experienced subjectively as threatening, and would be diminished if the threatening internal drive was made unconscious. Accordingly, many apparently dangerous drives are kept out of conscious awareness and result in a subjective experience of safety. If a drive is not experienced, as far as the individual is concerned it does not exist, and calmness prevails. Anything that tends to increase the likelihood that drives will become conscious presents a psychic emergency and brings about certain internal coping mechanisms that attempt to push the drives back into the depths of the unconscious.

However, unconscious components of the personality continue to exert an active influence on an individual's mental life and functioning. They account for many types of behavior, feelings, and thoughts that are otherwise without explanation. Many important drives, thoughts, feelings, and memories reside in the unconscious, but nevertheless play an important role in the development process. Material from the unconscious may appear in disguised forms, as in dreams and in everyday slips of the tongue or pen.[34]

FIXATION, REGRESSION, AND REPETITION COMPULSION

Clinical observations have led to the need to develop the concepts of fixation, regression, and repetition-compulsion. These observations include the following.

1 Adult conflict can usually be traced back to earlier conflicts in a patient's life. This does not necessarily imply causation from early life, but it implies some type of "linkage."
2 Under stress, an adult may resort to modes of behavior that had been used in earlier life. These modes of behavior are amazingly persistent and rigid.
3 The mode of behavior chosen to fall back on is usually associated with some previous developmental stress.
4 Some modes of behavior that develop during certain times of developmental stress become persistent behavioral styles, and the individual does not grow out of them.

Regardless of the theory of development to which one adheres, most agree that later behavior derives from childhood. The concepts of fixation, regression, and repetition-compulsion are used to explain these observations.

A *fixation* is a point along the developmental continuum where a stress has occurred, which results in arresting the developmental process or making it incomplete. The individual apparently develops considerable affect at that point in development, and this increases the likelihood of that behavior's persisting or recurring later. Fixation is the persistence of immature modes of coping. For example, a person with considerable stress in the first year of life may retain many characteristics of behavior from that phase, such as dependency, greediness, and oral interests. The fixated behavior is helpful to problem solving in the developmental period in which it arises, but it persists beyond the time of its appropriateness. The whole process of fixation remains unconscious.

Regression is related to fixation, and it means the employment of modes of behavior that were appropriate to earlier problem solving. Regression is unconscious, and is a psychological return to an earlier mode of function. The example of a retreating army is sometimes used. Imagine the psychological defenses of the adult under the bombardment of stress, and imagine that adult retreating back to the safety of a fort.

Repetition-compulsion refers to the tendency to repeat over and over old behavioral styles that had been associated with unsolved conflicts. It is unclear why there is a tendency to repeat behavior associated with unsolved conflicts, rather than to repeat behavior associated with mastery of conflicts.

In essence, these concepts explain that excessive stress and unsolved conflict during early development predispose the individual to certain behavioral styles in adult life, and the entire process occurs unconsciously.

ORGANIZATION OF PERSONALITY

Freud conceptualized the personality as being divided into three functioning parts, the id, the ego, and the superego. These parts were not concrete entities, but groups of functions. This continues to be a convenient way of describing functions of different personality components and their dynamic interplay.[35] Psychoanalytic theory emphasized the importance of developmental stages for the instinctual drives. That would now seem to be an incomplete way of viewing developmental stages, since multiple components of the personality go through a series of maturational stages that include instinctual drives, ego functions such as defense mechanisms, cognitive functions, and certain superego changes. A discussion of the three functioning parts of the personality will follow.

The Id

The *id* is the personality component that is comprised of the motivational forces stemming from innate biological drives. These drives motivate the individual toward action that results in gratification of the drives. The id provides the drive, the push, the motivation for the organism. The organism could not survive without drives. It is the innately given portion of the personality, and its impulses break into consciousness, and produce considerable discomfort.

The id's drives have been defined previously as innate biologic urges to action. The drives are initiated by a stimulus that is either external or internal, and leads to a state of central excitation. The state of psychologic tension pushes or urges the individual toward behavior that will reduce the tension.

The drives of the id operate entirely on the "pleasure principle." They urge action with the sole purpose of obtaining tension reduction and the subjective feeling of pleasure. The id has no reality testing, logical reasoning, or moral values. It can be visualized as a boiling cauldron of primitive drives seeking satisfaction without regard to the consequences. It remains for other personality components to add a sense of reality testing, logical thinking, and a control system so that id impulses cannot run rampant.

The patterns of behavior that are used to gratify the sexual and aggressive drives are influenced greatly by environmental experiences. An individual will learn different ways of gratification as development progresses. The importance of the sexual and aggressive instinctual drives as motivational forces early in life has been stressed by Freud. It should be repeated, however, that these drives in childhood do not resemble their adult counterparts, but they can be seen to provide motivation from birth into adulthood, when the more readily recognized sexual and aggressive drives are present.

Through a sequential series of developmental stages, these drives and the personality organization are altered in preparation for a stable adult adjustment. The type of gratification necessary for the instinctual drives varies according to the developmental stage, and the behavior needed to achieve it varies as well. For example, during the first year of life an infant is interested in "oral gratification," such as sucking and ingesting food. The importance of social contact with the nurturing mother is important during this stage as well. During the second and third year of life, however, there is an interest in motility, greater independence, and controlling certain body functions.

The Ego

The *ego* is the functioning component of the personality. It controls, coordinates, and negotiates compromise solutions intrapsychically. It mediates between different components of the personality, and relates to the outside world. As the ego develops, it gives form, direction, and order to the personality. This is in contrast to the disorganized behavior of the infant that is influenced mainly by id forces. The ego organizes behavior into realistic, mature patterns. It provides the individual with realistic perceptions, memory, logical thinking, feelings, skillful actions, and good judgment. The ego begins developing in infancy, and reaches its highest level of development in adulthood. It is essential to a person who lives in a civilized society. The disorganized, immature, irrational behavior of the infant must be altered in order for socialization and goal-directed behavior to occur. The ego contains the evaluating, judging, compromising, and problem-solving ability of the personality. In addition, it contains components known as mechanisms of defense. These components operate unconsciously, and are used to establish compromises between conflicting internal forces and to make certain that threatening id impulses are kept unconscious. The ego may be regarded as the executive agency of the personality and is responsible for appropriate adaptation to external reality. Major functions of the ego are: (1) perception, (2) consciousness, (3) memory, (4) attention, (5) thought, (6) intelligence, (7) speech and language, (8) motility and motor skills, (9) judgment and foresight, (10) capacity for the delay of needs and impulses, (11) mechanisms for defense, and (12) affects or feelings.

Development of the Ego Some ego functions (such as perception, consciousness, and motility) are present at birth. A second group develops as the infant matures, but they depend very little on learning. If the infant is healthy physically and the atmosphere is affectionate and appropriately stimulating, these ego functions develop in a predictable maturational sequence. Functions such as the ability to sit up, crawl, walk, and control bowel and bladder functions are examples. Another group of ego functions, the mechanisms of defense, develop under the influence of both maturational and environmental factors. They operate unconsciously and are important in alleviating anxiety and making extreme affective states more bearable. All developing ego functions need an emotionally nurturing environment. The development of the mechanisms of defense is highly dependent upon specific parent attitudes during different developmental stages. Failure of the parents to offer the appropriate response in any stage may lead to a developmental arrest for these particular ego functions. This arrest is referred to as fixation. Such an arrest may result in persistence of immature ego functions.

Ego functions in the cognitive sphere are more dependent upon experience and learning for their development. Higher intellectual functions, such as the ability to read, write, and do arithmetic, depend upon stimulation from experience as well as maturation of the nervous system. However, even with these ego functions, a child must have received adequate emotional nurturing before it will be possible to benefit fully from the higher intellectual stimulation.

A well-functioning ego will be able to modify and achieve gratification for its drives, alter and satisfy the demands of the superego, and make practical adaptation to the reality of the external world.

The Superego

The third functioning component of the personality, which is often equated with conscience, is the *superego*. It consists of internal moral and social values that are enduring and independent of external circumstances. It has both conscious and unconscious parts, and has two main functions. The first is an inhibiting, admonishing, and threatening function, giving internal advice regarding what the individual should not do. The second sets forth goals and ideals toward which the individual might strive, giving internal directions regarding what should be done.

The superego is formed during development by identification with important adults, mainly parents or their surrogates. These individuals and their values are incorporated into the personality to form the superego. This process begins early in life, and is well advanced by the age of 6. The developing individual continues to experience alterations in the superego as he or she comes into contact with other authorities and cultural influences. The superego that develops by the age of 6 tends to be a rigid, harsh, primitive, absolute force. It is uncompromising and inhibiting, and remains unconscious for the most part. It supervises the ego and the id and serves as a judgmental part of the personality. Conflict involving the id or ego in opposition to the superego produces considerable intrapsychic stress and discomfort. The rigid superego of childhood must be modified in order for an adult to have a comfortable, harmonious adjustment. Considerable modification occurs typically during the adolescent years. During this developmental stage, the second component of the superego undergoes its main development. This is the portion of the superego that advises an individual about what should be accomplished, and is referred to as the *ego-ideal*.

DEVELOPMENTAL STAGES

Important observations regarding innate characteristics and environmental influences have been reviewed earlier in this chapter. Development cannot be viewed as though these forces act independently. In fact, they influence each other repeatedly. For example, if an infant has the innate capacity to smile readily, this provokes a warm response from the mother. The warmth of the mother in turn aids in the healthy development of the infant. As the healthy infant progresses normally to each new developmental goal, the mother feels pride and warmth, which is reflected in her attitude toward the developing child. The important feature to emphasize is the interaction between the innate and the environment, between the child and the mother. The interactional approach emphasizes the mutual influence on each other in the mother-infant relationship. Henderson speaks of the "goodness of fit" between mother and child.[36] When the temperament and the attitude of the mother happen to match well with the temperament of the child, "consonance" is present, and optimal development occurs. Conversely, poorness of fit produces "dissonance" and distorted development occurs. Much more can be understood by studying the interaction between the mother and the child than by studying them independently.

Each person goes through a series of developmental stages from infancy to death. The distinction between stages is not clearly demarcated, since they merge one into the other. Many different components of personality undergo development simultaneously. For instance, cognitive skills are undergoing developmental changes parallel to instinctual drives, values, coping skills, and mechanisms of defense. The maturation of personality components may progress along parallel directions in a calm, even fashion, reaching adulthood with a well-integrated, mature, cohesive personality organization. However, stressful, frustrating experiences during critical developmental stages may lead to arrested development for certain personality components. As a result, development may proceed unevenly, and adulthood will bring with it problems of immaturity, lack of coping skills, and failure of adequate integration of personality components.

According to the epigenetic principle, certain maturational changes must occur during time specific developmental phases, referred to as "critical stages." The developing organism needs specific environmental responses during these critical periods. If these responses do not occur, development of particular personality components will be arrested.

Various classification schemes may be used in describing developmental stages. This depends upon which aspect of development is being emphasized. In fact, multiple changes are occurring at any given stage. Important factors undergoing maturational changes during various stages are:

1 Basic instinctual drives, motivational forces or needs
2 Methods of gratifying needs
3 Nature of relationships with others
4 Self-image
5 Conflicts between intrapsychic forces
6 Cognitive skills
7 Coping skills—ego strengths, including mechanisms of defense

These changing components of personality are integrated continuously with the physical maturational changes during each developmental stage.

Period of Infancy (First Year)

The human infant enters life with innately determined instinctual drives and a number of innately determined temperamental traits. However, little exists in the way of a true personality organization. Needs center around food, warmth, bodily comfort, certain types of sensory stimulation, and the need for maternal social contact. Basic physiologic satisfaction is provided to a large extent through the oral mucosa and the tactile-kinesthetic sensory system of the skin. Psychoanalytic theory has emphasized the need for satisfaction through the oral mucosa, and accordingly this period has been classified as the "oral phase." Sucking is an act of extreme pleasure, and breast feeding meets the need for both food and physical contact.

The relationship between the mother and the infant is very important in several ways:

1 Satisfying need for food.
2 Providing bodily comfort, warmth, and keeping the infant dry.
3 Providing stimulation of sensory system; this is an extremely important part of the mother-infant interaction. The importance of holding, rocking, and touching the infant has been demonstrated for both emotional and physical maturation. Stimulation of the oral mucosa and visual system are considered very important as well.
4 Meeting social contact needs.
5 Providing a sense of trust in the external world.

The attentiveness of a sensitive mother will result in the gratification of needs for food and basic bodily comfort. At the same time, the infant must learn gradually to tolerate some degree of discomfort, since continuous gratification of needs is not realistic. A healthy mother-infant interaction includes gratification of basic needs and also teaches the infant to gradually tolerate reasonable frustration. Maternal deprivation or overindulgence may create developmental problems.

The quality and quantity of sensory stimulation provided by the mother is important in early infancy. A highly developed sensory apparatus makes the infant acutely aware of the environment. Abandonment or severe neglect can lead to depression and physical wasting of the infant. Deprivation may lead to behavioral problems in adulthood. These include problems in forming intimate adult relationships, in parenting behavior, and a tendency toward depression.

Erikson has emphasized the development of "basic trust" in early infancy.[1] If the mother-infant relationship is dependable, consistent, and gratifying, a sense of basic trust develops within the infant. This is an important early building block in personality development. This early positive experience between mother and child has lifelong personality consequences. Confidence, optimism, security, and a positive self-image are related to the quality of the mother-infant relationship and the sense of basic trust that evolves. The dependent-receptive position of the young infant leads to an overall impression of passivity. This gradually gives way during the first year of life to a more aggressive approach, particularly at about 8 months of age. Sucking is replaced by biting, and it is hypothesized that aggressive drives increase in intensity at this time. Freud believed that the intense oral strivings of the infant constitute a forerunner of adult sexual urges. Accordingly, the pleasurable strivings of the infant undergo a maturational process through a series of stages which blossom into fully recognized sexual urges and feelings in adolescence. These "infantile sexual feelings" play a powerful motivational role in childhood behavior and in the way the personality is organized. To a large degree, personality organization is related to finding ways to modify, control, and gratify these instinctual strivings for pleasure.

Another important personality component is self-image, and early in life it is intimately associated with the body image. The infant experiences the self as being his or her body. A factor that contributes to some distortion in this regard is that the infant does not easily recognize where the infant's body stops and the mother's body begins. The two seem as one to the young infant. As awareness of the separateness of the mother increases, separation anxiety occurs and some vague awareness of extreme dependence on this powerful person develops. This lack of ego boundaries early in life facilitates the development of primitive ego mechanisms which serve the infant well at that point in time. However, they are maladaptive if used beyond early childhood. These defense mechanisms, projection, and denial will be discussed later in the chapter.

An important aspect of the self-image is gender identity, self-awareness of maleness or femaleness. By the age of 18 months to 2 years, a normally developing child has a concept of himself as a boy, or of herself as a girl. Normally, gender identity is fully differentiated between the ages of 3½ and 4½, after which it is relatively immune to change. The sense of maleness or femaleness develops mainly as a result of the attitude of the parents toward the infant. Parents relate very differently to male and female infants, and this attitudinal difference is much more important in the developing sense of gender identity than is the sex chromosomal picture. This attitudinal difference on the part of the parents starts at birth. Accordingly, the attitude of the parents during the first year is important in the ultimate establishment of a sense of sexual identity.[37]

A smooth, harmonious, gratifying first year of development allows the infant to move into the second year of life with a feeling of trust and·security. Excessive deprivation or other stresses, however, may result in various levels of developmental arrest and lead to excessive dependency, needs for excessive "oral gratification," self-centeredness, greediness, aggressive and demanding traits, avoidance of intimacy, adult problems in mothering, or a tendency toward depression.

A 36-year-old married female with three children came for treatment because of a recurring depression. She was a very dependent, clinging person who leaned heavily on her husband and children for emotional support. Her husband's business required a great deal of traveling. She became very depressed whenever he went on a business trip. This problem had recurred over several years and was getting worse. Past history showed that when the patient was 8 months old, her mother had become seriously ill and was removed from any contact with the patient for 1½ years. The infant experienced an "anaclitic depression," precipitated by the loss of contact with the maternal figure. This type of infantile depression was described earlier as a consequence of maternal deprivation and has been reported extensively by Spitz.[31] A fixation point developed in response to the stress and emotional upset experienced by the infant. Subsequently, when the patient experienced stress that was related to the loss of someone upon whom she depended, she regressed to the fixation point and became depressed as she had as an infant.

Late Infancy (2–3 Years of Age)

During later infancy, the infant develops new physical skills that influence the psychological development of this period. There is increased capacity for motility, manipulation of objects with hands, and walking and talking. Myelinization of the proper neuropathways allows for spincteric muscle utilization so that bowel and bladder control can be achieved. This is a period in which increased autonomy and independence are developed. Appropriate mothering allows for an appropriate amount of independence, autonomy, and separation without allowing the youngster to go beyond the developing physical abilities. A mother-child relationship that interferes with adequate separation-individuation may lead to developmental arrest which may present in adulthood as the so-called "borderline syndrome" (see Chapter 11). In late infancy there is a tendency toward negativism and the infant typically says "no" rather than "yes." The negativism is vital in the development of a feeling of individuation. During the first year of life, the infant does not experience the mother as a separate entity. This psychological fusion of mother and infant is referred to as symbiosis. As the child develops physically to the point of greater independence, there is parallel psychological development that gives the feeling of separation from the symbiotic relationship. After separation occurs, the individual then begins to recognize the uniqueness of his or her individual characteristics. Individuation promotes autonomy, independence, and a recognition of one's achievements and strengths.[38] Clearly, the tasks for parents during the late infancy stage change. They are required to be firm about the boundaries of acceptable behavior, while encouraging progressive emancipation.

One shift in instinctual drives that has played an important role in psychoanalytic theory is the maturational shift during which pleasure areas change from the oral mucosa to the bowel and bladder mucosa. Stimuli arising from the bowel and bladder mucosa produce central excitation, driving the individual toward behavior to obtain pleasure associated with these areas or mobilizing psychological defenses to deal with the inner tension. Infants seem to experience considerable pleasure in the eliminative functions. Freud considered that these "anal strivings" were part of the continuum of infantile sexual feelings. He stressed the importance of conflicts that develop between strivings on the part of the infant for gratification of these body parts and the social expectations of the mother. This is a period in which extensive socializing is taught by the mother. Gratification is not so easily achieved by the infant during late infancy, as more is expected in terms of self-control. The infant must learn to postpone bladder and bowel elimination until the proper time and place. Maternal demands interfere with strict pleasure seeking, and create conflict between the demands of the mother and the instinctual urges of the infant.

The child must struggle to resolve the conflict that develops between internal desires to gratify instinctual urges and the opposing demands of the powerful, loved, and frightening parent. However, observations of children indicate that this struggle between the desires of the infant and the expectations of the mother are much broader than just toilet training. Children in this phase are strong-willed about a number of their desires. In fact, if they are born with temperaments that include the easy establishment of physiologic rhythms, toilet training may proceed very harmoniously, and the struggle would be about other issues involving autonomous strivings. Adversely, overdemanding, rigid parents may produce parent-child struggles in several ways, and not solely in terms of toilet training. The struggle with toilet training would represent only one instance in an overall child-rearing problem.

The child has developed new tools with which to struggle against a parent. Maturational development gives the child motility, coordination, walking, and improved communication skills. Children within this age group tend to be "strong-willed," and to demand their autonomy. Yet, the demands of reality are powerful also. Some children resolve the power struggle by submitting to the parental demands completely, and develop behavioral patterns of submissiveness, clingingness, orderliness, and punctuality. Such traits may persist and dominate the adult personality. On the other hand, the infant may rebel against parental demands and become angry, obstinate, unreliable, and disorderly. These traits, too, may persist.

The self-image of the infant may evolve in different directions, depending upon experiences in this period. With positive experiences, the self-image that develops includes confidence in self-control, personal independence, and a sense of autonomy and pride. However, negative experiences emphasize feelings of shame and disgust. The infant comes to believe that he or she is always doing something wrong, should feel ashamed, and that bowels, bladder, and other bodily functions cannot be controlled in a way pleasing to the powerful parent. As a result, shame develops. If development is arrested at this particular phase with a negative self-image, the persistent negative effect may persist into adulthood and cause emotional problems. These individuals may have the persistent feeling of being viewed by others with feelings of disgust, regardless of attempts to please them.

Cognitive skills during this period play an important role. There is an increased ability to conceptualize the world and to communicate. Thinking tends to have an omnipotent, magical quality. The infant feels that inner thoughts are powerful, and finds it difficult to distinguish between urges as being equivalent to, or just as bad as, behavior. A desire to oppose the will of the parent may be viewed as totally unacceptable, and defensive maneuvers on the part of the ego go into action to repress or bury such urges or thoughts in the unconscious. Numerous defense mechanisms develop during this phase to deal with urges and thoughts that are so powerful and threatening to the infant. These include reaction formation, undoing, isolation, and rationalization.

Early Childhood (3-6 Years of Age)

Several personality components that have been developing simultaneously come together during this phase to give the youngster a feeling of confidence, mastery, and the ability to grieve and to worry. The child has growing cognitive skills and extensive fantasies and wishes. A considerable amount of omnipotence that is attached to fantasies continues, and these fantasies are seen by the youngster as extremely powerful. The child's reaction to wishes, fantasies, and urges may lead to defensive operations that play major roles. Freud emphasized the strong role that infantile strivings have during this phase, and especially the sexual strivings toward the parent of the opposite sex. Relationships take on the quality of specificity during this period. People are seen more as individuals, with differences and similarities, and intense attachments develop that are quite different from the generalized attachments that develop earlier in life.

Psychoanalytic theory emphasized that the development of these specific relationships is entwined with important shifts in the instinctual drives. According to psychoanalytic theory, pleasurable interest is directed more toward the genital area, and masturbatory play may occur. Intense attachment with a sexualized component develops for the parent of the opposite sex. The son wants an exclusive, possessive relationship with his mother, and the daughter an exclusive, possessive relationship with her father. Jealousy and rivalry develop with the parent of the same sex, and anger and fear often result. This creates a conflict for the young boy, for example, because the love he feels for his father conflicts with the anger and fear that are also felt. This triangular relationship involving child, mother, and father was described by Freud as the *Oedipal complex.* Feelings within the youngster consist of positive erotic feelings, anger, fear, and guilt. Discomfort develops because of the conflictual nature of these feelings, and the problem is usually resolved by the youngster's identifying with the parent of the same sex and renouncing the erotic attachment to the parent of the opposite sex. This process of identification lays the groundwork for a child's entry into the world, with an appropriate sexual identity but also the moral values, beliefs, and goals of the parent. In a sense, identification is an internal commitment to future goals. In this way, a parent's values may be perpetuated by the child.

Many believe that the Oedipal problem has been unduly emphasized. The theory was based upon the study of disturbed patients, and the problem itself may be aggravated in families that are disturbed but may not be as important in normal development. It may be more useful to conceptualize the problem as one of learning to share love and possessions. The child in this group has a hard time giving to or sharing with others, and has a highly competitive spirit that tends to produce rivalry and jealousy with others. Completing this developmental phase normally should set the stage for the individual's being a sharing, loving, giving person later in life. Failure to complete this stage normally may lead to an individual who is jealous, envious, and unreasonably competitive.

In this period the youngster shows initiative in thinking, fantasies, wishes, and behavior. If this period is traversed positively, the youngster will more likely have confidence in being able to approach future life situations with constructive initiative. If, however, the stress of this period outweighs the positive effects, tendencies toward guilt, inhibitions, and lack of initiative may develop in adult life. In essence, excessive stress during the early childhood phase leads to either unreasonable competitiveness or lack of initiative.

The intense feelings that the child develops for the parent during this period tend to be repressed into the unconscious. They may surface in adult life and be directed to others. These feelings are known as transference feelings. Transference is the unconscious transfer of feelings from childhood relationships onto someone in adult life. This may result in intense, irrational attachments that cannot be explained on the basis of current life situations.

Late Childhood (7-12 Years of Age)

During late childhood, there is socialization outside the family in the form of attendance at school, group play, and organizations. Identification with teachers or other important adults allows the child to adopt new, admired traits and to modify the superego by learning new moral values.

This is a development stage of great industry. The development of skills is extensive, with reading, writing, learning, and hobbies forming important achievements. Failure to achieve with peers can result in a deep sense of inferiority. Development of adaptive skills in this period facilitates adjustment in a number of ways. The skills themselves may be very useful in adulthood, and a self-image as a successful achiever is valuable.

During this time, instinctual drives appear to be diverted away from pleasurable gratification into channels of productive work. The term *latency period* has been used in describing this phase because of the relative inactivity of instinctual urges. However, latency is a misnomer because this is an extremely active stage for the development of essential skills. It is latent only if one focuses on infantile sexual strivings. It is very active in terms of the development of the skills that will be vital for adult adaptation. An important mechanism of defense that develops during this time, called *sublimation*, is valuable in channeling instinctual energy into constructive accomplishments.

Adolescent Phase (13-18 Years of Age)

Adolescence begins with puberty and is characterized at the onset by rapid growth and development of sexual organs, and a rapid upsurge in aggressive and sexual drives. An inner urge develops toward heterosexuality and genital sexual pleasure. The adolescent must go through an extensive personality reorganization in order to tolerate the internal sexual urges. The harsh, rigid, superego from childhood cannot tolerate such feelings and must be altered. This reorganization of the personality is a major struggle for the adolescent; a new self-image or identity must evolve. The development of a positive ego ideal is considered essential to a successful adolescent phase. It occurs by means of identification with various admired people with whom the adolescent has contact. The ego ideal promotes positive strivings, and gives the adolescent a new sense of being, identity, and character. Other important changes include new levels of abstract ability and cognitive skills, increased autonomy, decreased dependency on parents, and development of vocational and educational skills. To achieve this personality reorganization and to emerge with a new identity is a major struggle of the adolescent years.

Adulthood

Increasing chronological age does not mean maturity. The trauma and hardship during development may leave aspects of immaturity in the personality. These immature features may interfere with a healthy adjustment in adulthood. A mature adult should be essentially happy in love and in work, have a clear personal identity and the ability to form intimate relationships, be able to assume responsibility for rearing children, and be capable of working independently in a gratifying way.

Development does not stop at adulthood. Most psychological studies emphasize childhood and adolescent development and leave an impression of a static, mechanical adult. Observations of adults do not support this notion. Erikson emphasized the importance of developmental stages throughout life, but further clarification of adult developmental patterns is needed.[1] The formation of intimate relationships, satisfying family involvements, and adequate social support systems is crucial to mental health in adulthood. Status, achievement, and power are important. The interrelationship of physical and mental health is of nuclear importance. Essentially a changing, dynamic personality picture exists throughout adult life.

CONFLICT AND ANXIETY

The importance of intrapsychic conflict and its relationship to anxiety needs to be understood to appreciate the dynamic nature of the personality. The psyche is in a continuous state of flux, with various psychological forces always opposing or complementing one another. Id impulses are constantly striving for gratification, and the ego must coordinate these strivings with the demands of reality and the prohibitions and expectations of the superego. Id impulses invariably clash with the superego and reality. If an impulse is ruled unacceptable by superego dictates, an individual cannot tolerate awareness of the impulse. Conscious awareness of the intense intrapsychic conflict or impulse is unbearable, and a rapid solution must be found. The ego resolves this intrapsychic conflict by defensive operations that keep the id impulse and the superego prohibition unconscious. As long as the conflict with id and superego are kept unconscious, the individual is more comfortable. Anything that increases the likelihood of the conflict or the id components of the conflict's becoming conscious makes the individual uncomfortable. The discomfort occurs in the form of *anxiety,* a very important affective state, which is an uncomfortable feeling in response to internal threats. When an individual is threatened by external events, the affect is termed *fear.* Anxiety and fear are similar in subjective experiences. With anxiety, the individual is experiencing an internal threat and is often unaware of the nature of the threat. Anxiety may be subjectively perceived or it may be characterized by motor and visceral responses: hyperhidrosis, dryness of the mouth, anorexia, constipation, vomiting, diarrhea, gastric hypersecretion, and changes in heart rate and blood pressure. A person may become agitated, overactive, or show motor tension. The most acceptable theory about anxiety is that it functions as a signal of internal danger; anxiety is seen as a signal to the ego to use stronger control mechanisms to maintain id impulses and associated conflicts within the unconscious aspect of the mind. This ordinarily means the utilization of stronger defense mechanisms to achieve this control. Anxiety may remain unconscious and present itself only as motor and visceral experiences. Other painful feeling states that show evidence of underlying conflict include depression, guilt, and shame. Depression signals the actual or anticipated loss of love or approval from an outside person. Guilt signals the threat of disapproval from the superego because of immoral feelings, urges, or behavior. Shame indicates superego disapproval for failure to live up to expectations. Intrapsychic conflict and anxiety play important organizing roles for personality development. They occur at specific phases of development and precipitate certain defense mechanisms which may become permanent parts of the personality structure. To repeat, these defenses are activated to control id impulses from entering conscious awareness. Another feeling state, fear, alerts the individual to realistic external danger and mobilizes fight or flight responses.

Three special features of childhood mental life play an important role in increasing the intensity of the conflict and resulting anxiety during these years.

1 The immature evaluative functions of the ego. The ego of the young child does not discriminate among urges, thoughts, and behavior. They are all considered to be the same. The thought is, therefore, as bad as the deed. This literal, concrete thinking of the child results in an unacceptable wish or thought's being resisted as though it were behavior. Angry feelings toward parents might be perceived internally as being the same as, and therefore just as bad as, physically harming the parents; to wish death is to become a murderer. As a result, an unacceptable wish provokes intense ego operations to repress it.

2 The omnipotence of childhood. The ego of young children promotes an omnipotent view of themselves and their urges, wishes, and fantasies. They feel enormously powerful, and this adds to the threatening nature of their impulses. They view their urges and thoughts as magical, powerful, and a universal threat to others.

3 Harsh, punitive superego. The superego of the developing child is primitive, unyielding, and harshly punitive.

This combination of literal, concrete thinking that fails to discriminate between the thought and the deed; a self-view of omnipotent, powerful fantasies; and a harsh, punitive superego intensifies intrapsychic conflicts for children. Urges are seen as extremely threatening, and conflict with a rigid superego develops. Defense mechanisms keep the threatening urges out of awareness and thus decrease anxiety. However, this has the disadvantage of not allowing the immature evaluative functions of the ego to become more mature by interacting with reality. Any personality component that becomes conscious must interact with the world of reality and this has a beneficial, maturing impact upon the personality. Psychic forces that are buried in the unconscious stay there unchanged, without undergoing any maturation. Therefore, adults continue to react to immature, primitive impulses with the same anxiety experienced from these impulses as children. These immature, primitive impulses may continue to exert an impact on behavior and mental life in adulthood.

There are certain conditions that increase the threat of a breakthrough of an id impulse into conscious awareness. These conditions cause a sudden increase in anxiety and the mobilization of ego defenses to control the id impulses.

1 An increase in instinctual drives (at puberty)

2 Stimulation from without that stirs the instinctual drives (a highly stimulating festive occasion or a seductive relationship)

3 External events that impair ego functions (extreme stress such as the death of a loved one)

4 Physiologic impairment of ego functions (alcohol, fatigue, illness)

5 Ego deficits that are secondary to emotional stress during the formative years (neurotic illness or personality disorders)

When the id impulses threaten to break into consciousness, anxiety becomes extreme, and emergency ego maneuvers become operational. If the ego is mature, it can call upon adaptive defense mechanisms to control the id impulse, and maintain an adequate adjustment to the external world. An immature ego, however, relies upon less adaptive mechanisms of defense and may utilize pathological maneuvers to control anxiety. When the term *ego strength* is used, it refers to the ability to use adaptive, mature mechanisms of defense when stress occurs. *Ego weakness* is a term that refers to the tendency of an individual to utilize immature, less adaptive mechanisms of defense at times of stress. Anxiety is thus seen as a signal of impending ego breakdown and id impulse eruption. It represents an intrapsychic emergency that calls for rapid mobilization of whatever ego mechanisms are available once again to establish harmonious intrapsychic control.

There are other explanations for the occurrence of anxiety. Behaviorism explains anxiety as a conditioned response and supports a treatment approach that emphasizes deconditioning. Others would emphasize that anxiety is strictly related to an underlying biochemical abnormality of the central nervous system, and would support psychopharmacotherapy as the treatment approach. Still another explanation is more psychologically oriented and emphasizes the identification of children with unrealistic anticipatory fears of their parents; in essence, children learn to be anxious in the same way that their parents are anxious. The dominant view of anxiety continues to be, however, that it functions as a signal of threats to internal harmony.[39]

THE MECHANISMS OF DEFENSE

An important aspect of ego functioning is a system of special mental processes that offer protection from excessive anxiety and other unbearable affects. These processes are known as *mechanisms of defense,* which are defined as automatic, involuntary, unconscious mental processes utilized to prevent awareness of unacceptable impulses or urges, and to diminish the intensity of unbearable affect.

Mechanisms of defense may be utilized only briefly at times of stress, or may be ingrained into the character structure, and continue to be utilized long after the stress that activated them has subsided. While maintaining inner harmony by diminishing anxiety, mechanisms of defense may alter the individual's perception of internal and external realities and may compromise various aspects of cognitive thinking. In essence, psychic tranquility is achieved by some degree of distorted thinking.

Many different mechanisms of defense have been listed in the literature, one of the earliest outlines having been by Anna Freud.[40] No one list is agreed upon by all authorities in the field. The following outline presents a number of defenses that are frequently included in other lists.

Repression

Repression is the main mechanism of defense, and refers to the exclusion from awareness of urges, thoughts, fantasies, feelings, and memories that would be threatening if allowed into consciousness. The assessment of the dangerousness of the impulse is spontaneous, unconscious, and may be quite irrational. The irrational nature of the dangerousness of impulses should be emphasized. An impulse that was seen as dangerous in childhood may no longer be of any danger. Yet, the unconscious impression of dangerousness may have persisted into adulthood and will cause anxiety and mobilization of mechanisms of defense just as though a very real and serious threat existed. Repression pushes the dangerous urge, thought, or feeling into the unconscious. It is an automatic, spontaneous, unconscious ego action that prevents awareness of an intolerable internal state. Ideas and memories that might produce anxiety cannot be remembered because of repression. Experiences involving guilt or shame are buried in the subterranean region of the mind and cannot be recalled. Intolerable urges are not destroyed but are blocked from expression. The drives continue to strive for awareness, and the ego must supply continuous energy and effort in order to keep the forbidden urges buried. This depletes a certain amount of ego energy that could be used for other functions.

Repression is the basic mechanism of defense and many, if not all mechanisms, work in conjunction with repression. Other mechanisms of defense come into play to assist if and when repression fails to contain an intolerable state completely.

> An attractive 28-year-old female behaved in a highly seductive manner, but was unaware of the flirtatious aspect of her behavior. She was surprised and puzzled about the sexual interest shown in her by many men. She explained this to herself by forming an opinion of men along the lines of their animalistic instincts and constant interest in sex rather than in the whole person. Repression of her sexual urges made her unaware of these feelings and her sexually provocative behavior. She was inviting sexual advances, but superego prohibitions would not let her be aware of this. Conscious aspects of her sexual feelings had been repressed and were expressed through her behavioral style without her awareness.

Repression may lead to amnesia or frequent forgetting. Traumatic experiences in childhood are pushed into unconsciousness by repression. Repression occurs in normal individuals, particularly during childhood, when large segments of unacceptable, instinctual urges are repressed. Most of the elements of the Oedipal complex, for example, are repressed during childhood. Everyone experiences brief lapses of memory that are secondary to repression, such as forgetting a name or unpleasant past experiences.

Projection

Projection refers to disowning one's attitudes, feelings, and urges, and attributing them to some other person or external agent. An individual gives disclaimed and objectionable character traits, urges, thoughts, and impulses to others. Anxiety is diminished because one no longer is responsible for possessing the unacceptable urges. However, a high price is paid in terms of perceptual distortion when this mechanism is used repeatedly for diminishing anxiety. Projection, like denial, is one of the more primitive mechanisms, and when used in its extreme form, it leads to psychotic delusions and hallucinations.

This mechanism starts early in life, as evidenced by children's tendencies to identify good qualities as their own and attribute their undesirable traits to others. Retention of projection as a major mechanism of defense beyond early childhood years results in significant perceptual distortion that may predispose the individual to serious psychopathology.

During the developmental years, projection plays a major role in personality development. Feelings of anger are often personally responsible for such unpleasant feelings. This allows the child to develop a positive self-image since the "bad" feelings are cast out. However, the child then sees the parent as having the child's own powerful angry feelings. The child may then identify with these allegedly angry people and incorporate them into its personality in the form of an angry, harsh, punitive conscience. By this dynamic series of events, the child's own anger is transformed into a harsh, punitive conscience. This normal developmental occurrence accounts for the typically harsh, punitive conscience seen in normal children.

In the healthy adult, projection ordinarily does not dominate one's personality; it only occurs at times of stress, and then fleetingly. An adult who is angry because of sudden, extreme embarrassment as a result of a mistake may unconsciously project the blame onto someone else temporarily. The more a person relies on projection, the more distorted his or her perception of the external world will be. Beyond a certain point, paranoid delusional thinking will develop as a result of extreme projection. Less extreme forms of projection are involved in prejudice, unwarranted suspiciousness, and hyperalertness to external injustice. Individuals with such characteristics may be "odd," eccentric, and abrasive. The milder form is called *projection* and the more severe form of this mechanism is called *delusional projection.*

> An elderly widowed male had used projection as a major mechanism of defense throughout his life, and had achieved a neighborhood reputation as being eccentric and odd. He told neighbors strange stories about the dangers that abounded in the community, warning them to carry a gun with them if they walked to the shopping center, because someone might try to harm them. (In fact, the neighborhood was safe and walking to the shopping center was common.) He carried several guns in his car in case of an attack and had obtained "stink bombs" from the Army for riot control. He believed extreme measures should be used to stop law breakers. On one occasion, he pushed his lawn mower in front of a passing car that he considered to be going over the speed limit. He complained bitterly when he was fined $25.00 by the city commission, because he felt his act had been honorable and on the side of the law. His anger was handled by projecting it onto several outside agencies, and he then reacted to the threats around him.

Denial

Denial refers to excluding from awareness some aspect of disturbing reality. It occurs normally in young children and is a mechanism whereby a young and immature ego delays awareness of a threatening world until greater levels of maturity are reached. As the ego matures and can tolerate reality issues more comfortably, the use of denial diminishes. Denial goes hand in hand with a weak, immature ego. Children show considerable denial as they engage in extensive fantasy life, which they believe at times to be true. However, as the individual reaches adulthood, the ego should have matured to a point where denial is used minimally. Extensive denial results in massive perceptual blind spots and can impair mature functioning to the point of psychosis. Denial occurs in normal individuals in certain fairly transient circumstances, and can be corrected in due time by factual information. A normal person facing severe stress, such as a fatal illness or severe injury, or death or illness in a loved one may use denial to deal with the overwhelming feelings that occur suddenly.

Also, highly motivated individuals can be trained to use denial in times of stress such as times of war, where the realistic risk of injury cannot be perceived accurately if a soldier is to function well in the battlefield. To avoid the realistic fear of injury or death, one denies the danger of the situation.

A 35-year-old married female with three children had a coping style with immature features, but had managed to make an acceptable life adjustment with the support of her husband and other family members. One of her children became acutely ill and died suddenly, through no one's fault. The sudden, natural tragedy was extremely stressful. After being in a shocklike state for a few days, she began talking and acting as if nothing had happened. She began talking to others as though the child were still alive, and went through a daily routine that included attending to the deceased child's daily needs. She cleaned the dead child's room each day, prepared the child's meals, and washed his clothing. She had denied the child's death to the point of psychotic thinking, and would not respond to any attempts to correct her thinking.

The unbearable feelings at the time of the child's death could not be tolerated, and the mother regressed to a developmental level of extreme denial. This protected her feelings, but grossly distorted her perception of reality and her functioning.

Distortion

Distortion is defined as a mechanism of defense that involves reshaping external reality to suit inner needs. This defense is seen in children before the age of 5 and is similar to denial. Distortion, however, emphasizes the changing of reality and not simply denying the existence of reality. It may include unrealistic thoughts of one's omnipotence, wish-fulfilling thoughts, or an unrealistic superior self-image. Distortion is seen normally in young children, in dreams, and in fantasies. It may lead to delusional thinking in an adult.

A 30-year-old single male was convinced that he was a superior musician and could make a fortune by singing and playing his guitar. He sent tapes of his music to recording companies and distorted the rejection of his offerings in ways to preserve an unrealistic superior self-image. He convinced himself that the companies were jealous of his superior abilities and did not want him to capture the entire music market. He would not obtain a regular job, for he was convinced it would be a waste of valuable, talented time. In reality, his musical abilities were mediocre, at best. Inwardly, this individual had serious doubts about his value as a person and found this feeling of worthlessness unbearable.

Hypochondriasis

Hypochondriasis is a defense mechanism that transfers aggressive, critical feelings that are felt toward others into complaints of pain and somatic illness. The individual cannot tolerate anger toward others and hides these feelings through the development of hypochondriacal symptoms. This may occur especially when there are feelings of reproach arising out of bereavement or loneliness. The individual is angry at being left alone and not having dependency needs met. The anger felt toward someone else is redirected inwardly in the form of self-reproach, and then transformed into physical complaints. The individual with hypochondriasis suffers considerably, feels afflicted, and appears to be in physical misery. Often, others have to attend to the suffering person, and in this indirect way dependency needs may be gratified.[41]

A 50-year-old married male had been a productive worker, but had also been cynical and pessimistic throughout his life. He had multiple somatic complaints, saw doctors frequently, and never really achieved a state of self-acknowledged good health. His wife had developed a number of outside interests, both socially and vocationally, which increasingly took her away from home and her husband. His anger at having less contact with her was converted into increasing hypochondriacal complaints. When she would arrive home after being away pursuing her outside activities, she would find him in physical misery, with severe constipation, headaches, blurred vision, and chest pain. He was unaware of any anger at her despite her increasing absence from home, since the anger was hidden from awareness or converted into hypochondriacal symptoms.

Passive-Aggressive Behavior

Passive-aggressive behavior is a frequent defensive style of dealing with internal aggression. Feelings of aggression toward others are expressed indirectly and effectively through passivity, masochism, and turning against the self. Passive-aggressive behavior may convert anger at others into silly, provocative behavior or failures that bother others more than the individual. Procrastination and underachieving may be forms of passive-aggressive behavior. The individual may use failing behavior as a means of expressing anger at someone else. The anger felt toward the other person is threatening to the individual and is quickly converted into behavior that hides it from awareness. Passive-aggressive behavior is classified by some as a personality disorder and not as a mechanism of defense.

> A 14-year-old male was experiencing considerable stress from multiple sources. His internal biological drives were seeking gratification, and were accompanied by intense fantasies. He was anxious because he was not convinced that he could control the increasing drive forces. In addition, problems with a number of close friends had disrupted his usual friendship pattern. His father was gone most of the time on business during this part of the year. He needed emotional support, but his mother had focused on his making good grades, and hoping that he would get an academic scholarship to college. She put enormous pressure on him, and he experienced extreme anger toward her. The multiple stresses led to some degree of regression, and he began using passive-aggressive behavior to deal with his anger at his mother. He had used this behavior during an earlier developmental stage, and he returned to it from time to time when under stress. He would not read his homework assignments, turned his school work in late, and began failing tests. The more aggressive the mother became in her demands, the more he underachieved in school. This behavior was most upsetting to the mother, but allowed him to make his angry feelings for the mother more bearable. He expressed his anger at her indirectly without having to be aware of the feelings.

Rationalization

Rationalization is the act of giving logical, believable explanations for behavior that is, in fact, irrational. It is motivated by unconscious urges that are unacceptable, and rationalization provides an acceptable, tolerable reason for the behavior. This is a familiar psychological process and is used by everyone to some degree. Each person has a strong need to view one's behavior as coherent, organized, and logical. Rationalization allows for the maintenance of this self-view through times of inexplicable behavior. It should be emphasized that rationalization, like other mechanisms of defense, is unconsciously motivated. This is in contrast to conscious lying or excuse giving.

Rationalization is generally used with other defense mechanisms that have led to behavior that cannot be easily explained. It provides the explanation for behavior, further disguises other defenses, and reduces the anxiety. For instance, repression can be seen as a front-line defense against unacceptable urges, and if repression fails, displacement might be used to disguise the urge from awareness further. If the behavior that results from displacement is unusual and illogical, rationalization might be called upon as a third line of defense, to give coherence to the behavior.

> A 39-year-old male employee of a large company ordinarily was a passive, unaggressive individual who had difficulty asking his supervisor for a promotion. When he finally mustered the courage, he met with a strong refusal from the supervisor. Following this disappointing interaction, he became angry and insulting in an uncharacteristic way toward several fellow employees. He quickly rationalized his behavior as relating to errors that others were making in their work, and was totally unaware of his anger toward the supervisor. This situation was made possible by means of repression, displacement, and rationalization.

Reaction Formation

Reaction formation refers to the conversion of attitudes, behavior, and feelings to those that are exactly opposite to one's disturbing, unacceptable drives. This defense is seen most often in individuals with obsessive and compulsive behavior.

This defense is called into action when repression begins to weaken. Reaction formation starts early in life, when the conscience begins to form and demands are placed on the child to conform. After the age of 3 demands on children to conform increase, and punishment is delivered to children who do certain unacceptable things such as scream, kick, hit, or throw food. Some children, in an attempt to conform, overshoot the mark and conform to an extreme degree by utilizing reaction formation. In general such youngsters become unduly clean, neat, orderly, and have difficulty in recognizing and expressing aggressive impulses.

This defense is related to a rigorous self-discipline needed for achievement in many professions, such as medicine, science, and architecture. The self-discipline that seems to evolve from reaction formation can be useful vocationally in normal individuals, but in its extreme forms reaction formation can become emotionally crippling.

> A married woman could not tolerate it if things were disorderly or unkempt. Her early developmental history revealed difficulty in toilet training and conforming in general. At her job, her insistence on order, promptness, and attention to detail served her well. At home, her insistence on extreme neatness and excessive orderliness made her family and friends uncomfortable. The entire household was dominated by her controlling attitude. Her instinctual desire to "dirty up" her surroundings had been defended against by reaction formation and had thus been retained as a part of her character.

Isolation

Isolation is a mental mechanism in which there is an involuntary separation of the idea of an unconscious impulse from its appropriate affect. The idea then enters conscious awareness, but the affective component is repressed. As long as the feeling part of the impulse is kept unconscious, the individual feels no responsibility for the impulse. This diminishes anxiety for an otherwise unacceptable impulse. The idea without the associated affect is experienced by an individual as strange, unreal, foreign, and something from the outside. This mechanism is used when repression breaks down and cannot keep all components of an impulse hidden. Isolation allows the idea part into conscious awareness, but keeps the feeling part unconscious. The protective value of isolation rests in the repression of affect.

The mechanism is involved in the formation of obsessional thoughts. An obsessional idea seems unreal because of the absence of conscious affect. Frequently, the thoughts have aggressive or sexual connotations. A person may think, "I want to kill him, I want to kill him" over and over, without having any feeling. The anger associated with these thoughts remains unconscious, and the thought seems strange. The person with such thoughts may not be able to prevent their recurrence. They may take on a tormenting, guilt-engendering quality, but the discomfort is not nearly as great as it would be if the underlying affect were suddenly made conscious.

In addition to being an integral part of obsessional thinking, isolation may occur normally. It may occur during certain life events, following the death of a loved one for example. In the initial stages of grief, a person may be devoid of feelings, or "numblike," because of isolation. The overwhelming feelings that accompany sudden, severe life crises, may be protected against temporarily by isolation. The individual is consciously aware of the sudden tragedy, but it seems strange, unreal, and foreign. In time, the feelings associated with the event are allowed into consciousness, when the individual is better able to cope with them.

A 35-year-old Army sergeant consulted a psychiatrist because of recurring thoughts that his wife was going to die. At times the thoughts came frequently despite his attempts to prevent them. He felt tormented by the thoughts, and became extremely agitated on occasion. An examination of the relationship between the patient and wife revealed considerable friction in their relationship. However, he was unaware of his angry feelings, which were intolerable to him. He separated his feelings from the idea and experienced recurring ideas about her death that seemed strange and foreign to him.

Displacement

Displacement is a defense mechanism that transfers an emotional feeling from its actual object to a substitute for that object. The feeling is first repressed and then displaced to a safer substitute. This occurs when simple repression is not sufficient to keep the threatening urge under control.

A 40-year-old male became angry with his wife and was upset by his unacceptable rage toward her. He had a long-standing unconscious fear of experiencing any anger toward someone upon whom he was dependent, because he might lose their love. This fear originated from interactions with his mother early in life. He dealt with this anger for his mother early in his childhood by displacing the anger onto toys, other inanimate objects, and pets. As an adult, he displaced the anger toward his wife onto the family dog and kicked it. The dog happened to be a favorite pet of his wife. Anger at his dog was less threatening, slightly gratifying, and most importantly, could be tolerated within his conscious awareness.

Angry feelings for one person may be displaced onto another person who has some degree of similarity. Unacceptable feelings toward one's father may be displaced onto some other authoritarian male. This mechanism occurs in normal individuals, and on occasion in certain neurotic conditions such as phobias.

Undoing

Undoing refers to acts which magically cancel out or reverse a previous act or thought. The previous act or thought must have been motivated by an unacceptable, unconscious urge, and the act of undoing serves the psychological purpose of temporarily abolishing the intolerable impulse. Like reaction formation, it is characteristic of obsessive-compulsive states.

Undoing usually has two parts. In the first, an unacceptable impulse is expressed in thought or action. The expression may be symbolic, trivial, and even unconscious. The fear that the forbidden impulse may erupt into consciousness and take over brings forth the magical second step, which symbolically undoes the first step and thereby eliminates the fear of retaliation for having allowed an unacceptable urge to escape into awareness and action.

A strong fixation to magical thinking is necessary for this defense to be potent. This type of thinking stems from early childhood, when thoughts are seen to be powerful and magical. Many individuals have certain ritualistic practices which serve no apparent useful purpose. Often they have an unconscious, magical purpose and undo certain unacceptable practices or thoughts.

Before going to school each day, a 13-year-old male went through an elaborate series of rituals that served no practical purpose. He checked his closet and checked under his bed exactly three times before leaving his room. On his way out of the house, he always straightened a picture on the living room wall until it looked just right. On his way to and from school, it was important to him to walk in definite pathways in relation to several telephone poles he passed. If he deviated from this routine, he became quite anxious. He was sexually inhibited, and experiencing guilt about masturbatory fantasies. His ritualistic behavior served the purpose of decreasing guilt and anxiety by magically undoing his unacceptable sexual fantasies and urges.

Dissociation

Dissociation is a mechanism through which certain mental functions are split or divided in a way which allows for expression of forbidden impulses without having a feeling of responsibility. The behavior and feelings involved may not be remembered. With dissociation, there is a lack of integration of various components of the personality in order that certain impulses can be repressed.

There may be an entire set of unacceptable personality traits buried unconsciously that erupt into expression through dissociations. During a period of dissociation, this set of traits may function as a unitary whole. The fictional account of Doctor Jekyll and Mr. Hyde, in which two totally opposite personalities operated within one person, can be cited as an example of dissociation. Multiple personalities result from dissociative mechanisms.

The behavior that occurs during a period of dissociation is repressed, and the individual is left with no memory of the episode. The behavior is ordinarily brief and poorly organized, but at times may take on a more organized quality if that is part of a second personality. The separate personality may even assume a different name.

Dissociation does not occur in normal individuals except during extreme stress. Survivors of concentration camp experiences report episodes of dissociation under conditions of life-threatening stress. Individuals who have experienced other life-threatening experiences report episodes of dissociation. Dissociation is seen in a variety of psychopathological states such as fugue states, episodes of amnesia, and some neuroses, as well as multiple personalities. Multiple personalities have been described by Thigpen and Cleckley in *The Three Faces of Eve*[41] and by Schreiber in *Sybil.*[42]

> A 16-year-old adolescent female attended a picnic with a group of high school classmates. Some teenage boys had recently discovered the technique of hypnosis, and were experimenting with hypnosis on their friends. One of the young men hypnotized the 16-year-old girl. During the hypnotic trance, with her eyes closed, she was encouraged to go into a state of deep sleep. Unexplainedly, she suddenly opened her eyes and expressed no interest in continuing the hypnotic session. A few minutes later, she began behaving peculiarly. She acted like a young child, babbled incoherently, chased mosquitos, and was disoriented and silly. An attempt to rehypnotize her and bring her out of this new personality failed. She was then taken for a walk down a secluded path by one of her girl friends, and one of the teenage boys jumped out from behind a bush and said "boo" in a loud, frightening way. The girl suddenly snapped out of her altered personality state and started crying as she regained her usual senses. She had amnesia for the entire event. On one occasion not related to any hypnotic attempts, this young lady spontaneously moved into this altered personality for several minutes.

Identification

Identification is a defense mechanism which refers to internalizing attitudes or behavior patterns of significant people in one's life. It is important early in life in assisting the maturation of the ego, and many aspects of identification become deeply entrenched in the individual's character. For example, a developing child identifies with the values, attitudes, and behavior of the parents, and these memories become a part of the personality. This mechanism operates more actively during the development years, but may also be active during adulthood.

Identification provides the means whereby a constructive influence may be provided for the developing child by a parent. This requires that the environment consist of healthy, desirable people. A child may identify with undesirable or maladaptive traits if repeatedly exposed to them. In early infancy, a loving, warm, caring mother offers a good identification model for the infant. The internalization of basic traits of love and caring will serve the infant well later.

During the Oedipal conflict, the boy identifies with his father out of fear of harm from the father (whom he views as a competitor for the mother) and guilt for his anger toward the father. The boy is saying, "I would rather be like you than afraid of you." Identification ends this father-son conflict and results in the child's taking in many features and values of the father.

The counterpart of this is the Electra complex, in which the daughter has strong positive feelings for her father, and feelings of jealousy and fear insofar as the mother is concerned.

When individuals are frightened by hostile attitudes and actions of people in their environment, they may take on the characteristics of the threatening group. This "identification with the aggressor" decreases anxiety and fear because it gives an inner feeling of being strong like the aggressor.

People who have recently lost a loved one may start acting like the deceased. Identification with a dead person decreases grief because it gives unconscious assurance that the loved one still lives, even though it is only in the unconscious mind of the grieving individual.

Identification is an important mechanism in development, and is also seen in times of stress. It may also be seen in a variety of pathological states, such as severe depression, schizophrenia, regression, and states of multiple personality.

Reports from concentration camps indicate that the prevailing mood of fear contributes to the formation of seemingly strange behavioral patterns. Some prisoners in a concentration camp may take on the characteristics of their captors. In German concentration camps, certain prisoners began to behave arrogantly, just like their German captors. They would goose-step and in general behave in a way that would seem unappealing and undesirable to them. They were identifying with the feared aggressor. By taking on the traits and qualities of the feared German captors, they produced an inner feeling of comfort, as though they had assumed the power and confidence of the captors.

Altruism

Altruism is a mature defense mechanism that transforms an id drive into behavior that is a vicariously gratifying, constructive service to others. Many do not consider it a mechanism of defense but rather a coping style, perhaps representing a composite of several defense mechanisms. It includes philanthropy and service to others. The service rendered to others offers real benefit, and the id impulse involved is at least partially gratified by the behavior.

A 44-year-old successful businessman was a leader in several organizations that offered help to poverty-stricken children. He was raised as a poor youngster, and experienced frustration and anger at his deprived state. However, he learned early to be polite around people who were economically advantaged, in the hope that they would reward him financially. Much of his anger was channelled into polite behavior that did not allow for self-awareness or direct expression of angry feelings. After having achieved considerable success in business, he began to devote time to philanthropic and altruistic organizations, especially those that assisted underprivileged children. His leadership skills were excellent, and he successfully promoted several badly needed programs for children in his community. He enjoyed seeing the children's lives improved through his efforts. In a sense, he was righting many wrongs that he had experienced as a child. Clearly, he channelled many aggressive feelings into this work. His altruism, in addition to offering intrapsychic assistance in dealing with his aggressive drives, served him well in terms of his community reputation, for public relations for his business, and for self-satisfaction.

Suppression

Suppression is a defense mechanism defined as a conscious or semiconscious decision to postpone paying attention to another impulse or conflict. Because of the conscious aspect of suppression, some would not classify it as a true mechanism of defense. It allows a person to pace the working through of difficult conflicts and avoid being overwhelmed with excessive worry at any one time. The person says, "I am busy with other concerns at the moment, so I will deal with this problem tomorrow." It is to be emphasized that the conflict is not avoided, merely postponed until a more advantageous time.

A 25-year-old female graduate student was completing some extremely difficult and time-consuming studies. There was a deadline for completing the work. For some time, she had been involved in a romantic relationship with a young man, but had developed serious questions about her feelings for him. She wanted time to reflect on her feelings and attitudes toward him before making a decision that would have lasting effects. It was not possible in terms of time and energy to deal with this important personal issue while completing the academic assignments. She postponed dealing with the relationship question until the graduate studies were behind her. This was accomplished in a reasonable period of time, and allowed her to deal more effectively with the important personal issues with the young man. The problem was not avoided, but had been postponed to a more advantageous time.

Anticipation

Anticipation is an ego-adaptive mechanism which involves realistic anticipation or planning for future discomfort. It includes goal-directed thinking, planning, and worrying about unpleasant future happenings. For instance, anticipation would include realistic planning about death, separation, or serious illness. It provides for realistic problem solving at a time when the individual is not under great stress, so that when the unpleasant event occurs, much of the planning has been done. Anticipation provides the opportunity to deal with unpleasant affective responses to a life crisis before the crisis actually occurs.

A 53-year-old married male with three children and four grandchildren had anticipated the possibility of serious illness at some point in life, and the problems that would be created on an emotional as well as a practical level. He had made good, common practical arrangements in terms of medical insurance, sick pay benefits, and other financial necessities. As well as he could, he had thought through the emotional conflicts he would face if serious illness occurred. When he did develop a serious medical problem requiring surgery, he was naturally upset, but not nearly so much as if he had not anticipated the many facets of this type of life stress. Reassured by his financial arrangements and not totally shocked by the illness and treatment since he had considered such a possibility, he weathered a serious life crisis fairly well. His physical recovery was assisted by his emotionally mature way of dealing with the illness.

Sublimation

Sublimation is a mechanism of defense which transforms energy from repressed instinctual urges into socially useful and constructive goals. It is conceived as the most complete, mature, and effective defense. It is the process whereby the forces motivating the sexual and aggressive drives are transformed into useful social work. This is a complex mechanism and obviously is presented here in simple terms. It is more of a channelling mechanism than a defensive mechanism. It is a loose conceptualization of the many psychic processes that lead to behavior of a higher social order.

Sublimation is especially active in the latency-age child who learns mechanisms for transforming sexual energy into school work, hobbies, and other achievements. These activities become incorporated into the individual's lifestyle. Various sublimations represent patterns of behavior that originated as defenses against forbidden urges, but the defensive behavior is so valuable and socially useful in its own right that it is retained as a valuable part of the personality. The behavior no longer serves a defensive purpose, but achieves an independent value of its own. Aggressive impulses may be transformed, for example, into sports or other games, and the social and personal value of athletic success may be rewarding enough to perpetuate the behavior pattern. Vocational pursuits, arts, science, religion, and other activities that promote cultural enrichment are made possible by the mechanism of sublimation.

A 35-year-old female artist had a reputation in her community for being an excellent, prolific painter. She was highly successful and amazed others with her abundant work output. Her work was widely exhibited and bought by many. She was in an automobile accident and broke both arms, which stopped her artistic output for a period of time. During the rehabilitative phase, when painting was not possible, she developed intense sexual fantasies, urges, and some degree of restlessness and anxiety. It became difficult for her to refrain from sexual acting-out behavior. She had intense urges to become involved sexually with several older men, whom she had known as acquaintances or friends for several years but for whom she had not had sexual urges before. Her background revealed that she had had a fairly traumatic developmental period from age 3 to age 6. There had been marital discord between her parents, and the patient usually sided with her father. She developed considerable anger and jealousy toward her mother, and retained very positive, erotized feelings for her father. She had repressed this entire conflict involving her mother and father and had channelled many of these unacceptable feelings into artistic endeavors. At the age of 8, several teachers praised her for her natural skills at painting. This skill served her well in many other ways and provided an outlet for some unacceptable feelings, especially sexual feelings for her father. When she was unable to continue with her painting, an important outlet for the unconscious sexual feelings was removed, and these feelings began to present themselves in other ways, in the form of fantasies, urges, and a desire to become involved in sexual behavior. Once she resumed her painting, the problem resolved itself quickly.

HIERARCHY OF DEFENSES

Vaillant has devised a theoretical hierarchy for mechanisms of defense that classified them according to their degree of maturity.[43] This is a useful way to view the ego defenses, as it ties them into maturing life adaptation. Defenses used early in life evolve into mature defenses as development proceeds. For instance, denial can be conceived as evolving toward repression, which may be replaced in adulthood by suppression or sublimation. Immature defenses are replaced by more mature defenses in a sequential series of developmental stages. Theoretically, immature defenses may persist because of developmental arrests, or recur later in life during severe stress. Early in life, the immature ego and central nervous system are not capable of employing more mature mechanisms. They evolve with maturation. Vaillant's follow-up study of 30 men suggested that the defenses selected were correlated with life adjustment in occupational, marital, and medical spheres. Individuals who use more mature mechanisms of defense had better life adjustments than those who used more immature defenses. This included better physical health as well as better work and marital adjustment. Vaillant's studies indicate that the maturity level of mechanisms of defense that are utilized by individuals has considerable impact on the degree of life adaptation.

This concept has important implications for evaluating patients. The examiner should be acquainted with the mechanisms of defense and their position in the maturational hierarchy. Individuals who rely heavily on immature defenses have poorer life adjustments and increased vulnerability to emotional illnesses. An assessment of the maturational level of defenses is an aid in assessing levels of psychopathological disturbance. During recovery from psychotic decompensation, changes in maturational levels of defenses can be observed to parallel the healing process. A seriously disturbed psychotic patient may rely heavily on the primitive mechanisms of denial, distortion, and delusional projection. As healing occurs, the more mature mechanisms of rationalization, repression, and reaction formation may take their place. In essence, more mature defenses appear as healing occurs.

An outline of ego defense mechanisms in accordance with their level of maturity (adapted from Vaillant's outline) is as follows:

Level 1: *Narcissistic*
          Delusional projection
          Denial
          Distortion

Level 2: *Immature*
          Projection
          Hypochondriasis
          Passive-aggressive behavior

Level 3: *Neurotic*
          Rationalization (or intellectualization)
          Repression
          Reaction formation
          Isolation
          Displacement
          Undoing
          Dissociation
          Identification

Level 4: *Mature*
          Altruism
          Suppression
          Anticipation
          Sublimation

Narcissistic defenses are normal in young children before the age of 5 and are common in adult dreams and fantasies. These mechanisms distort the perception of reality considerably. When seen extensively in adult life, they are associated with serious psychopathology (psychosis), and indicate the necessity for strong treatment intervention, frequently requiring major tranquilizers, decrease in environmental stress, or developmental maturation.

Immature defenses are normal in individuals from age 3 to 16. They tend to be used by those who are threatened by interpersonal intimacy or the loss of interpersonal intimacy. Such individuals behave in a socially undesirable way. They benefit from improved interpersonal relationships, realistic helpful deeds, and prolonged psychotherapy with forceful interpretations.

Neurotic defenses are commonly seen in healthy individuals from age 3 to 90. They appear frequently in neurotic disorders or in adult acute stress. For the individual they alter internal feelings of instinctual expression, making the individual appear to have selected pecularities or "hang ups." They tend to respond to conventional psychotherapy.

Mature defenses are commonly seen in healthy individuals from latency-age years (6 to 12) to 90. They may actually be well-integrated components of simpler mechanisms. They emerge during adolescence probably as a result of successful identifications and the replacement of the primitive conscience with a more tolerable conscience and a positive ego ideal. In the literature, all of the defense mechanisms in level four have been lumped under the heading "sublimation."[44]

Some are not considered defense mechanisms, but are referred to as healthy coping mechanisms. Under stress they may change to less mature mechanisms.

In summary, ego mechanisms of defense may be normal or abnormal. They may be a persistent part of an individual's coping style, or may occur in response to acute stress. Defenses develop along a continuum that is parallel to maturing life adaptation. Some defenses are more mature than others. Defenses may become fixated at an immature level, or they may undergo regression back to immature levels under stress. The level of ego-defensive functioning can be used to assess patients in terms of successful life adjustment, vulnerability to psychopathology, degree of recovery from serious psychopathology, and general level of maturity.

HEALTHY RELATIONSHIPS

A study of the dynamic forces that shape personality development leads logically into a discussion of healthy adult relationships. When all of the psychologic theorizing has been completed, what people really want to know is how to involve themselves in intimate, gratifying human relationships. What can be said about the correlation of developmental accomplishments with healthy interpersonal alliances? Much of the literature regarding psychologic health focuses upon the individual rather than upon relationships. Psychoanalytic writings have emphasized that health comes when there is freer access to the unconscious and freedom from infantile conflicts.[45] An important study on the psychologic health in family systems was done by Lewis et al.[46] Though the study focused upon healthy families, it says much about healthy relationships between individuals. The pertinent findings were:

1 The role of many variables. There is no one single quality that healthy families demonstrated. Many variables are associated with health, and impressive differences among healthy families exist. There is no "one way" to achieve family health—no single thread running through optimal families to explain their success.

2 An affiliative attitude toward human encounter. Optimal families demonstrate strikingly affiliative attitudes about human encounter. There is an expectation that human encounters are apt to be caring, and this encourages reaching out to others. This observation appears related to Erikson's concept of basic trust.[1]

3 Respect for subjective views. These families show the characteristic of respect for one's own world view, as well as that of others. Individual differences are tolerated, and respect is taught for the values of others. Each individual's opinion is respected, and authoritarianism or patterns of dominance and submission are incompatible with the pervasive respect described.

4 A belief in complex motivations. The behavior of healthy families shows a willingness to explore numerous options in approaching problems within the family. If one approach does not work, another is tried. The families believe in the complexity of causes for problems, in contrast to dysfunctional families who

often persist in a single approach to problem solving, which suggests a belief in a single or linear causality.

5   High levels of initiative. The families demonstrate much initiative in responding to input. They show constructive reaching out, and most had many interests: recreational, athletic, artistic, or educational. They interact with the community and receive a tremendous variety of stimuli.

6   The structure of the healthy family. Healthy families demonstrate flexible structures, whereas dysfunctional families show rigidity and severely dysfunctional families show chaotic structure. Healthy families show a strong parental coalition, with a marriage that is effective in meeting the needs of both parents. Leadership is provided by the parents and shared between them. This healthy, egalitarian marriage is in contrast to the patterns of dominance and submission or conflict in dysfunctional families. The power of the parents is not experienced in an authoritarian way. The opinions of the children are considered and negotiations are common. Even so, power is clear.

The strong affectional bond between parents serves as a model for relating that is of great learning value for the children. The marriage reveals a high degree of complementarity, and shows a good fit between the parents' individual skills. They take pride in one another's assets, and are not torn by competitive strivings.

These families show interpersonal closeness, but no blurring of ego boundaries. Separation with closeness is the norm.

7   The healthy family and personal autonomy. Healthy families contain individuals who demonstrate high levels of personal autonomy. Personal autonomy is encouraged by the family. Beavers describes this as the family's ability to "self-destruct."[47] Children are encouraged to express individual feelings and thoughts, and are trained to feel as individuals. There is encouragement to accept responsibility for one's feelings, thoughts, and actions. A strong belief seems to exist that basic human needs and drives are not evil. Therefore, shame is diminished and there is no need to hide feelings and thoughts.

8   A congruent mythology. Healthy families see themselves much as they are seen by others. Dysfunctional families often see their functioning at a much higher level than others do.

9   The healthy family and feelings. An important need is that of sensing that one's feelings are understood, and that one may express feelings openly. The expression of affect is central to human interaction. Healthy families are open in the expression of affect and demonstrate high levels of empathy. Children who spend formative years in healthy families learn that it is safe to talk about feelings, and that understanding will occur. Feelings are seen as human, and expressiveness is seen as normal.

Although this study is about healthy families, parallels can be drawn with the characteristics of healthy adult relationships of any type, whether family or nonfamily relationships. Clinical observations and research studies support the connection between good child-rearing practices and the establishment of warm relationships in adulthood,[48] though the specifics are not well understood. Furthermore, healthy personality development does not guarantee healthy adult relationships. It seems likely that the potential for warm adult relationships is enhanced by the quality of childhood development, but is not assured or fixed by it at an early age. Much happens in adulthood that affects the success of that phase, as evidenced by the ongoing nature of dynamic interactions in healthy adults.

What can a physician advise parents about child-rearing techniques? First, there is no cookbook approach to parenting that guarantees a psychologically healthy child. There is no one way of parenting, any more than there is one way of relating. However, general knowledge of the different psychologic needs at various developmental stages may help a caring, sensitive parent relate more effectively to a child. For instance, the child's needs for close contact with the mother early in life, and a different need for gradually developing autonomy within firm limits in late infancy, are examples of helpful parent information. The nature of the interaction between mother and child should be emphasized as perhaps being more important than any specific technique. In addition to attending to the specific needs of each developmental period, it would seem helpful, based upon healthy family interactions, to instill these important attributes:

1   A positive feeling about meeting others
2   Respect for others
3   An appreciation of human complexities
4   High levels of initiative
5   Willingness to share power with others and be affectionate
6   Encouragement of autonomy
7   Positive attitudes about expression and understanding feelings
8   A feeling that much hard work must be done in adulthood to achieve and maintain gratifying relationships

SUMMARY

This chapter has reviewed the development and structure of personality. Personality development is a complex phenomenon involving many complex factors over a long period of time. Simplistic explanations based upon a limited number of hereditary or environmental factors do not pass the test of close scrutiny. A major criticism of Freud's psychoanalytic theory of personality development is that it is too limited in the factors considered and places too heavy an emphasis on instinctual drives. A newborn infant begins life with a number of innate characteristics, and immediately begins interacting with the environment. The interaction between innate characteristics and environmental influences must be emphasized, since one affects the other repeatedly and continuously. Parents mold infants, but infants also mold parents. In the long run, the interaction, or "fit," between infant and parents may relate much more to personality development than any isolated set of factors. Experiences that occur earlier in life have the most lasting impact on the child.

Personality organization has been conceptualized in psychoanalytic terms such as id, ego, and superego. This formulation has enjoyed traditional, widespread acceptance, and despite many weaknesses, has yet to be replaced by a superior theoretical construct. A person starts life with certain innate characteristics, including instinctual drives (id) that motivate behavior. The controlling (ego) and value-orienting (superego) components develop with maturation and are greatly influenced by environmental experiences. Much of the personality remains in the unconscious realm of the mind. Many immature personality functions that remain unconscious do not undergo maturation because they do not interact with reality factors. As a result, these unconscious immature functions exert a disturbing influence in adult life that can be explained only in terms of childish fears, immaturity, and misconceptions.

Development proceeds along a continuum through a series of sequential stages, with each succeeding stage being more advanced and complex. Under stress, an adult may revert to earlier modes of functioning and repeat patterns of behavior established in childhood. Falling back to earlier adaptive patterns is known as regression. A person may be visualized as moving up and down a developmental continuum. Regression is an important concept in explaining the appearance of inexplicable behavior in adults. Development proceeds from birth to death, though obvious changes are more common earlier in life. Multiple personality components mature in a parallel fashion.

Conflict and anxiety play important roles in development. Realistic demands of society will not tolerate complete gratification of instinctual drives. Ego mechanisms that control drive gratification evolve. Anxiety may be conceived as an intrapsychic alarm conveying a threat to integrated functioning. Defense mechanisms develop to bolster the ego's attempts at controlling id drives and intolerable affect. They develop along a maturational continuum, with the more mature mechanisms being much more adaptive and associated with more success, better physical health, and a more gratifying personal life. Ego strength can be viewed as a tendency to use mature adaptive mechanisms rather than immature ones under stress.

A basic goal during adulthood is the establishment of intimate, caring relationships. Characteristics of such relationships include mutual affection and respect, sharing of power, sensitivity and responsiveness to one's needs, the encouragement of autonomy, and the expression of and empathy for feelings. Successful childhood years prepare an individual for important tasks in adulthood, but they do not guarantee health. Regardless of the quality of a person's developmental years, adult success is not "fixed" early in life. Interactions during development are important to adult emotional health, but are not the only consideration. Active work within adult relationships is essential to their success.

REFERENCES

1   Erikson, E. H.: "Identity and the Life Cycle," in *Psychological Issues, Monograph 1,* New York: International Universities Press, 1959.
2   Freud, S.: *New Introductory Lectures on Psychoanalysis,* New York: W. W. Norton, 1933.
3   Freud, S.: "On the History of the Psychoanalytic Movement (1914)," in *Collected Papers,* vol. 1, New York: Basic Books, 1959, pp. 288–359.

4   Hoffer, W.: "The Mutual Influences in the Development of Ego and Id: Earliest Stages," *The Psychoanalytic Study of the Child,* **7**:31–41, 1952.

5   Mahler, M. S.: "On Child Psychosis and Schizophrenia: Autistic and Symbiotic Infantile Psychoses," *The Psychoanalytic Study of the Child,* **7**:286–305, 1952.

6   Jackson, John Hughlings: "Croonian Lectures on the Evolution and Dissolution of the Nervous System," *Lancet,* **1**(1884), p. 555.

7   Anonymous.

8   Wordsworth, William: "My Heart Leaps Up When I Behold," *William Wordsworth Selected Poetry,* New York: Modern Library, 1950, p. 462.

9   White, R. B. and R. M. Gilliland: *The Mechanisms of Defense: Elements of Psychopathology,* New York: Grune and Stratton, 1975.

10 Allport, G. W.: "European and American Theories of Personality," in H. P. David and H. von Bracken (eds.), *Perspectives in Personality Theory,* New York: Basic Books, 1961.

11 Gesell, A., and L. B. Ames: "Early Evidences of Individuality in the Human Infant," *Journal of Genetic Personality,* **47**:339, 1937.

12 Shirley, M. M.: *The First Two Years: A Study of Twenty-five Babies,* Minneapolis: University of Minnesota Press, 1931 and 1933.

13 Thomas, A., and Stella Chess: *Temperament and Development,* New York: Brunner/Mazel, 1977.

14 Brazelton, T. B.: "Early Parent-Infant Reciprocity," in V. C. Vaughn and T. B. Brazelton (eds.), *The Family—Can It Be Saved?* Chicago: Year Book Medical Publishers, 1976.

15 Redlich, F. C., and D. X. Freedman: *The Theory and Practice of Psychiatry,* New York: Basic Books, 1966.

16 Lorenz, K.: "Über das Sogenaunte Böse," *Zur Naturgeschichte der Aggression,* Wien: Barota Schoeler, 1963.

17 Maslow, A. H.: *Motivation and Personality,* New York: Harper, 1954.

18 Freud, S.: "Three Essays on Sexuality," in *The Standard Edition of the Complete Psychological Works of Sigmund Freud,* vol. 7, London: Hogarth Press, 1953.

19 Brenner, C.: *An Elementary Textbook of Psychoanalysis,* New York: Doubleday, 1955.

20 Sheldon, W. H., and S. S. Stevens: *The Varieties of Temperament,* New York: Harper and Brothers, 1942.

21 Jensen, A. R.: "How Much Can We Boost I.Q. and Scholastic Achievement?" *Harvard Educational Review,* **39**:1–23, 1969.

22 Watson, J. B.: *Behaviorism,* New York: W. W. Norton, 1924.

23 Riesen, A. H.: "Effects of Stimulus Deprivation on the Development and Atrophy of the Visual Sensory System," *Am. J. Orthopsychiatry,* **30**:23, 1960.

24 Crelins, Edmund, Yale University School of Medicine, New Haven, Connecticut: personal communications, 1977.

25 Benjamin, J. D.: "Some Developmental Observations Relating to the Theory of Anxiety," paper presented at the American Psychoanalytic Association, December 1958.

26 Spitz, R. A., and K. M. Wolf: "The Smiling Response: A Contribution to the Ontogenesis of Social Relations," *Genetic Psychology,* **34**:57–125, 1946.

27 Harlow, H. F., and M. R. Harlow: *The Affectional Systems in Behavior of Non-Human Primates,* in A. M. Schrier, H. F. Harlow, and F. Stollnitz (eds.), vol. 2, New York: Academic Press, 1965.

28 Bowlby, J.: *Maternal Care and Mental Health,* 2d ed., Monograph Series No. II, Geneva: World Health Organization, 1952.

29 Goldfarb, W.: "Emotional and Intellectual Consequences of Deprivation in Infancy: A Reevaluation," in P. H. Hoch and J. Zurbin (eds.), *Psychopathology of Childhood,* New York: Grune and Stratton, 1965.

30 Spitz, R. A.: "Hospitalism (1946)," *Childhood Psychopathology,* New York: International Universities Press, 1952.

31 Spitz, R. A.: "Anaclitic Depression," *The Psychoanalytic Study of the Child,* New York: International Universities Press, 2:313-342, 1946.

32 Levy, D. M.: *Maternal Overprotection,* New York: Columbia University Press, 1943.

33 Masterson, J. R.: *Psychotherapy of the Borderline Adult,* New York: Brunner/Mazel, 1976.

34 Freud, S.: *A General Introduction to Psychoanalysis,* New York: Garden City Publishing, 1938.

35 Freud, S.: *The Ego and the Id (1928),* translated by J. Riviere, London: Hogarth Press, 1927.

36 Henderson, L. J.: *The Fitness of the Environment,* New York: Macmillan, 1913.

37 Money, J., and A. A. Ehrhardt: *Psychosexual Differentiation,* Baltimore: John Hopkins Press, 1972.

38 Mahler, M., F. Pine, and A. Bergman: *The Psychological Birth of the Human Infant,* New York: Basic Books, 1975.

39 Freud, S.: *The Problem of Anxiety (1926),* translated by H. A. Bunker, New York: W. W. Norton, 1936.

40 Freud, A.: *The Ego and Mechanisms of Defense,* New York: International Universities Press, 1946.

41 Thigpen, C. H., and H. M. Cleckley: *The Three Faces of Eve,* New York: McGraw-Hill, 1957.

42 Schreiber, F. R.: *Sybil,* Chicago: Henry Regnery, 1923.

43 Vaillant, G. E.: "Theoretical Hierarchy of Adaptive Ego Mechanisms," *Archives of General Psychiatry,* **24**:107-118, 1971.

44 Fenichel, O.: *The Psychoanalytic Theory of Neurosis,* New York: W. W. Norton, 1945.

45 Offer, D., and M. Sabshin: *Normality: Theoretical and Clinical Concepts of Mental Health,* New York: Basic Books, 1974.

46 Lewis, J. M., et al.: *No Single Thread: Psychological Health in Family Systems,* New York: Brunner/Mazel, 1976.

47 Beavers, W. R.: "Family Variables Related to the Development of a Self," Dallas: Timberlawn Foundation Reports, 1973.

48 Grinker, R. R., Sr., et al.: "Mentally Healthy Young Males (Homoclites)," *Archives of General Psychiatry,* **16**:405, 1962.

Chapter 4

The Family of the Patient

Jerry M. Lewis, M.D.

EDITORS' INTRODUCTION

How strange and upsetting it is for a family to be interviewed together as a unit! So much depends upon the comfort or discomfort of the physician who conducts the interview. When has the family ever sat down with an outside authority? Isn't it natural for its members to wonder how the doctor will perceive them together, whether or not they will be liked? Maybe the family will be questioning whether there are new developments, and will wonder why the physician decided on a family session. Such concern may precipitate an initial reluctance to be open, and may even result in deliberate distortion of some aspects of family life.

To be effective in what can be a tremendously valuable therapeutic experience, the physician must first believe in the process. The second step is to sense the subtle interplay between those forces in the family that reach out for help, and those that wish to avoid or minimize the anticipated pain of family disclosure. Unless trained and familiar with the techniques of family interview, the physician may also experience anxiety related to the newness of the situation. But it is surprising how, with experience, empathetic physicians may soon become comfortable in the situation and may find themselves using family interviews more frequently.

Most physicians are comfortable with single-patient situations in which the physician directs and controls the quality, length, and direction of the doctor-patient interaction. To ask a family to share its personal problems, to allow the material to evolve spontaneously from the family itself, may seem curiously unstructured and unlike the physician's usual activities.

There is, however, another possible source of anxiety for the physician. Being with a family, observing the relationships which unfold in the physician's office, may stir up in the physician a variety of feelings about families in general and about his or her own family in particular. Most physicians have intimate experience with only two families, their family of origin and their current family. For many, the experiences in both these families were basically positive, in which case the physician has a core attitude about the family in general that is positive and optimistic. Other physicians, however, have been less fortunate in their two-family experience, and being with a family may evoke a general reaction of displeasure, painful memories, and a pessimistic attitude.

In addition, some families are struggling with problems that, on the surface, appear to be identical to problems in the physician's own family. A depressed spouse, a rebellious teenager, a college dropout, chronic marital conflict—each of these may hit close to home, and the superficial parallels may be distressing enough to interfere with the physician's capacity for helpfulness. The recognition that all families have problems and that most struggle with the same issues can be helpful. Often, physicians can be more objective and helpful with other families than they can be with their own.

Families who turn to their physician for help at times of crisis can also teach the physician much about the nature of life in families, the struggle to find both meaning and intimacy in the connectedness of human existence, and the remarkable human capacity for change and growth.

There are two important reasons for the physician to develop an ability to make reliable clinical observations about the patient's family. The first is that what goes on within the family may play an etiologic role in the patient's illness. Certain patterns of family life may predispose family members to high levels of all illnesses, or may be associated with specific illnesses. The second reason is that the response of the patient's family to illness may influence the course of the illness. The family's response may sustain or deter the progression of some illnesses.

This chapter presents findings that suggest the importance of the family in illness and disease, and reviews briefly the basic concepts of the family as a system. A series of discrete family system characteristics, including typical responses of families at different levels of competence, will be presented. Finally, the ways in which these observations and research findings can be used in clinical medicine will be discussed.

THE FAMILY AND ILLNESS

Two lines of investigation suggest the role of the family in individual illness. The first and broadest involves observations about the role of family factors in psychiatric illness. The second involves observations regarding the family and its role in so-called physical illness.

Psychiatry, as part of its current understanding of psychiatric illness, has generally accepted the concept of multiple causation. For example, a particular schizophrenic patient may have an inherited tendency to develop the signs and symptoms of the illness when exposed to certain developmental stresses and ongoing patterns of family relationships. The illness may be understood with equal validity from the viewpoint of aberrations in neurotransmitter chemistry, developmental events, or the family's patterns of communication. The impact of family factors must be understood within the context of accepting the role of multiple factors in etiology.

Initially, the major focus of interest was in the early mother-child interaction; more recently, emphasis has been on the entire family's characteristic ways of communicating and relating. All family members are seen as participating in a system which has consequences for each individual member. From this perspective, there are no villains, and no heroes or heroines. The role of patient may be assigned to, and accepted by, a family member for a variety of reasons. At times, for example, if one member becomes a patient, it may offer the family system a tenuous equilibrium that prevents its dissolution. For example, it has been noted that the improvement of a seriously disturbed adolescent patient is occasionally followed by a parental divorce; the concern that the family focuses on the disturbed youngster may be all that is allowing it to avoid facing other problems. In this sense, an adolescent's illness may keep the family from dissolution.

In other circumstances, the development of an illness may best be understood as an attempt by the patient to separate from the family system. This is seen at times in families that are dominated by one powerful parent's rigid authoritarianism. An adolescent family member may develop significant symptoms that take him or her out of the family and, at least in part, out from under stifling family controls. Often, several purposes appear to be served.

The role of family factors has been studied most intensely in regard to schizophrenia, but more recently this perspective has widened to embrace other forms of individual patienthood, including delinquents, neurotics, and patients with psychosomatic disturbances. There have been two major approaches to the study of families containing a psychiatric patient. The first is *family therapy,* in which a therapist meets with the entire family and attempts to help the family, as an interacting system, change its characteristic patterns of relating. Out of this therapeutic movement have come numerous observations about the ways in which the family is involved in the development of a family member's illness. This type of observation may produce rich clinical insight, but it is difficult to quantify; one family cannot be compared and contrasted easily with others that contain patients having similar illnesses.

The second approach has been designated *family systems research.* Investigators have devised a variety of tasks for the whole family to accomplish. These range from specific problems that they are asked to solve, to standard ink blot cards that they are asked to interpret. The family's responses are recorded and analyzed for clarity of expression, patterns of interruption, distribution of power, response to feelings, and other specific interactional variables. These kinds of observations can be quantified, and the results enable a more ready comparison of one family to others. Both family systems research and the family therapy movement have greatly increased our understanding of the role played by family factors in the development of psychiatric illness.

It is now generally accepted that the family is often involved in the development of a member's illness. Research has demonstrated that the severity of illness in psychiatrically disturbed adolescent family members is correlated directly with the degree of family dysfunction.[1] The adolescents studied were suffering from psychotic, neurotic, and personality disturbances of sufficient intensity to necessitate hospitalization. Although it is possible to consider the development of an individual illness as occurring in a member of an otherwise healthy family (the result of strong genetic loading or a particularly traumatic initial year of life, for example), there are no published family studies of such circumstances. This may reflect a variety of factors: for example, the disinclination of family researchers or therapists to search for or attend exceptions to their usual findings. Another possibility is that the patterns of family life found with such consistency in the families of a wide variety of psychiatric patients are either themselves genetically determined, or are responses to the presence of severe disturbance in a family member. Longitudinal, predictive studies are necessary to weigh the validity of such interpretations. There is little doubt, however, that individual psychiatric illness is correlated strongly with disturbed patterns in family relationships.

Perhaps the most impressive evidence that such correlations have causal significance is found in the responses of individual illnesses to interventions that alter the family system. Skynner, for example, presents a number of examples of impressive and rapid changes in the individual patient's symptomatology following brief family therapy[2] (see Chapter 27). Although treatment in psychiatry, as in the rest of medicine, need not be etiologically based in order to be effective, it is difficult not to conclude that the family plays a significant role in the mental health or illness of its members. At this stage of our knowledge, it appears reasonable to conclude that disturbances within the family may play a necessary, but not sufficient, role in determining whether there will be a patient in the family. After that consideration, individual traits (genetic, chemical, developmental) may be crucial both in deciding which family member becomes ill, and the nature and quality of that illness.

When one turns to the part family interactions play in an individual's physical illness, the evidence is weaker but suggestive. In part, this may reflect the fact that so little attention has been paid to the possible role of family factors in physical illness. For several decades, there has been an accumulation of evidence that stressful life circumstances are one factor in the development of individual illnesses. Life change, unusual life stress, and the recent loss of a loved one have been found to correlated with higher than usual prevalence of illness.[3,4,5] Schmale and Engel suggest that it may not be the life circumstance per se, but a person's deep and prolonged response of helplessness or hopelessness to the circumstances that precipitates illness.[6,7]

The vast majority of these studies focus on individuals and do not concern the family specifically. Many years ago, however, Richardson called attention to the fact that the family may often be the appropriate unit of disease and illness.[8] He was impressed by the fact that, in some instances of chronic or acute repetitive illness, the illness could best be understood as being responsive to disturbed patterns of family life. In another study of 25,000 illnesses in 100 families over a 10-year period, Dingle, Badger, and Jordan found that many families had relatively stable rates of illness, with variations between high and low rates of family illness over long periods of time.[9] Although these investigators were not psychiatrists interested in family systems, they concluded that there may be family factors involved in the establishment of both high and low illness rates. In England, Kellner, a family practitioner, noted that in his practice, illnesses in a family were not distributed randomly in time, but tended to cluster.[10] Different family members' diverse illnesses would often occur within the space of several months, and then there would be a period of freedom from illness, to be followed by another cluster of illnesses. Recent research suggests that the way in which a family deals with loss may be correlated with its illness rate, and that those families who deal openly with their feelings reveal fewer episodes of all illnesses.[1]

Another line of inquiry has been the search for particular patterns of family interaction that correlate with a family member's specific disease. Jackson, for example, studied families containing patients with ulcerative colitis.[11] Meissner has compiled the literature and presents a composite of the findings for families with members suffering from one of the "classical" seven psychosomatic diseases.[12] This search for specifity is in its early stages, and the results of such studies must be understood from the perspective of family factors that may play a role in the determination of family members' general resistance and susceptibility to all diseases.

Evidence that family interactions may play a role in all illness and disease is growing. At this time, such factors seem more clearly established for those diseases considered psychiatric than for those considered physical. In part, this may reflect the greater attention (both clinical and research) paid to the family by psychiatry than by general medicine. The evidence in both areas, however, seems a sufficient mandate for the physician to have available a practical method for studying the families of those patients cared for in the office or hospital. Systematically evaluating the families of patients will give the physician competence in deciding whether treatment efforts should be directed at the individual or at the family system as a whole in order to achieve maximum therapeutic leverage. It will also encourage the physician to recognize with greater clarity those occasions when a referral to a specialist with greater or different expertise should be made.

THE FAMILY AS A SYSTEM

There are a number of ways to think of the family, and the manner in which the clinician conceptualizes the family will influence the techniques or approaches used to study the family. If, for example, the family is seen basically as a collection of individuals who share some type of living arrangement, the clinician may study the individuals within a family and put together a composite of what the family must be like, based upon observations of the individuals. For many years, this has been the approach used most often, and it does lead to valuable insights. It is, however, more or less restricted by what individuals can or will tell the clinician about life in their families. This "content-bound" approach cannot reveal those aspects of family life (such as family rules) about which the individuals within the family are not aware. It poses an additional problem for the clinician who cannot decide which individual to believe, because members often describe family life in terms that are strikingly different.

A second, and in many ways complementary, way of looking at the family is as a system. This conceptualization focuses primarily on the whole family as a unit, with characteristics that are greater than the sum of its parts—that is, the family system as more than the simple sum of the individual family members' personalities, attitudes, values, or other individual traits. Metaphorically, the family is like an individual organism; it has a distinct boundary that separates it from the surrounding environment, with which, however, there is constant interchange. Since the larger surrounding social system has greater ability to influence the obviously smaller family systems that comprise it than the smaller family systems do to influence it, the individual family system must adapt to the larger social system.

The family as a unit has a well-defined structure with its own particular ways of maintaining viability and performing routine tasks. The cornerstone of this structure is the nature of the parental relationship to which much that occurs in the life of the family is directly related.

A central premise of the family system viewpoint is that a family must develop certain patterns of system behavior, both responsive and initiating in type. It is impossible, for example, to imagine any system that responds to each input or change from within or without as if that situation were novel. Rather, the system develops certain more or less automatic responses to different types of stimuli. Family system research studies point the way for family therapy to intervene in those characteristic family processes that have proven to be dysfunctional.

The notion that certain family patterns are clearly dysfunctional is based on a value judgment regarding the purpose of the family. Throughout history, the family's cardinal purpose can be understood as a survival mechanism. The chances of individual (hence, species) survival have been augmented by living in a family. Although this physical surviving function may be understood with greater clarity when the family is seen in primitive circumstances (that is, in a hostile and untamed environment), it continues to operate in the here and now. People who live in families generally live longer and better than those who live outside families. There are, of course, many exceptions, and the causal relationships are complicated; for, on the average, stronger and more fit individuals may have a greater tendency to marry and live within a family. Nevertheless, a strong case can be made for the family as a survival mechanism.

However, beyond the family's function in helping its members to survive, there are other purposes for the family. These purposes are influenced by cultural and historical factors. In the Western world, the family may currently be seen as having two central purposes: the stabilization of adult family members' personalities (and, it is to be hoped, their continued growth and maturation), and the production of autonomous children.

Each individual comes to adulthood with certain personality vulnerabilities occasioned both by genetic temperament and by the difficult process of growing into adulthood. These vulnerabilities may be seen as soft spots in the individual's personality, and they can include, for example, excessive dependency upon others, unusual fear of closeness, heightened aggressive responsiveness, a tendency to impulsive behavior, and many others. These vulnerabilities are not necessarily translated directly into disabilities. Whether or not they become disabilities by being converted into symptoms and reduced effectiveness, is influenced strongly by the nature and quality of the social systems that either support or pressure the individual participants. The social system of greatest impact for many individuals is the family. Some research data suggest that individuals of comparable vulnerability may either perform relatively well or experience severe symptomatology depending upon the quality of their marital and family life.[13]

Marriage and family enable many individuals to grow and mature throughout their lives. When a couple has children, they have an opportunity to retrace developmental stages and to evolve further themselves as they foster their children's growth.

The second major function of the family is the production of autonomous children—children who can experience their own individualities, become entities separate from the family, and continue the cycle of family life. Children of healthy families are well prepared for this life task. Other families produce children who demonstrate autonomy and can separate from their families of origin, but lack the interpersonal skill of loving and being loved. Some unfortunate families, however, fail completely in their tasks; they produce children who cannot be autonomous, cannot separate, and begin their own lives, but remain in their families of origin instead.

Currently in the Western world, the extent to which a family succeeds in accomplishing these two central tasks may be considered a measure of its competence. It is possible, therefore, to consider families as falling somewhere along a continuum of family competence. At one end are those families which accomplish the central tasks effectively, and at the other end are those which fail miserably. For descriptive purposes, the levels of family competence at different points on the continuum can be designated by phrases. *Optimal families* accomplish both tasks well. *Competent but pained families* do less well. *Midrange dysfunctional families* have significant difficulty accomplishing the tasks, and *severely dysfunctional families* fail miserably.

Certain variables have been found to correlate with differing levels of family competence. These will be described and brief examples of families at different levels will be presented.

VARIABLES INVOLVED IN FAMILY COMPETENCE

The structure, the way in which power or interpersonal influence is distributed, is of major importance in determining a family's level of competence. "Who has the right to decide what?" is a question that is seldom articulated openly. Yet each family (or any more or less enduring social system) evolves a set of rules or guidelines regarding how decisions are to be made. In discussing rule systems with families, one most often hears that the rules "just happened." When studying families, a physician will find a number of different patterns of varying degrees of effectiveness. The most competent families have a clear structure in which authority is solidly in the hands of the parents, who do not use it in an authoritarian way, but take into consideration the feelings and wishes of their children. Under most circumstances, they negotiate decisions: they obtain a consensus, or work out a compromise. In these families, the parents provide leadership and share the power between them. Each parent sees the other as competent, and the context determines whose expertise provides the leadership. This pattern of family organization is best described as one of clear structure with flexibility.

A less effective organizational structure is a pattern of stable dominance and submission. Here, one family member, most often one of the parents, has a disproportionate amount of power, exceeding by far that of other family members and influencing decisions unduly. There is little, if any, negotiation, search for consensus, or compromise. The submissive family members appear resigned to the unchangeability of the family structure. There may be considerable underlying dissatisfaction, but there is little open rebellion. Any resentment is muted and does not influence the balance of power. This type of family may appear to be effective in solving problems, but such solutions reflect the will of the dominant individual, not of the family system. The marital relationship is, of course, dominant-submissive, and the dominant partner has the final say in all matters. This pattern of stable dominance and submission is not found in the most competent, healthy families, but it occurs often in families containing a disturbed individual. Usually, the disturbed family member is either the submissive spouse or a child. This is the pattern of family organization known as midrange dysfunctional.

In the second type of midrange dysfunctional family, the individuals are neither dominant nor submissive consistently, but rather are openly and chronically conflicted, and no family member is able to achieve the upper hand. The parents fight constantly. Each wishes to be dominant, and neither is willing to accept a submissive position. They are not able to resolve who has the right to decide any particular matter. The children may be drawn into the fray on one side or the other, or they may seek to distance themselves from the parents and search elsewhere for a more peaceful, gratifying group to which they can belong. Such families are ineffective, and the same problems tend to persist over periods of time. This conflicted pattern of midrange dysfunctional families is often seen in clinical settings, and the designated patient is usually one of the children.

At the farthest extreme of family structural organization are chaotic, severely dysfunctional families. In these families, members clump together in a murky formlessness that obliterates individual boundaries. This type of family has been described as having an "amorphous ego mass."[14] It is difficult for the observer to know who thinks what, and there is an aimless, drifting quality to family conversations. Family rules are often impossible to ascertain because there is no clear structure. This most incompetent type of family is rare, and is associated with severe psychiatric disturbance in one or more of its members.

To summarize, family competence on the continuum of overt power ranges from a clear structure with flexibility in the healthiest families, to either a dominant-submissive or chronically conflicted pattern in midrange dysfunctional cases, to the chaos of severely dysfunctional families.

Another variable associated with the different levels of family competence concerns *coalitions,* which are strong alliances between two people for a specific purpose. These occur naturally in all groups and are not necessarily destructive to the goals of the group itself. For example, the strong parental alliance in a healthy family serves to strengthen and reinforce each parent in the task of family leadership. It also serves as a model of complementarity and cooperation for their children. However, other kinds of coalitions that are less beneficial may exist either within the family itself, or with a person outside the family group. One of the internal types is a parent-child coalition that either has greater power, or is more charged emotionally, than the parental coalition. Coalitions with someone outside the family commonly are of three types: a powerful, close coalition between a parent and his or her own parents; a consuming alliance with a friend; or an intense bond with a lover.

In healthy families, the parental coalition is strong, and there are no alliances that compete with it, either within the family or outside it. In midrange dysfunctional families, other powerful coalitions occur frequently. The submissive parent may seek an alliance with one or more children, or an outside coalition with a parent, friend, or lover. Coalitions in the severely dysfunctional families are difficult to detect because the entire family structure is so blurred. Nevertheless, within this context, one may at times observe parent-child coalitions which appear to reflect a fusion of individual identities in a symbiotic relationship.

Another variable related to family structure is closeness. Healthy family members, with their clear individual boundaries (easily recognized by how little difficulty the clinician encounters in discerning what each member thinks and feels), are obviously very close to each other. They maintain eye contact, touch often, and are clearly intimate and devoted. Midrange dysfunctional families generally demonstrate clear individual boundaries, but there is considerable interpersonal distance. This may range from politeness to open dislike, but the emotional remoteness of members from each other is clear. In severely dysfunctional families, the undifferentiated obscurity of individual boundaries precludes emotional closeness, which can occur only between individuals who are separate and equal.

Several other variables that distinguish different levels of competence in families involve communication characteristics that encourage autonomy: clarity and expressiveness are particularly important. Healthy families express themselves clearly. Individuals express their own thoughts and feelings and take responsibility for them. Most midrange families articulate thoughts, ideas, and opinions clearly enough, but not feelings. In the dominant-submissive type, feelings are avoided or masked. In the chronically conflicted type, anger is expressed openly, but other feelings rarely. In the severely dysfunctional family, individuality is unclear, and expressiveness is lost in a type of "we-ness" in which all members feel and think the same way.

Feelings are handled differently at different levels of competence. Healthy families are more open to all kinds of feelings, and the baseline family mood or tone is one of harmony, with warmth, affection, and humor. Each person's feelings are met with an empathetic response. Midrange dysfunctional families may express anger, but they usually avoid expressions of warmth or closeness. The baseline family mood is one of estrangement, with tension, depression, and anger. There is little empathy. Severely dysfunctional families seldom express feelings, and the baseline family mood is one of alienation, with pessimism, cynicism, or hopelessness.

Another family interactional quality that varies at different levels of competence involves the efficiency with which problems are solved by the family. Healthy families do have problems, of course, but they recognize them early and approach solutions most often through negotiation. Midrange dysfunctional families usually seek solutions in one of two ways. Problems may be solved by the dominant individual, with little or no participation from other family members. In the chronically conflicted midrange dysfunctional family, the amount of internal conflict seems to preclude any reasonable approach to problems, making all efforts ineffective. Severely dysfunctional families are grossly inefficient, and often tend to deny the very existence of problems. For example, members may describe a psychotic child as "a little nervous" when, in reality, the child may be delusional, hallucinating, and grossly disorganized.

Since the organizational variables of structure, coalitions, closeness, clarity, expression of feelings, and problem-solving effectiveness have been found to differentiate various levels of competence in families and to have a resulting clinical usefulness, a brief description of a typical family at each of four levels of competence may assist the reader.

Jack and Joan Smith, and their 14-year-old son, Ralph, were seen by their physician. Ralph had requested that his parents make the appointment because of his concern about lack of pubic hair and a persistently high voice. Both parents had reassured Ralph, but acquiesced quickly to his request. All three were seen together initially by the physician, who noted that both parents encouraged Ralph to describe his concerns. Jack and Joan appeared serious, but not overly anxious. Ralph appeared to have no difficulty in expressing himself, and told the physician that his parents had explained that changes would be forthcoming and that different young people matured at different rates. He was aware, however, that all other boys in his gym class had pubic hair, and he felt both worried and somewhat embarrassed. Following a physical examination which revealed that he was entirely within normal limits, the physician met again with Ralph and his parents and indicated that he felt Ralph was one of those normal youngsters who mature slowly. Two options were presented to the family. The first was to do nothing for six months to see whether evidence of puberty would appear during that time. The second involved having additional studies done by a specialist in endocrinology. These studies could have been conducted immediately, or 6 months later if puberty changes still had not occurred by that time.

The physician noted that in the family discussion Ralph was encouraged to express his thoughts and feelings. These were treated with respect by both parents, who seemed united and in no conflict about the issue. Their attitude was one of shared concern about Ralph's feelings. Ralph seemed reassured by the physician's examination and presentation of options, and decided to wait 6 months before proceeding with further studies.

There were many clues that suggested to the physician the likelihood that the Smiths were a competent, healthy family. The parents appeared to have an effective coalition, Ralph was encouraged to express himself, each spoke with clarity, there was an openness about the importance of feelings, all were involved in decision making, and there was no suggestion of underlying conflict.

The Jacksons brought their 13-year-old twin daughters to their physician because both girls wanted their ears pierced. Mr. Jackson was adamant in refusing them permission to do this, and had only agreed reluctantly to "let the doctor decide" when he had been faced with the combined pressure of both the twins and their mother. In the office Mr. Jackson dominated the conversation, interrupted everyone, and clearly stated that pierced ears were a sign of immorality. The twins and their mother were subdued, but looked expectantly to the physician to take their side.

With this family, after only a short interview, the physician could note evidence that the Jacksons were a dominant-submissive midrange dysfunctional family: there was no evidence of an effective parental coalition, the twins and their mother seemed in alliance against the father, yet were not able to fight with him openly. Although the boundaries of each family member were clear, there seemed to be an angry undertone to the family. Characteristically, they made an appeal to authority as a way out of an interpersonal conflict.

Helen and Marshall Toliver brought their 17-year-old daughter, Mindy, to see Helen's gynecologist. Mindy insisted that she wanted to be on the "pill" and her mother was in favor of this, but her father was opposed. In the physician's office, Helen and Marshall were soon in open conflict, arguing, calling names, and making irrelevant accusations. For long periods, there was no mention of Mindy, the pill, or what advice the doctor might have.

The Tolivers presented themselves in a way that suggests that they are a chronically conflicted midrange family. The parents' open warfare, which seemed to have little to do with the issue of Mindy and the pill, is the most pronounced clue. Both parents were clear in their accusations and counter-charges, and the family was dominated by the angry, conflicted parental relationship.

> The Antonios brought their 14-year-old son, Harold, to the pediatrician because the school nurse had told them that he could not return to school without medical clearance. When the physician inquired about the problem, the parents were unable or unwilling to define it. They thought their son seemed fine, but they were vague and difficult to follow. Harold stared straight ahead in a fixed way, did not answer questions, and was seemingly unaware of his surroundings.

There are clues here that suggest that the Antonios are a severely dysfunctional family and that Harold is seriously disturbed. The parents' grossly inappropriate denial of Harold's problems, along with their vagueness and a tendency toward disorganization, reflects their chaotic family structure.

These brief examples are used to illustrate the kinds of clues to a family's level of competence that the physician may note. In order to arrive at a full clinical appraisal, the physician must accomplish a more thorough investigation of the family system.

EXAMINING A FAMILY

In their education and in their practices, most physicians have focused almost solely on the patient as an individual and have shown little interest in considering the family as a whole. Many, therefore, experience considerable discomfort in their initial efforts to conduct a family interview. Chapter 27 presents clear and practical guidelines for an initial family interview that can be useful when read in conjunction with this chapter. A somewhat more structured approach to examining the family may be useful when it is employed with a method for exploring the presenting problem as suggested by Skynner. Rather than directing the flow of the conversation by asking a series of questions, the physician encourages families to discuss among themselves the matters that concern them. In this way, the physician can play a smaller role and make observations of the family processes. An analysis of the family dialogue can give many clues to the level of family competence.

Often, however, the physician needs more data, and it may be helpful to involve the family in a special examination. Each family member may be requested to write the answer to a question on a piece of paper. One of two questions may be particularly useful. They are "What is the main problem in your family?" and "What would you like most to change about your family?" After reading the answers, the physician can explain to the family that they do not agree on the answer to that question (there is usually disagreement in every family). Then the physician may suggest that the family take 10 minutes to discuss and resolve their disagreement, while the physician observes but does not participate. This is difficult for some families, whose members resist with questions like "But, Doctor, how can this help Jane?" or "That's what we want you to tell us." It is necessary to explain that this procedure is an important part of the evaluation.

As the family tries to resolve its differences, it is crucial that the focus of the physician's attention should be on the process of family communication rather than solely on the content of what is said. It is helpful to keep in mind separately the variables involved (overt power, coalitions, closeness, clarity, expression of feelings, and problem-solving effectiveness). Judgments of the family communication variables have been of great importance in understanding the level of family competence. Because most clinicians focus naturally on the content of the family conversation and follow it as a whole, the ability to focus on process and to follow a series of discrete variables systematically requires an evaluation structure and practice.

This interactional task takes only a few minutes and opens the family system for examination. It is of great value in making a clinical appraisal. In some ways it is parallel to the mental status examination of an individual patient (see Chapter 2). Findings may corroborate the clues coming from the initial family interview, as well as reveal additional information about the system. When the family is faced with a problem of their own creation and given the opportunity to work on it, their characteristic style emerges without their being inhibited by knowing what the physician is observing. This supplement to the initial family interview grew out of family research in which such problems were presented to families, the families were left alone to respond, and their subsequent conversations were videotaped. The data obtained in this way were not obscured by the presence and personality of a clinician, two particularly potent factors when there is an active, directive examiner.

The initial interview and the structured problem-solving exercise generally produce sufficient data to allow an initial formulation of the family's level of competence. Most of the families seen in psychiatric practice are at the midrange dysfunctional level, a few are severely dysfunctional families, and only rarely is there a healthy family in the midst of a crisis. The clinician must consider whether the initial formulation describes the family's characteristic level of competence or whether the family's effectiveness is hampered by its being in the midst of an emergency. Anthony's work with families facing one member's severe physical illness suggests that during crises the family system may regress from its usual level of effectiveness.[15] He noted that families with clear and flexible structure (healthy) sometimes move toward a more rigid structure, with a single family member in charge (midrange dysfunctional). If the crisis is not resolved, the family system may regress further to an aimless, drifting, and chaotic lack of organization (severely dysfunctional). The physician must keep in mind that a family in a severe crisis may have temporarily diminished competence. Often, however, the families interviewed are not caught up in a severe crisis, and the clinical data will indicate the family's customary level of functioning.

Of what value is an assessment of the family's level of competence? To a considerable extent that depends upon the individual physician and his or her major interests. As Skynner (Chapter 27) points out, it is important for physicians to enlarge their repertoires of therapeutic skills, and competence in family therapy can greatly increase the physician's capacity for helpfulness. Without such specialized training, however, a formulation of a family's level of competence can offer the physician some rough guidelines. Basically, families which are healthy but are caught in crisis can be helped by their primary physicians to weather the crisis and learn from the experience. Often, one or two family sessions, in which the physician basically supports its strengths, are all that is necessary. Many problems of midrange dysfunctional families can be helped by the primary physician. On the other hand, severely dysfunctional families often are extremely difficult to treat, and the physician may need to consider referring such families to a skilled and experienced family therapist.

When individual patients are referred, some therapists now insist that a family appraisal be made as part of their initial exploration of the individual's problems. Often it may be concluded that the primary focus of treatment should be the family unit or the marital couple. On other occasions, individual therapy is the chosen treatment. This clinical flexibility is a great advantage, for the decision about treatment is based on first hand knowledge of the individual's family and its capacity to support the patient, or on clear evidence of its inclination to make the patient feel stress.

The psychiatrist in private practice sees all types of patients, but most commonly it is the middle-aged woman with depression and anxiety. She is often overweight and takes antianxiety agents on prescription from her physician. Her complaints often focus on her marriage. She reports that she doesn't "get enough" from her husband—that he is remote, preoccupied, and that she feels isolated and rejected. Before the advent of marital and family therapy, this woman would most often be seen in individual therapy, and the psychiatrist would explore the historical antecedents of her "problem with men." Although this is often a useful approach, to focus solely on the individual patient may underestimate the role of current, here-and-now family factors in individual symptoms. Research has identified a group of families termed *competent but pained.*[1] In the range of family competence, they fall between the healthy and the midrange dysfunctional. There is much that is healthy about such families. They produce healthy, autonomous children, have clear structure, and solve problems well. The husbands and wives fail, however, to evolve a relationship that meets the needs of both partners. The husbands may be preoccupied, may not spend much time with their wives, and may not be able to reveal their deeper feelings. The wives, whatever their historical difficulties with men, are deprived, and their depression, anxiety, and obesity are, at least in part, responses to this deprivation. The description, however, suffers in the sense that it omits the wives' roles in the disturbance. They may whine, eat too much, and in general behave in ways that invite neglect. As a consequence, the failure is a shared one. Whom should the physician treat? Should it be the wife, the husband, the couple, or the family unit? The answer varies with the clinician and the specifics of each situation. The development of techniques that allow the physician to ask and to answer that question is a movement toward a pluralism that enables the physician to make better decisions. Knowledge of the therapeutic leverage available at various levels of intervention—individual, marital, or family—lets the physician choose more specific techniques and enhances the ability to heal.

REFERENCES

1 Lewis, Jerry M., W. Robert Beavers, John T. Gossett, and Virginia Austin Phillips: *No Single Thread: Psychological Health in Family Systems,* New York: Brunner/Mazel, 1976.

2 Skynner, A. C. Robin: *Systems of Marital and Family Psychotherapy,* New York: Brunner/Mazel, 1976.

3 Rahe, R. H.: "Life Change Measurement as a Predictor of Illness," *Proceedings of the Royal Society of Medicine,* **61**:1124–1126, 1968.

4 Wolfe, S.: "Life Stress and Patterns of Disease," in H. Lief et al. (eds.), *The Psychological Basis of Medical Practice,* New York: Harper & Row, 1963.

5 Rees, W. D., and S. G. Lutkins: "Mortality of Bereavement," *Brit. Med. J.,* **4**:13–16, 1967.

6 Schmale, A. H., Jr.: "Relationship of Separation and Depression to Disease: A Report on a Hospitalized Medical Population," *Psychosom. Med.,* **20**:259–277, 1958.

7 Engle, G. L.: "A Life Setting Conducive to Illness: The Giving Up-Given Up Complex," *Bull. Menninger Clinic,* **32**:355–365, 1968.

8 Richardson, H. B.: *Patients Have Families,* New York: Commonwealth Fund, 1945.

9 Dingle, J. H., G. F. Badger, and W. S. Jordan, Jr.: *Illness in the Home: A Study of 25,000 Illnesses in a Group of Cleveland Families,* Cleveland: Western Reserve University Press, 1964.

10 Kellner, R.: *Family Ill Health,* Springfield, Ill.: Charles C Thomas, 1963.

11 Jackson, D. D.: "Family Homeostasis and the Physician," *Calif. Med.,* **103**:239–242, October 1965.

12 Meissner, W. W.: "Family Dynamics and the Psychosomatic Processes," *Family Process,* **5**:142–161, 1966.

13 Rogler, L., and A. B. Hollingshead: *Trapped: Families and Schizophrenia,* New York: Wiley, 1965.

14 Bowen, M.: "Family Concept of Schizophrenia," in D. D. Jackson (ed.), *The Etiology of Schizophrenia,* New York: Basic Books, 1960.

15 Anthony, E. James: "The Impact of Mental and Physical Illness on Family Life," *Am. J. Psychiat.,* **127**(2):138–146, 1970.

Chapter 5

Reactions to Physical Illness and Hospitalization

Eric J. Cassell, M.D.

EDITORS' INTRODUCTION

What is it like to be a successful businessman who is secure as a person, competent as an executive, is constantly being looked to for advice and leadership, and then suddenly to find oneself a patient in a coronary care unit? What is it like to feel helpless and totally dependent upon others?

The author delineates the cardinal features of illness. The loss of a sense of indestructability, the loss of a feeling of connectedness to one's supportive interpersonal networks, the failure of logic when thinking about the disease, and the disappearance of a sense of control over one's life are all central to the experience of illness. The mix differs from patient to patient, but all four features can be found to one degree or another by the physician who observes, listens, and thinks. By means of clinical material and brief vignettes, Cassell brings to life that which the sensitive physician may discern. This chapter provides the physician with much to reflect upon, and a framework upon which to construct the understanding of illness. More than just illustrating a cognitive structure, however, the author illustrates the many ways in which physicians may use their understanding in the service and humanistic care of patients.

It has often been said that all physicians would be better physicians had they experienced hospitalization, a significant illness, or an operation—a full indoctrination into patienthood. Some physicians have their encounter with "the other end" of the physician-patient relationship. Even if it is as simple as a sigmoidoscopy, barium enema, examination of the genital area, or repeated blood surveys "for some reason," something can be learned about patienthood. More frightening experiences, such as a lymph node biopsy, often strain the physician-patient's need to be calm. Major surgical procedures, fever of unknown origin, a small infiltration picked up on a routine chest x-ray, "suspicious" cells in the Pap smear—the list of truly frightening possibilities is endless.

Most upsetting, however, is the experience of either severe or chronic illness. Here the physician may understand something of shattered omnipotence, disconnectedness, illogicality, and feelings of loss of control.

As Cassell brings it all together for the reader, it may become more "real." Some physicians have the capacity to place themselves in the patient's situation, others do not. A basic premise of this book is that this capacity can be developed or improved upon in most physicians.

What about the person who has abdominal surgery and has the need to show the surgical scar afterwards? How different it is for the attractive, slender woman who loves her bikinis and is undergoing abdominal hysterectomy! Readers may also reflect on how the patient with a permanent colostomy may feel. How important it is for the physician to take time to explain carefully to the patient not only about the care of the orifice, but also what can be expected in day-to-day functioning, including sexuality, exercise, and "noise."

Some physicians are uncomfortable in talking about sex, suicide, dying, or any emotional problem. Some even have difficulty discussing excretory processes with patients. It is hoped that the basic attitude throughout this book will enable the physician to talk with patients appropriately regarding all body functions, physical or emotional. Cassell's vivid way of bringing the reader into the patient's room with him should be a great aid in their regard.

Recent research on the psychological results of cardiac surgery noted that while 90 percent of the patients who survived showed improvement in physical status, more than one-third developed psychological problems that strongly impaired their functioning. Even those with less serious difficulties appeared to be limited in one or more spheres; they did not return to work, resume normal activities, participate normally in their families, or return to normal sexual function. The surgery had improved the hearts, but apparently had not benefited the patients equally.

All physicians have had similar experiences. A man with a myocardial infarction may return to normal cardiac function. But after going home he may experience numerous symptoms, including sticking chest pains, easy fatigue, and poor exercise tolerance. His wife may complain that he is not the same as before the heart attack and not only because he has lost interest in sex. Such a patient may become more placid, but in any case he may lack his former drives and interests. His symptoms may be attributed to depression, and he may respond to antidepressant agents when they are used in proper dosage for a sufficient period.

Or perhaps he may settle down to a career of illness, and become preoccupied by exaggerated fears and crippling concern about the heart.

Why do these things happen sometimes to patients who have been seriously ill, and why did those patients not get the same benefit from surgery that their hearts did?

Every disease has features that are unique because of the physiology or anatomy of the organs involved. The heart can malfunction as a muscle pump, hydraulic system, or electrical system, and the symptoms of heart disease reflect these malfunctions. As that is true of the heart (or the liver, uterus, muscles, colon, and so on), it is also true of the whole person. When a person becomes ill, there may also occur a distortion of his or her relationship to the body, to other people, to work, and to the other aspects of being a person, a private individual, and a member of society. Such behavioral changes are often as much a part of illness as the disease itself. It follows that when sick patients get better, it is not only the diseased organ system, such as the lungs in pneumonia, that returns to normal, but also those activities that are involved in being a normally functioning person in the day-to-day world. We know much more about what happens when organ systems become diseased and then return to health than what happens when people get ill and return to health. Perhaps such a lack of knowledge was acceptable during an earlier period in medicine. Now, when we can do so much more for terribly complicated diseases, and when patients are less likely to die but may be sick for long periods of time before they recover, our lack of knowledge often hampers our patients in returning to their former selves. With a little more help, they could return to normal functioning. It is as simple as that.

Just as a heart or a liver can malfunction in only so many ways, the psychological changes that accompany illness are also limited, and can be described in an orderly and useful manner. The big difference is that our language for describing disease is more precise than the language for describing the "disorders of person" that accompany illness. For the former, we have objective measurements, while for people, our terms are subjective and thus seem "softer" and less real. To put it another way, sick people, no matter what the cause of their sickness, have certain characteristics that are different from those of people who are well. These characteristics are not chance or random events, but are definable, diagnosable, and relatively constant in occurrence. For this reason, the apparently illogical or difficult behavior of the sick is not at all illogical, but is the result of internal and external forces acting on the sick person. The physician must often manipulate these forces to return the patient to health in the same way drugs or other modalities are used to return a diseased part to health.

THE CHARACTERISTICS OF ILLNESS

Sick people suffer a disconnection from their usual world, a loss of their sense of indestructability (omnipotence), a loss of the competence and completeness of their reasoning, and a loss of control over themselves and their world. These features, which will be explored in depth, *are* illness. When they are absent, no matter what the state of the body's integrity, illness *is not present*. Similarly, when one, another, or all these features (arising in the course of disease or for some other reason) are present to whatever extent, then illness continues, again without regard to the body's state of integrity. Furthermore, the effect of each or all of the features of illness on the patient is dependent upon the patient's personality, surrounding social forces, and the nature of the disease or situation that causes them. The features of illness will be discussed separately, but they are inevitably intertwined. For example, problems of reasoning interfere with the perception of the disease process and social relations, and thus reinforce or diminish the force of those features. Similarly, the boundaries among physical, emotional, and social contributions to the illness are also blurred. Keeping these regions separate, while a necessary task in writing about the sick, may interfere with understanding both the patient and the illness.

The Loss of Connection

What I am going to discuss is best illustrated by the cases of actual patients.

> You would have no difficulty guessing what disease Wallace Black has. Sitting up in his bed, he looks somewhat like a white-haired, partly bald, and plucked turkey, because of the wasting of his face, neck, and shoulder girdle. That muscle wasting, which is not quite the cachexia of terminal malignancy, in addition to obvious ascites, is the hallmark of late-stage cirrhosis with portal hypertension. He has been in the hospital for almost 3 weeks. The first 10 days were occupied by diagnostic studies, and in the last week or so a good diuresis has been obtained. The present difficulty is not ridding him of more ascites, but rather that he insists on going home in a few days. Since he is finally making progress, that would be an error. He has offered the usual justification about the bad food and how he would rest better at home. But the real reason is that he is having trouble keeping his business going from the hospital room. While it is often true that a patient's business does suffer during illness, and that should not be dismissed lightly, such is not the case here. Mr. Black is 70 years old and in good financial condition. He has told me that he is a self-made man who has had little education, and that he has been very successful as a broker. Almost no visit to his room goes by without some reference to an important person who just called, or to some business situation in which he alone was able to solve the problem. Mr. Black prides himself on his work and on his social connections, and there lies our difficulty. While he is sick and in a hospital bed, Mr. Black cannot be the person he knows and admires. He knows who he is in part by his relationships to other people and to the world of his business. When he is cut off from those associations he ceases to exist, at least on one level, and that is profoundly disturbing to him.

We are all connected to the world by our relationships with other people and our place in the social scheme. To some, as to Wallace Black, that connection is more important than it is to others; but our interaction with others is vital to the maintenance of our person. In sickness, all these things change. As illness deepens, patients become more and more withdrawn from their usual world, their previous interests, friends, and even their families. We can learn how important this characteristic feature of illness is to our patients by observing how they defend themselves against its effects. (Indeed, that is true of all the characteristics of illness.) It is difficult, if not impractical, to ask patients whether they feel disconnected. They may not know themselves, or be able to verbalize it in that way. But by watching their behavior in the hospital (Mr. Black is always on the telephone), seeing the visitors, and listening to the small talk, we can construct a picture of what is important to the patient. Mr. Black lives near my home, and in the weeks preceding his admission, I would occasionally see him going toward his office. He walked slowly, with 15 liters of ascites sticking out in front of his wasted frame, but he was erect, impeccably dressed, and a figure of respect. I know what effort that continued presence must have cost.

The disconnection of illness is not only social. It may take place over the entire spectrum of being. We exist to the extent that we are connected. Some of the connections are physical, such as the senses, postural reflexes, and proprioception. Even the tearing eyes and the loss of sense of smell that accompany a cold may be disruptive to some. Patching one eye for 24 hours is often associated with irritation, nervousness, difficulty concentrating or coping—disruptions of normal thought and function, despite the fact that sight remains in the other eye. The loss of balance of true vertigo is also profoundly upsetting past the degree of purely functional loss, which is why patients with this sickness may be helped by small doses of phenothiazines in addition to antimotion sickness medication.

Patients are not used to calling these disruptions *symptoms.* They simply do not feel like their usual selves, and when asked about it will point to the eye, ear, or other malfunctioning organ. However, universal recognition of the profound disconnection that can occur is part of the dread of blindness. The losses of connection that accompany interference with the senses are poorly understood when each sensory modality is seen as standing only for itself, like the individual ropes that hold a boat to its dock. Think instead of the empathy one feels for the deaf Beethoven, who has to be turned around so that he can see the audience acclaim the Ninth Symphony. Has he lost only his hearing?

In order not only to understand their behavior better but also to reduce their discomfort, it is necessary for us to know that patients are reacting not only to the physical symptoms or disease, but to the disconnection itself. Further, since patients may not know why they are irritable, depressed, anxious, fearful, angry, or whatever, they may react to their own seemingly inexplicable behavior by externalizing the source or projecting blame for their feelings onto others. That is why we hear Mr. Black complain about the food and cite the behavior of the nurses and house staff as the reason he must go home. Or, he may say to me that I never explain what is wrong with him, just after I have finished answering his questions in detail. He does not know why he feels the disquiet that he does, and must seek some outside reason for it. Often, the patient's distress will subside as a result of just being reassured that it is normal to feel irritable when, for example, vision is acutely impaired. On occasions, it may be necessary to stress the other ways in which the patient is concerned. The doctor should never simply brush aside patients' concerns about business, work, or social relations as being unimportant, no matter how serious the disease, because to do so is to brush aside the importance of the people themselves. Think how badly you would feel if, because you were ill, you were unable to hold up your part of the duty schedule or do your part of the work, or see patients who had been given appointments. When patients have as little insight as Mr. Black does, explanations may be useless. Then one must balance the danger that the disconnection poses against the need for further hospitalization.

But what threat is posed by something like disconnection? First, it is not too strong to say that anything that threatens the integrity of self, self-concept, or the patient's ability to function as an intact person endangers the patient's physical well-being. *Physical integrity cannot withstand the dissolution of the social personality.* The most extreme example of this is the phenomenon of voodoo death, where the individual is cut off from the group. Friends and relatives share the victim's belief that he or she is doomed. The community withdraws, and on every occasion and by every action suggests to the victim that he or she is indeed dead. Torn from family and social ties and excluded from all the functions and activities through which self-awareness is experienced, the victim yields, and in time dies.

Many of us have seen patients who, when cut off from their world, family, friends, and social ties, simply give up and die from diseases for which recovery might otherwise have been expected. Furthermore, there is increasing evidence that the phenomenon of "giving up"—when the person experiences a sense of helplessness, hopelessness, and deprivation of love or support—may antedate the onset of important organic disease. More commonly, we see an apathetic or depressed patient lying limply in a hospital bed, or we see a patient who will not take medications, refuses diagnostic studies, or insists on leaving the hospital even when obvious danger is involved. The irritation of the staff and its counterarguments merely increase the patient's sense of isolation and disconnection from others, and thus heighten the problem.

But how can we be sure that Mr. Black's complaints about the food and the staff are not the issue, that indeed he is suffering from disconnection and isolation from the people and environmental props that help maintain his integrity of self? As with any other diagnosis, the first thing needed is a high index of suspicion, and the next is listening for the clues. Mr. Black insists that he is going home this weekend—as a matter of fact, on Friday. I cannot, in conscience, discharge him on Friday, but I think I could on Sunday. We talk back and forth for a while, and I ask him why those 2 days are so important. He says, "Doc, I need those 2 days to rest up." Now I know. Rest up? Rest up for what? I turn to his wife and say, "Charlotte, Wallace is going to work on Monday, isn't he?" And that turns out to be the case. He has been working on a deal by telephone, and the papers will be signed Monday. Perhaps they could be signed in a hospital room, but that would not serve the purpose. Wallace Black does not need the money, but he does need the setting and the people around him to tell him that he is Wallace Black. And to him and to many others who are sick, hospitalized, and disconnected from their world, that is more important than merely being alive. We will try to work out something that can meet both objectives: diuresis and improvement of hepatic function, as well as the restoration of his person.

Disconnection may occur rapidly, as in such acute emergencies as myocardial infarction or severe trauma. Suddenly the patient is among people who, well meaning as they may be, are nevertheless strangers. While the patient is lying on a stretcher in a hallway or being moved like an object from place to place, the sense of isolation is heightened. It is also worsened by the lack of privacy in intensive care units, where even the markers of individuality that are usually found in hospital rooms—family pictures, get-well cards, or what-have-you—are absent. It is very common for patients in these circumstances to try to identify for the strange doctor some connection, common acquaintance, or place that connects them. The small talk made while waiting can be used to establish such ties and relationships, thus diminishing the patient's stress. In those settings, there is no such thing as meaningless conversation. It can always be used to serve a purpose. In emergency situations, few needs are as important and as simple to satisfy as making patients feel that they are known.

In chronic diseases or long-term illness, the withdrawal from the world may be gradual. Connection to friends and associates may be replaced slowly by new friendships and relationships that are drawn from within the world of illness. The patient may be alternately frightened by the perception of withdrawal, or disinterested as the horizon shrinks. Leaving the outside world, the sick person begins increasingly to build a new reality that is shared exclusively with the other sick. In the beginning, friends and family may have abandoned the patient, but now the sick person actively begins to reject those from the outside. Even the relationship with a spouse or children may change radically, as everything becomes oriented around the illness. This phenomenon has been compared to the social consequences of aging, with illness producing the social equivalence of premature aging. Thus, in a sense, sickness spreads into the family, causes disruptions, and causes relationships to change in ways of which the members may not be aware. As one must learn to deal with the disconnection of the patient, so must the needs of the family be tended. Once again, from the patient's point of view, these changes may be seen as originating in others and as being directed toward the ill person, rather than, as is often the case, starting with the patient's behavior. Psychotherapeutic intervention may be desirable to diminish the impact of the patient's withdrawal on the family and on the patient. *But it may be an error to attempt to reconnect the patient to his or her former world, since the reality of the illness and its physical and social impact often cannot be overcome.* The new world of the chronically ill exists because it allows patients to reconstitute a self, a sense of their own persons that is appropriate to their new circumstances. In former times the tuberculosis sanitorium, which was described so well by Thomas Mann in *The Magic Mountain,* was an example of the society of the sick. *The Magic Mountain* is worth reading, if only for its superb insight into that society. Today, kidney dialysis and transplant units provide better examples. It is interesting how many patient associations have arisen, associations such as Ostomy Associations, Reach for Life, or Run for Your Life groups that serve the purpose of reconnecting the sick to the world of the well through the mediation of others in the same situation.

The fact that the dissolution of the social personality is often the basic element in the *suffering* of a patient cannot be overemphasized. The sick will tolerate, or even adapt to chronic pain, dyspnea, weakness, or other symptoms without considering themselves to be suffering. If you ask those patients whether they are suffering, they will say that they have pain (or whatever), but are not suffering. But if they perceive themselves as losing their connection to their group—friends, family, or peers—then they will consider themselves to be suffering.

That point was central in the case of Annette Landy, a 53-year-old woman with increasingly severe chronic obstructive pulmonary disease. Despite severely compromised pulmonary function, she managed to go shopping occasionally, visit friends, or even go to the movies from time to time. She seemed to have adapted well to her considerable disability. Then office visits began to become too difficult for her, and it was evident that her pulmonary function had decreased even further. However, repeat studies, while dreadful, were not worse than previously. She felt, and I concurred, that going out of her apartment had become too difficult, so an oxygen "walker" at home was arranged for her. I was troubled because, despite her taciturn manner and no objective evidence of worsened disease, she seemed sicker. Within a week of my return from vacation, she reported increased cough, phlegm, and dyspnea. I admitted her to the hospital. Her pO_2 on admission was 50mm of Hg. There was little evidence of infection. What had precipitated her respiratory failure? While examining her I noticed shiny, brownish, palm-sized patches about both knees. They came from resting her hands on her knees while urinating—30 to 40 times, day and night! Urinary frequency started about the time I perceived her as worsening, before she could no longer leave the apartment. She urinated so often because she was afraid she would be incontinent. Indeed, that had happened on several occasions. Respiratory failure was probably precipitated by exhaustion. However, both the urinary symptom and her lack of desire to leave her apartment occurred when she began to feel that it was simply too difficult to keep up appearances any longer. She said, "I just decided I didn't give a damn anymore and I didn't care anymore what anyone thought." A devastating idea for someone as well bred and ladylike as this patient—the equivalent of deserting a lifelong mode of behavior and interaction with the world. As in all instances, it is the meaning of the behavior to the patient that counts, not what others believe.

Cystometrics were normal. First desire to void occurred at 15 ml, but her bladder capacity was 350 ml. There was evidence of mild trignotis, but infection was not present.

In the hospital, with indwelling catheter, adequate rest, increased bronchodilators, and steroids, she began to feel much better. Even though she felt better and was optimistic about going home (although, as usual, slightly apprehensive in anticipation of discharge), her arterial blood gases at discharge were not appreciably better than on admission (although her steroid requirement was increased). Her pulmonary function was marginal at best, and the probability of early death had not diminished. Yet the patient returned home better in her eyes and in mine. What had treatment accomplished aside from teaching her to control the desire to void? She was again one of us, a part of her social group and no longer alone.

It is sad but inevitable when patients die from diseases that we cannot control, but it is an absolutely unnecessary tragedy when the same patients die alone and disconnected from their social world, like a sailor fallen overboard at night.

One other facet of the disconnection of the sick is symbolized historically by Hansen's disease. Here, the sufferer is not only ill, but a threat to the healthy. Venereal diseases are often seen in the same light, even when treatment is simple. With these and other infectious diseases, the bond of the patient to the group is disrupted by the patient's fear of causing sickness in others, which would be a deep breach of social convention. Sometimes one must temper the zeal of hospital epidemiologists when they isolate patients for questionable reasons. The fact of isolation can be an added stress for a patient and should not be done without good reason and without active and continued reassurance.

The tie of the sick to their world, then, may be menaced by the effects of the disease on them or by the danger of their disease to others. Thus, the loss of connection that happens in illness can occur at any or all the places where we connect to our world: physically, as with the sensory disturbances; emotionally, in our connection to those close to us; or socially, where we are connected to the wider world. The physician must be aware of these losses of connection and their danger to the patient's well-being. Dealing with them may mean simple reassurance in conjunction with other treatment, as in the case of the patient who loses vision temporarily, or may be one of the most important aspects of treatment, as with the patient whose ventilatory failure I just described.

The Loss of the Sense of Omnipotence

The next patient, Mr. Fred Bortman, came up from the cardiac care unit a few days ago. He was admitted with a typical history of myocardial infarction, which had been confirmed by the evolution of his electrocardiograms and enzymes. His chest pain subsided rapidly, with no evidence of failure or important arrhythmia. He is 48 years old, white, and a relatively successful middle-level manager for a large corporation; my "typical" patient with a myocardial infarction. He appears healthy, and that is part of the problem in caring for him. In his behavior and in his reaction to the heart attack, he demonstrates another feature of illness, the loss of the sense of omnipotence—a failure of the person's belief in his or her own indestructibility. In health, we take our bodies for granted. Even when one does not like his or her body, its intactness and readiness to go and do are prized. The fact that the world can be a dangerous place that threatens injury or death is known to everyone, but that knowledge is no match for the sense of omnipotence that denies the possibility of bodily damage or death. If there were no sense of omnipotence, who would cross a busy street? Certainly no one would ride a motorcycle. Some individuals have a more strongly developed sense of omnipotence than others, and they are frequently described as fearless, while others who are more fearful have a sense of omnipotence that seems less protective. All physicians have patients who are racked by body fears; every symptom seems to them the ticking of a time bomb.

That was not Fred Bortman's problem. He worked and acted as though nothing could happen to him. But it did. When I see him now, he is talking as if nothing has happened. He tells me that he is not sure that he had a heart attack; he feels fine now. He never felt better. The chest pain that made him call me was not that bad. When I remind him of how severe his pain seemed to be on admission, he tells me that he was "overreacting."

We do not have difficulty identifying his reaction to the heart attack as denial. Indeed, the conversation is reminiscent of many similar interactions with men who have had heart attacks. (Women behave this way less often.) The threat that illness poses to the sense of omnipotence must be met, and denial is one of the most common defenses. A sense of omnipotence, of indestructibility, is essential to *normal* functioning, just as the normal person must feel connected to others and to the social world. Just as the heart muscle heals, so, too, must the sense of omnipotence regenerate. There are, however, some ways of reconstitution that are better than others. The degree of denial displayed by Mr. Bortman is going to get in the way of his return to health.

What this patient is doing is not unusual. I am sometimes awestruck by the power of denial in the face of the most dire symptoms. Patients will occasionally alter their entire life-style to avoid the activity that produces the symptom. Denial is often the mechanism that keeps patients from going to a physician in the first place. Further, denial may be selective—present for one symptom or disease, but not for another. A 58-year-old woman came because of episodic abdominal pain, which was quite typical of gall bladder disease. No other complaints were offered. During physical examination, I was shocked to discover a large fungating carcinoma of the left breast. She said, "To tell the truth, I forgot all about that." Her sister had died of breast cancer (the patient also had cholecystitis).

Angina pectoris and dyspnea are examples of symptoms that are so distressing, not only in themselves but for the meaning they convey about the vulnerability of the body, that patients may go to great lengths to deny their existence. History taking from someone you are sure has angina can be difficult, because occasionally the patient denies not only the symptoms, but also any activity that might produce the symptom. For the same reason, exercise programs for rehabilitation in cardiac or pulmonary diseases have the difficulty that the therapeutic regimen produces symptoms of these diseases, thus constantly reminding the patient of the disease.

On occasion, a patient may report a worsening of symptoms when there is no objective evidence that the disease has worsened. What has happened is that previous denial has failed, and the patient perceives now what was concealed previously.

Symptoms of central nervous system disease are more shattering than most others. Difficulties in speech or memory, hallucinations, and interference with thoughts may strike at the sense of oneself as a person. They are person symptoms rather than body symptoms. In the same manner, disturbances of thought or perception may make patients feel that they are losing their sanity. The same worry about losing their sanity may disturb patients with organic symptoms of disease, such as myalgias, arthralgias, weakness, or fatiguability, when physicians do not believe what the patient reports. The patients are first distressed at the failures of their bodies and then, when they are not believed by physicians, they begin to doubt their own perceptions. Patients with insidious onset of, for example, thyroid disease, myasthenia gravis, or multiple sclerosis, will often report such occurrences as part of the very distress of their illnesses.

The sense of omnipotence is protected by denial even in the language that patients use to describe their symptoms or disease. During a second-year class on interviewing, the demonstration interviewer asked the patient (who was unknown to him) what his problem was. The patient said, in almost so many words, "acute lymphoblastic leukemia." The interviewer never quite recovered, but the patient then proceeded to give the stunned class a lecture on his own inevitably fatal disease. After he left, we all wondered how he could be so calm and self-assured despite his fate. After we had listened to the recording of the interview, the mechanism became clear. All the symptoms and signs of disease were preceded by impersonal pronouns. For example, "you get these spots on your skin" or "one gets bleeding from the gums" or, referring to patients with leukemia, "they often feel weak and listless." On the other hand, all manifestations of health were preceded by personal pronouns, as in "I worked hard all fall" or "we went sleigh riding in the country in February" or "I expect to go home next week." It was as though his internal conception of self was still healthy and intact.

The sense of omnipotence is like a shield around the integrity of the person; it preserves intactness. The symptoms of illness are the enemy of that intactness, and denial is one of its defenses; the completeness of a person extends past the physical boundaries of the body. A person is also his or her beliefs and ideas, as well as usual activities, habits, and patterns of behavior. That is why sometimes, when you are about to hospitalize someone who has been taken with serious illness suddenly, the person will say, "I can't go to the hospital. I have to go to my exercise class tomorrow." The comment is inappropriate to the seriousness of the situation, but the patient does not seem aware of how silly it sounds. Going to the exercise class is part of the weekly routine. It is not so much the content of the activity that is important—although exercise may play a significant part in the image of self—as it is the loss of part of oneself. Nonetheless, patients are usually aware of the symptoms they deny, but to accept the symptoms would demand a change in self-image, in the sense of self. Thus, if you listen closely, you will hear patients depersonalize their symptoms by doing what the patient with leukemia did—using impersonal words. The pain, not my pain. A woman with a pulmonary embolus was giving the history of the thrombophlebitis that preceded her present illness and said, "My left leg" (the patient's own leg, part of herself) "which is the bad leg" (no longer "my leg," but a bad leg that is not part of myself) "from the vascular point of view," (not bad from her point of view but from some outside, abstract position) "had a thrombophlebitis in it." (She did not have thrombophlebitis—a leg had it.) She could have said, "I have vascular problems in my left leg and I got thrombophlebitis." You will have to listen very carefully because such impersonal usages are so common that they are difficult to hear as distinct entities. The difficulty in picking up the language attests to the normalcy of the phenomenon. The language distances the patient's intact self from the phenomenon that threatens the self. Women virtually always refer to their breasts as "my breasts," but when about to have a mastectomy, they will commonly talk about "the breast." More strikingly, after the mastectomy, they usually refer to the remaining healthy breast as "the breast" rather than "my breast." Months after the mastectomy, the healthy breast again becomes "my breast." The fundamental point is that the self, the person as seen by oneself, must be preserved at all costs, and illness threatens that sense of self. Thus, the sense of omnipotence functions to maintain certain aspects of self-image.

Ultimately, as sickness becomes worse, all defenses fail and the patient is forced to acknowledge the body's failure. Previously powerful and now helpless, previously sure and now untrustworthy, the body is seen for what it is: fragile and defenseless against injury.

The problem with denial as a defense against the recognition of illness is that its opposite face is frequently panic. The sick person has refused to accept or even consciously recognize all symptoms of disease, even the trivial, but when illness overwhelms, the patient begins to react with great fear to all the symptoms that had previously been denied. The panic comes not only because of the sudden awareness of illness, but *also because of the loss of the major defense mechanism*. To be both sick and defenseless is terrifying. Denial can cause major problems for a physician. The patient does not accept the facts of the illness, and thus may not take medications, go for needed diagnostic studies, or return for the follow-up. I am sometimes uncertain what to do when a patient behaves in this manner. I know how dangerous it can be to breach the denial forcibly by telling the patient in no uncertain terms what the situation is. I do not want to use stark language that would be avoided with the most stable person. If I use it, the patient will not act, but will be paralyzed with fear by what I said, and that was hardly my original object. Furthermore, by using such straight language I become the enemy (after all, I frightened the patient, not the disease).

In these situations, I try to provide an alternate defense for patients. Overintellectualization is a useful substitute that can be encouraged by long intellectual discussions of the disease or symptom, as though we were talking about someone else's body, and that can point the way to the desired action. In engaging in such discussions, I am employing the same mechanism described above—depersonalizing the body part of symptom by using impersonal pronouns. I might say, "Fluid in a chest like that often comes from the reaction of the chest lining to an inflammation. It is important to find out what the chest wall or the lining is reacting to in order to prevent the lining from making more fluid and compressing the lungs." The fact that what afflicts the lungs afflicts the person is not mentioned.

At other times I let more time pass, when that can be done safely, because I know that sooner or later the patient will be forced by the symptoms to recognize the illness. Panic may follow, but now I am not the one whose bad tidings caused the panic, but rather the one who offers safety.

After Wallace Black, the patient discussed earlier, went home, his diuresis continued. One day he called, weak-voiced, from his bed. His weight that morning had been 116 pounds. (His weight when leaving the hospital was 126 pounds, and his normal weight about 155 pounds.) He said he was dying—wasting away and dying. I saw him at home. The abdomen was flat, almost free of ascites, but there had been no further muscle wasting. He went on for awhile about his pitiful state. He was finally ready to listen as he had not been for all the months of his illness. So frightened was he by the sudden awareness of his condition and by his interpretation of its fatal meaning, that what I had to say about his cirrhosis seemed to be a reprieve. Together, we could plan a realistic therapeutic regime. Fred Bortman is not yet there.

Denial is by no means present in all patients with myocardial infarction or other serious illness. On occasion, patients appear to be completely aware of the danger of their situation, or the bleakness of their future. Not surprisingly, such awareness is frequently followed by depression. Those patients may appear agitated, apathetic, or merely bland. It is distressingly common to find every emotion that patients evidence labelled as "anxiety" and treated with antianxiety agents. In the first place, all emotion does not have to be "treated away," as though it is inappropriate to be sad or depressed after serious illness. Rather, the reasonableness of the response and its reasons should be acknowledged by the doctor. As will be discussed later, the patient is beset by uncertainties about the future, many of which can be put to rest by the doctor in a few minutes of conversation. False optimism is neither desirable nor desired by patients who are alert to their situation—they see through it quickly. But what is necessary is an attempt to elicit the concerns that are *specific* to each patient, followed by information that the patient needs in his or her own terms. Second, sedative drugs may depress the patient further by restricting psychic and physical activity, which may increase the patient's sense of being in a straitjacket.

When speaking with Mr. Bortman, I discovered that his heart attack had occurred one year to the day after his wife died. His relationship with his wife had been extremely close, and he has felt lost since her death. One of his two children fled the home and married unexpectedly two months after her mother's death, and the other daughter left college to come home and care for him. Aside from telling me these facts, he does not want to talk about his wife, the emotional impact of her death, or the possibility that he might be depressed. The anniversary timing of his myocardial infarct is to him "coincidence." Mr. Bortman's denial, then, extends beyond physical illness and into his emotional life. When denial is present in psychological matters, we often speak of a patient as having no insight. But the problems presented in caring for such patients are the same as those presented in other cases of psychological denial. Just as it will be difficult to get Mr. Bortman to accept a program of cardiac rehabilitation, so too are the chances minimal that he will seek needed psychiatric help.

A number of studies have reported the anniversary phenomenon—death or illness occurring on the anniversary of the death of a loved one, who is most commonly a parent or a spouse. The finding is interesting in itself, but it points to something of broader significance: the association of illness in the patient with illness in other family members, who are generally the parents. Patients commonly tell us that they know that their joint pain is arthritis because their mothers or fathers had arthritis. As I said earlier, the boundaries of a person do not stop at the limits of the body. We often speak of identification with a parent as though the connection to the parent occurred solely in thought. In fact, however, the person may think or behave as though his or her body were a literal extension of the parent's, and display the same physical strengths or weaknesses, or be prone to the same diseases, as the father or mother. (A child may identify with either parent.) We acknowledge this, generally, by inquiring specifically for a family history of heritable disorders. But it is important to go beyond such diseases and inquire whether the patient knows of any diseases or health problems that "run in your family or which are of concern to you because of your family history." Unless specifically asked, patients will often not offer such information because they are unaware of its importance, or even on occasion because they are embarrassed at what they perceive to be a "nonrational" influence on their behavior. On the other hand, the link of their illness to that of a parent may offer comfort. A 49-year-old physician had what he thought was an inexplicably prolonged upper respiratory infection and finally went to see his own doctor. When told that he had hay fever (a diagnosis that should have been obvious to him) he said "But that's impossible, I'm 49." He did not seem satisfied when told that it did not matter how old he was. But then he said, "What's the matter with me, I forgot all about it—my father and sister had hay fever." Now hay fever was acceptable.

While that is a trivial example, more serious situations exist when patients act as though history is prophecy, as though if the parent died of (say) congestive heart failure, it is inevitable that they, too, will die of congestive heart failure. Because of that belief, they may not carry out simple and obviously effective treatment. Since the patient may not be aware, for whatever reason, of the association with the parent's disease, the information must be actively sought. Often merely pointing out the association and showing what can be done for patients to change their future is sufficient to avoid an otherwise fatal outcome—it is often a matter of a few minutes conversation.

Fred Bortman's illness extends to his family. Indeed, he was referred to me by his sister-in-law prior to his heart attack (but he did not call until he developed chest pain) out of her concern for the disruption of the family following the death of his wife. His heart attack has compounded the family problem. The wife on whom he was so dependent is dead, but her place has been taken by the daughter who left college to care for him. With his illness, the burden on the daughter has increased and I suspect that she will have difficulty leaving her father again and resuming her own life and career. Similarly, the flight of the other daughter suggests trouble. I call it flight because the period of mourning for the death of a parent is usually longer than two months; usually families draw together rather than disperse during that period. Furthermore, she married someone whom she had not known prior to her mother's death. This added to my belief that her actions were precipitous. One may speculate about the reasons for her departure and marriage—that she was escaping the burden that ultimately settled on her sister. But those would be speculations that could neither be confirmed nor acted

upon. Indeed, what action is possible, even after we recognize how physical illness has caused widespread family disruption? Frequently, perhaps usually,
serious illness in an individual leads to difficulty in the family unit, but often all
the family members are not our patients, or they do not seek our assistance, or
they may even be unaware of the extent of the problem or its source. Where possible, referral to a psychiatrist or family agency may be very helpful. But when that
is not possible, we are left treating the only family member to whom we have access—the patient. In Mr. Bortman's instance, his family will be best served if we
are able to rehabilitate him to the point where he feels whole again—not just from
the heart attack, but from the death of the wife. Because of his denial and his lack
of insight, the best approach, referral for psychotherapy, may not be
possible—he does not think he has an emotional problem. Nonetheless, such
treatment should be suggested when appropriate. Using psychotropic drugs, such
as tricyclic antidepressants, probably is also not feasible. To be of value, these
agents must be used in adequate dosage for a long enough period. Drug side effects are inevitable, if they are only dry mouth and some initial lethargy, and Mr.
Bortman will not tolerate symptoms produced by drugs whose aim is to relieve a
depression that he does not even think he has. Here, as in so many instances, if we
are to be successful *we must start where the patient is.* In planning his treatment,
we are forced to work from his point of view of himself, his illness, and his family, since he will not accept our view. We are left, then, with only his body to work
with and somehow, by doing that, we hope to have an influence not only on his
heart disease but on his family unit.

What is Mr. Bortman's understanding? He tells us that he does not believe
that he has heart disease. Rather, he thinks that he was very upset after his wife's
death and because of that he worked himself into exhaustion. His present illness
resulted, he says, because he was "overtired." Furthermore, he used to be very
active physically, and after the death of his wife he stopped playing squash and let
himself get "out of condition." In the subsequent discussion I use his viewpoint.
I do not stress his heart disease, which would further weaken his failed sense of
omnipotence and breach his denial (in addition to providing more reason for him
to be dependent on his daughter). Rather, I lay stress on his physical vanity and
his view of himself as a powerful man on whom others depend. That, after all,
was the image he used to pretend to himself that he was not so dependent on his
wife but rather vice versa. In outlining an exercise program for cardiac rehabilitation, I emphasize the state of fitness he used to enjoy, and make it clear that he
can be in even better condition in the future. In the months to come I will stress
the same points repeatedly. As he achieves maximum fitness in a regular running
or other aerobic exercise program, there is a high probability that his body will
tell him that he is what his body is: strong, trim, functional beyond others of his
age and medical background. Body pride based on real achievement has a powerful effect on self-image. We know the task will be difficult. Keeping him running,
and handling the symptoms that arise without either reinforcing his physical fears
or allowing him to go beyond prudent limits will test my ingenuity. But the alternatives are increasing dependency, cardiac fears, and a trapped daughter—to say

nothing of recurrent myocardial infarction. With Fred Bortman, as with other patients, we must start where he is and work within his own worldview to achieve the goal of a return to health for both him and his family.

The Failure of Reason

These patients asked many questions about their illnesses. Some of the questions I had answered during previous visits, and yet they came up again. Your own experience will confirm that, even after you have provided lengthy and apparently lucid explanations in response to patients' queries, the patients will ask the same questions again, as though you had never spoken to them. With good reason, we believe that patients should know what is happening to them. Informed patients work better with their physicians. Yet these experiences make us wonder, occasionally, whether sick people are capable of understanding the complexities of modern medicine. Indeed, it is true that the ill have problems in reasoning. The difficulties arise for two reasons. The first is that sick persons cannot, because of the nature of thought, stop thinking about their illness, but they lack the knowledge about the body and disease that is essential to understanding their circumstances. The second problem is that in profound illness, the very nature of the thinking process changes without the patient's being aware of the change.

Normal thought strives continually to understand events even when the dynamics cannot be controlled and the real significance of those events refuses to reveal itself. An event is merely something that happens, a change from one state to another. Illness also is an event, or series of events. Thus, patients attempt to understand what is happening, but their knowledge is inadequate, and the things that are happening seem beyond control. One of the ways we maintain control of our world is by knowledge. Certainly, as physicians, we maintain control of our cases in part by knowing what is happening. Consider a patient who is getting sicker, in a case where death seems inevitable. Think of how differently you would feel if you understood the disease and what was happening to the patient, as opposed to having no idea what was going on. Where your knowledge was adequate, you might feel sad that the patient was dying, but you would accept it and consider yourself in control. On the other hand, if you had no idea what was transpiring, you would probably feel desperate. The crucial difference between the two alternatives is not what is happening to the patient, but your sense of the adequacy or inadequacy of your knowledge. Our knowledge is part of ourselves. When it is incomplete, we feel incomplete. In abstract matters or those of little concern, where information is inadequate, one can merely stop thinking or change the subject of thought. But in illness that is not possible. Each symptom, each body sensation or event demands thought. Because the presence of symptoms maintains a threat, thought cannot stop, nor can the subject be changed. Rather, new information must be sought, and where that is lacking, repeated reinterpretations of existing material are constructed, with new content from memory and emotion added to make up for a deficient reality. Rather than moving away from danger, each new interpretation seems to increase the patient's fears and sense of threat. It is as though some force was always pushing toward an abyss.

The next patient will demonstrate the importance of understanding the relationship between the reasoning of the sick, and the phenomenon of illness. Further, this case will illustrate how such understanding can be used to reduce the sick person's burden.

Mr. Fanton is 24 years old, and he is here for the second hospitalization for an undiagnosed illness within a month. About 3 months ago he developed generalized, tender lymphadenopathy, accompanied by malaise, intermittent headaches, and transient and variable pains in the lower extremities. He was seen by several physicians before he consulted me, and he had received two adequate courses of tetracyclines. Laboratory studies at that time were extensive, appropriate, and uniformly negative. He was admitted for an axillary lymph node biopsy, which also was not diagnostic. Two weeks later his condition had not changed and he was readmitted for further diagnostics and repeat biopsies. Again, all the very extensive tests and biopsies were negative. Even his sedimentation rate was normal. As he had reported, he was not febrile, and moderate generalized lymphadenopathy (no longer tender) and mild splenomegaly were present. He had been informed of his negative test results as they became available, and yesterday he was told of the negative biopsies. He has been becoming increasingly depressed since the first hospitalization, and now the depression is obvious. He tells me how frustrated he is, and how much worse he feels than he did when he came to the hospital a week ago. His appetite is poor, and he is occasionally nauseated. He reports an inordinate amount of pain from the biopsy wounds.

He says that he would be better off if he had a lymphoma and was receiving chemotherapy. He knows about lymphoma because his father has lymphosarcoma and is receiving chronic chemotherapy. Further, his father has had repeated complications in therapy. Why would that state be better than his? "Because anything is better than not knowing, and besides I know that's what I have." Clearly, the uncertainty is a major source of his distress, not only because that is what he says, but because virtually all patients with undiagnosed disease and confirming symptoms behave similarly. Furthermore, he, like many patients, continues to question all the doctors in a way that increases his uncertainty by exposing theirs. As the conversation continues, he says that perhaps I believe he is making it all up, that he is not ill. Or perhaps the illness is psychological, that deep down he wants to be sick like his father (the modern patient is often very sophisticated). On the other hand, he thinks perhaps the disease is from the damage he did to his body when he used to take hallucinogens. Or possibly it is a virus that is still in his system from a previous illness. At each almost contradictory step, he pays little attention to my answers or reassurances, and tells me that I do not know whether he is wrong because I do not know the diagnosis. When we discuss his return to work (he had been on sick leave for almost 2 months), he insists that he cannot return to work. I point out that if he did have a lymphoma, and was on chemotherapy, I would be urging him to return to work. It compounds his problems to lie in bed at home when his symptoms do not warrant that. He says he would return to work if he had a lymphoma, but he cannot because he does not know what is the matter with him. Unless his symptoms and signs subside promptly and completely, I will indeed have greater difficulties caring for him without a diagnosis than I would if he did have a lymphoma. He and I both know that the possibility of lymphoma remains despite the negative studies.

How interesting that this patient conceives himself to be more disabled without a diagnosis than he would be if he had a lymphoma, the disease he fears! While the problems raised by this patient are extreme, they provide an opportunity for a closer look at the thinking of the sick patient.

Notice the number of possible causes for the illness that he raises almost simultaneously. He proposes that it came from damage to his body from previous drug usage. Patients will suggest other behaviors that they conceive of as being "bad" or "wrong"—overwork, poor diet, stress, or sexual practices, for example. He suggests "A virus that remains in the system." Other commonly expressed causes are toxic exposures—food additives, air pollution, work-site exposures, and so forth. Fear of malingering may be expressed as "perhaps there is nothing wrong with me at all," which is sometimes said in the presence of undiagnosed high fever or other obvious abnormality. Other psychogenic etiologies that may be either sophisticated, as in this instance (identification with the father), or quite simple are sometimes offered as possibilities. In advancing this glut of possible causes, Mr. Fanton is doing what all patients do, seeking cause.

It is important to realize that when we think of events we must inevitably think of cause at the same time. When I enter a room that is well known to me, and see the furniture arranged in its typical fashion, I do not "think" about the room. I merely recognize it. Should I return home one evening when no one has been in the room and see a piece of furniture in a different position, recognition is not sufficient. The change is an event, and I must search for cause. Finding none, I might think of an intruder. Similarly, a strange sound can drive someone wild until its source is identified. In illness, symptoms always represent a change whose cause must be sought. Generally, cause will be looked for outside the person—infection or trauma, for example. When such causes are not obvious, patients will inevitably look within themselves for cause, as did Mr. Fanton. Often more than one cause will be attributed, and will always include something the person did, including what the unconscious may have done. That is why we so commonly hear patients ask whether their disease is due to "nerves." Cause, in other words, may be seen by the patient to occur at several levels: the outside world, the patient's behavior, or within the patient's mind.

The one unacceptable cause is fate. That some things just "happen" is an intolerable blow to the sense of omnipotence, because acknowledgment of that fact would render the person helpless. Remember that the biblical Book of Job is occupied in large part by Job's friends' explanations that he was being punished because of something he did wrong, whether or not Job wanted to acknowledge that. A capricious God or fate is intolerable.

In short-lived, acute, or unimportant diseases, the doctor does not have to know what is occupying the thought of the patient, although questioning will reveal the same processes I have described. In chronic disease or in serious long-lasting illness, however, *the patients' reasonings and the behavior that is based on them influence the course of the illness.* Compliance with instructions in regard to medication, bed rest, activity, return to work, and other aspects of therapy is influenced by what patients believe to be the cause of their illness and its manifestations, and equally by their understanding of the disease process.

The question is simple. Do you want patients to act on their understanding of diseases and their causes or on your understanding? If you want their thinking and actions to be based on your knowledge, then matters must be explained to them in detail. Patients in this era do not undertake complicated regimes or alternatives in life-style simply because they are told to do something (if, indeed, they ever did). For your explanations to be effective, they must start with the patient's existing concepts, and the information you provide must relate to the patient's existing knowledge. For that to be possible, you must question patients about their concepts of the disease and its course, and respect their answers, no matter how odd they sound. Simple questions, like "What do you think brought on your condition?" or "Do you have some ideas about what makes your pain (or shortness of breath, weakness, swelling, or what-have-you) worse?" are often sufficient to produce enough information on which to base other questions. Some beliefs or fears, such as the fear of cancer, recur commonly and will allow you to offer some suggestions when patients are hesitant to voice their concerns. The following example is typical of how the patient's beliefs about cause can become the basis for continuing illness, and can provide the point at which the doctor may intervene.

A 67-year-old man was admitted to the hospital because of an old urethral stricture with secondary urinary symptoms. The work-up was given urgency because of continuing abdominal pain and progressive weight loss of several month's duration. A barium enema before admission had shown diverticulosis. Intravenous pyelography, cystoscopy, and retrograde pyelography revealed no new disease, although on the basis of the history of significant weight loss, a malignancy was suspected. Because of the negative findings, a medical consultation was called.

One brother had died of cancer "all over," but otherwise his family history was not helpful. His wife was alive, and he had children and grandchildren. Originally he had been quite heavy, but he had lost more than 20 pounds during the illness. Earlier, he had noted that the pain, which was quite severe and cramping and more prominent in the left lower quadrant, was clearly aggravated by eating. Because of that, he ate smaller and less frequent meals. Recently the pain had become much less severe and less frequent, but he had continued to avoid food. During the month before admission, he had slept poorly and had become less interested in things and less active.

How prominently the pain figured in the history and in his discussion of his situation, despite the fact that at present it was quite minimal! Indeed, it took many questions to establish how little pain he now had compared to months ago. In his thoughts, in other words, the pain was still a prominent symptom although in fact it was now minor. He had been told that his x-rays and tests were negative. There were no findings on examination, and the only evidence of weight loss was the change in belt notches. This patient is no different from any of us; because of persistent abdominal pain and weight loss, he was sure he had cancer. In fact, what had happened was this: The abdominal pain was aggravated by eating (quite typical in diverticulitis), so he ate less and less often. Because of that he lost weight. He attributed the weight loss to the disease, not to his change in eating habits, and after adding things up, became convinced that he had cancer. But why did he not improve when told that the tests were negative? Because his think-ing included another belief common among patients, particularly those of his age and background—doctors do not tell patients the truth about cancer.

When I asked him what he thought had been the cause of his condition, he answered that he did not know. He was not a doctor. I suggested that most people with his symptoms would think they had cancer. Had that not entered his mind? He admitted that the possibility worried him. I told him that I had examined him and reviewed his x-rays, and that he did not have cancer. But saying that was not sufficient, so I related what I believed to be the chain of events, including the fact that patients often believe that doctors do not tell the truth about cancer. I also pointed out that his pain had subsided, which would have been unlikely if the cause had been cancer. But why had he not been able to reassure himself with the same information? Because once his thoughts had seized on cancer as the cause, all other information was used to serve that belief. What did not fit his fears was dismissed. He, like all of us, believed the worst. When I saw him the next day at lunch time he was a different man. His appetite had become voracious, which served to reinforce my point. Often such patients will not acknowledge overtly that they have had the fears that I suggest were present. They are afraid that the doctor will consider them a "mental case." As in this instance, one can suggest that other people in the same situation, or even you, the doctor, might have felt that way. It is sometimes difficult in the setting of physical illness to suggest to patients that you know what they are thinking; they may view that as an intrusion on their privacy. Other patients will feel very comforted to know that you under-stand them. But even in the patient who denies that he or she ever had such a fear, the effect of correct interpretation will usually be beneficial. It is not necessary that patients agree with you; it is only necessary that they get better.

The case should make clear that what the patient thinks and how the patient reasons are as much a part of the illness as is the disease. Consequently, what the doctor says and how it is said can aggravate or ameliorate the illness process.

What we have been discussing is similar to the problem of truth telling that is discussed in Chapter 30 on the care of the dying—the problem of uncertainty. Both Mr. Fanton and the man with weight loss and abdominal pain demonstrate the effect of uncertainty on patients. When patients do not know the cause of their illnesses, they do not know how to act. Furthermore, lacking any defined understanding of the process of the illness or its outcome, they begin to associate symptoms with events in their lives or in their thoughts, events that have no basis in fact. Because these associations have no factual basis, they do not hold true from day to day, and uncertainty increases. Ultimately the patient becomes trap-ped in all the contradictions, and a sense of helplessness ensues. The feeling of helplessness can be extremely dangerous. It has been repeatedly documented that patients' sense of helplessness can precede the worsening of their diseases and lead to the "giving up" complex from which, in serious disease, death may follow. Furthermore, a sense of helplessness is not unique to illness, but occurs in many life situations. Here, too, there is considerable evidence showing that illness can arise in the previously well when they become overwhelmed by helplessness.

The role of physicians in the face of uncertainty and helplessness is clear. In providing knowledge of cause, process, and outcome, they provide both certainty and a basis for actions. Doctors are overly aware of their own uncertainties and of the fact that decisions in medicine are based on competing probabilities. Because of that, they are hesitant to reveal those facts to patients. But the patient is in an endless sea of contradictions, which is much worse than that of the doctor who faces perhaps two or three possibilities. Thus, even the doctor's doubts and questions seem like a rock of safety to the patient, because each possibility entertained by the physician opens an avenue to action. And each action is based on reasoning and evidence—things that are outside the patient. It is not necessary for doctors to make statements that falsely hide the uncertain future. It is possible to stress what is most probable at the same time that other possibilities are mentioned. If the other possibilities are serious or unpleasant and must be discussed, then the patient should be told at the same time what will be done if the serious alternative occurs. To the patient the dangers are unlimited, so that whatever the physician says *must put limits on the threat.* Statements that point out that the future is unpredictable should be avoided. It is rare that the future for a particular patient is totally unpredictable. We should not worry that the future will prove our statements wrong. Patients know that doctors are fallible, and even an incorrect prediction (within limits) is often better than no prediction at all.

A common example would be a conversation with a patient who has had a myocardial infarction, like Mr. Bortman. Such patients want to know what their future will be but we may not be sure whether they will have angina or congestive heart failure after they resume their activities. However, we usually have a pretty good idea from their past history and their course in the hospital. I might say, "It looks to me as though you will be able to resume your life pretty much the way you did before, and that your heart disease will not limit your activities. I want you to start an exercise program, in which case you may be in better shape in a year or two than you have been in many years. Sometimes people who have had a heart attack get chest pains, or angina on effort, afterwards. I don't think that will happen to you, but it is possible. If it does, I will be able to give you medication that is effective in controlling the symptoms and may still allow you to participate in the exercise program. Another possibility is that your heart may not work as effectively as it did in the past, in which case I will be able to give you drugs that strengthen the heart and reduce its workload and allow you to get on with your life." That is, of course, a monologue in a situation where there is usually a dialogue. A dialogue is necessary for the patient to make clear his or her questions, life demands, or understandings, and for the doctor to make sure the patient understands not just the words but the meanings. Not uncommonly, patients will seize on the worst possibility, no matter how unlikely, and act as though you had told them it was their inevitable fate. The importance of something to all of us is not how likely it is but how threatening. (Think back to your fears of flunking out of medical school.) When as part of your discussion it is necessary to relate some remote danger, and the patient acts in that manner, you can say that although some people just have to have something to worry about, the realities are those you have just listed. Do not get driven to denying that the danger exists. If it is said and then denied, its importance is heightened. The principles here are clear, as in the case of the dying (see Chapter 30). Information should reduce uncertainty, increase the patient's ability to act in his or her own best interests, and strengthen your relationship with the patient.

Reason fails the sick for another important reason. When Piaget's tests for the conservation of liquid and area are administered to the profoundly ill, their responses are similar to those of children who are 7 or 8 years old. In Piaget's tests, two short squat containers are filled with an equal amount of water and are shown to the patient, who is told that the volumes are equal. While the patient watches, the content of one of the containers is poured into a tall, thin tube. Then the patient is asked which contains more liquid—the tall, thin tube or the short, squat container. The patient will usually respond that one of them, often the thin tube, has more liquid! Sometimes patients will say that they know that both *must* be the same but that the tall thin tube *has* more fluid. These patients may be completely oriented in all other dimensions. The same findings have been reported for the aged.

If one looks further at the psychology of children of age 7 or 8, other similarities with the ill are apparent. The most evident is the inability of very sick patients to *decenter*—to see themselves and their actions objectively in relation to their physicians, families, other people, objects, and events. Simply put, ill patients often interpret every action of others as being directed toward them. If the nurses are slow, it is because the nurses do not like them. Patients commonly ask whether I am angry with them or whether something is wrong between us when I appear irritable, even though the irritability has nothing to do with them. The self-centeredness of the sick is not within their control. It is an inherent characteristic of the state of serious illness, just as bronchoconstriction is part of obstructive pulmonary disease. For this reason, doctors must learn to be aware and consciously choose their words and actions in the presence of the sick patient. Their words will never be taken casually. They will be interpreted by the patient in relation to him- or herself. It is not a novel observation that regression occurs in illness, but it is vital to understand that regression is not an abstraction. We must wonder whether patients who are reasoning in the fashion described are best able to understand complex medical information, make definite decisions about their treatments, or sign truly informed consents. How then to square the importance of providing knowledge to patients with the limitations of their ability to reason?

As I have shown, the ill are continually attempting to understand cause and outcome, and because of their need to understand and their self-centeredness, they interpret almost all information in terms of their situation. It is all the more important, therefore, that they be provided with the facts by their physician. Furthermore, these explanations must be concrete, as detailed as is necessary for the patient to understand, as free of abstractions as possible, and ideally should be accompanied by a sketch or other graphic. Simple and clear does not mean simplistic, nor does it mean talking down. Sick people may not be aware of the change in their reasoning, but they are more than usually aware and insulted when they are treated like children. The explanation to a patient with preexisting heart disease, who develops congestive heart failure because of fluid overload after common duct exploration, would sound like this: "Because of the heart trouble you have had for years and which you know about," (the reference to something known limits the danger—nothing new has occurred) "the extra intravenous fluid you received during and after your operation was too much for your heart to pump. Because of that, some of it has backed up into your lungs, and that is why you are short of breath. We can easily make that better by giving you this drug to make your kidneys get rid of the extra fluid. You will be better in a couple of hours." That, or some variant, is better than "You've gone into congestive heart failure from fluid overload and an inadequate cardiac output. The diuretic will increase your urine output." The words congestive heart failure, fluid overload, and cardiac output are not merely technical terms, they are abstractions. Diuretic and urine output are technical terms.

Similarly we are all aware of the need for informed consent but also of its difficulties. Therefore, the patient must have the necessary information presented in a manner best calculated to achieve understanding. A mere recitation of the facts does not meet the overriding moral, legal, or clinical demands.

The Loss of Control

The patients' perceptions of their altered physical being, and perhaps never-before-experienced sense of fragility, loss of connection to others, and altered patterns of thought, add to the sufferings of illness. These features of the sick are not abstractions. They are concrete changes that alter the very rules of human existence. It is this perception that adds to the next and perhaps most potent fact of severe illness, the loss of control.

To be or to perceive oneself as helpless is one of the most frightening of human experiences. Yet helplessness is the cardinal fact of severe illness. The sick do not *do*. They are done to. It is not merely that the infirm body will no longer obey commands, but rather that at every interface of the person with his or her world, there are obstacles to the control of that world. The characteristic features of illness that have been discussed are contributors to the loss of control, while psychological defenses and coping mechanisms such as denial, suppression, regression, rationalization, projection, sublimation, intellectualization, and so on, are attempts to protect the patient from the helplessness or its perceptions.

Throughout this chapter, I have tried to show how the disability of the sick comes not only from specific disease manifestations, but also from the changes that occur in the relation of patients to themselves and to their self-concepts, to their social existence, and to their ability to control their own existence. To understand this, one has to break down, or at least set aside the usual distinctions between physical, psychological, or social.

Mr. Black's muscle wasting, ascites, and weakness clearly result from altered hepatic function, and can thus be seen as organic or physical. Dietary or diuretic interventions may improve his situation. But when he leaves the hospital and returns to work prematurely because he is trying to maintain intact his sense of himself as a person, and as a consequence his ascites increase again, will that be a psychological, physical, or social problem? As the distinctions become blurred, our knowledge of how and when to intervene to make Mr. Black better becomes much sharper. We can do something to diminish ascites. We can intervene at the level of his altered reasoning by making cause, process, and outcome clearer (in the light of his wasting and weakness, he too was sure, as was his family, that he had cancer), and thus reduce uncertainty. Or we can teach him how to obtain maximum social function by appropriate use of rest, medication, and diet in order to preserve his sense of himself. All levels of intervention will make Mr. Black better within the ultimate constraints of his liver disease, by returning to him as much control as possible. And return of control will not be accomplished by merely treating his liver or by treating only his psychological or social problem. Obviously, in acute diseases such as pneumococcal pneumonia or appendicitis, the best way to return control to the patient is to cure the disease. But today we are more often faced with the kinds of cases discussed in this chapter, where no easy or permanent cure is possible. We have three kinds of tools available to make these patients better: (1) our knowledge of disease and medical technology, the things usually associated with the doctor's job; (2) our knowledge of the effects of sickness on the person, which is what we have discussed in this chapter; and (3) the thing that allows the other two kinds of knowledge to have an effect, namely, the doctor-patient relationship. Throughout this chapter I have used the personal pronouns *I* and *we* to refer to me and to other doctors, and I have discussed actual cases. We all know enough by now to treat each patient as an individual—to individualize care. But each doctor is also an individual, an *I*. I stress this because the illness phenomena presented here are subjective and are not easily measured, except indirectly, and therefore they depend on the person of the perceiver, unlike the reading on a sphygmomanometer. The process of returning control over their circumstances to patients requires a physician who is in control. That is, the doctor is the patient's surrogate—returning the connection to the world, supplying an alternate method of reasoning, and acting for patients where they cannot act for themselves. Control for physicians comes in part from being able to see what the patient sees and know what the patient knows, and from being able to put themselves in the patient's position without being overwhelmed by fear or sadness, and without dying with each patient who dies. The process of learning that control starts with using yourself to know and feel what the patient knows and feels, and learning to distinguish within yourself what comes from the patient and what comes from you. That is a difficult task that takes time, but it takes no more time to learn the basics than it does to learn to use a stethoscope, or teach one's hands to feel pelvic organs. The first and necessary condition is understanding that the information gained is as important as that coming from a stethoscope. With that in mind, let us return to the patient's loss of control.

Some symptoms, such as the loss of bowel or bladder control, are worse than others because, harkening back to infancy as they do, they symbolize for the ill the sorry, helpless things they have become, likened to babies by themselves and by others. We are often not aware of how the everyday world is adapted to the needs of the normal body. The height of the bus step, curb, or table; the way typewriters work; the way food is served; bathrooms; the length of meetings; doorbells; doorways; and countless other details in the world around us are invisible only to those who are well. Let a knee joint stiffen or give pain, a hand wither or tremble, or even chronic itching appear, and the world no longer works so well. Then those invisible details become obstacles to be surmounted.

In the same manner as the other factors that make up illness, the loss of control extends past the physical into the social and emotional life of the sick person. When the ill patient can no longer work, not only is his or her income threatened, and with it control of the world and image of self associated with economic power, but more importantly, that patient may no longer feel needed or important to others.

In emotional relationships as well, the helplessness of illness can be destructive. We know ourselves not only by our work and by our place in society, but also by those whom we love and by those who love us. But loving relationships, to whatever extent they may be possible in each individual, demand the ability to give as well as to receive. Helpless people, who have no sense of their own presence or power, feel that they are valueless, that they are objects neither deserving of love nor able to give it. Indeed, they may feel diminished by the love of others as it emphasizes, in its necessary one-sidedness, the patients' likenesses to a child.

It is obvious that helplessness and loss of control, in common with the loss of connection to the world, the diminished sense of omnipotence, and the sense of the incompleteness of reason can be imposed by things other than disease. The environment in which the sick are cared for adds to the physical losses of illness. Beds that are too high, side rails, unnecessary wheelchair or stretcher transportation, even the bed and pajamas for people whose disease does not require the bed, all emphasize the patient's impotence and reinforce the helplessness. For the limited view of illness and the care of the sick that are provided by the concept of the sick role, we can understand the apparent utility of emphasizing the patient's helplessness. It would seem to make the job of the health personnel easier, by making the patient more compliant and more receptive to the constraints imposed by treatment. But the advantage is more apparent than real, since it only makes treatment easier, without facilitating a return to health. Since the object of treatment is to make the patient well again, the paradox in the previous sentence must be resolved.

It is clear that before one can become well from an illness, one must first become ill. Since potent psychological defenses work against an inner recognition of illness, those things in the therapeutic environment that reinforce helplessness help force the patient to accept that illness is a fact. When that has been accomplished, many things, from the acceptance of imposed pain to the taking of medication, would become easier. Indeed, in certain diseases in which no symptoms are present, such as diabetes, it may be difficult to get a patient to comply with therapy, especially if the therapy is unpleasant. In such instances, the amount of sugar in the urine can be made to cause the same lack of a sense of wholeness that physical symptoms do, and thus can substitute for symptoms. But those are examples of less common situations.

Social scientists have suggested that physicians, other caregivers, and the actual settings of medical care emphasize the helplessness of the patient, because in treatment the status and power of the caregivers are elevated. Sickness is an inevitable fact of existence, and becoming well is usually desirable. Role relationships and the functions of individuals such as physicians may organize around those essential facts, and even acquire a social configuration that almost hides their initial determinants. The paradox that the treatment situation may reinforce illness is not resolved by understanding social role conflicts, but by recourse to a simpler truth. The focus of Western scientific medicine is disease.

When doctors treat patients, they do so to get at the disease. Put another way, unfortunately too many doctors do not treat patients, they only treat diseases. Given the long history and successful development of our ideas of disease, it could be no other way.

The answer to the paradox that the environment of the care of the sick may actually potentiate or worsen some of the features of illness lies in the fact that the patient is not in the hospital or other medical setting for the treatment of illness. The patient is there so that the disease that produced the illness can be treated. *Illness* is something that affects a person; *disease* afflicts an organ. They are two distinct phenomena. A disease can be present when there is no illness at all. Hypertension is an example of a disease that may, for the greater part of its life history, result in no symptoms. It may never make its owner ill. Or, even in the absence of hypertensive symptoms, which are generally alien body sensations, the person with hypertension may become ill. Suppose, for example, that someone has high blood pressure and knows it. Suppose that both of this person's parents, who were also hypertensive, died of strokes in their middle years. Such a patient may, indeed probably will, interpret each headache or episode of tingling of the fingers, anything that suggests a weakness of a limb, as an impending stroke. The relationship between that person and the body will be altered: the sense of omnipotence will be damaged slightly. The person will be ill.

You may protest that the patient is hypochondriacal, that the illness is psychological. "Psychological," used in this fashion, usually implies that the illness is not real or that the symptoms are fancied. The hypertension is certainly real. So too are the headaches, tingling fingers, and even questions of weakness. Such transient symptoms occur in virtually everybody. One might suggest that such a person has a vivid imagination or exaggerated fears. In the face of the family history, are the fears really exaggerated? We hope that the individual will not duplicate the parents' fate, but even in this day of effective antihypertensive medication we can offer no such promise. The illness is psychological only in the sense that the mind must process all present experience in the light of past experience and preexisting conceptions. It is psychological also in the sense that without the hypertension's getting worse, the patient's fears could be reinforced by the thoughtless words of a physician ("What do you see in my eyes, Doctor?" "Well, the blood vessels are a little tortuous, show a little arteriosclerosis—the kind of thing, you know, that happens with high blood pressure.'') Or, the patient's dread could be at least partly relieved by reinforcing those features of behavior, physical condition, or conceptions of the disease that demonstrate that the family history need not be a prophecy. I find it difficult to distinguish the illness as psychological or physical, but I am capable of speaking of certain manifestations of the illness as primarily physical, psychological, or even social. Since, as was noted earlier, all the features of illness can occur in the absence of any demonstrable disease, it is certainly true that the initiating event in the illness could be social or psychological. Many studies over the years have demonstrated unquestionably how frequently physical illness (appendicitis, for example) occurs during periods of life stress. It is not necessary to point out the well-known effect of the emotions on the body, but rather to make it clear that when we are considering sickness, distinctions such as social, psychological, and physical, while real in themselves, may not clarify but may confuse.

Finally, of course, disease can be the cause of, and can be associated with, the illness. Still it is possible to dissociate the manifestations of the diseased organ from those things that occur in the person as a result of the loss of function. Those manifestations of illness have been the subject of this chapter.

Recognizing the features of illness and the part they play in patients' disability makes our job clear. We are not finished until we have helped the patient to once again gain control over the environment and over self. The degree to which physicians can accomplish this will depend upon the disease, the life situation, and the nature of the patient. But the goal is clear. Details of rehabilitation cannot be left to the physiotherapy department, and are not complete when the patient can step up onto a curb. The task is more global, but the tools are readily available. In this discussion of the factors that make up illness, I have tried to provide an understanding of the places where interventions are possible. The primary agency by which control is returned to the patient is the doctor-patient relationship, which includes the actions and words of the physician who is utilizing that relationship. Skill and experience are required here as in every other aspect of medicine, but the results make the effort worthwile.

The report on postcardiac surgery recovery with which I opened this chapter detailed improvement in the patients' hearts, but not in patients. Attention to the features of illness and to the job of helping patients regain control over their lives will finish the doctor's job. Then the patients, and not just their hearts, will be better.

REFERENCES

1 Heller, S. S. et al.: "Psychological Outcome Following Open Heart Surgery," *Arch. Intern. Med.,* **134**:908–914, 1974.
2 Schmale, A. H.: "Giving Up as a Final Common Pathway to Changes in Health," *Adv. Psychosom. Med.,* **8**:20–40, 1972.
3 Singer, E.: "Premature Social Aging: The Social Psychological Consequences of a Chronic Illness," *Soc. Sc. & Med.,* **8**:143–151, 1974.

BIBLIOGRAPHY

Abram, H. S.: "The Psychology of Physical Illness As Portrayed in Thomas Mann's *The Magic Mountain,*" *Arch. Intern. Med., 128*:466–468, 1971.

————: "The Psychology of Chronic Illness," *J. Chron. Dis., 25*:659–664, 1972.

Allander, E., and E. Hakanson: "The Layman's Medical Vocabulary," *Scand. J. Soc. Med., 4*:31–40, 1976.

Antonovsky, A.: "The Image of Four Diseases Held by the Urban Jewish Population of Israel," *J. Chron. Dis., 25*:375–384, 1972.

Arce, L.: "Somatopsychic Disease," *Psychosomatics, 13*:191–196, 1972.

Banks, F. R., and M. D. Keller: "Symptom, Experience and Health Action," *Med. Care, 9*:498–502, 1971.

Barsky, A., III: "Patient Heal Thyself: Activating the Ambulatory Medical Patient," *J. Chron. Dis., 29*:585–597, 1976.

Croog, S. H. et al.: "The Heart Patient and the Recovery Process," *Soc. Sci. & Med., 2*:111–164, 1968.

Engel, G. L.: "Personal Theories of Disease as Determinants of Patient-Physician Relationships," *Psychosom. Med. Res., 35*:184, 1973.

Fabrega, H., Jr.: "Culture, Language and the Shaping of Illness: An Illustration Based on Pain," *J. Psychosom. Med., 20*:323–337, 1976.

Friederich, M. A.: "Psychological Aspects of Chronic Pelvic Pain," *Clin. Obs. and Gyn., 19*:399–406, 1976.

Gardner, R. A.: "Guilt Reaction of Parents of Children with Severe Physical Disease," *Am. J. Psychiat., 126*:82–90, 1969.

Gentry, W. D., and T. Haney: "Emotional and Behavioral Reaction to Acute Myocardial Infarction," *Heart and Lung, 4*:738–745, 1975.

Gerson, E.: "The Social Character of Illness: Deviance or Politics?" *Soc. Sci. & Med., 10*:219–224, 1976.

Glaser, J. R.: "Is It Obvious Why Patients Ask Questions?" *JAMA, 235*:1223–1224, 1976.

Hurtado, A. V. et al.: "Determinants of Medical Care Utilization: Failure to Keep Appointments," *Med. Care, 11*:189–198, 1973.

Hyman, M. D.: "Social Psychological Factors Affecting Disability among Ambulatory Patients," *J. Chron. Dis., 28*:199–216, 1975.

Imboden, J. B.: "Psychosocial Determinants of Recovery," *Adv. Psychosom. Med., 8*:142–155, 1972.

Kahana, R. J.: "Personality and Response to Physical Illness," *Adv. Psychosom. Med., 8*:42–62, 1975.

Katz, J. et al.: "Psychological Variables in the Onset and Recurrence of Gouty Arthritis," *J. Chron. Dis., 8*:51–62, 1975.

Kaufman, R. V.: "Body-Image Changes in Physically Ill Teenagers," *J. Am. Acad. Child. Psych., 11*:1, 157–170, 1972.

Kennedy, D. A.: "Perceptions of Illness and Healing," *Soc. Sci. & Med., 7*:787–805, 1973.

Kiely, W. F.: "Coping with Severe Illness," *Adv. Psychosom. Med., 8*:105–118, 1972.

Koch, M. F., and G. D. Molnar: "Psychiatric Aspects of Patients with Unstable Diabetes Mellitus," *Psychosom. Med., 36*:57–68, 1974.

Lipowski, Z. J.: "Physical Illness, the Individual and the Coping Process," *Psychiatry in Med., 2*:91–102, 1970.

Livsey, C. G.: "Physical Illness and Family Dynamics," *Adv. Psychosom. Med.,* **8**:237–251, 1972.

Markson, E. W.: "Patient Semiology of a Chronic Disease: Rheumatoid Arthritis," *Soc. Sci. & Med.,* **5**:159–167, 1971.

Mayou, R.: " The Nature of Bodily Symptoms," *Brit. J. Psychiat.,* **129**:55–60, 1976.

Parsons, T.: "The Sick Role and the Role of the Physician Reconsidered," *Milbank Mem. Fund Quart.: Health and Society,* Summer:257–278, 1975.

Pilowski, I., and M. D. Spence: "Pain and Illness Behavior: A Comparative Study," *J. Psychosom. Res.,* **20**:131–134, 1976.

————: "Pain, Anger, and Illness Behavior," *J. Psychosom. Res.,* **20**:411–416, 1976.

Rutter, B. M.: "Measurement of Psychological Factors in Chronic Illness," *Rheumatology and Rehabilitation,* **15**:174–178, 1976.

Schmale, A. H.: "Giving Up As a Final Common Pathway to Changes in Health," *Adv. Psychosom. Med.,* **8**:20–40, 1972.

Segall, A.: "The Sick Role Concept: Understanding Illness Behavior," *J. Health & Soc. Behav.,* **17**:162–168, 1976.

Schontz, F. C.: "The Personal Meanings of Illness," *Adv. Psychosom. Med.,* **8**:63–85, 1972.

Shuval, J. T. et al.: "Illness: A Mechanism for Coping with Failure," *Soc. Sci. & Med.,* **7**:259–265, 1973.

Singer, E.: "Premature Social Aging: The Social-Psychological Consequences of a Chronic Illness," *Soc. Sci. & Med.,* **8**:143–151, 1974.

Sternbach, R. A.: "Psychological Aspects of Pain and the Selection of Patients," *Clin. Neurosurg.,* **21**:323–333, 1974.

Tagliacozzo, D. M., and K. Irna: "Knowledge of Illness as a Predictor of Patient Behavior," *J. Chron. Dis.,* **22**:765–775, 1970.

Thurlow, J. H.: "Illness in Relation to Life Situation and Sick-Role Tendency," *J. Psychosom. Med. Res.,* **15**:73–88, 1971.

Verwoerdt, A.: "Psychopathological Responses to the Stress of Physical Illness," *Adv. Psychosom. Med.,* **8**:119–141, 1972.

Wadsworth, M. E. J.: "Illness Behavior and Studies of Communications between Doctors and Patients," *J. Psychosom. Res.,* **20**:317–322, 1976.

Waitzkin, H., and J. D. Stoekle: "The Communication of Information about Illness," *Adv. Psychosom. Med.,* **8**:180–215, 1972.

Chapter 6

The Physician and Social Issues

B. Perry Ottenberg, M.D.

EDITORS' INTRODUCTION

What is it like to be black, be referred to a prominent specialist who is white, and have no idea about his or her position on racial issues? What is it like to be a woman who is happy with a life centering around marriage, family, and home, and be the patient of a woman physician who strongly urges her patients to become actively involved in the women's rights movement? How must it feel to be poor, sick, and a patient at a teaching hospital where one is to be presented at grand rounds? What is it like to wait for hours in the emergency room to be examined? How must it feel to be poor and a member of a Spanish-speaking minority group, and realize that all the doctors and nurses seem to come from a world that is different by virtue of its whiteness and affluence?

What is it like to be the husband or wife of a patient who has suffered a massive stroke and is being kept alive by newer technologies? How does it feel to try hesitantly to discuss the issue with your spouse's physician? Is the mixture of shock, sadness, and confusion helped by the physician's manner and words? What is best for your loved one?

What is it like to be a physician who is a member of a church vestry and believes strongly in a moral code that permits sexual intercourse only in marriage, and to see many patients for whom sex is a recreational activity? Must or should this physician fit a colleague's 18-year-old unmarried daughter with the intrauterine device she requests?

What feelings are provoked in the staunchly conservative physician as he or she takes a medical history from an unkempt radical campus leader who espouses revolution? What is it like to be a devout Catholic physician and be elected president of the medical staff in a hospital where abortions are performed? How does it feel to be a young doctor in a large medical group, see nothing wrong with the recreational use of drugs, and know that the other physicians in the group disagree emphatically?

What is it like for a physician to feel that a patient's condition is hopeless and that he or she will die soon after support mechanisms are turned off? How much should the wishes of the family be considered? Some physicians may be requested by the family to turn off the machine or stop hydrating the patient. Is there a legal risk for the physician either in following the family's wishes or in refusing them? What if the family's desires conflict with what the doctor believes is right?

All people have beliefs about what is "right" and what is "wrong." Often, these are clear and conscious thoughts and are very much a part of the person's daily life. Frequently, however, these beliefs lurk in the shadows of the person's mind and their influence on daily events is subtle. Whether or not a person is fully conscious of basic personal beliefs or values, they are a part of every experience and color each relationship. It is, however, in the area of social conflicts that a person's values are apt to dominate. These conflicts, by their very nature, involve the issue of "right" and "wrong," and most often do not yield to scientific investigation.

In this chapter, a prominent psychiatrist with a long history of involvement at the interface of medicine and social issues presents information about the ways in which the doctor-patient relationship may be compromised by the physician's value orientations toward current social issues.

All people are caught up in the conflicts of social issues. The nature of the issues changes from period to period. Whether it is the prohibition of alcoholic beverages in the 1920s or legal abortions in the 1970s, there are topics about which strongly conflicting feelings are expressed. These issues are part of the process of living together, and often can be understood as reflections of opposing ideas regarding the nature of man and the meaning of life. For some individuals, participation in social issues is the passionate core of life, while for others they are experienced as a distant and trifling nuisance.

Although physicians may be either intensely involved with or relatively disinterested in social issues, the actual practice of medicine may be influenced profoundly by physicians' attitudes and feelings regarding the value judgments which underlie conflicts about social issues. Their deeply held and often unconscious values about the nature of man and life are always present as a part of their personalities, diagnostic skills, and technical proficiency. However, it is when science provides no clear answers to medical problems that the physician's values are most apt to influence medical decisions. Scientific knowledge rarely coincides with the needs of a specific patient, a fact which leaves the door wide open for distortions.

This chapter reviews some of the ways in which the practice of medicine can be influenced by the physician's value judgments regarding a few current social issues. Its purpose is to illustrate rather than review all the current social issues which may impinge on the practice of medicine.[1]

Lewis Thomas has written that a visitor from another planet would marvel at the degree of individuality exhibited by the people in this world.[2] They would, he points out, be equally astonished by our social connectedness. Humans are social animals, and much of human life is lived in relationship with others. A large part of what makes us human involves incorporated social experiences, cultural heritage, and primary socialization in the family. To use a different model, people live in systems: families, neighborhoods, towns, cities, and countries. People have impact on what occurs in their systems, but the influence of most individuals on the large systems is hard to detect. The systems, however, profoundly influence the participating individuals and often shape the nature of their perceived reality. The mother and child—born or unborn—may be conceived of as a social system just as any hospital, clinic, or dyadic doctor-patient relationship may be.

Many persons wish to minimize or deny the numerous ways that feelings, thoughts, and behavior are molded by the structure of the large social systems in which they are raised and educated. The concept of individual determinism—the ability of people to shape their own lives—seems to many to suffer from an emphasis on social forces as significant determinants of human behavior. In reality, it is not an "either-or" situation. Each individual's behavior is influenced significantly by biologic, psychologic, and social forces, but the individual, within certain limits, has much to say about the conduct of his or her own life. There remains, however, a tendency to polarize the question. Often, for example, the "conservative" position is said to place particular emphasis on the role of the individual, and the "liberal" position to stress the impact of social factors in determining behavior. During the campus upheavals in the 1960s, one "expert" would place sole emphasis on the individual participant's presumed mental illness or immorality. Another "expert" would describe the phenomenon only in terms of social forces. Rarely would an analysis incorporate both perspectives and search for the relative influence of both individual and social factors.

The emphasis of this chapter is on social factors, their relationship to personal values, and the ways in which broad socioeconomic and historical values may influence the practice of medicine. The emphasis is deliberate, but this is not meant to minimize the important role of personal contributions to individual behavior. Medical education and practice often focus only on individual variables and technological issues, and frequently leave the physician with minimal appreciation of social forces.

The large social system, which is American culture, influences the individual in both explicit and implicit ways. The explicit influence is transmitted through education, family life, television, group membership, and legal systems that teach what the individual may or may not do, to and with others. Laws evolve and often lag behind what comes to be assumed as acceptable behavior. Current examples are sexual relationships and the use of certain mind-altering drugs. In many parts of the country, for example, homosexuality and the use of marijuana are illegal, although they are increasingly accepted forms of behavior. Although laws may lag behind the social acceptance of certain behavior, there is generally considerable clarity about what the law says.

The culture's implicit influences on the behavior of individuals are also important, but operate with much less clarity. Of particular importance to the practice of medicine are the many implicit influences that are profoundly shaped by social class status. The middle- and upper-class values held by most professionals are applied, for example, to lower income groups, without due consideration of the contextual differences that often make the application grossly unfair. If the current status of this country's value orientation is analyzed by using the format of Spiegel and Kluckholm, the following questions would be asked:[3]

1   What is the relation of humanity to nature?
2   What are the temporal forms of human life?
3   What is the ideal form of human activity?
4   What is the optimal form of interpersonal relationships with other men?

Despite rapid change, this culture continues to teach that the human race is the master of nature; that the future is more important than past or present; that "doing" is more important than "being"; and that relationships are highly individualistic in nature. Although these values may well represent the underlying assumptions of the white, middle-class majority, they are difficult to apply to a poverty-level minority population. The real-life circumstances of such a population may involve such deprivation, prejudice, and exclusion from the mainstream of American life as to instill value orientations that are more closely related to actual physical survival. The importance of this idea is that medicine, in addition to its professional values, participates in the middle- and upper-class cultural value orientations. Although there are exceptions, many physicians accept mainstream values and apply them without awareness to the practice of medicine. If their patients are of the same social and ethnic background, the implicit assumptions are shared and emotionally gratifying. If not, there is a strong likelihood that the conflicting values will interfere with the doctor-patient relationship and result in an authoritarian doctor-patient relationship which neglects actual sharing in decision making.

The practice of medicine is based on the physician's capacity to achieve a balance of empathy and detachment in his or her relationships with patients. Empathy, the ability to temporarily place oneself in another person's predicament and feel as he or she feels, is the foundation of humanism. Without it, the physician may become a remote, detached figure whose skills are technological. But detachment is equally necessary in order to apply scientific knowledge about disease processes to patients with a variety of illnesses. Empathy without detachment leads to unscientific quackery. Detachment without empathy often results in dehumanization. If physicians are unaware of the subtle ways in which unarticulated mainstream values can influence relationships with some patients, there is little likelihood that a reasonable balance can be achieved. Physicians' values concerning the quality of life ultimately determine who gets what kind of care, how much, how long, and where.

Other social forces have an impact on the doctor-patient relationship. As a part of a rapidly changing technological society, expectations about health care have changed dramatically. Often physicians are expected to do the impossible. The problems are particularly pressing in cases of chronic illness. Many such illnesses result, in part, from faulty health habits (sedentary life-style, obesity, tobacco, alcohol) and probably will not yield to the "silver bullet" approach that works well with infectious disease. People cannot smoke and drink too much and lead sedentary lives and then expect that medicine will provide a simple solution. Yet they do.[4] There is a quandary: if one eats, smokes, and drinks excessively to counter unemployment, poverty, or lack of education and skills, how is one to correct the defect medically without modifying the social reality?

An increasing number of people have come to feel that proper health care is a right with which they must be provided. Whatever the arguments for or against this proposition, health care comes to be equated with health for many, and when physicians cannot provide health, disappointment results, even when the individual faces social conditions of overwhelming adversity.

Many physicians become part of larger institutions—hospital staffs, group practices, teaching facilities—which may interfere with the doctor-patient relationship. The physician's loyalty to the values and goals of the institution may, on occasions, conflict with the individual patient's best interest. As institutions grow in size and complexity, there is a movement toward a rigid bureaucracy that may lead to dehumanization. Patients are not seen as individuals with illnesses, fears, hopes, and uncertainties, but as "cases" of one or another disease. Not only are patients dehumanized, but physicians and other staff may gradually be robbed of their humanism by rule-oriented procedures.[5]

Repetitive procedures may also impair the doctor-patient relationship. The physician who does only a small group of procedures (proctoscopy, coronary bypass surgery, insurance physical examinations, ophthalmological examinations, etc.) may come to have only a "part" interest in the patient, much as the assembly-line worker may care little about the total product. This side effect of increasing specialization can lead to increasing dehumanization of both patients and physicians.

In dealing with patients of different social class or ethnic backgrounds, it is too easy for the physician to rely on cultural stereotypes. A demanding black male patient, for example, is apt to be seen as expressing a genetic trait rather than as an individual who is dealing with personal fear. Designations of "pushy," "aggressive," "passive," "loud," and "uncouth," are often social stereotypes used for distancing others.

There are, then, countless ways in which underlying values can impair the development of the doctor-patient relationship. These may be seen more clearly in the following clinical vignettes which have been selected because each represents a social issue met often in the practice of medicine.

CLINICAL VIGNETTES

Patient A

A 14-year-old black adolescent girl arrived at the emergency room with a complaint of abdominal pain. Physical examination revealed that she was 14 weeks pregnant and in danger of aborting. She indicated that this was her second pregnancy, the first having terminated spontaneously at 9 weeks.

The resident physician asked her whether she wished to consider an abortion and she replied that she wanted to have the baby and raise it herself. The decision about her medical care had to take into account the options of hospitalizing her and treating her intensively in an effort to salvage the pregnancy, or sending her home with a clinic appointment in several weeks.

There are several social issues involved in the resident physician's dilemma. Consequently, there are obviously different ways for personal values to influence the process of medical decision making. First, there is the issue of abortion. What is the resident's position regarding the value of unborn life and the question of when human life begins? Of particular importance, what is the physician's stance about a woman's right to decide whether she is going to carry a pregnancy to term? Does a 14-year-old girl have the right to make that decision for herself? What does the physician feel about the right of the unborn child to have an accepting and nourishing environment, which could be related to its future health? Although there may be data about the outcome of pregnancy in groups of 14-year-old black girls, there are no scientific data that provide clear answers to these questions for this particular patient.

Another group of questions might deal with the impact of values relating to the issue of race and socioeconomic status. What does the physician feel about racial differences? Are carefully camouflaged notions of racial inferiority still present? Is a black pregnancy less valuable in the physician's eyes than a white pregnancy? What will be the impact on the child's health of being raised by a 14-year-old mother under welfare circumstances? What are the physician's assumptions about the causes of poverty? How does the physician react to the patient's lack of guilt and apparent pride in her pregnancy? Would the prescribed treatment be significantly different if the patient were white, middle-class, and expressing guilt? Would it be different if she were married?

This is the type of situation in which the physician's values may influence profoundly his or her medical decision making. If this occurs, there is a strong likelihood that the patient will neither be presented with all the available options nor be allowed to participate fully in the solution. The approach to treatment may reflect the physician's hidden values more than anything else. All of this may occur without the physician's awareness and with no conscious malicious intent.

Predetermined social attitudes override the individual issues between doctor and patient.

A preponderant number of physicians are products of middle-class white families. They have completed an ardous educational experience successfully and, for the most part, have done so with similar people. The educational experience itself reinforces the values characteristic of a doctor's position in mainstream America. It comes as no surprise, therefore, to find that most physicians think that the individual can overcome all but a few obstacles; that competing with others is valuable; that nature can be modified; that accomplishing is important; and that the individual should always look to the future. Such values find confirmation in the successful life experiences of most physicians.

The 14-year-old pregnant black girl, however, on the basis of her experience, might well feel that an individual cannot overcome obstacles (racial prejudice and poverty, for example); that "just living" is more important than "doing"; and that the present is much more important than the future. Her pregnancy may reflect genuine love of life, a repetition of a family pattern, and the onset of meaningful growth as an individual. The assumption by the physician that the patient shares the physician's view of life is apt to lead to a failure in the doctor-patient alliance that is so necessary for effective treatment of patients with alternative life-styles, a situation that increasingly confronts the middle-class point of view.

Patient B

> A 59-year-old white male was admitted to the hospital because of carcinoma of the pancreas and multiple metastases. He was experiencing severe pain, vomiting, and jaundice. The decision was made to treat him both with irradiation and chemotherapeutic agents. When the resident physician outlined this treatment approach to the patient, the patient refused and stated that although he wanted as much relief from pain as possible, he did not want to be treated. He stated further that he did not wish to eat nor to be fed intravenously, but wished to die as painlessly as possible.
>
> The patient's wife and grown children felt differently. They wanted the physician to treat the patient and prolong life in the hope that a "miracle" would occur and the cancer would disappear.

In this instance, the physician is faced with several social issues. The first involves the question of the termination of life. Although the issue is often discussed in the context of "pulling the plug" on life-support machines, it often happens that there is no such dramatic step. Who has the right to decide when an individual is going to die? Is it the patient, the family, or the physician? How rational is the patient? How rational is the family? In this type of situation, how does the physician evaluate rationality? What is the doctor's orientation about the value of life? Is death always an enemy? What if the patient asks the physician to do something actively to hasten death—for example, write an order to discontinue intravenous feeding? What is the physician's liability if a patient's wishes are not responded to? Will the family sue for malpractice?

Although with such patients medical decision making may involve considerable complexity, there is often uncertainty on the part of the physician, which in turn makes it difficult for the patient and family to express their wishes. The physician's indecision may accordingly result in a course of action which is strongly influenced by the physician's orientation about the value of life. During their educations many physicians are exposed to nothing but technological medicine. When technology does not give clear answers to questions like those above, the physician may respond only in ways that feel "right" to him or her. Disease and death are often experienced as the physician's enemy, and the principles outlined by Cassell (Chapter 30), which emphasize the patient's need to feel in control of dying, may be experienced by the physician as antagonistic to his or her childhood, group, religious, or unconscious beliefs. The situation may be even more complicated when the patient's condition precludes any clear understanding of his or her wishes as, for example, in coma or delirium. Such a situation makes it even more likely that the physician's unchallenged values will play a decisive role.

Usdin has reviewed five cardinal factors that influence the physician's attitudes and actions in confronting death and dying.[7] First, there is the physician's attitude toward his or her own death. A second factor is that physicians are educated to believe that death is an enemy and that life is to be maintained as long as possible. Third is the impact of family and close friends, often with a bewildering diversity of feelings about the impending death of a family member. A fourth factor is the changing social and community attitudes about death. Passive euthanasia, for example, has been openly and comfortably discussed only for a few decades. Finally, there is the realistic concern about legal action against the physician for allowing a patient to die without the use of heroic measures to prolong life. As physicians discuss issues about rational choices in treatment, they are often the object of distortions about playing God, omnipotence, genocidal authority, and other unconscious fears of death, pain, and separation in the public mind.

Several recent developments are relevant to this complex issue. One is the establishment within hospitals of committees that have the responsibility for decisions regarding the termination of life. Although such committees may be helpful in formulating general guidelines and in offering individual physicians consultation upon request, they should not substitute for the physician's personal involvement with specific patients, diseases, illnesses, and families in an approach that allows the individual patient to participate in the writing of his or her own final chapter. To give up this individual responsibility may dehumanize the patient and, ultimately, also the physician.[8]

The living will is a legal innovation in which the patient writes how he or she wishes to be treated when dying, particularly when dying under circumstances in which such wishes cannot be spoken clearly. The legality of such living wills has not been determined as of this date.

Patient C

A 37-year-old physician colleague and friend appears to be depressed and drinking excessively. It is no secret among the hospital staff that he is a homosexual and is currently living with a 21-year-old man. The hospital administrator informs you that your friend's hospital privileges are to be suspended.

Situations of this type present the physician with uncertainty and anxiety. What does he or she owe to a friend and colleague? Will trying to be of help to the colleague be interpreted as meddling? Would it make any difference if the friend's lover were female? If the physician were heterosexual, would the administrator have dealt with the drinking and depression differently?

Such very human considerations cannot fail to affect the physician. There are no clear guidelines, although the responsibility of friendship surely requires an attempt to be of help with the depression and drinking. The friend's homosexuality, however, may provoke such strong feelings in the physician as to prevent helpful intervention.

The past decade has seen much social change regarding homosexuality. There is increasing awareness that homosexuality in itself may be considered an alternate life-style rather than invariably an illness. Although homosexuality may be associated with clear evidence of emotional disturbance, it is not always so. The laws in many states are being changed to make homosexual acts between consenting adults no longer a crime. Despite change, many, if not most, Americans continue to respond to homosexuality as if it were either immoral or a disease. Physicians, as members of the mainstream of America, often share these value judgments.[9] This fact can influence the physician's ability to offer homosexual patients an atmosphere of medical care in which there is a reasonable balance of empathy and detachment. It is often difficult for the physician to empathize with the homosexual patient. The reasons for this are multiple, but they often include the physician's personal anxiety about his or her own earlier homosexual experiences or fantasies. The greater the difficulty the heterosexual physician has in identifying with the homosexual patient, the more the likelihood that the physician will either stereotype the patient or allow personal value judgments to influence the treatment of the patient. As alternative types of family living emerge, there are growing numbers of same-sex couples with children. The people in such families will need, at times of illness, the care of a sensitive physician.

Patient D

A 29-year-old woman attorney who had been active in the women's rights movement was admitted to the hospital for biopsy of a hard nodule in her breast. In discussing her condition, the male surgeon told her that if the mass was malignant, he would do a radical mastectomy. She refused, and vigorously quoted statistics suggesting that less extensive surgical procedures had equally good results.

A social issue of importance to a growing number of men and women involves the redefinition of woman's role in this culture. Many women wish to correct not only economic inequalities, but also a wide variety of discriminatory practices that they feel are part of medical treatment. One common criticism has been that male physicians often treat women patients as children rather than as equal adults capable of effective decision making when presented fairly with options and clinical probabilities. There is validity to this generalization, although, of course, there have always been exceptions.

Physicians can develop strong authoritarian tendencies and react to any question about their recommendations with increased authoritarianism, pompous retreat, or the labeling of women who question their authority as "terribly neurotic." Many physicians grew up in a period when there was little question about the role of women or their own authority. It was "natural" for women to be wives, mothers, homemakers, and little else. Career women were often seen as strange or deviant. These attitudes often become core values about judging what is "right" or "wrong" for women. Sometimes these attitudes toward women are strongly held, conscious opinions, but often they are subtle beliefs about which male physicians are not consciously aware. They can influence drastically the nature of the doctor-patient relationship and cause many women to seek care from members of their own sex.

The case of the 29-year-old woman attorney raises a number of questions for the surgeon. If alternate treatment approaches are available, is it his role to discuss them with his patient and allow her to decide? Should any patient, male or female, have that much to say about the nature of his or her treatment? Is the vigorous response of the patient to be understood as "neurotic penis envy," or as the sign of an adult woman who insists on being treated as a responsible adult? What should be the physician's response if he feels that the treatment he recommends has a distinct advantage for the patient? A slight advantage? A questionable advantage? Does it make any difference that his wife divorced him several years ago and employed a woman attorney who, he felt, fleeced him aggressively?

There are many medical emergencies in which the physician must take over and do what he or she considers best, but a great many patients desire to participate in a collaborative way in reaching decisions about their health care. The physician who adheres to an older role model for women may be unable to function comfortably with such patients, and may report seeing an increasing number of "difficult" patients in the practice of medicine.

Patient E

A 17-year-old white male was seen in the emergency room for scalp lacerations resulting from an automobile accident. He was obviously "stoned," and his behavior was sufficiently inappropriate to make the surgeon's efforts to suture his scalp difficult.

The use of drugs for pleasure has been a social issue of considerable intensity. The conflict about their use was particularly intense a few years ago, although there is now less hue and cry. Some drugs, such as marijuana, have found increased acceptance or tolerance. Marijuana is now second only to alcohol as this culture's favorite intoxicant. Large numbers of young people of diverse backgrounds prefer marijuana to alcohol and are encouraged by the inability of scientific investigation to document its dangers as equal to or as great as those of alcohol. Many states have modified their laws to make possession of small amounts of marijuana a misdemeanor rather than a felony.

Although the hard-line crusade against marijuana use has softened, a conflict remains as to whether or not it is "right" for people to use drugs in an effort to feel different or better. Science does not provide a clear answer. It is apparent, for example, that many individuals can use marijuana without apparent injury, but that for a few it can lead to serious behavioral consequences. The absence of conclusive scientific data leaves the door open for the physician's own value orientation about drug use. One position is that marijuana is not "right" because people should not need drugs to feel good, that "feeling good" should result from good relationships with people and the satisfaction derived from productive work. The opposite position is that life is difficult, complicated, and often absurd, and using marijuana to feel good is appropriate as long as it doesn't hurt others. These polar positions—here deliberately simplified—involve very different stances regarding values. The former emphasizes obligation to the collective efforts of society. The latter suggests an underlying commitment to "being" rather than "doing," the present more than the future, and the self before the collective social effort.

It is too easy, therefore, for the physician to allow personal values to influence the doctor-patient relationship and the nature of treatment. Negative attitudes regarding recreational use of drugs may be more likely to occur in older physicians, who grew up at a time when alcohol use was "right" and other intoxicants were "wrong."

The 17-year-old stoned boy is not so cooperative as he might be. Attempts to help him lead to mounting frustration and, in that context, the surgeon is apt to become judgmental which, in turn, can lead to a hostile and even punitive series of actions. The physician may experience the adolescent as "just another damn pothead who has gotten what he deserves" rather than as a confused, toxic, difficult, and bleeding patient. The physician's value judgment about the use of drugs has added to the very real problem presented by the boy's toxic state. Often, the deprivation associated with a medical career in its delayed gratifications and prolonged period of self-sacrifice during the many years of training are aroused by the seeming self-indulgence involved in "getting high."

Patient F

A 51-year-old white male consulted an internist because of sadness, insomnia, anorexia, and diminished libido. The physician, recognizing the presence of major depressive symptoms, elicited the following clinical material. The patient was single and in good physical health. He was self-employed in the business of pornography and owned two "X-rated" theaters and several "adult book stores." The physician recalled a recent newspaper account of the city's attempt to close the patient's theaters, an account in which the patient had been described as the "king of smut."

The internist's customary approach to depressed patients was to see them weekly for 30 minutes of supportive psychotherapy and to prescribe an antidepressant. With this patient, however, the physician began to contemplate an immediate referral to a psychiatrist.

Pornography is a social issue that elicits strong conflicting opinions. Scientific studies regarding the impact of pornography on individual behavior are insufficient to justify a factual stance. The problem of obscenity versus freedom of the press is not resolved by our U.S. Constitution. Two conflicting ideologies are often presented. One, the catharsis concept, maintains that sexual tension, energy, or conflict are "drained" by exposure to pornographic material; proponents of this view suggest that potential sexual offenders are relieved of whatever propels them, and that the incidence of sexual offenses declines. The other concept, "provoke the devil," suggests that the stimulation provided by pornography actually incites individuals to sexual behaviors that would not occur otherwise. Proponents of each view may cite isolated and unreplicated studies to support their specific thesis and fail to attend those which contradict it.

The issues are complex, but there is much to suggest that basic value orientation regarding the nature of man plays a role in polarizing the issue. Physicians, despite professional familiarity with the human body, are not immune. The case of the 51-year-old "king of smut" suggests that the internist's underlying values about the rightness or wrongness of pornography may have influenced him or her to consider a plan of treatment that was different from the customary approach to this type of clinical problem. Even if the physician decides not to refer the patient to a psychiatrist, personal underlying feelings about this man's occupation may, regrettably, interfere in the evolution of a helpful doctor-patient relationship. There are numerous other occupations that evoke powerful physician reactions and may lead to punitive referrals, occupations such as loan sharking, numbers writing, prostitution, rackets, drug selling, and marginal trades.

Patient G

A 57-year-old physician with offices in the same building appears in your office late in the day. He is obviously distraught and unsteady on his feet. He indicates that he has been injecting himself with demerol for several years and requests a prescription from you in order to withdraw himself.

The impaired physician is a social issue of growing public concern. Physicians have an ethical mandate to offer care to fellow physicians and, at the same time, are criticized for protecting the public inadequately by not ensuring basic levels of medical competence. The impaired physician often cannot provide patients with good medical care. The nature of the impairment varies, but alcoholism, drug addiction, mental illness, aging, and disability due to organic disease are some of the more common examples.

Under many, if not most circumstances, at least one other physician is aware of the colleague's impairment. The impaired physician may be a patient formally and the nature of the impairment discovered within the context of the doctor-patient relationship. Often, however, the impairment is noted by observing the physician's care of hospitalized patients, from hearing secretaries' comments, through direct reports from patients, or in social circumstances.

What is the physician to do under these different circumstances? It is often easy to minimize or deny the evidence that suggests the impairment and hope that the behavior will "go away" or be dealt with by others. Some physicians are most comfortable talking directly with the impaired colleague, but hesitate to do so if the colleague is not a close friend. Calling the behavior to the attention of the hospital medical staff committee or local medical society is sometimes seen as "going behind the back" of the impaired colleague or as a form of disloyalty. It can even provoke fears of retaliation in the form of a legal action by the impaired physician.

There is often great stress for physicians in deciding what to do about an impaired colleague. The issue of what is "owed" to a colleague and what is one's responsibility to the public may impinge on the physician's basic values about individual rights and the rights of the social system. It is, however, a historical truth that, as a profession, medical practice has often paid inadequate attention to the public's right to be protected from incompetence. However, unless physicians adequately police their own ranks, this task will be taken over by others. This possibility has prompted medical organizations to pay greater attention to the impaired physician, and there is currently much more professional attention given to the subject. In some hospitals and medical groups, it is possible to find the best friend of the physician, discuss the problem with him or her, and allow the friend to act as an intermediary in facing the problem. Often, the intervention of the staff comes as a relief to the involved doctor and to the family, which has been unable to cope with the problem. A friend acting as an intermediary is not the same as the threat of a legal or medical review board, which will eventually be called if the issues are not faced.

THE INTRUSION OF THE PHYSICIAN'S VALUES INTO MEDICAL PRACTICE

The brief clinical vignettes are only examples of the many ways in which the physician's values may interfere with establishing helpful treatment alliances with patients. It is impossible, however, for physicians to be free from their value orientations. What is to be hoped for is an awareness of the physician's personal value orientations that can minimize their destructive and insidious impact on the doctor-patient relationship. On some occasions, the physician's feelings about a social issue involved in a patient's care will be so clear and strong as to necessitate referral to another physician. This positive action clearly is in the best interest of the patient. The personal values of the physician cannot be expected to allow the development of a helpful doctor-patient relationship with every patient. Clear recognition that some patients present the physician with one or more social issues about which the physician has feelings so intense as to make the treatment relationship difficult or impossible is preferable to the failure to recognize the harmful impact of value judgments on the relationship.

The impact of hidden value judgments does the most damage. These judgments can seriously distort the doctor-patient relationship. Operating out of the physician's awareness, they significantly influence the quality of the relationship. Of even greater importance, however, hidden value judgments can lead to subtle behavioral changes in the physician which provoke responsive patient behavior that reinforces these judgments. A male physician, for example, may have an internal model of what is "right" for a woman to be. The physician may have some awareness of this value judgment, but may be hiding the strength of his feelings when consulted by an aggressively competent women's rights advocate (e.g., Patient D, the 29-year-old female attorney). However subtly, he may demean her opinions. Simply not answering all her questions may communicate lack of respect. She, in turn, may respond to these subtle messages with increased aggressiveness. Their interaction may escalate to the point that, considering only her behavior, he can conclude comfortably that "all career women are a little sick." He behaves in a way that confirms his hidden hypothesis or value judgment.

Several clues suggest that a physician's behavior is influenced by hidden value judgments. The first is taking a strong stance about a patient's treatment in the absence of either firm scientific data or strong medical consensus. The question, "Why do I feel so strongly about this?" is crucial for the physician to ask.

A second context that suggests the impact of hidden value judgments is a situation where the physician finds that he or she is departing from a customary approach to patients. The internist considering a quick referral of the depressed pornographer (Patient F) is an example of this.

A third situation involving a high likelihood that underlying values are intruding would be an occasion when the physician uses stereotypes to describe individual patients. "Just another damn pothead" (Patient E) is a typical example. Referring consistently to an individual patient as a member of a certain group (e.g., rigid Catholic, smart Jew, angry black, dumb Polack, etc.)[10] strongly suggests that the patient's individuality has been lost in the physician's value orientation. As such, the treatment alliance will almost certainly suffer. Full awareness of another social class, culture, religion, and style of life requires long-term, intimate contact that often lies outside a physician's experience.

A fourth clue suggesting the role of the physician's value judgments involves the arousal of strong feelings which seem disproportionate to anything that has actually happened in the doctor-patient relationship. Each physician will, at times, note unusually intense feelings about a particular patient. Often, the reasons for the feelings are clear and relate to some aspect of the patient's behavior. Occasionally, however, the feelings do not "add up" and the thoughtful physician will need to consider whether or not a hidden value judgment is responsible.

Physicians, like all other people, carry value judgments that often are not clearly articulated. These judgments concern answers to questions about the nature of man, what is "good" and "bad," what life is all about, and a host of others. They are an essential part of being human and influence the way each person perceives and responds to the world. In the practice of medicine, they are particularly apt to be influential when scientific data fail to provide clear guidelines for medical decision making. Even when the data seem clear, however, they influence and often distort the decision-making process. Value orientations are inescapable and, therefore, ubiquitous in the practice of medicine.

Social issues are topics of group concern that polarize individuals into conflict about the "right" and the "wrong" way to deal with the subject. Advances in science and medicine both provide new social issues and recharge old ones. Physicians differ in the extent to which they wish to participate in the public resolution of conflicting social issues. When they do participate, many physicians find it easier to be aligned with mainstream values which usually emphasize tradition and the status quo and are cautious about rapid social change. In this sense, organized medicine often occupies a conservative position. This chapter's intent is neither to support nor attack the position of organized medicine on social issues. Rather, it is to emphasize the role that individual physicians' value systems have upon relationships with patients and their families. There is no "cure" for this phenomenon. Many feel that the practice of medicine has an inherent political aspect, in that medical decisions influence the distribution of care in this country. Out of this grows the suggestion that physicians should tell patients directly about their stances concerning charged social issues. This may burden most patients with information they neither want nor need. However, it is important for physicians to know what their basic values are and to recognize how frequently these reflect participation in the reasonably affluent and white segment of this country. This type of insight may diminish the distorting impact of the physician's values upon relationships with patients from different social or cultural groups.

REFERENCES

1 Ginsburg, S.: *A Psychiatrist's Views on Social Issues,* New York: Columbia University Press, 1963.
2 Thomas, Lewis: *The Lives of a Cell,* New York: Viking Press, 1974.
3 Spiegel, J.: *Transactions: The Interplay between Individual, Family, and Society,* New York: Science House, 1971, p. 162.
4 Eisenberg, L.: "Psychiatry and Society," *N. Eng. J. Med., 296*(16): 903–910, 1977.
5 Ottenberg, P.: "Bureaucratic Attitudes As a Psychosocial Defense," *Psychiatric Opinion,* 11(1): 26–35, 1974.
6 Bernard, V. W.: "Some Principles of Dynamic Psychiatry in Relation to Poverty," *Am. J. Psychiatry,* 122(3):254, 1965.
7 Usdin, G.: in "Symposium: To Live, to Die—Who Decides?" *Southern Medicine,* 65:2, April 1977.
8 Group for the Advancement of Psychiatry: *The Right To Die,* New York: 1973.
9 Marmor, J.: *Psychiatry in Transition,* New York: Brunner/Mazel, 1974.
10 Jahoda, M.: *Race Relations and Mental Health,* Paris: UNESCO, 1960.

Part Two

Children and Adolescents

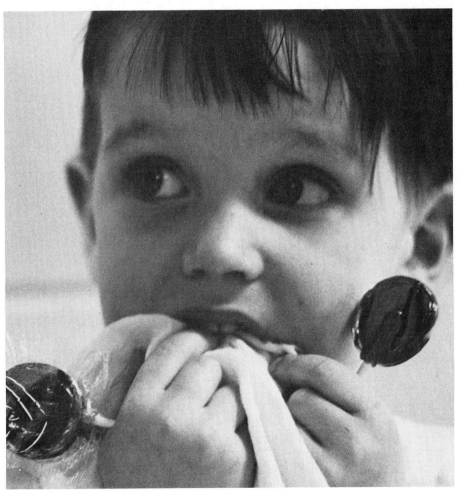

Chapter 7

Children and Their Emotional Maladies

Henry H. Work, M.D.

EDITORS' INTRODUCTION

What is it like to be 4 years old and have a urinary tract infection requiring examination and treatment? What is it like to be 5 and have your stomach hurt every morning before you go to kindergarten? How must it be at age 7 to be so frightened of a darkened bedroom that you are unable to sleep? What is it like at age 9 to hear your mother and father shouting and arguing night after night? What are the concerns of the 10-year-old admitted to the hospital for a tonsillectomy?

What is it like to be the parent of a child with leukemia? How must it feel to be told an only son is mentally defective, has a congenital heart defect, or has a convulsive disorder? What must it be like to watch one's 5-year-old daughter being wheeled to surgery? What feelings are involved in parents whose children have phobias?

The physician's involvement with children and their parents is often one that is charged with feeling. It may be difficult for some physicians to identify empathetically with a child—the feelings, thoughts, and experiences of childhood are far away and cannot be retrieved. It may be difficult to remember that these youthful patients are not adults, and their being terrified of an injection may be appropriate to their experience. How do you handle the clergyman whose child has a behavior problem? The realistic need to be objective and analytic may dominate the physician's response and be interpreted by the child as remoteness, coldness, or disinterest. The concerned parents of the child may also provoke a wide variety of feelings in the physician. Some feelings reach back to the physician's relationship with his or her parents, and others may impinge on the physician's relationship with his or her own children. Even if the physician is relatively free from such impeding carry-overs from his or her personal life, there is an urgent need to understand the child's developmental timetable, to know where the child is and, as a result, be able to understand the child's response to illness as influenced by specific developmental tasks and mechanisms. In this chapter, Henry Work, who is both a pediatrician and a psychiatrist, presents a concise overview of what the physician should know about child psychiatry. He does so against a backdrop of normal growth and development, and suggests, therefore, a complete way of thinking about the children who come to us as patients.

CHILDREN GROW

An appreciation of the concept that children grow provides a framework for looking at the emotional and behavioral problems of children and is crucial to an understanding of those problems. Both the failure to grow and deviations in growth cause concern as well as misunderstandings. The symptomatology of childhood is intimately linked to the changes that development brings about, and the manifestations of a child's adjustment to development become the day-to-day issues of pathology in the child.

In an infant, emotional problems are diffuse; difficulties in sleeping, changes in bowel habits, and uncontrolled crying characterize anxiety at that age level. In the toddler, emotional disorders become more organized. The child is then subject to fears, temper tantrums, and at times, frequent accidents or recurrent illnesses.

After the advancement to school age, learning problems, as well as resistance to attending school, become manifest. For many years the classic expectation of a child in psychiatric treatment was a 9- or 10-year-old boy who manifested aggression by lying, stealing, or harming other children.

Growth Is a Process

The growth of children does not proceed with an absolute evenness, but occurs in spurts and plateaus. More importantly, growth is occurring in several planes at the same time.

Physical growth is easy to measure. The most massive physical growth occurs during 9 months prior to birth, but rapid changes in size and shape continue throughout the first year of life, and only slowly settle down to a constant level of change. Parents and others are caught up in the phenomenon of physical growth during the first year of life. They pour fantastic amounts of concern into their observation of the child's progress, and experience intermittent anxiety that the child is not changing as rapidly as he or she should be. Physical growth during the first year is not only measured in pounds and inches, but in the impressive motor development that changes a supine newborn, totally dependent on the environment, to a walking, babbling, active 1 year old in such a short span of time. Never again will physical growth be so dramatic.

This physical growth is matched by *intellectual growth,* which is often measured by the same tokens. With a neurologic process that is represented by changes from head to tail (cephalocaudal), children hold up their heads, smile, use their arms, sit, pull to a stand, maneuver about, and finally walk. The outstanding human capacity for talking caps the measurement of intellectual development for the first year. The arrival of speech makes it possible to measure more fully the child's cognitive gains throughout the rest of the growing years.

There is a *behavioral level of growth* that is comparable to the physical and intellectual changes. An intriguing measure of this is seen in the capacity to delay. The newborn is entirely selfish, demanding, and seemingly insensitive to the surrounding world except for responses to pain or hunger. Changes in the child's demand for food appear to parallel the changes in sleep patterns that are so obvious during the first year of life. Just as the child moves from an intermittently sleeping being to an individual who sleeps in measured periods, mostly at night, so the demanding nature of the child begins to modify with age. Instead of crying for food immediately after awakening, as at the beginning of the year, the child who is a few months old wakes, plays, smiles, and babbles with an appreciation that food will come.

With subsequent growth, the control and organization of the mind react more and more to the world in which the child lives. Depending upon the manner in which the child is being reared, control expresses itself in either compliant, organized, or "disobedient" behavior.

While the physical growth and development of the child are the easiest to measure, it is aberrations in the intellectual and behavioral development that cause the most concern to parents and provide the basis for symptomatology of children as presented to the physician.

Children and Their Parents

The truism that children do not develop in a vacuum is painfully obvious when one listens to parents' complaints about their children. It is equally patent that the pathology and symptomatology which are brought to the physician to be unraveled often consist primarily of those things that *bother* the parents in the child's process of growth and change. The mother of an infant seeks help from the pediatrician because her child is fussy and restless and, in the process of not sleeping well, keeps the parents awake. The mother of a 15-month-old child who has not yet begun to stand or walk, reacts to her own appraisal as well as the criticism and anxiety of others in the family and seeks medical help.

A 4-year-old who spends her time at nursery school sitting in a corner sucking her thumb and refusing to join the others in play, provokes worry on the part of both teachers and parents, and again professional help is sought. The characterization of the 9-year-old boy who aggressively assaults his schoolmates reinforces the concept that the effect of a child's behavior on others is often the starting point for seeking help.

Seeking Medical Help

In the introduction of this book, it was pointed out that things that annoy a patient lead, at times, to medical consultation. It was also noted that annoyances on the part of the physician many either emphasize the need for help or interfere with it because of the subjective reaction of the physician. All these principles are applicable to the care of a patient who is a child, but the problems are more often manifested by the guardians who bring the child for help than by the child.

THE FIRST YEAR

Expectations

The nodal point of birth is critical, and not just for the physiologic phenomena and the hazards that may attend that process. From the point of view of emotional and psychological development, it represents the point where the child joins the family, is recognized by the family, and begins to establish a host of relationships both with the family and with others. The expectations (particularly those of the parents) that surround this moment are critical.

Consider the example of a pair of young parents anticipating the birth of their first child. In addition to the pressures built up by the hopes and fears of their own life experiences, there are all the pressures of grandparents and society in general that call for the production of a perfect child. The parents may have strong (and even conflicting) expectations about the sex of that child. More often than not, the child meets these expectations, although disappointments are bound to occur with even minor deviations from perfection. When, by virtue of genetic pathology or intrauterine pathology related to the pregnancy itself, expectations are not met, the entry of the child into the family can predictably be seen as presenting a potentially difficult relationship problem. A severely damaged child, such as one with obvious mental retardation or gross physical anomalies, poses hardships that are difficult for parents to cope with; such problems demand immediate, continuing professional care. The anxieties that build up around the child's failure to meet the maternal or paternal expectations may well demonstrate themselves in a host of difficulties when the parents are caring for the child. These difficulties can be seen in less severe forms in many other children, depending upon the capacity of the parents to cope with the child's demands and needs.

Developmental Progress

Most children satisfy their parents, or the latter adjust quickly to minor aberrations. Then begins the process of matching the child's growing capacities to the caretaking abilities of the parents. It is at this interface that parents seek help from physicians during the first year of the child's growth.

We have already sketched the motor development of the child as a series of progressive steps from supine to upright behavior. Sensory growth patterns are equally important and must be responded to. We now know that infants have much greater sensory capacities, manifested by organized development of sight and hearing patterns, than was formerly thought. These changes are normally responded to through the parents' active care, fondling, and stimulation of the infant. Smiling is an especially active demonstration of a child's progress, and parental encouragement and response. While hearing and vision are easy to appreciate and measure, a critical aspect of the growth of a child is offered by kinesthetic and skin sensations. Children who are not adequately stimulated in the normal course of handling may well suffer a general deprivation. This may be manifested later on (at the end of the first year or at the beginning of the second) by withdrawal and apathy. This is evidenced to an extreme degree in the condition of infantile marasmus, which is manifested by failure to eat, irritability, poor sleeping, and general difficulties in thriving.

The focus of parental complaints during the first year tends to center around physiologic mechanisms. Failures or difficulties in eating, excessive or inadequate sleep with consequent irritability, and aberrations in elimination make up most of the complaints that parents bring to physicians who are caring for their child. At mid-year and later on, the process of development of teeth gives rise to complaints about the child's pain and the expressions of the parental response to it. Reactions may well range from genuine concern to frank annoyance.

A child, therefore, may be brought to the physician because of vomiting or diarrhea, but equally because of parental concern about failure to eat or about constant hunger. Sleeplessness or failure to change from the intermittent sleep pattern of the newborn to a more comfortable pattern of daytime naps and nighttime sleep can plague the parents and upset their schedules. Crying and irritability are the most demonstrable indications of pain, but they can also be indications of an anxious or otherwise poor relationship with the parents.

The Physician's Role

A host of physiologic problems are best met by careful and calm understanding of the situation. A physician who continues to see the child from birth through early hospital days and then into the home has an advantage in understanding the parents and consequently may understand their approach to the child. Interfering factors, such as the duties of the home, care of other children, or grandparental concerns, can be appreciated objectively.

To deal with the mother, it is good to recognize her needs and capacities. Mothers, particularly at this time, need both reassurance and a calm understanding. A description of the common problems with which any mother is faced serves as an alleviating mechanism in itself. At times, the problem may be as simple as the mother's misunderstanding of the normal developmental stages. Overanxiety may cause the mother to do too much for the child or to respond too quickly to the child's cries and demands. At other times, it may well be the mother's desperate efforts to prove herself a good mother in the eyes of her husband and relatives. She may be distraught because, without an adequate model of care, she is unfamiliar with the simple handling of a child. This deficit is most easily corrected by supplying such a model of care through a competent nurse or other experienced technician.

Depression

A particular concern of young mothers is the so-called "blues," or postpartum depression. While it is found in an extreme form only infrequently, even its milder stages affect many mothers and interfere with their interest in, concern for, and approach to their children. The failure to respond to a child increases the child's irritability. This may well increase a mother's guilt and set up a cycle of poor care at the beginning.

Crucial to all these problems is the intervention of the physician by way of clarifying, and elaborating upon, the situation. While it is important to make sure that the child is functioning properly and has all the appropriate equipment, internal and external, it is equally important to understand the manner in which the mother handles the child, her schedule, her competing pressures, and other responsibilities.

Abnormal Expectations

A particular problem is that of parents who dramatically and energetically anticipate their child's growth. This may manifest itself initially as constant checking for change during the first year. It may involve looking ahead to such an extent that the child is felt to be ready for school at a time when he or she is only learning to sit. Such anticipation leads to anxiety and a search for minor, or even major, defects. It is extremely important to clarify these unusual expectations.

The anticipations may be coupled with attempts to "discipline" the infant. The problem of child abuse, which will be discussed later, is merely an extreme manifestation of parental concern about the child and the child's response to the parents. There is increasing evidence that some children seem to provoke abuse, and that some parental expectations demand more of a child than the child can produce. When the parent is irritated by forces external to the child, the child may be the most likely target of parental demands, punishment, or even extreme physical abuse.

The Complication of Fear

There was a time when pregnancy was beset with a host of fears related to "old wives' tales." Many of these carried over into the early stages of child rearing, with a consequent group of superstitions about growth and about the handling of this growth.

We have not moved too far from these tales, as evidenced by our increased knowledge of the hazards of pregnancy (gene patterns, rubella, etc.) and the conflicting knowledge presented in the many books advising parents about child rearing. This poses a double problem for the physician who must first alleviate both the reasonable and the unreasonable fears of a parent, either about genetic difficulties or environmental casualties during pregnancy. The physician must then assist parents to have a clear and honest knowledge about development to counteract the superstitions and patterns of advice given. Many mothers read each new "baby book" avidly. They may, however, fail to understand the message. The task of the physician may very well be to interpret and help the parent understand what it is he or she is doing, and relate this directly to both an understanding of, and help for, the child.

Summary

If the task during the first year of the child's life is to grow motorically, sensorily, and behaviorally, the task for the parent is to appreciate this growth, to accommodate to it, to support the child in such simple things as feeding, playing, and talking. The child is building a picture of the world which includes understanding of sounds, sights, feelings, and the temperaments of those who care for her or him. The task of the mother is to support the child's physical growth, to stimulate his or her sensory input, and to ensure both the child's comfort and her own availability. Through this process, the child achieves greater control of self, is able to tolerate delays in parental response, and becomes capable of distancing self from parent, a process that is even more critical during the second year.

The physician's task is to observe, to describe clearly what is occurring, and to point the way to better methods of support and stimulation on the part of the parent. The physician will be alert to specific physical aberrations, both in the child's body and in the development of the body. His or her knowledge of these aberrations, however, will be used to help the parents understand the meaning of these changes and to project, without undue anticipation, into the future.

New Approaches

In the last quarter-century, certain phases of the first year of life have been looked at more critically than others. One of these is the phenomenon of birth itself, either in the hospital or at home. A quarter of a century ago, leading pediatricians and obstetricians made vigorous attempts to enhance the process of caring for the child in the hospital. Alterations in hospital nurseries allowed the mother to care for her child under the supervision of the hospital staff, and encouraged her to offer breast feeding whenever possible.

Related to these earlier efforts were the subsequent attempts to modify the whole process of pregnancy. Precepts of earlier ages and other cultures were used to make natural childbirth a thing in itself, with greater involvement of both parents both during the pregnancy and at the time of birth.

From the point of view of psychological development, such efforts have paid valuable dividends in the manner in which parents are introduced to their children, made comfortable with them, and begin to establish an easy relationship. The hazards lie in a risk of fetishistic overinvolvement in such activities. The role of the physician is that of objectivity in the face of sensationalism. To strike a balance between parents who are so diffident that they avoid their children, and those who get so locked up with them that they become inseparable, will strain the capacity of the physician's objectivity.

THE SECOND YEAR

Growth Includes Independence

If the process of physical growth is impressive during the first year of life, the process of development and its consequences demand special attention during the second year, which begins with the child's standing, forming a few words, and being ready to explore. The year ends with the child's being able not only to walk but to run, with a competence in handling things, a vocabulary of from 50 to 500 words, and an awareness of his or her role in the family.

A host of new studies in the last three decades has been impressive enough to result in changed and better-organized concepts of cognitive growth; the manner by which the child's capacity to learn and the learning process itself are known to expand rapidly during this second year. We are equally aware of the profound impact that all this development has on the family. If, indeed, the child does rapidly develop sensory skills, language, capacity to handle his or her own body, the child is moving from a late stage of dependence toward one of considerable independence during this second 12-month span. Progress in motor and social development, however, is not free of cost. It patently involves more than an intrinsic mode of developing. Profound changes in relationships between the child and the parents, siblings, and family begin to take place.

In general, motor development is permitted a fairly free expansion. Walking is encouraged, and at times, pushed. Speech in most parts of our society often meets with a response (at times it is corrected), but it is generally encouraged. A number of studies have highlighted deprivation in this particular area and have led to such societal plans as Headstart and parent-child centers to encourage the use of speech and language.

Roadblocks on the Way to Independence

Despite changing cultural patterns, two areas of potential conflict are apparent throughout many levels of American society. One of these relates to the feeding experience. While the smaller child is fed of necessity, the advent of his or her independence and newfound capacity urges the parent to turn eating over directly to the child. A variety of cultural norms, including parental concerns about manners and "dirtiness," may inhibit the child's capacity for self-feeding. Thus, the easy manner in which the child learns to walk and run is in direct contrast to efforts at training him or her to eat properly, have some manners, and fit into a societal pattern.

The other area that may well bring forth a potential conflict is that of the child's elimination habits. While the pressure to "train" or even "break" a child has diminished, there is still a strong push to have a child establish toilet habits which are in keeping with those of the family. Natural development of muscular and sensory control may be grossly interfered with by this process. More importantly, conflicts over teaching manners and teaching toilet patterns may only be a reflection of a wider concern on the part of parents about development of the child during this particular year. If motor and sensory accomplishments of the child lead toward independence, there may be a considerable concern about this change on the part of some parents. Many mothers prefer the dependent infant to the independent child who can not only walk, but walk away from them, talk, and talk back to them. Potential struggles develop. The "who-is-in-charge" attitude is enhanced.

Discipline

The extent, duration, and form of parent-child conflicts play a large part in shaping subsequent personality patterns. Such conflicts set up new patterns of relationships between the child and parents, and considerable elements of anger and even hostility may be in the new patterns. Some of this is reflected in the concept of discipline. Indeed, the need to discipline a child, depending upon the personalities and backgrounds of the parents, is one of the outstanding manifestations of child rearing in this age period.

> Consider the example of a 2-year-old boy who was brought to the physician because of nightmares, destructive behavior toward toys and, at times, toward other small children. The parents characterized all these actions as "disobedience." The child had a comfortable first year, but at about 15 months of age began to demonstrate a general increase in activity which the parents felt needed to be curbed. One method of handling the child was to shut him in his room. This merely led to destructive behavior toward furniture, toys, etc. On the advice of grandparents, the parents instituted patterns of physical punishment that grew in number as the year went by, until both parents and child were exhausted by the process. The father felt that physical punishment, in the form of spankings, was the only way to control a child. The mother was more inclined to be lenient, but out of her own fear of the father, she too complied. The result was a family at terrific odds with one another, with an anxious, fearful, and at times, hysterical child demonstrating a pattern that would possibly lead either to violent behavior or to a severe obsessional personality disorder.

Similar patterns can be seen when parents put a tremendous focus on cleanliness in eating and in toilet habits. At times, a standoff position about the phenomena of toilet training, and particularly of bowel training, becomes so great an issue that it involves both parents and becomes a focus of all disciplinary activities in the parent-child relationship.

Customarily, attempts to modify development by curbing independence, demanding perfection in social skills, and insisting on docility and compliance mark most of the struggles in the second year. Occasionally one sees parents who solve the problems of their child's growing independence by fostering an infantile form of dependence. While such attempts to curb activity in the child are only occasionally successful, they may at times lead to a whining, clinging type of dependent attitude that persists over the years and interferes with the child's social and integrative capacities as she or he moves away from home and family.

Separation

The growing independence of the child is a preparation for a life apart from the parents. This requires a break from the close ties that the young child has had from the moment of birth, particularly with the mother. Separation thus becomes a pervasive aspect of life throughout the first few years. It begins to demonstrate itself during the middle of the first year and it becomes particularly evident during this second year.

While it is normal for parents to cling to, and foster dependence in, the infant, pride in the child's growth sets the stage for a separation of the parent-child pair which allows each of them a comfortable and mutually satisfying existence. The bond, however, is not easy to break. A child's exposure to others outside the family can be most frightening. This is seen in its clearest form during the second year, when a child is taken abruptly (or even at times in a planned fashion) into a hospital setting. Such a change in environment is reacted to with irritability, intense crying, and ultimately, if it is protracted and not adjusted to, with apathy.

In a less dramatic way, however, the problem of separation occurs on a daily basis throughout the months from 6 to 30. The capacity of the parent both to protect the child and to lead him or her slowly into new situations is an important one. A special problem is faced by the immature parent who is unable to give up the child and who, in a sense, becomes dependent on the child. As the child achieves some independence, the parent views it as a rejection and, in response, may turn away from the child.

The Medical Role

Once more, knowledge of development, knowledge of the development of a specific child, and knowledge of the family's way of dealing with the development are important. It is worth noting, on the basis of the descriptions above, that parents may do extremely well with a child during the first year of life and yet have considerable difficulty as a child begins to establish independence and separate. Both problems combine to make the parent anxious and the response may be critical. The complaints which parents bring to physicians are outlined in the example; namely, difficulties in sleeping, especially with nightmares; difficulties in habit patterns; and difficulties with what the parents view as bad behavior. All the complaints are expressed in a manner that sugests that the child is "willfully" doing things, either against the parents' wishes or to punish or act against the parents' pleasure. The child is described as having a "temper," or as being subject to temper tantrums, varying in degree and quality. For some parents, these tantrums are frightening. For others, they merely manifest willfulness, stubbornness, and a need to be "broken."

The task of clarification, therefore, becomes critical. Parental complaints often are not brought to physicians. Parents may prefer to talk the problems over with neighbors or with relatives, or they may turn to child-rearing manuals. The critical ingredient for the physician to supply is objectivity. The ability to recognize and outline the problem, and then to clarify the parents' response to the difficulty or the perceived difficulty in the child, can lead to new parental approaches which are hopefully more comfortable both for parent and for child. The physician may be drawn into the role of marriage counselor, or into supporting the parents against pressures from grandparents, other relatives, and even neighbors. The physician who is known and respected for ongoing care of the family has the most to offer in such situations. These problems are not to be superficially assuaged with sedatives, but rather analyzed on the basis of developmental knowledge and an appreciation of family and marital tensions.

THE PRESCHOOL YEARS

Birthdays are notable events in a child's life, but as sociobiologic milestones none can compare with the first. As a child moves through the third, fourth, and fifth years, growth is steady, development proceeds at a pace determined by the stimuli that the environment supplies, and cognitive gains become the most important measuring device. During the second year, children learn what capacities they have. During the ensuing years, they learn what to do with these capacities.

The years from 2 to 6 are therefore marked by great curiosity. The curiosity starts with self and the exploration of self; it extends to curiosity about others of the same and of the opposite sex, and ultimately it leads to all kinds of concerns about size, space, speech, and how to get along or not get along with others. At times, the curiosity about the outside world only reemphasizes the smallness and impotence of the child. Thus, fears which are becoming noticeable during the second year, may become a critical aspect of this period's pathology.

At times, a child's curiosity leads him or her into situations of which the adult world disapproves. Sexual explorations may very well be limited or even punished. If parents are bothered by "old wives' tales," so the child is bothered by a host of admonitions that come in this period: "Behave yourself," "Don't touch," "Mind what you say." Contradictions abound, "Act your age" versus "Why don't you grow up!" Threats of isolation may very well lead to projecting fears onto the dark, the outside world, and various other special phenomena.

Fantasy is the compensatory aspect of life that is most commonly found during this period. A child who is impotent and small may well visualize himself or herself as big or grown-up, and play out the fantasy in all sorts of activities. These fantasies are especially apparent in the dream productions of children. Obviously these games serve as compensatory mechanisms for all the slights and disabilities that the child feels during this particular period.

Play becomes an important aspect of demonstrating and utilizing the thought processes which we call fantasy. Play begins in infancy, develops during succeeding years, and is at its peak during the years just prior to school. Later, play becomes a much more organized phenomenon, but true play can best be observed among preschool children. Nursery schools and other teaching institutions take advantage of this fact and use it to build language and other skills.

Another tangible aspect of play is the child's use of a transitional object. This is a highly personal phenomenon whereby the child uses a toy, blanket, or other object as comfort against the vagaries of a frightening outside world. Taking an object to bed serves to ward off the terrors of the night. Some children rely heavily on this. They become wedded to the transitional object, and its serves as a barrier to ordinary relationships. The child who withdraws, develops thumbsucking habits, clings to an object constantly, and shuns the company of peers should be of real concern to the physician caring for the family. Such withdrawal demands explanation. It signifies an important disruption in normal development, probably having to do with the phenomena of independence and separation.

Problems

There are other important problem areas during this period. The most common presenting complaints are:

1 Chronic irritability, temper tantrums, and violent behavior
2 Inability to socialize
3 Specific failures of development: speech, hearing, etc.
4 Cognitive delay

As noted above, some parents are loath to bring children to the physician for problems which they see as relatively minor or transient. It is not until a child assaults others violently or is critically withdrawn that such parents seek help. Often parents are pushed by nursery schools or others to get assistance in managing a child who demonstrates severe temper tantrums and violence; or they may be urged by the school to find out why the child withdraws, plays very little, and is apathetic and listless. Developmental delays, unless gross, are often missed during this period and come to light only when the child goes to school.

In clarifying these difficulties, it is important that the physician not only see the child and observe the manifestations of the difficulties first-hand, but also understand a relatively complete pattern of the child's development and relationships in the home. This would include not only the mother/child and father/child relationships, but the relationships of the parents to each other and the child's relationship to siblings.

Treatment through the Family

A critical development in the practice of child psychiatry has been the use of a family approach to problems. One sees this coming into play with the difficulties described for children in this age period. Unless the physician has a picture of what goes on in the family setting, it is not easy to understand the complaints of a teacher. Unless the teacher can understand the parental systems of punishment, discipline, and control over habits such as sleep and eating, and can get a clear picture of how the parents handle the child's sexual and general curiosity, it is not easy to approach these problems. While an understanding of the family situation is not a de facto solution to the problem of handling a child, it is awesome how much can be accomplished by means of a thorough, extensive review of the child's developmental history and the observation of parental management tactics. Obviously, the physician will be concerned about the physical condition of the child as well as her or his disabilities. Specific disabilities in terms of learning, sight, and hearing may need extensive testing. It is important to recognize, however, that focusing on the child alone will rarely give a clear picture. The child's developmental disabilities take on their full meaning as they are viewed by the parents, in the light of parental tactics for exaggerating, minimizing, or understanding them.

The Value of Early Schooling

An outstanding manifestation of developmental change is the child's capacity to engage with others. Instances of children who shun the company of their peers may appear in medical practice. Normal development, particularly in the presence of siblings, accustoms a child to peer relationships. Such relationships are well documented in the scientific literature, and it is obvious that, despite the stress they pose, siblings often give strong support. The same is true of peers. A great deal of learning takes place in the presence of peers; strong, effectual knowledge comes out of such relationships.

The physician's task is to see that these relationships are fostered. Schooling in early years enhances such relations, but only if teachers are aware and concerned about the growing complexity of the child's relationships with companions. It is apparent that many children profit greatly from such schooling. Good peer relations are especially helpful for the only child or the child whose home life is disrupted by parental conflict or divorce. Once more, the physician becomes both an observer and a manager in trying to develop an optimal climate for the normal socialization and peer contacts to be established.

Hospitals and Their Meaning

Children at this age are especially prone to accidents and acute infectious conditions. Regression is the most common response pattern. Such regression is manifested by a return to simpler and earlier habit patterns. It may include changes in bowel, eating, and sleep patterns. It may involve the giving up of learned speech and the adoption of a simplified baby talk. It is demonstrated often through whining and through clinging behaviors that are distressing to the adults caring for the child.

Such symptoms are often understood and accommodated to in a modern child hospital practice. When they are not, one may see the development of a severe form of withdrawal, apathy, and infantilism, all of which may lead to profound difficulty in the healing process. Children in hospitals are there to get well. When the psyche is altered, the process of healing may be grossly hampered. The physician would do well to be aware not only of the child's condition, but also of the condition of the hospital setting.

Many advances in the provision of care for such children have been made, but all of them are based on the clear understanding of the disability which the child demonstrates. Increased visiting on the part of parents, increased solicitude on the part of other adults, congenial surroundings, lack of restriction, and other modifications of hospital setting are crucial. It is equally crucial that the child be stimulated properly to move away from the depressive elements of withdrawal. Schooling becomes as important in the hospital setting as it is in the child's regular setting; play and contact with other children are equally crucial. It behooves the physician to be aware of these factors which influence the child's experience.

THE SCHOOL YEARS

From the point of view of teachers, all that happens to a child during these first five or six years is merely a preparation for the phenomenon of learning. From the point of view of the child (and of the parent as well), entry to school is a critical event to be either welcomed or feared, depending upon past parental experiences and the actual stage of development in the child.

Both parent and child face three problem areas. The first is separation, the second is accommodation and adaptation to the new culture (the school), and the third is the whole business of academic learning.

Earlier it was noted that separation begins early and is normally handled by an ever-expanding series of contacts outside the family. Children who go to nursery school have usually made a major break and accommodate themselves easily to the elementary school exposure. Other children may find that first grade or kindergarten is the point where separation becomes a clear-cut phenomenon. Many children experience serious difficulty in separating and demonstrate fears both day and night with, for example, episodic crying. Similarly, the accommodation to the world of school may be a difficulty in itself for some children.

These children are frequently a source of major concern to the teacher, in that they lack attention to their studies, hamper the studying of other children, and in general are disruptive elements in school. By testing the tolerance of teachers, they may very quickly be labeled as disobedient, bad, or truant, and referred elsewhere for help. "Delinquency," a common school opprobrium, is easily attached as a label.

Learning

The most serious demand that a school imposes is the demand for learning itself. Placing this demand on a child who is unprepared, either by virtue of a lack of intellectual capacity or because of not having learned how to learn, may present a very severe strain. The process of schooling begins to sort out these capacities quickly. Unfortunately, a major delay frequently exists between the teacher's recognition that a child is not learning and the issuance of a warning or expression of concern to those who might be of assistance. Thus, the physician is often confronted with a complaint from the school that the child is not learning and, therefore, needs to be evaluated, but this complaint may not be presented until the child is well into the second grade.

Medical Care

The medical role at this point is twofold: (1) to assess the physical condition of the child in order to ascertain that nothing about the state of physical health is interfering with learning, and (2) to make sure that proper studies determine the intellectual and sensory capacities of the child. Here, the knowledge of the child's past history, including responses to previous learning experiences, adds an important dimension to the study of the child that cannot be obtained through a spot diagnosis.

The Hyperactive Child

In recent years, in addition to the problems of irritability, restlessness, difficulty in learning, and disobedience in school, a syndrome known as the "hyperactive child" has been prominent in the literature.[1] The syndrome, which is characterized by the evidence of more than usual activity on the part of the child, may be apparent from infancy and persist through school years. In the classic picture of this syndrome, the child during preschool and learning years is clumsy, awkward, and at times has a difficulty in learning which is characterized chiefly by difficulty in reading.

Observations of these children has led to a whole host of diagnoses, many of which are seemingly contradictory, and all of which are confusing. "Hyperactive child," "dyslexic," "primary dyslexia," "slow-learning child," and "minimal brain dysfunction" epitomize the diagnostic categories. Patience and skill are required to sort out those children who are overreacting to the disciplinary or school situation from those who have an intrinsic neurological difficulty, minor in nature, which leads to specific difficulties in the learning sphere, and especially in learning to read. It calls for the best of psychological examinations, in addition to an understanding of the physical condition of the child and of the home situation. The physician's task relates more to the latter investigation. Any child presenting the syndrome of hyperactivity and learning disability warrants a thorough psychological examination by someone competent in this area. Very often, the physician serves chiefly as an expert referring agent to make sure that the testing is the best that can be found.

Medication

A brief word about medication. Once the physician has been satisfied that the pattern of hyperactivity is chronic and that counseling or other efforts will not serve to ameliorate the situation, a certain group of drugs, particularly the stimulant drugs, have often proven efficacious.

The most common of these are the amphetamines which have been used for hyperactive children since the 1930s. Many parents are concerned about the development of drug dependence. This danger has not been confirmed. The response of a very active child who had been unable to learn, to the use of such drugs as dextroamphetamine or methylphenidate hydrochloride, is sometimes very dramatic. The results in terms of learning and changed behavior may become a source of solace both to parents and to the hyperactive child.

SPECIAL SITUATIONS

Adoption

Out of common cultural practices, society has evolved the legal phenomenon of adoption, which serves a dual function: placing seemingly unwanted children in homes where they can be cared for, and providing a family for parents who are unable to procreate. It is a civilized and yet complicated procedure involving the giving up of a child by the natural mother on the one hand, and on the other hand the rearing of the genetically unrelated child by parents who have felt deprived or cheated in their own efforts to have a child.

The advantages of the placement are usually great. Children are taken into homes and supplied with parents who hopefully are capable of guiding them through their early years, supporting and cherishing them, and providing opportunities for independence and a place in the world. However, there are hazards.

There is increasing difficulty in finding children for adoption. This and other cultural changes have led to the adoption of children of mixed racial parentage, as well as of children who are coming from countries where war has destroyed the family pattern. The most recent example of this is the large number of Vietnamese children adopted, a wave that followed an earlier wave of the adoption of Korean children in America.

Another factor in decreasing the number of available children relates to recent cultural changes that encourage young mothers who formerly might have given their children up for adoption to keep the children with them instead. The difficulties faced by mothers who do give up their children is a separate issue that becomes important as the practice of adoptions changes to allow more open records of the children's biologic parents. The possibility that a child given up for adoption may one day confront the natural mother is frightening to many.

Customarily, the physician is faced with the problems of the child growing up in the adopted family. Adoptive parents often wait lengthy periods of time before deciding that they are not capable of procreation, and then seek to adopt a child. This period of waiting has inherent disadvantages. The family patterns have become fixed and sometimes rigid. There are often anxieties about adoption, and these are frequently enhanced by delays in the adoptive process. Furthermore, the child comes, often abruptly, into an organized family. The classic 9 months' preparation that natural parents have before a family becomes complete is not always available.

The literature about adoptions demonstrates clearly that the former focus of adopting agencies was on the capacity of the parents, particularly the mother, to care for a very young child. In the last several decades, there has been a growing number of scientific studies of this process. Some of these demonstrate very clearly that the care of a growing child involves far more than the care of an infant. Parents selected on the basis of their capacity for dependent care may not adapt easily to the problems of a child's growing independence.

Other recent studies have suggested that the incidence of behavioral and emotional disturbance in adopted children is considerably higher than in the population at large. The extent of this discrepancy remains to be determined, but it is apparent that help is sought for such children more often than it is for nonadopted children. Such help is nearly always sought during the latency age period (the school years), and the common complaints are those of aggressivity, hyperactivity, and poor socialization. A physician treating such a family over a period of time, however, may well see difficulties much earlier in the life of the child. While the period of adjustment is often bumpy for the infant, it is usually not outstandingly stormy. Difficulties frequently do not emerge until the second year.

Here the classic problems concerning parents' adaptations to the independence of the child are noticeable. Many of these parents have set and comfortable lives. Some are highly concerned about the child's changed behavior. Thus, the struggle between parent and child, which was described in the earlier discussion of the second-year period, becomes accentuated. A physician who sees this can take steps to prevent the situation from going on to the aggressive, acting-out behavior of the school years, when the situation will be more difficult to cope with. Generally speaking, once symptoms of a severe nature, such as an extremely poor school adjustment, have appeared, the situation calls for specialized care. The task for the primary physician is to anticipate the coming trouble and to make the appropriate referrals.

Medical Role   Long-time observations of children in adoptive families suggest that the medical focus should be on the second year, with the physician evidencing a comforting and reassuring attitude toward the adoptive parents. One should look for early signs that the parents see the child as something totally alien. The ''bad seed'' phenomenon is a very persistent shibboleth in the pathology of adoptions. Parents can easily distance themselves from a child who is not born to them. The role of the physician in looking for and trying to make explicit this situation becomes one of the major parts of therapy.

The Search   The patterns of social work agencies are changing. An observation made many years ago is that the adolescent adoptee very frequently indulges in a "search" for the "real" mother. The convention of closing the records and sealing them from parents and children alike is changing. It is too soon to know how critical the phenomenon of open records will be. It is at least apparent that many young people and young adults who start the search for their mothers end up only discovering their names and going no farther in making contact. So new is this practice that it will take time to evaluate the clinical meaning of the search phenomenon.

Divorce

It has recently been noted that if one assumes the traditional American family consists of a pair of young parents and two children, a boy and girl, then only 8 percent of American families fit this pattern. Divorce is the most common social action disrupting families. However, divorce does not occur in a vacuum. The parents who ultimately come to the conclusion that a total break and legal separation is necessary have usually been at odds over a period of time. During that period, the child or children are subjected to undue pressures. Loyalties are pulled in one direction or another, and the standard patterns of relationships to both parents are distorted. The assistance that the child needs from the mother or father may be unavailable.

It is scant wonder that the children of divorced parents find themselves struggling in the midst of a sea of parental passions and conflicting pulls. It is equally no wonder that the resiliency of children is strained. The actual occurrence of divorce, with the legal complications of custody and visiting rights, only strains the ties and feelings of the children further.

We have listed previously the classical behavior mechanisms that children demonstrate when under strain. Acting-out and violence on the one hand apathetic and withdrawn behavior on the other hand, and difficulties in learning, constitute the major triad of children's psychopathology. All these may become manifest at various times in children of divorced parents. Regression is common, nightmares are frequent, and asocial behavior occurs.

The physician has a different role in these settings. In addition to helping clarify the parents' attitudes toward the children, the critical objective may be to serve as a stable element in a situation that is marked by flux and unrest. Children cling to sameness and consistency in their lives. When these factors are upset by a major conflict between their parents, they turn to others. The school may very well be a haven. A doctor's office may be a place of solace. A physician who can offer something different as a model to the child may very well be of major assistance throughout a stormy period of life.

Psychosomatic Disorders

The complaints that parents bring to the physician about the growing child include a host of concerns about the body. This is a matter of generalities during the first year, but focuses on specifics very quickly. The primary areas of concern about the child are those related to the respiratory tract and the G. I. tract. The infant can demonstrate tension only through nonverbal clues. Crying, fussiness, irritability, vomiting, diarrhea, coughs, and chronic infections are part of this repertoire. The older child can point to parts of the body that hurt, can complain about them, often in infantile fashion, and can make bodily concerns clearer.

Much of the physician's time is spent sorting out these complaints. Of the complaints that bring children to physicians most often, a tremendous number relate to tensions and anxieties in the family situation.

"Bellyache" A strikingly clear symptom in the school-age child is that of abdominal pain. Occurring more often on those days following holidays or in relationship to stress in the family or school situation, complaints of "bellyache" plague the physician. Such complaints, however, are only paradigms for a host of other phenomena. A parent with an irritable, fussy child (age 7 to 9 months) is likely to assume that the child has an earache. Prompt help is sought from the physician. The problem may well be a change in sleep pattern that irritates the parent. Throughout childhood, complaints referrable to the throat, lungs, and belly serve as dramatic indices of other disturbances. All the tools of medical practice are useful in ferreting out the underlying cause. Critical, however, to the general physician are certain principles:

1 Pains or other symptoms that persist
2 Pains that seem totally out of proportion to any of the physical or physiologic findings
3 Dramatic changes or alterations in physical symptomatology

While all these serve as guidelines for parents in bringing the child to the physician, the physician must separate those symptoms which seem to have a physical basis from those which do not. Long-standing, persistent, severe physical complaints without a physical basis suggest referral to, or at least consultation with, a psychiatric practitioner.

It is important to note that, although physiologic symptoms make up a huge bulk of medical practice, many of them defy the ordinary reassurance and therapy that are customarily available. Unfortunately, many psychosomatic disorders begun in childhood may carry on with exaggeration in adolescence and a fixed pathology in adult life. They warrant early and skilled intervention at the earliest possible opportunity.

Clear-cut psychosomatic disorders are less common in early childhood than in adolescence and early adult life, where dramatic examples may be seen. However, the child with a chronic gastrointestinal disorder, the child with chronic asthma, and the child with any of a host of urticarial skin disorders, warrant consideration as examples of the effects which emotional disorders can have on bodily functions. It is critical at this time to consider the parents, the environment, and other aspects of the child's living conditions, in order to come to an adequate conclusion about the influence of emotions on the disorder presented in somatic form. Severe and lasting illnesses may well necessitate hospitalization in addition to psychiatric referral.

Death

While the incidence of acute infections which cause rapid death and high death rates has changed, the incidence of those illnesses which produce death in a slow and lingering fashion seems to be on the increase. This is particularly true of children with various forms of carcinoma, especially the leukemias. The care of such children, in cases where death seems inevitable, is largely a problem of hospital care. The principles of this care are becoming more evident.

One of these is truth. Physicians and others only fool themselves in concealing knowledge either from children or from their parents. While it is often difficult for parents to accept such diagnoses, ignorance or untruth only makes the problem worse.

A second principle is the sharing of knowledge. Parents, children, and others profit by group activities of all sorts. An interesting description of children on a chronic burn ward expressing their feelings in song has appeared in the literature. It demonstrates the value of shared group activities in hospital settings, where illnesses can give rise to chronic tension. Relief of anxiety through discussion groups is equally beneficial. Skill in leading such groups needs to be combined with a knowledge of the disease process involved.

The third principle relates to the attitudes of the hospital staff. Just as we expect children and parents to know the truth and to share, so the burden of caring for sick children warrants an open attitude that has not always been present. The burden of caring for children is a heavy one for staffs. They become attached to and identified with, the dying child. To assist them, the principles of group discussion, with open and free approaches to the problem, become critical.

It may well be of major importance to remember the lesson learned in the introduction to this chapter. Physicians, nurses, and others are human. Many of them are parents; all of them have been children. The problems, concerns, worries, and complaints that parents present to physicians stir up old feelings, especially guilt. All of these have to be coped with. In an ideal world, physicians themselves would have human sounding boards with whom to discuss their problems. In a somewhat less-than-ideal world, groups of physicians are banding together not only for peer review but also to offer each other solace and understanding.

Child Abuse

In discussing the disciplinary aspects of the parents' relationship with the growing child, it was noted that in many families a struggle begins very early in the child's life. The struggle is often expressed in terms of control. The growing body of knowledge about children who are abused physically and emotionally suggests an exaggeration of this all-too-common process.

The complexities of rearing children are great. For some parents, the process of child rearing is a burden that they are ill-equipped to handle. Such individuals are often described as immature. It is also important to recognize that parents have had their own needs, starting in childhood, which may or may not have been fulfilled. For some parents, the mere presence of a child in the home and the opportunity to care for it satisfies needs which were previously unmet. At times, however, one sees parents turning to the child for help and assistance. When this burden is too great for the child and the child becomes angry, irritable, or otherwise annoying, the parents turn on and punish the child, often brutally.

For three decades we have recognized the fact that children who are brought to emergency wards and other medical settings with severe injuries might be the victims of abusive actions on the part of their parents. These angry parental outbursts are often hidden. While medical skill can cope with the child's physical disabilities, to ferret out the disturbed relationship between the child and the parent is often an extremely complicated process. A great deal of denial, overt and covert, is evidenced by these parents. When accused of having damaged their child, they become defensive and belligerent.

Society's concern about child abuse has been so marked recently that special units in police departments, social agencies, and hospital clinics have been set up on a cooperative basis to deal with these battered children and their parents. Physicians would do well to know the resources for handling such problems in their own communities. Such resources warrant continued and intensive attention. The physician's role may include a healthy and legitimate suspicion of those instances where a family seems to be punishing the child excessively or where there is a repetitive injury that cannot easily be explained. Once more, the physician's knowledge of the family may prove to be the critical factor in leading to an appropriate diagnosis.

Infantile Autism

In the 1930s, several clinicians began to suspect that certain children who exhibited withdrawn and highly disturbed behavior might be suffering from psychoses similar to those seen in adults. Out of these suspicions has come a massive literature about psychotic, schizophrenic, and autistic children. The term *infantile autism,* first used by Kanner in the early 1940s, described a rather specific type of childhood psychosis, one which is usually present at an early stage yet is not always recognized.[2] The psychosis is characterized by withdrawn behavior, avoidance of parents and others, the unwillingness to be cuddled or cared for closely, and subsequent speech and language difficulties. Many autistic children do not develop language skills, and those that do often develop repetitive echolalic patterns of speech which are usually unrelated to the current situation. Many of these children develop strange, repetitive habits such as running about in circles.

The diagnosis, by virtue of the child's withdrawn behavior and unwillingness to be held and cuddled, can be made early. Unfortunately, many of these children are not diagnosed until well into their second or third year of life. It is not necessary to await the customary onset of speech to diagnose an infant who is aloof, noncuddly, or preoccupied.

The critical problem for the physician who is caring for the child and family is early diagnosis. There continue to be differences of opinion among leading authorities about the optimal treatment procedures for autistic children. all, however, agree that treatment should begin as early as possible, often in a hospital setting and involving parents as well as child. The prompt referral of such children is one of the critical phases of care and may lead to a modification of the disorder.

SPECIAL PROBLEMS

This section might well be entitled: What moves parents to seek help for their children? Children do not go to a physician complaining of anxiety states, misconduct, or even bed-wetting. They are brought to a physician's attention because the symptom bothers someone else, either a parent or teacher, and frequently both.

For many years the most common referral to a child psychiatrist or guidance clinic has been a 9- or 10-year-old boy who has been acting out in school. As noted before, school places a special set of stresses, involving both learning and conforming, that may give rise to a symptomatology that subsequently disturbs the teacher, interferes with the learning of others, and is generally considered to be both inappropriate and a cause for concern. In the past, such behavior was called an "adjustment reaction of childhood."

These conduct disorders come to the attention of physicians because of the concerns that they stir up in the adults who must cope with such a child. As we have already suggested, such problems do not arise in the school situation *de novo*. For that reason, the general principles of clarification, understanding within the family, elucidation of the learning problem, and understanding of the specific child and his or her response to the situation, stand as guidelines to the resolution of the difficulty.

Enuresis

In the preschool years and sometimes extending into school age, bed-wetting is a symptom which drives parents to seek help for their child, both through general medical channels and, at times, through psychiatric care. Enuresis is a symptom that extends back to antiquity; it has been known in the medical world for well over 3000 years. The variety of treatments for bed-wetting reflect prevailing medical thought concerning the cause of all disorders.

For the past 100 years the syndrome of enuresis, marked not only by the child's failure to control his or her urine, especially at night, but by all the attendant circumstances of wet beds, rotting mattresses, and foul smells, has been coped with primarily by mechanical methods and psychological approaches. The mechanical methods relate to the use of electricity to set off an alarm when the child's urine makes a connection with a device in the bed. This form of modification of behavior has more recently been utilized to fit into the general pattern of "behavior modification."

Within the last two decades, there has been an increased interest in drug therapy. Imipramine has been used with considerable success to modify the wetting pattern. It should be noted that earlier use of purely psychological approaches, which involved the child and his or her own concern about the symptoms along with reward efforts, also led to some success. Some believe that a combination of one of the electrical devices, plus the appropriate use of drugs, is the best approach to the problem.

Encopresis

Encopresis, or soiling, is generally considered to be a more serious problem of psychological disturbance than enuresis. Parental concern about encopresis often reaches a higher peak because it tends to be a daytime phenomenon, and the child becomes a pariah in the home, with friends, and in school. Drug treatment of children who soil has not been so successful as in the treatment of bedwetters, and therefore it is generally felt to be a more serious symptom requiring deeper psychiatric exploration.

By and large, children who soil have been doing so for some time prior to coming to the physician, and the symptom or syndrome is usually well ingrained. It is, therefore, considered more appropriate to make a referral for psychiatric exploration in these cases.

There are a variety of theories about this disorder, some of which relate to physical conditions such as *Hirschsprung's disease* or other diseases causing megacolon. In the uncomplicated case where there is no demonstrable bowel change, psychiatric evaluation, exploration, and family therapy have been of considerable efficacy.

Attention Deficit Disorders

This new diagnostic coding for children's disturbances marked by hyperactivity and difficulties in school has been described earlier. The approach is similar to other conduct disturbances and requires the unraveling of the family situation, as well as a clear understanding of the stresses posed by school. In addition, certain of these children were found through psychological testing to have difficulties in perception. Such difficulties are at times considered to be related to minimal brain damage, and the perceptual deficit is considered to be a developmental one. These children may respond to drug therapy, as noted. The response may be enhanced by a clear understanding of the stresses felt by the child and the manner in which the family is coping with the child's distress and concern about the learning difficulty (see Chapter 22).

Stuttering

Like enuresis, stuttering has a long and respectable history in medical care. Once again the number of theories about stuttering match the eras through which medical care has moved. From the point of the physician, the primary concern is evaluation rather than detailed speech diagnosis. This can be left to those with specialized training in the area. The physician who sees a child at an early stage in the development of this symptom is indeed in an important position since he or she has an opportunity to seek out the stresses and strains within the family and to see whether these can be alleviated promptly.

Once the symptom has become ingrained, it is often an intractable phenomenon, persisting into adult life. Theoretical knowledge and pedagogic approaches have grown so extensively that there is an entire professional field of speech and learning problems. Most pediatric centers have such centers available for diagnosis, evaluation, and therapy. It is important that a child with stuttering, stammering, or other manifestations or misarticulations, be referred as soon as possible for such diagnostic and evaluative care and treatment.

Phobias

As in all stages of life, the fears (both real and neurotic) of children match their age period. Early in the second year, children begin to express fears that are generally related to their immediate situation: fear of going to bed, fear of the dark, or fear of punishment. While it is obvious that some of these fears are tangible and real, often they persist beyond the immediacy of the situation that created them. The anxiety of separation (noted in earlier sections) may be manifest in a set of concerns that seem to be directed outward as the child grows. For example, parents may bring a child to the physician because the child seems afraid of the dark. Further investigation may suggest that what the child actually fears is the separation that occurs at the end of the day—leaving the company of adults and being placed in a room away from all the activity of the family.

Serious manifestations of fears are common in the preschool period. Some of these seem to relate to those aspects of growing up wherein the child feels incompetent, unworthy, small, or useless, and therefore resorts to fantasy. Sometimes these fantasies develop into worries about the outside world or other members of the family or friends. At times, such phobias are translated into worries about the child's own conduct. This leads to stereotyped behavior that becomes obsessive or even ritualistic. We are all well acquainted with children who worry about stepping on cracks. At times, however, worries about one's own conduct become so enormous that the child becomes paralyzed with the fear of doing anything outside a special ritualized procedure. Such rituals are usually highly specific to the child and to the individual environment. When parents seek help for such a child, the process has usually been going on for quite some time. It has become a focus of family concern and the approaches of evaluation and clarification within the family setting which we have described elsewhere become the first line of approach. Persistence of such symptoms suggests that referral for more extensive psychiatric care is warranted.

Eating Disturbances

One of the earliest concerns that often has a clear psychological aspect is that of a child's failure to eat. This is usually found during the second and third years of life. The physician who has followed such a child and the family will be aware of great parental concern about food, eating habits, or cleanliness. The child's active refusal to eat then becomes part of an overall pattern which must be looked at not only so far as the child is concerned, but in the family setting. Such children are often quite healthy, and a physical exam reveals no particular disabilities. The approach, then, is an understanding of the parents' need to force the issue of eating and an attempt to help them understand what the child is doing by presenting the symptom of failure to eat.

More serious complaints focus around abdominal pain or pain related to the digestive tract. These need a much more intensive and, at times, very comprehensive sorting-out process. Here again, however, the child may very well be using the symptom of pain to avoid some other situation in his or her daily life or within the family setting. The physician who has had an opportunity to follow such a child will be aware of the types of things that the child is seeking to avoid. At this point, direct counseling with the parents becomes the logical approach.

A very severe disorder of young children is that of *pica*. This disorder is manifested in abnormal eating patterns, particularly chewing on nonedible items, such as paint or metal. It is often of such severity that it requires intensive investigation. It may result in death (e.g., from lead poisoning). The syndrome has been attributed to a variety of circumstances, but it apparently occurs more often in lower socioeconomic settings where children are less stimulated, less involved, and are frequently left entirely to their own devices without adult attention. Obviously, investigation of the family setting and the mode in which the child lives is critical. Very often such children, understimulated and uninvolved, profit greatly from settings outside the home, such as day care centers or nursery schools, where the child may receive more attention.

Toward the end of the childhood period, one begins to see in some girls the severe symptom of *anorexia nervosa*. This symptom, usually appearing in early adolescence, is characterized by a near or total abstinence from food. It is a serious and severe syndrome that can be fatal. Prompt attention, hospital care, and extensive psychiatric intervention are warranted.

Depression in Childhood

Despite a host of fictional presentations about unhappy children, the concept of depression as a clear-cut childhood syndrome has only recently begun to appear in the psychiatric literature. The normally evanescent state of children's feelings, with quick ups and downs of affect, has mitigated against an understanding of the depths of unhappiness that can be manifested in childhood. The picture of depression as seen in adults, with complete sleep disorders, difficulty in eating, withdrawal, and chronic inability to respond, is not, however, common in childhood.

It is apparent that many children, particularly those in the 6- to 12-year-old range, in addition to a presenting complaint of conduct disturbance, learning disorder, or enuresis, show profound worries and anxieties about themselves. Such anxiety is quickly seen in the consultation room as a mixture of both sadness and anger. The predominance of the angry symptoms often masks the sense of aloneness that is characteristic of such children. Many children do feel isolated within the world of their peers as well as within their families. Many children express anger toward their parents by entering a sullen, withdrawn state. They are characterized as "loners" by their peers. They are often ignored by teachers (who are more concerned about the child whose disturbance is manifested in aggressive activity) and are, therefore, left completely alone. For years, it has been pointed out that in school, boys tend to misbehave, and girls to withdraw. These withdrawal symptoms are now being seen more clearly to be manifestations of both anger and depression and should be treated in such a fashion.

Depression is an excellent example of a symptom which needs detailed investigation, either in an individual setting through psychological tests, or as part of a family evaluation. Such evaluation may lead to a recognition that the child is not only fighting outwardly in an aberrant form, but is also withdrawing and becoming more and more angry. As with its care in adults, the treatment of depression in childhood is very often a matter that demands time and extensive care. Some children's symptoms are severe enough to warrant care in a residential setting.

Care outside the Home

The use of residential care is most appropriate where circumstances within the family seem to be of a nature that will lead to persistence of the symptoms, rather than offering the child an opportunity to improve. Deeply depressed and angry children often need to be taken out of a specific home situation and placed in residential care, where their immediate symptoms can be understood and dealt with quickly. The trend in psychiatric care is generally to try to avoid hospitalization or residential care for children. To accomplish this, however, requires a great deal of professional work with families, often in the homes, and the use of group work as well as family-centered therapy. A decision to place a child outside the home usually comes about when symptoms persist. Depressed and angry feelings are particularly important clues to the presence of a severe internalized disorder of the child that may warrant extensive care, often outside the family setting.

Referral

Giving up a patient is not always an easy thing for a physician to do. The rapid changes that occur in the child's development make it at times difficult to focus on the intensity and importance of any single symptom. The concept of growth inspires the feeling, "He'll grow out of it" or "She won't do that for long."

It is true that symptoms do change with the passage of years. However, the appreciation of unhealthy family situations, abnormal school settings, and poor socioeconomic environments often does not change, and the child merely progresses from one symptom to another with increasing anxiety, concern, anger, and depression. Simple rules of thumb concerning the time for referral relate primarily to the intensity and chronicity of any single symptom. All the symptoms and syndromes which have been outlined above may not reach the physician's office until after they have been present for a long period of time. It is important to try to understand, to evaluate, to clarify these symptoms as quickly as possible. A noticeable response to such intervention suggests that improvement may well occur.

Very often, however, symptoms are chronic in nature and resistant to such exploration. When this is the case, it may be necessary to seek help elsewhere. The current body of psychological and mental health knowledge is broad and has been embraced by a variety of professionals. Psychologists perform testing procedures to help understand the child in the family context. Social workers assist with the evaluation of the family in its environment. Teachers, speech therapists, and a host of other allies have positions of importance in dealing with children's problems.

Children's therapeutic settings have tended to be multiprofessional. In a team approach to health, the focus is on the child and the family, as well as on the home and community setting. Such a principle is both efficient and rewarding. It is incumbent upon those in the treatment setting to keep in touch with the referring physician, teacher, or parent not only in order to alleviate the child's difficulty, but in order to pave the way for the child's resumption of normal life patterns.

Fortunately, the focus of interest in professional mental health care has shifted from the clinic and the hospital to the community. The newer methods of care match more closely the approach which has always been part and parcel of good medical care. Efforts on the part of professionals in the mental health field to understand the child in his or her family context, in the school setting, and in a natural setting have paid dividends in more efficient care of children. The newer involvement of professionals in the community has meant a shift in patterns of mental health care which has tended to be more economical in the long run. The individual physician who knows the family, has followed the child's progress, and is prepared to understand the child in a very natural setting may well make the role of the mental health consultant more useful.

POSTSCRIPT

Most of the references to medical care in the field of emotional and behavioral disorders in childhood suggest that the physician's greatest medical tool is his or her own abilities. Much depends upon a broad knowledge of development, understanding of family relations, and a true concern about the emotional stability of the child as well as the child's position in the family. Physicians are only human, and they too have gone through all these stages of growth. At times, our own memories, whether conscious or unconscious, of certain phases of our own growth make us uncomfortable in dealing with parents who bring a disturbed child to us. It is a truism that the more a physician knows about his or her own past, the better the physician will be able to deal with presenting problems in the emotional and behavioral area.

The physician may also wish to have special knowledge of certain treatment procedures. Pharmacological approaches are widely used but should be thought of as supportive actions in relation to most childhood pathology. More recently, a host of uses of "behavioral modification" or "behavior therapy" have become available to those who deal with children. They are not necessarily difficult therapeutic tools, but they do require some special training before being used.

A common feeling in dealing with children is that if one waits long enough, the problem will go away. While this is not an unwarranted approach, the concept "He'll grow out of it" is a useful solace that is not necessarily true. There is a definite tendency toward maturation in the developmental process which has its own healing power. On the other hand, the physician who is confronted with a family where the tensions are overt and continuous must consider whether or not the child is going to respond to these tensions by developing behavioral symptoms. Brief, episodic variations from normal development are common; development itself occurs in a steplike process including continuous relationships with others. However, when one is confronted by a behavioral symptom, it is better to look for the causes rather than to sit back and wait for it to go away.

Children grow.

This chapter started with this admonition. Normal growth is a productive process. To support, to stimulate, to redirect at times yet try always to undestand, may be the most valuable contributions that the physician who is dealing with the family can possibly offer.

REFERENCES

1   Wender, Paul H.: *The Hyperactive Child,* New York: Crown Publishers, 1973.
2   Kanner, Leo: *Child Psychiatry,* 3d ed., Springfield, Ill.: Charles C Thomas, 1957.

BIBLIOGRAPHY

Adams, Paul L.: *Obsessive Children,* New York and Baltimore: Penguin Books, 1973.
Advisory Committee on Child Development, Assembly of Behavioral and Social Sciences, National Research Council: *Toward a National Policy for Children and Families,* Washington, D.C.: National Academy of Sciences, 1976.
Allen, R. P. et al.: "Behavior Therapy for Socially Ineffective Children," *Am. J. Child Psychiatry,* **14:**500–509, 1975.
———: *A Primer of Child Psychotherapy,* Boston: Little, Brown, 1974.
American Medical Association and the American Academy of Pediatrics: *Growing Pains,* Chicago: American Medical Association, 1969.
Cantwell, Dennis P.: "Genetic Factors in the Hyperkinetic Syndrome," *Am. J. Child Psychiatry,* **15:**214–223, 1977.
Cohen, D. J., and J. G. Young: "Neurochemistry and Child Psychiatry," *Am. J. Child Psychiatry,* **16:**353–411, 1977.
Committee on Adoption and Dependent Care: *Adoption of Children,* Evanston, Ill.: American Academy of Pediatrics, 1973.
Committee on Child Psychiatry: *Psychopathological Disorders in Childhood: Theoretical Considerations and a Proposed Classification,* New York: Group for the Advancement of Psychiatry, **6:**62, 1966.

Committee on Children with Handicaps: *Pediatrician and the Child with Handicaps,* Evanston, Ill.: The American Academy of Pediatrics, 1971.

Guttman, H. A.: "The Child's Participation in Conjoint Family Therapy," *Am. J. Child Psychiatry,* **14**:490–499, 1975.

Lidz, Theodore: *The Person: His Development throughout the Life Cycle,* New York: Basic Books, 1968.

Looff, David H.: *Getting to Know the Troubled Child,* Knoxville: University of Tennessee Press, 1976.

Rexford, Eveoleen N. et al.: *Infant Psychiatry: New Synthesis,* New Haven and London: Yale University Press, 1976.

Strauss, Susan: *Is It Well with the Child?* Garden City, N.Y.: Doubleday, 1975.

Wing, Lorena: *Autistic Children,* New York: Brunner/Mazel, 1972.

Chapter 8

Adolescence

Robert Michels, M.D.
Everett P. Dulit, M.D.

EDITORS' INTRODUCTION

What is it like to be an early pubertal girl with budding breasts and to wait in an examining room for the new doctor to whom your mother has brought you for your precamp examination? How does it feel when the physician makes some offhand joking remark about changing body characteristics? What about the early adolescent boy with a cracking voice and a need to prove he is really a man when he is entering a hospital for surgery and is ashamed to admit he is terribly frightened? To most adolescents, these and other events present threats which evoke strong and mixed feelings. The treating physician who is sensitive to the needs and problems of adolescents is in a key position to aid these patients in treading difficult pathways. This is particularly so if physicians refuse to get caught up in the stimulus responses that adolescents especially are able to elicit, and if they recognize that the "fight" in adolescents is actually "fright" in adolescents.

In dealing with adolescent patients, physicians should be aware that we often have our personal conflicts of many years past stirred up; the adolescents may revive the feelings that we experienced as painful social ineptness or frightening tumultuousness. Too often the physician carries into the room a third person—the physician as an adolescent.

Physicians are products of their past. They have grown up in a culture that no longer exists, a culture as remote as that of a foreign land. As Michels and Dulit point out in the following chapter, many adults, including physicians, may have difficulty accepting the present, seemingly open culture with its bold and vivid media and dramatically changing mores, including dress, innovative language, styles of commitment, and "hanging loose." To attempt to "get with it" can only result in a sham performance played against the screen of a physician's lingering and unresolved personal conflicts. Adolescents value genuineness, even if it is from a position of the "way it used to be."

For these and many other reasons, the adolescent, who is often caught on the ledge between childhood and adulthood, is difficult for professionals to handle. The formation of an effective treatment relationship, actually a treatment alliance, may founder because of the rapid, frequently indecipherable changes in the adolescent patient's mood, thought processes, and behavior, and the physician's reaction to them.

In addition to the global impact of adolescence on many of us, there are themes that peak during adolescence that can impinge selectively on some of us. The struggle of dependency versus autonomy as an either/or situation, the impulse gratification, and the need for emancipation may indeed be disturbing.

Another variable of potential impact is the physician's age. How close is he or she in time to these normative conflicts? How much influence is the physician's current struggle with his or her own children having? How much does the adolescent provoke "what might have been"? So often the physician expresses a sense of "if only now were then" regarding the greatly increased sexual freedom.

Michels and Dulit have brought the reader with them into their clinical practice. This chapter not only relates to the most frequent emotional disturbances experienced by adolescents, but should also help physicians to be mindful of the rather unique stresses that the adolescent experiences when faced with physical examinations and medical illness.

INTRODUCTION

Adolescents can be difficult—for parents, for teachers, for physicians, for anyone who has to work with them. They are beyond the charm and the compliance of childhood, but not yet into the control and the conventional courtesy of adulthood. They can come on as frosty and sullen, or they can suddenly turn uncontrollably giggly, especially when talking about bodies or sex. Often emotional and given to emotional swings, they can be enormously concerned about things that seem to adults like minutia, and be completely indifferent to much more serious issues relating to their health, their bodies, and their welfare. They can be acutely uncomfortable in having to deal with adults, and that discomfort can be so hard for adults to tolerate or dispel that it may block all effective communication. They can approach encounters with an "official adult" with so strong an expectation of being misunderstood, criticized, and patronized as to generate reactions in adults that make things happen exactly that way. They can be smug, irreverent, disrespectful, outrageous, scornful, contemptuous, and, what is worse, enjoy it.

Armed with a belief about what is right and what is wrong, they can become fanatic in their zeal, and ride roughshod over what most adults would regard as plain realities. Armed with some freshly discovered belief, they can be intolerably patronizing. And while they may not yet be willing or able to function as adults, neither are they willing to be "treated like kids."

Whence comes this creature? From what combination of circumstances?

PUBERTY

Adolescence has a well-defined beginning and an ill-defined ending. It begins with a biological event, puberty. It ends by shading off gradually into young adulthood.

The onset of puberty is programmed internally in the hypothalamic-pituitary-gonadal system. The entire process takes about 2 to 4 years, from the first signs to completion of physical growth and other associated changes. The age of onset is distributed over a statistical curve, with some youngsters beginning early and others beginning late. The growth spurt, a significant middle point in the process, is on the average about 13 years for girls and about 14.5 years for boys. Thus, girls mature on the average about 1½ years earlier than boys. This is strikingly apparent in the sixth and seventh grades, where a goodly proportion of the girls begin to look like young women, and most of the boys, by sharp contrast, still look like children. The majority of boys and girls reach puberty within a year or two of these averages.

Most youngsters who mature early or late represent nothing more than extremes of normal statistical variation. A small proportion of youngsters who mature very early or very late represent cases of endocrine pathology, and only some of those can benefit from hormonal therapy. Distinctions are best made, when indicated, by the experienced adolescent endocrinologist. Very early and very late puberty are, regardless of cause, psychological hazards. *Precocious puberty* (for example, puberty before age 10) introduces into childhood an element that tends to be experienced as "freaky" and embarrassing, which complicates the experience of living and growing up for a youngster, and can linger long thereafter in fantasies and feelings. One 35-year-old woman, a stable, effective person who was in treatment for marital difficulties revealed that she had had breast budding and menarche at about 8 and 9, and remembered feeling "terribly weird, like some kinda freak, like I was being dirty or something. My mother was obviously terribly uncomfortable with it." Some of these feelings persisted as a core element in the pronounced sexual self-consciousness from which she suffered, with resulting difficulties in the marriage. Slightly early puberty can also be awkward, but usually the associated feelings are more readily converted into a kind of pride at having been "first on the block," especially after the others have begun to catch up and one is not alone.

A delayed puberty places the youngster in an exceedingly difficult position, especially in a society that further intensifies already intense adolescent preoccupations with the body, secondary sexual characteristics, and competitive comparison. As Tanner has pointed out, physical development may take place more rapidly during its initial surge *in utero* and in early infancy, but it is only in this final surge of growth and change during puberty that "the subject himself is the fascinated, charmed, or horrified spectator that watches" the proceedings.[1] Late puberty deserves to be regarded as a major psychological trauma for adolescents. It behooves parents and physicians to do their best, with grace and tact, to soften the impact of that trauma by telling such youngsters in ways they can hear and believe that by the time they complete puberty, they will "be the same as anyone else." However, to have to live in a child's body for months that seem like years while everyone else your age has long since acquired a much more interesting and impressive body is hard to endure. Worse, it is an organizing experience that attracts to itself fantasies and feelings, with effects on self-esteem that linger long past adolescence. One 16-year-old boy had a brother 2 years younger who had matured earlier and looked older than he did. The patient came into treatment after a suicide attempt precipitated by finding out that a popular girl in the school who had been unexpectedly open to him had really been trying to wangle an introduction to his "good-looking older brother." Another patient, a man of 28, was still struggling in his social life with the conviction that he "wasn't as good as the others" in a way he related directly to the painful experience of a strikingly late puberty.

The question often arises as to whether or not the onset of puberty can be influenced by psychological factors. Although menstruation can be suppressed by emotional factors and physical growth can be affected by faulty nutrition related to general neglect, the evidence is that this particular internal clock is minimally or not at all vulnerable to the influence of psychological factors.

It usually takes a youngster about 2 to 4 years to go through puberty. The component features of the process, in the order in which they usually occur, are:

For girls: breast budding, straight pigmented pubic hair, maximum growth rate, kinky pubic hair, menstruation, axillary hair
For boys: beginning testicular growth, straight pigmented pubic hair, penile enlargement, early voice changes, first ejaculation, kinky pubic hair, maximum growth rate, axillary hair, marked voice change, development of beard

Note that breast budding is usually the first sign of puberty in girls, that maximum growth rate and first menstruation or first ejaculation all tend to come somewhere in the middle, and that lush axillary hair tends to mark an endpoint.

There is a quality of finality to the ending of puberty. Physical characteristics directly related to bone growth, such as facial features, principal body proportions, and overall height become what they will remain "forever," a real-life embodiment for the late adolescent of "all ye who enter here, abandon hope" of any subsequent change. One becomes locked into one's frame, for better or worse. That can make the ending of puberty a life event with major psychological repercussions, particularly for the child who has been constantly hoping for something distinctly better or different, and now has to accept that "this is it."

STAGES OF ADOLESCENCE

Given the rapid rate of change through these years, psychological development in adolescence is conveniently and usefully subdivided into early, middle, and late stages. These categories are not sharply defined at the edges, but are well enough defined at their centers, with each representing a recognizably different cluster of psychological trends and central themes.

Early adolescence occurs roughly at ages 12 through 14, the junior high school years. Middle adolescence is at about ages 15 through 17, the high school years. Late adolescence is roughly at ages 17 through 20, and shades off gradually into young adulthood. These ages are intended only as approximate. Early, middle, and late are best defined by the following characteristics.

Early adolescence is dominated by the biological event of puberty and its immediate psychological repercussions. It is a time of emotional lability, of "normal abnormality." For most youngsters, the relative calm of the latency years is shattered by the impact of puberty, and the calm is replaced typically by the much more edgy quality of inner turmoil that is barely held in check, that is under strain and regularly breaking through. The easy vitality of childhood, which is laced through with good feelings bubbling up, changes its character, and is now more often frantic and frenetic, now more often shot through with anxiety and tension. These are the years of tears and tantrums for no apparent reason, of overreactions and of rushing off in a huff, of mysterious moods understood by no one, including the adolescent. Emotions run rampant; unpredictability is the rule. This is the age at which one may see episodes of frank cruelty that are much less common earlier or later. Because these youngsters are past the compliance and openness of the childhood years and are not yet into the appreciably greater sense and stability of middle adolescence, this age range is probably the most difficult to work with psychologically. In many ways, the young adolescent is the quintessential adolescent; betwixt and between, very much in turmoil.

Middle adolescence is marked by a distinct settling down, a greater capacity for composure and compromise, and the advent of a more civilized and complex way of relating to adults. Feelings come under control better. Thinking is noticeably more mature, and encompasses much more of the all-important capacity to appreciate the inner logic of a point of view that is not one's own. Self-absorption begins to give way to a greater capacity to become absorbed once again in work. The defensively charged total commitment to "my peer group, right or wrong," so characteristic of early adolescence, begins to give way to a more differentiated response and to a greater capacity to cope with pressures from the group and from individuals within the group, including the critically important capacity to stand separate from the group. In general, it becomes easier to work things out with middle adolescents—in the family, in school, and in the office (not easy, but easier).

Finally, building on the more stable platform represented by middle adolescence, young people begin to work at "getting themselves together," a phrase nicely evocative of what is probably the single most important psychological task of *late adolescence,* that is, *identity formation.* This refers to putting together into one relatively unique, coherent package, which we call the "psychological self," all the diverse strands of constitutional givens, developmental experiences, patterns of coping, stylistic preferences, partial iden- tifications, characteristic defenses, and chosen roles that have been developing rather more separately through a couple of decades of living. This is psychological work that comes to the fore in late adolescence. The self and sense of self, the identity that emerges can be conceptualized as the public and private answer that each person works out to the question so characteristic of these years: "Who am I?" The best answer to that question, which is a fully realized and stable identi- ty, is (like most of the achievements of later development) achieved partially by many, and achieved fully only by some.

Late adolescence is a time of making choices. Work and career lines begin to take shape in ways that are increasingly difficult to reverse. Personality structure begins to crystallize into forms that are likely to endure through the remainder of life in a way that is mostly a happening but partially a choice. If middle adolescence is, as one scholar expressed it, a time of "omnipotentiality," then late adolescence is a time of closing doors, of going one way and not the other, and of having some sense that fateful choices are being made, fateful turns being taken. The feeling is expressed by Robert Frost:

> Two roads diverged in a yellow wood
> And sorry I could not travel both
> And be one traveler, long I stood
> And looked down one as far as I could
> To where it bent in the undergrowth
> . . . .
> Then took the other as just as fair
> And having perhaps the better claim
> . . . .
> Oh, I kept the first for another day
> Yet knowing how way leads on to way
> I doubted if I should ever come back.
>
> I shall be telling this with a sigh
> Somewhere ages and ages hence:
> Two roads diverged in a wood, and I—
> I took the one less traveled by,
> And that has made all the difference.[2]

What forces lie behind the stages just described? It is the *biological event* of puberty that initiates the process, *psychological reactions* to that event that dominate in early adolescence, *psychological work* done through early and mid- dle adolescence that brings about the characteristic settling down of middle adolescence, and *social forces* that play a critical role in pressing the late adoles- cent to "get it all together" into a package that will work in the outside world of adulthood. The study of adolescence provides a good example of a behavioral phenomenon within which one sees an interaction of biological, psychological, and social forces, with each playing a major role, and no one factor dominating the others appreciably. It represents an example in which the mix is uncommonly even. Let us trace a few of the important subthemes within that process.

Psychoanalytic perspectives on adolescent development stress the impact of the sudden surge of sexual and aggressive drives riding the crest of the wave of the hormonal events of puberty, with the characteristic moderating effect of ego functions so characteristic of the years of latency temporarily overcome in early adolescence by the surge of inner events. In the Freudian metaphor of id as horse and ego as rider, the horse bolts and the rider is left behind. Ego is running to catch up, but remains a poor second through early adolescence. Associated with this surge of sexual and aggressive feelings is a reactivation of forbidden unconscious Oedipal fantasies, which were previously active in early childhood, were much less so during latency, and are now to the fore again. This time they are all the more real for being in a body that is increasingly adult in size and capacities. Because it is intensely threatening to ego and superego, this provokes a defensive counterreaction, which contributes to the sense of inner strain so characteristic of this time of life. These defenses against Oedipal fantasies motivate the adolescent to seek distance from the parents. Being close stirs up too much discomfort. It is at this time that parents get hit with the classic stream of accusations: "old-fashioned," "impossible," "unfair," "You just don't understand," "How did I ever get stuck with—" etc. It is a process that is notoriously hard on parents, but it is a normal, even necessary one to some degree. It tends to simmer down, to everyone's relief (adolescents included) by middle and late adolescence.

Another key casualty of the upheaval of early adolescence is the superego, that cluster of moral standards that is internalized during childhood out of love and identification with the parents and parental surrogates, and that becomes subject, as the parents do themselves, to the same process of scornful questioning, reevaluation, and sometimes precipitous abandonment. Both superego and parents are replaced for a while, at least partially, by the standards of the peer group.

Another perspective on development through these years is provided by the study of the development of intelligence. Adolescence brings the potential for a vast expansion in the capacity for abstraction, and for hypothetico-deductive, logical thinking. The forms of thinking mastered by the latency-age child stay rather close to the concrete facts of experience, and tend to organize those facts in terms of the very basic concepts of class and serial order. New and much more powerful cognitive forms begin in early adolescence, especially for about one-third of the normal population, for whom this form of thinking becomes particularly well developed. Thinking in this stage comes to be cast in terms of a network of the full range of possibilities that are implicit in a problem. This network is generated by abstracting from the real-life situation all the essential variables, and then running them through all possible combinations of values. These are the years when one sees the shift from thinking mostly about things (*concrete stage* of thought, characteristic of childhood) to a vastly expanded capacity for thought about words, concepts, hypotheses, ideas, and systems (*formal stage* of thought, characteristic of adolescence and adulthood). With the expansion of mental horizons to include the full range of "what could be," the formal-stage adolescent begins to think of concrete actualities as "mere special cases," a reversal of priorities from the situation that prevailed in childhood, where facts and concrete actualities have top priority in the learning and thinking process. That crucial shift of emphasis from "what is" to "what could be" provides cognitive underpinning to phenomena as diverse as the familiar surge in adolescence of interest in ideas and ideology, as the special commitment to things that "could be, but are not" basic to adolescent idealism, and the difficulty even the experienced clinician sometimes has in distinguishing incipient schizophrenic thought disorder in adolescence from extreme but basically normal adolescent flights of abstraction.

Sexual development in adolescence merits special attention. For girls, the onset of menstruation is a physical and psychological landmark of paramount importance. For most girls in our culture, the first menstrual period rarely comes as a surprise, and seems to be taken in stride more often than some of the older literature would suggest. Yet at deeper levels, it invariably is an event with profound psychological implications. There are the pitfalls inherent in the troublesome fantasies inevitably associated with blood, with discharge from one's "bottom," and with any uncontrollable event in one's body. Above all, there is the enormous range of feelings and fantasies about the transition from girlhood to womanhood, and about the suddenly real possibility of actually being able to have a baby born from one's own body.

For boys, first ejaculation plays a somewhat similar role and marks the transition from boyhood to sexual manhood. Studies suggest that this takes place most often in the form of masturbation and somewhat less often in the form of a nocturnal emission (a "wet dream").[3] Parents are not so likely to talk in advance with their sons about nocturnal emissions as they are to talk with their daughters about menarche; nor are physicians and nurses. They should. Yet most boys do not seem to experience nocturnal emissions as unsettling, probably because it is either preceded by ejaculation deliberately sought through masturbation, or is discovered the next morning in the form of "something starchy" on the pajamas, and is sometimes not connected with "what it must have been" until some time later. If the discovery takes place while the semen is still wet and sticky, it may be more unsettling, and an associative link with bed-wetting can be troubling if that has been an issue.

For boys, masturbation to orgasm usually begins in early or middle adolescence. Failure to have begun by late adolescence tends to be associated with conflicts about the body and about sexuality that are often quite responsive to consultation. Normal frequency of masturbation varies widely from a few times per week to daily. Unusually high rates (e.g., many times per day) suggest the syndrome of *compulsive masturbation.* An even more reliable sign of that syndrome is masturbation that is more driven than gratifying, more a search for relief of anxiety than a search for pleasure. Among adolescent girls, older data show about 20 percent masturbating by middle adolescence and 60 percent by late adolescence. Modern studies suggest a moderate rise in those percentages.[4] But lower frequencies and percentages remain the rule among young women, by contrast with males. As a consequence, the information that a young woman has never or hardly ever masturbated is much less reliably associated with sexual anxiety. Nonetheless, the physician is in an excellent position to be a benign and supportive voice regarding sexual self-exploration by adolescents, male and female. Although most adolescents do not feel comfortable bringing up the subject, or making an "incriminating" admission even if the doctor is the one who brings the subject up, some passing benign remark like: "Most kids sooner or later . . ." and "Some people still have the idea that maybe it's harmful in some way, which of course it isn't," or even "It's a very private thing of course, but something most people your age do and enjoy" are usually mildly helpful, especially if the doctor is comfortable and sounds that way.

According to some recent data, 5 to 10 percent of young people have begun to have intercourse in early adolescence, about 30 to 40 percent by middle adolescence, and about 50 percent by the age of 18 or 19.[5] Physicians are in a key position to be helpful with information, advice, and practical assistance regarding contraception, venereal disease, pregnancy, and abortion, but only if they are able to develop a working relationship with adolescent patients, and are accepting of and comfortable with adolescent sexuality. Most young people can be expected to be wary and uncertain of discussing their sexuality with an adult; it is up to physicians to be comfortable, skillful, and knowledgeable enough to make it possible for a useful interchange to take place.

To summarize this section, early adolescence is thus a time of tumult, middle adolescence a time of settling down, and late adolescence a time of making choices and of forging an identity with which to move forward to young adulthood.

The psychological work of adolescence can be conceptualized as a series of tasks that one works through to get from early to late adolescence: mastering the surge of sexuality and aggression, working through the progressive separation and increasing independence from the family while yet maintaining a necessary and meaningful connection with it, developing cognitive skills and other talents to a level of significant accomplishment, and moving into young adulthood by forging some relatively coherent and unique sense of personal identity.

These are the main themes, and they are a useful beginning for a framework within which to order the data presented by adolescents who are seen in practice. But main themes are only a beginning. The physician must also develop, through experience and reading, a working sense of the range of normal variation, and a sense of the distinction between pathological exceptions and benign exceptions. For example, for most youngsters the main theme of tumult and turmoil in early adolescence is markedly present only intermittently, and is effectively moderated much of the time by the operation of normal adaptive functions that help them to "roll with the punches." For some youngsters, coping skills and defensive capacities operate so effectively that they present a moderated picture all the time, even though good interviewing might disclose that much inner work is going on to achieve that outcome. Though some degree of strain and breakthrough is commonplace for the broad range of normal adolescents, when that turmoil seems exaggerated or unrelieved, one may be dealing with a disturbed adolescent, with an impaired capacity to do the psychological work of moderating essentially normal inner surges. When the tumult is altogether absent, one may be seeing pathological repression and suppression of the normal inner surges of adolescence, as in the highly obsessional child who goes through adolescence as a tightly overcontrolled automaton, and is sometimes described as "perfectly behaved" by parents or teachers, although often more perceptively identified by others as "a bit too well behaved" or "too good to be true." Such youngsters essentially bypass the growth experience of psychological adolescence and are at risk for a constricted adulthood lived within obsessional armor. In differentiating normal from pathological adolescence, it helps to look at the course of development over time, which the physician can do by seeking developmental past history, and by making a point of encouraging brief follow-up reports and visits. Where there is a sense of forward movement and progressive mastery, one can be hopeful despite the presence of difficulties. Where the situation seems stalled developmentally and there is minimal adaptive effectiveness in many key areas, notably in the areas of family, friends, and school, there are ample grounds for concern, and it is best to seek consultation.

THE ADOLESCENT AS PATIENT

Adolescents do not think that they should be patients, and most of us agree with them. The patient role is contradictory with the new identity that they are in the process of forging, and this contradiction is central to adolescents' experience as patients and to our experience in treating them. They know that their bodies are changing; they are involved in consolidating new images of their physical selves and do not want to have to worry about defects or diseases that are affecting their bodies. They are just negotiating the transition from dependency on parents to relative autonomy, and are distressed by any threat to that autonomy that pushes them back toward dependency. The adolescent is immensely private, and being a patient is like inviting caretakers to invade one's privacy. Adolescents are concerned about preserving their omnipotentiality, and disease threatens to limit it.

The first consequence of these themes is that adolescents avoid being patients, and the clinical significance of that avoidance is important. They will often disguise or conceal symptoms, ignore treatment, defy prescriptions, and act in accordance with an inner personal idea of health rather than a painful reality of disease. The doctor may have to reach out to an adolescent who ought to be a patient in order to coax, urge, or persuade him or her to accept the patient role. For example, an astute family practitioner noted that an adolescent girl who occasionally accompanied her diabetic grandmother to his office began to come more regularly and to ask casual questions about her grandmother's disease, especially whether or not it ran in families. One day the physician invited her to come in for a minute after her grandmother's appointment, and learned that she was frightened that a mild burning she had developed upon urination was a symptom of diabetes. She had told no one about her symptom, and as a result had received no treatment. The physician was able to reassure her, make the diagnosis of cystitis, and treat it. Later, after she had recovered, he arranged to talk with her again and begin a process of health education by teaching her something about cystitis and diabetes and, perhaps more important, something about how to be a patient with a doctor.

This reluctance about becoming a patient means that the adolescent often comes to the doctor as a result of being brought by parents or perhaps referred by a school. This is routine for younger children, and the physician characteristically establishes a primary relationship with the parents of the young child, with the child as the locus of the illness but not really as the client of the caretaker. It is particularly important not to do this with the adolescent. The parents or other escort may be seen purely as a route into treatment, but the physician must establish a primary therapeutic relationship with the adolescent. This is not only because to do so recognizes the phase-appropriate striving for autonomy, but also because of the much more pragmatic reason that the adolescent patient has the capacity and often the motivation to obstruct treatment. If the physician fails to be sensitive to this and to deal with it directly, the likelihood of the patient being helped is diminished. The doctor can establish this relationship in little ways from the very first minute of contact. For example, the patient should always be seen alone as well as with parents, and, frequently, seen alone before being seen with parents. The history, the diagnosis, and the treatment plan should always be discussed directly with the adolescent patient, although the parent may be present and may participate. Many parents will try to establish the primary interaction between themselves and the doctor, and many doctors are more comfortable with such an arrangement. However, its effect is to give the adolescent patient only one way to express independence and maturity, and that is by defying both parent and doctor and refusing to accept the childish role they are both offering him.

INTERVIEWING THE ADOLESCENT PATIENT

The interview with the adolescent patient requires the doctor to cope with some-one who is not simply halfway between child and adult, but is also both at the same time. Flexibility is a central requirement, as the patient shifts in seconds, with maturity varying from moment to moment as, for example, the voice of the pubertal boy shifts within a single sentence. An example is the pregnant, unmar-ried, late-adolescent girl who in the same meeting with her doctor tried to decide whether or not she was going to have an abortion and disclosed that she still went to sleep each night with a treasured toy animal.

Adolescence has a distinguishing language, with slang terms and phrases that differentiate it from the language of adults. An immediate question results—in what language should the health professional speak to the adolescent patient?

Some doctors who work extensively with adolescents learn and talk their language because it has become part of the doctor's natural behavior (a participant observer in a foreign culture always develops traits and mannerisms of that culture). For the rest of us, the question is whether we should try to talk and sound like adolescents when we are working with them. The doctor should be interested in the language and customs of the patient, and in this respect the adolescent is like any other patient. However, one striking general characteristic of adolescents is their intolerance of sham or hypocrisy, and the high value they place on authenticity. The doctor who feigns comfort with adolescent language is more likely to be experienced by an adolescent patient as a fake or as insincere rather than as "one of the gang." Since adults frequently try to penetrate the generational barrier with adolescents in order to gain their trust, this behavior is in fact typically adult rather than adolescent. The doctor should show regard for adolescent culture by accepting its highest value, being true to oneself. The adolescent patient has little difficulty with the stuffy or old-fashioned doctor who is genuinely, spontaneously, authentically, and honestly stuffy and old-fashioned. The adolescent is far less comfortable should this same doctor try to use contemporary slang by asking whether he or she is "letting it all hang out" or "getting it all together," or perhaps whether the adolescent has smoked any "reefers." One of the problems with trying to use slang is, of course, that last year's slang is far more out of date than Chaucerian English, and the slang the doctor knows is likely to be last year's.

The interview with the adolescent patient raises more difficult problems of confidentiality than does the interview with either child or adult. With the child, there is seldom a question, there is little the child is likely to disclose that the parents have an interest in knowing and that the child has an interest in withholding—the child's secrets are more likely to seem trivial than shocking to parents, and the unconscious meaning of the secrets probably would not be believed anyway. With the adult patient, the rules of medical ethics are clear and compelling. But what does a doctor do when a 13-year-old reveals that she is having sexual intercourse without her parents' knowledge and wants contraceptive advice, or when a 15-year-old indicates that he is involved in the use of addictive drugs and criminal behavior in order to obtain the necessary money? The discussion of the ethical problems raised by these examples goes beyond the scope of this book, but they illustrate the special problems of treating adolescent patients, problems experienced by both doctor and patient. From the point of view of the interview, it helps to keep in mind that these are shared problems, and that they should be shared with the patient. This will often initiate a discussion of the patient's relationship with parents and, if indicated, of adjustments in that relationship that might be appropriate in view of the adolescent's problems. Even if this suggestion about adjustment is not successful, it promotes an open and honest discussion between doctor and patient, and gives the patient an opportunity to recognize the doctor's dilemma. In doing so, the patient may come to see the doctor's respect for the patient's rights. The doctor accepts the patient's right to confidentiality, but recognizes that that right has limits. However, the doctor also recognizes that the patient has a right to know the limit of his or her rights to confidentiality. When the doctor believes that the patient's confidentiality must be violated to protect the patient's health or life, it should be done only after explaining the reasons as thoroughly as possible.

EXAMINING THE ADOLESCENT PATIENT

The physical examination of the adolescent patient is an emotionally charged experience. Adolescents are concerned with their bodies, and particularly concerned with how others will respond to their bodies. They have only recently acquired the right to privacy, and value it highly. They have only recently entered the world of sexuality, and are unsure how to act in possibly sexual situations. Should they take off their clothes and feign nonchalance, or cover the private parts of their bodies and refuse to expose them? Their anxiety leads to the question, and they try to find an answer that will help to control and to conceal that anxiety.

The physician is of a different generation from the patient, and accordingly may at times misinterpret the patient's experience. Young adult male doctors examining early adolescent girls commonly experience the event as highly charged sexually, while the girls' conscious experience is that of a child with an adult, since a 20-year-old medical student may seem little different from a 40-year-old doctor. However, if the girl is uncomfortable because of her shyness in exposing herself to an adult, the doctor may detect that discomfort and mistakenly translate it into male-female terms.

It is particularly important that the doctor examining an adolescent patient maintain a comfortable social context for that experience. This is, of course, important for any patient, and it is sometimes difficult for a medical student or inexperienced physician who is new to the skill and engrossed in the technical aspects of what he or she is doing. The adult patient is more likely to recognize and accommodate, while realizing that the physician is concentrating rather than being unfriendly. The adolescent, who typically has greater anxiety about his or her body, and who at the same time is less accustomed to differentiating young, inexperienced adults from older, more authoritarian ones, is more likely to interpret the doctor's silent concentration in personal terms. The doctor can avoid this problem by maintaining social contact during the examination. Perhaps he or she may ask about the patient's health and bodily experience, conduct a "review of systems," or comment in a positive way about the patient's physical growth and maturation ("Your shoulders are broader than when I saw you last year" or "Your figure is filling out nicely"). A matter-of-fact, neutral, interested, but professional attitude toward the patient's body makes it easier for the patient to introduce thoughts, feelings, or questions relating to it. As a general rule, the doctor can assume that adolescents are less certain about their body functions than they are revealing. The doctor should overexplain, and not force the patient to reveal ignorance. Knowing about one's body is associated with maturity, and adolescents are likely to pretend more maturity than they feel in this as in other things.

With adolescents, as with other patients, the more chronic the illness, the more important it is that the doctor develop a truly symmetrical "partnership" with the patient. This means that the acutely ill adolescent is more likely to be experienced and treated by the doctor as a child, with no great harm coming from this as long as the illness is brief and the patient returns to the expected path of development upon recovery. In fact, such brief "vacations" from the challenges and responsibilities of increasing maturity can be comforting, by reassuring the adolescent patient that it is safe to grow up because in time of crisis the securities of childhood are still potentially available. In effect, response to illness is viewed as an illustration of the general principle that psychological maturity is an adaptive mode that is never permanent, and is always doomed to failure or even disaster if it cannot be set aside temporarily and replaced by more primitive patterns of behavior in time of life crisis, strong emotion, or great intimacy.

The adolescent patient in the hospital responds not only to illness and to the treating physician, but like anyone else in a hospital, also to the complex social structure of the treatment setting. What is somewhat special for adolescents is that hospitals, like schools, have authoritarian hierarchical structures that are likely to provoke defiant "antiestablishment" response patterns in someone who is just emerging from a dependent involvement in his or her own family. Adolescents may see hospitals as adult institutions against which they must rebel at the risk of being swallowed up. One solution is to develop hospital programs that are designed for adolescents, or special units and special staff who are trained in the psychological problems of caring for patients in this age group. In this way, peer support can help a sick adolescent cope with illness, rather than the more customary process of hospitalization compounding the problem by separating the adolescent patient from the peer group just when its support is most essential.

If adolescents should not be sick, certainly above all else they should not face death. However, cruelly, at times they do. The problems of treating sick adolescents are multiplied many times when treating dying ones. Staff distress often leads to avoidance of the patient and the patient's problems, undoubtedly the worst possible outcome. Here adolescent peer group support is particularly important, since the patient's family may be even less able than the staff to cope with the overwhelming sense of injustice that we all experience with a dying adolescent.

Adolescents are troubled by death, but surprisingly are often less so than adults, and are certainly less troubled than adults imagine in their fantasies of adolescence. Adolescence is the time of heroism, of the triumph of ideal over reality, and the importance of ideals can help to sustain the dying adolescent's sense of personal value. Adults are more likely to experience their self-esteem in terms of concrete realities of personal productivity and specific human relationships, realities that come to an end when their physical existence terminates. In a sense, the treatment of a dying and despairing person is to instill in him or her the adolescent's view of the universe. The caretakers of dying adolescents can be helped if they understand the special strength that their patients possess.

PSYCHOPATHOLOGY IN ADOLESCENCE

The forms of psychopathology in adolescence are almost as varied and diverse as are all the forms of psychopathology in general psychiatry. A useful way of distinguishing them follows.

1 *Disorders primarily associated with childhood that persist into adolescence.* Important illustrations would be (1) the pervasive developmental disorders of childhood, such as autism and childhood psychosis, which almost invariably lead to a markedly atypical adolescence; and (2) the attention deficit disorders (synonymous with minimal brain damage, commonly including specific learning disabilities), when the difficulty in adolescence is a combination of current interference superimposed on deficiencies accumulated through childhood and carried forward into adolescence.

2 *Disorders primarily associated with adulthood that can begin (early) in adolescence.* The most important example here would be adult schizophrenia, where age of onset commonly ranges from late adolescence through early adulthood. Another example, less familiar but of intense current interest, would be early cycles of manic-depressive illness. Looking back into the adolescence of recognized adult cases, one can often get a history of states of elation and depression that had been identified as "merely adolescent mood swings."

3 *Disorders present through the life span.* These are cases where the disorder in adolescence is basically the same as at any age, although its expression may be shaped by the stage-specific features of adolescence. Examples here would be most of the personality disorders, the anxiety disorders, mental retardation, and some of the depressive disorders.

4 *Disorders especially associated with adolescence.* This category includes disorders that can be present through the life span, but are included here rather than in the previous category because they tend to be especially intense or frequent in adolescence. Examples of the latter would be the conduct disorders (juvenile delinquency) or the identity disorders. A disorder frequently associated with adolescence would be anorexia nervosa.

Five disorders have been selected for special attention and brief summary. Depression and schizophrenia are included because they are major psychiatric disorders that are studied throughout the life span, and also because in adolescence they may present themselves in forms that are different from their adult forms. Anorexia nervosa, conduct disorder, and identity disorder are included because all are highly associated with adolescence. Anorexia nervosa is a behavior disorder that almost invariably calls for medical attention. Conduct disorder and identity disorder are less "medical" in character, but both are sufficiently common and sufficiently distressing to parents for them commonly to seek help from the family physician.

Depression

Depression in adolescence represents a cluster of rather different conditions that need to be understood separately and treated somewhat differently. A useful subdivision would be:

1 Acute reactive depression. The emphasis here is on the depressive reaction to a real event, or to the psychological significance for the person of the real event. Classic examples would be a depressive reaction to the sudden loss of a boyfriend or a girlfriend; to the sudden loss of a parent or of family through illness, death, separation, divorce; to the sudden loss of self-esteem through some sort of setback in school or athletics; or to illness. The typical reaction here tends to be intense and acute, in keeping with the characteristic emotional intensity of adolescence. However, chronic and smouldering forms can also occur. Reactive depression is probably the most common form of depression in adolescence. Although the emotionality of the reaction may be more intense on the average in adolescence than in adulthood, it is similar in its essentials to reactive depression of adulthood.

2 Chronic deprivational depression in adolescence. This is a syndrome of devitalization and blunted emotional expressiveness, with a quality of "emptiness" in activities and in the mental life, with few real interests and little pleasure in living. Usually it occurs in continuity with a similar childhood, and derives from a family or institutional experience of "psychological impoverishment" (i.e., a marked deficit through the years of childhood of ordinary caring and vital interactions between parents and child). It has to be distinguished from the similar picture that can prevail with mild retardation or with process schizophrenia. The use of the word depression in this case does not carry the usual implication of a dip from a previously normal mood state; in this form of depression, a normal level has never been established. This form of depression is particularly common among institutionalized children, or among children from severely pathological families.

3 Depressions related to schizophrenia. When a syndrome of severe withdrawal and isolation is seen in adolescence, with markedly blunted affect, similar to what one might call severe endogeneous depression if the patient were age 50, the likelihood is that the depressive state in adolescence will prove to be the initial or most evident manifestation of an underlying schizophrenic process, rather than primarily a severe mood disorder. In principle, a trial of treatment with a nonsedating phenothiazine such as trifluoperazine would be consistent with consideration of this diagnosis.

4 Bipolar manic-depressive depression. This is a subject of active, current interest, largely because of the recent emergence of an effective treatment modality (lithium carbonate). The study of this biologically cyclic mood disorder in adults has brought to light from the adolescent history of some patients depressive episodes that were almost certainly the beginning of manic-depressive cycling, but understandably were identified then as "merely adolescent mood swings." This is a difficult differential diagnosis to make with confidence, but a combination of severity, evidence of cyclic recurrence, and a positive family history would warrant a referral for further evaluation.

5 Unipolar endogenous depression. The emphasis here is on biological vulnerability to depressive states. Primarily, this is an illness of middle and late adulthood. However, recent work suggests that some small percentage of depressions in childhood and adolescence may be essentially the same illness earlier in life. These depressions may also respond favorably to antidepressant medications, as do the endogenous depressions of adulthood. They are not like the reactive and deprivational depressions of adolescence, which generally do not respond to antidepressant medication.[6]

The emphasis in reactive and deprivational depressions is on psychological causation, whereas emphasis in the schizophrenic, manic-depressive, and endogenous forms of depression is on the biological roots. Psychological factors, however, do play a role and do become caught up in the predominantly biological disorders, and biological vulnerabilities may be an important contributing element in the depressions that are primarily reactive to psychological causation. Treatment of depression in adolescence would depend critically upon differential diagnosis, would include trial of specific medications only where indicated (e.g., antipsychotics for schizophrenia-related depressions, antidepressants for endogenous depressions), would include general nonspecific psychological support for all the forms of depression, and might well include insight-oriented psychotherapeutic work in the reactive and deprivational forms. Although reactive depressions tend to be acute and often resolve on their own, treatment during or after the episode may be indicated as a preventive measure, especially if there are repeated episodes. By helping the adolescent to understand and to master some sources of his or her vulnerability, subsequent episodes may be prevented, and the depressive reaction converted into an opportunity for facilitating psychological growth. The treatment of chronic deprivational depressions usually goes beyond what the physician or even the psychotherapist can provide. What is commonly required is helping the patient to find in adolescence some source of the ordinary psychological input from adults and/or peers, an input that has been absent throughout that young person's life. That input usually has to come from some person, agency, group, or social movement in the adolescent's real life. But the physician or psychotherapist may be able to provide critical help in guiding the adolescent toward finding and making such a connection.

Suicide in adolescence may be an outcome of severe reactive depression. Although suicide in adolescence is an infrequent event (only 4 per 100,000 in middle adolescence, in comparison with numbers twice or four times as high in middle age and ten times as high for males over 60), suicide does rank high as a cause of death among adolescents because their mortality rate from other causes is so low.[7] Thus, suicide is the second most common cause of death among college students, and the fifth most common among adolescents in general (exceeded only by accidents, neoplasm, cardiovascular-renal disease, and homicide). Furthermore, postmortem investigations regularly confirm that a sizable proportion of deaths in adolescence that are identified as accidental (particularly auto accidents) or homicide are deliberate or unconscious suicides related to a depressive attitude within which one does not "take care" because "nothing matters much anyway." Suicide in early adolescence is exceedingly rare, and is almost always associated with marked psychopathology in the child and family, a psychopathology that notably includes a family "tradition" of suicide attempts and gestures as a way of controlling others. Although the curve of committed suicide versus age keeps increasing with age and thus has no peaks in adolescence, the curve of attempted suicide versus age does tend to peak in late adolescence and young adulthood, particularly among young women, where the most common precipitating factor is distress over a failed or disrupted love relationship. In adolescence the ratio of *attempts* to *actual* suicide is 50 to 100:1, by comparison with a ratio of about 10:1 in adulthood. In adolescence, the ratio of female attempted suicides to male attempted suicides is 3:1, whereas the ratio for completed suicide is 1:3.[7]

In evaluating suicidal potential, all attempts and gestures in adolescence should be taken seriously. It is better to err on the side of caution. The stakes are too high for a casual attitude. A certain proportion of gestures succeed "by accident." Failure of the family to respond emotionally is a bad prognostic sign, and often sets up a situation in which the adolescent gets even more depressed and hopeless and makes an even more serious attempt to get people to hear the cry for help. All possible suicide attempts seen in the office (e.g., ambiguous overdoses) deserve evaluation by an experienced person, who might be a psychiatrist or a general physician with above-average experience and background in this area. In making an initial evaluation, it is important to find some comfortable middle course between asking too abruptly about suicidal intent (and getting a quick reflex denial) and not asking at all. Good technique here begins with sympathetic questions about mood ("Sounds like you've been pretty down lately. From what I hear about what's been going on in your life, that's not so surprising"), leads into a question about the quality of life ("Life not much fun lately?" or "Hardly worth living?"), and then into a direct question ("Ever actually thought about just ending it?" or "Even actually planned anything?" "Or done anything?"). Above all, the physician should convey a serious attitude that bespeaks real interest, and sufficient comfort with this highly charged subject so that the patient can feel that the doctor really wants to hear and will not overreact to the truth.

Schizophrenia in Adolescence

The understanding of schizophrenia in adolescence is basically an understanding of schizophrenia. However, the context in adolescence does create some special circumstances that bear special emphasis:

1 Some schizophrenia in adolescence is childhood schizophrenia carried forward into adolescence. Some is early onset of adult schizophrenia. Although there are similarities and continuities, the two forms tend to differ in symptom picture, prognosis, and treatment. Childhood schizophrenia tends to be chronic, progressive, and marked by withdrawal and failure to thrive psychologically, a failure that is partially related to the disease itself and partially to accumulated interferences with the necessary work of normal development over earlier years. Adult schizophrenia can take the same form, but is more often marked by florid episodes ("breaks"), which are separated by intervals of remission to improved levels of functioning that can vary from moderately impaired to virtually normal. The more intense, acute, and episodic the symptom picture, the better the prognosis (both short-term and long-term), and the more likely that medications will be able to have a useful role in the treatment. Antipsychotic drugs can be very effective for moderating the acute episodes, but much less helpful in countering the chronic impairments of the illness (not surprising, since some of them are not related directly to the disease but derive from earlier interferences with the psychological work of normal development). Furthermore, chronic use of anti-psychotic drugs is complicated, and has become of significant concern because of increasing current awareness of the frequency of tardive dyskinesia, a late-developing, severe, as-yet-untreatable neurological side effect of long-term use of antipsychotic medications.

2 It can be notoriously difficult, even for the experienced diagnostician, to distinguish milder forms of disorganization and disordered thinking, which are associated with schizophrenia from similar overabstract or overconcrete think-ing that can be associated with nonschizophrenic disorganized thinking in adolescence. There is no great difficulty in making the diagnosis when the psychotic process is marked. And the more experience one has with normal adolescents, the less likely one is to mistake ordinary adolescent overabstractness or overconcreteness for schizophrenic thought disorder. However, there is an ap-preciable intermediate zone of cases within which even the experienced clinician and the experienced psychologist, armed with a battery of systematic tests, can re-main uncertain of the distinction. Usually only the passage of time will tell, but fortunately the same psychotherapeutic approaches (directed toward fostering development and adaptation) are usually appropriate and potentially helpful, regardless of the roots of the disorganization. Sometimes a trial of antipsychotic medications will help in making the diagnosis, for which referral to a consultant would usually be indicated.

Anorexia Nervosa

Anorexia nervosa is a disease of adolescence; cases where age of onset is in childhood or adulthood are quite rare. Essential features of the syndrome include marked weight loss (the American Psychiatric Association[8] uses a 25 percent weight loss as a criterion); other criteria are intense fear of gaining weight, unusual preoccupation with food, and peculiar patterns of behavior in handling food (hoarding, concealing, discarding). Roughly 95 percent of the patients are female. Remarkably high energy levels are frequent, even against a background of cachexia. Disturbances of body image are typical, including a conviction of overweight despite a manifestly emaciated appearance. Amennorhea is frequent, and may be an early sign. Severe cases are a psychiatric emergency. Death by star-vation is a real possibility, and mortality rates are in the range of 15 to 20 percent. Treatment includes hospitalization and forced or intravenous feeding when medically indicated, and early referral for psychotherapy. One principal psychodynamic trend involves intense conflicts about womanhood, with the female patient often symbolically equating plumpness with a womanly body and with pregnancy. No single causal or predisposing factor has been identified. The syndrome is probably best understood as a cluster of varying etiologies leading to a similar outcome.

Delinquency

Delinquency is perhaps the most prominent of all the characteristic psychological disorders of adolescence. This cluster of clinical conditions is called variously juvenile delinquency, "acting-out" behavior, or conduct disturbance. Behavior of this sort will often be brought to the attention of the physician by parents seeking help or advice. Such behavior may also be the background of medical difficulties that are the direct result of the behavior pathology (e.g., pregnancy or venereal disease may be secondary to promiscuous or careless sexual activity, physical injury may be secondary to dangerous or criminal activity, or any of the many possible medical consequences of drug abuse). The diagnosis of conduct disturbance would tend to rest on the finding of persistent and repetitive misconduct, including destructiveness; stealing; violence; lying; truancy; or vandalism at home, at school, in the community; it may also rest on such associated personality characteristics as impulsivity, irritability, low frustration tolerance, and impaired capacity for forming close age-appropriate relationships with peers. This behavior can be regarded as a pathological exaggeration of trends seen to a lesser degree in some varieties of normal adolescence. A fair proportion of mild-to-moderate versions of this disorder tend to be transient and "settle down" by late adolescence, especially those that rest heavily on support from a delinquent peer group. But where this behavior seems to have become structured and established as a basic and recurrent trend in the life of the adolescent, that youngster deserves a referral for evaluation and possible treatment.

Much work has been done in this area, and understandably so, considering the stake society has in the subject. The literature is vast, and ranges over such diverse areas as sociology, child rearing, personality development, psychoanalysis, and biology. One can appreciate some of the key themes in the study of delinquency by noting that this form of behavior can represent the outcome of markedly different lines of prior development, with differing implications for treatment and prognosis, as follows:

1 For the youngster from a poverty background, an antisocial stance may be behavior that is essentially learned and subculturally supported. Indeed, participation and membership in a gang may be necessary adaptive behavior for survival on the street, while nonmembership or nonparticipation may be indicative of incapacity. Although for some such youngsters this behavior may become deeply internalized and may lead to seriously impaired capacities either for self-control or for effective ego functioning, this group also includes an important fraction of youngsters with intact and even impressive capacities for adaptive functioning, which can be turned to socially productive ends as well as to criminal ones (e.g., capacity to think, to plan, and to defer gratification in the service of some desired goal).

2 Some delinquent youngsters from middle-class and working class backgrounds prove to be distinctly impaired in their capacity to "make it" in their peer group in the ordinary socially approved ways. These are youngsters limited by some sort of intellectual and/or personality disorder, who escape from the pain and shame of failure in school, in social life, and/or in athletic competition into the excitement and status of a delinquent peer group. Getting such youngsters on a better track usually includes trying to help them with their impairment, and trying to help them to find some way to get pleasure and status out of socially approved activities that are within their capacities.

3 For some adolescents, delinquent activity represents a neurotic resolution of internalized struggles around such issues as independence, masculinity, femininity, defense against depression, and the search for self-esteem (better to be a bad somebody than a good nobody). Where this sort of neurotic conflict seems to be at the heart of the matter, psychotherapy would be strongly indicated.

4 Sometimes the delinquent behavior is the manifestation of a psychotic process. Treatment here may properly include antipsychotic medication.

5 Some delinquents, perhaps the most seriously disturbed of all, are young people with a pervasively disturbed capacity for human relations, and are seemingly incapable of feelings for others. This could be considered the archetypal psychopath. Such patients are notoriously difficult to engage or to help through psychotherapy of any type. A fair proportion of youngsters from this group end up in penal institutions and lead lives of crime. Present studies of the treatment of severe narcissistic personality disorders and borderline personality organization may contribute to a psychotherapeutic approach. Often these youngsters require institutionalization before a therapist gets an opportunity even to begin working with them.

Identity Disorder in Adolescence

Only partial success at forging a stable, coherent identity is the rule in late adolescence and young adulthood, and is not defined as psychopathology. But a conspicuous failure to be able to form a stable and acceptable identity is defined as a form of psychopathology characteristic of this stage of life. The essential feature is a marked incapacity to put together a sense of self that is experienced as acceptable to oneself and that also "works" and is recognized by the outside world. This manifests itself most typically in difficulty with making choices about career, values, loyalties, and long-term goals. Frequently the individual is immobilized by conflicts, doubts, and indecision. Anxiety and depression are common and are related to preoccupation with these issues. Negative or oppositional patterns may be chosen to define a life-style that is conspicuously different from derogated family or community life-styles, and sometimes these patterns take the form of extremes of experimentation. The foregoing can sometimes be the surface aspect of what could really be a much more pervasive underlying psychopathological process, such as schizophrenia or borderline personality organization. The diagnosis of identity disorder should be reserved for cases where the syndrome is not the presenting aspect of a more pervasive underlying disorder. In cases of identity disorder in late adolescence, a brief psychotherapy that focuses on the central psychological conflict may be particularly helpful, and referral should be considered.

CONCLUSION

Adolescents can be difficult, but they can also be unusually responsive to the physician's active interest in a very special way. Memories of adolescence, recalled from adulthood, so often include the experience of one or two fateful encounters with a valued adult, encounters that one identifies as having left an unforgettable imprint on one's view of oneself, and of the world. That adult may be a teacher, a coach, a counselor, a minister—or a physician.

REFERENCES

1 Tanner, J. M.: "Twelve to Sixteen: Early Adolescence," *Daedalus,* Fall 1971:907–930.
2 Frost, Robert: *Complete Poems,* New York: Holt Rinehart Winston, 1949, p. 131.
3 Kinsey, Alfred C., W. B. Pomeroy, and C. E. Martin: *Sexual Behavior in the Human Male,* Philadelphia: W. B. Saunders, 1948, pp. 313–326.
4 _____: *Sexual Behavior in the Human Female,* Philadelphia: W. B. Saunders, 1953, pp. 132–190.
5 Zelnik, Melvin, and J. F. Kantner: "The Baltimore Study," *U. S. Commission Report on Population Growth,* Washington, D.C.: vol.1, no.3, pp. 355–375, 1972.
6 Klein, Donald, and John M. Davis: *Diagnosis and Drug Treatment of Psychiatric Disorders,* Baltimore: Williams and Wilkins, 1969, p. 309.
7 Weiner, I.: *Psychological Disturbance in Adolescence,* New York: Wiley, 1970, pp. 176–178.
8 The American Psychiatric Association Task Force on Nomenclature and Statistics, DSM-III: Operational Criteria Draft, April 15, 1977.

BIBLIOGRAPHY

Group for the Advancement of Psychiatry (GAP), Report no. 68, "Normal Adolescence," G.A.P. Publications, 1968.
Hofman, A. D. et al.: *The Hospitalized Adolescent: A Guide to Managing the Ill and Injured Youth,* New York: Free Press, 1976.
Meeks, J.: *The Fragile Alliance,* Baltimore: Williams and Wilkins, 1971.
Weiner, I.: *Psychological Disturbance in Adolescence,* New York: Wiley, 1970.

Part Three

Psychiatric Syndromes in Adults

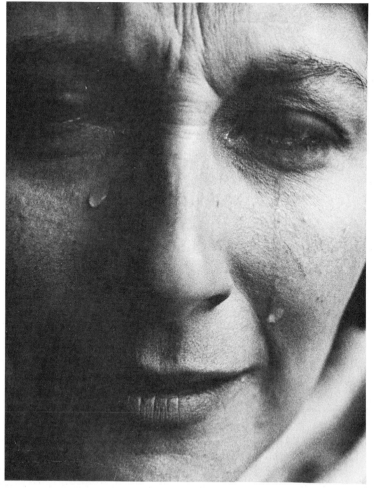

Courtesy of Richard Frieman/Photo Researchers, Inc., NYC.

Chapter 9

The Response to Life Stress

Ransom J. Arthur, M.D.

EDITORS' INTRODUCTION

What is it like to be a middle-aged female physician with cystic disease of the breast and one day discover a nodule that just does not feel or seem the same as two other cysts did before they were surgically removed? What is it like to wait several months because you are concerned you may seem too alarmed or stupid if you consult a colleague about the nodule? What is it like for the same woman to have consulted a physician, who reassured her that it was "just another cyst," but then begin to wonder whether the physician might be wrong and whether the cyst may be increasing in size since the consultation? What is it like to be a physician who appreciates the frequency of functional chest pain, and yet realizes that despite a recent examination, the pain which has been persisting for several days may be an early coronary occlusion?

These two examples seem all the more poignant because the physician has more medical knowledge than the layperson, but the episodes are repeated with many patients who, under considerable emotional stress, worry about the possibility of a fatal illness.

How does the physician aid the patient in the prevention of a chronic stress reaction to realistic emotional or organic pathology? Many people may be competent and seemingly well adjusted. The stress of the symptoms (or, more precisely, patients' interpretation of their symptoms) may, however, lead to less than rational behavior.

As Arthur points out, stress is ubiquitous. The physician is in an advantageous position for observing the ways in which life stress correlate with the onset of illness. Out of such observations may come suggestions and treatment programs aimed at lessening, whenever possible, the role that life stress plays in increasing vulnerability to illness.

In addition, however, the physician must be sensitive to the stress involved simply in consulting the physician. Many patients arrive with diffuse complaints and obvious fears that there is something dreadfully wrong. There may be considerable apprehension that the illness will be a serious or even fatal one. In this regard, the physician can make use of his or her own experiences with personal stress.

In addition to personal experiences with life stress and the stress of personal illness, many physicians allow their practices to become sources of stress. For some, it is the reality of too many patients wishing to be seen, but for others it can reflect the impact of the drive for economic success or for prestige. Some such physicians try to do more and more, and often sacrifice the quality of their practices, their home lives, and their own health.

Although to live is to experience stress, the physician can read the following chapter both as a means of understanding patients' illnesses better, and as a structure with which to evaluate the stress in his or her own life.

INTRODUCTION

To live is to be under stress. To be human is to experience humiliations, rebuffs, changes, departures, disappointments, triumphs, successes, and failures. The events of life reverberate in the mind and in the brain which is its physical embodiment. These reverberations spread throughout the body and impinge on health itself.

History affords us some striking and terrible examples of how massive stress can have deleterious consequences on the health of large numbers of humans. The concentration camps of Hitler's Europe were the setting for barbaric and inhumane cruelties carried out on an unprecedented scale.[1] Beatings, wholesale executions, starvation, endemic diseases, and the constant threat of death combined to provide an incredible set of stressors. The individuals who survived such experiences have continued to have many symptoms such as difficulty in thinking, difficulty with memory, sleep problems, chronic dysphoria, anxiety, and gastrointestinal symptoms. This combination of phenomena is known as the *KZ syndrome,* from the German word for concentration camp. Virtually everyone who spent any length of time in these institutions has continued to have KZ symptoms for decades afterwards.

In the remote past the black death that swept Europe in the fourteenth century was followed by psychological illnesses on a mass scale, including lycanthropy, ritual whippings, mass dancing, and other forms of hysteria, which represented attempts to come to grips with an experience of the most gruesome sort, in which literally millions of individuals perished of a scourge which was inexplicable by means of the knowledge of biological phenomena available at the time.

The horrifying experiences of the concentration camps and the black death seemed to affect virtually all the individuals involved. On the other hand, we have examples of stressful phenomena on a mass scale which increase the incidence of illness only in certain individuals. During the German air attacks on London from 1940 to 1941, there was a very sharp rise in the incidence of intestinal perforations secondary to peptic ulcers as compared to previous and subsequent years.[2] When the air attacks ended, the incidence of perforations quickly returned to baseline levels. Large numbers of individuals experienced stress as a result of the bombing experience, but only a certain proportion developed this particular stress response. Similarly, data from studies of released prisoners of war, including those who had undergone experiences second only to the concentration camps in ferocity, indicate that while some of the prisoners developed stress-related illnesses of a persistent character, others seemed able to handle the demands of the prisoner of war camps without developing any diagnosable illness of either a mental or physical type.[3] It is clear that maximal stresses, especially those that involve the constant threat of imminent death, seem to be the ones which lead to severe, chronic impairment of physical and mental health. On the other hand, submaximal stress affects different individuals in a nonuniform manner. Some may succumb, but others are able to carry on without apparent impairment.

The striking historical examples were chosen to illustrate the well-documented thesis that life events and the setting in which they occur can have a profound and deleterious effect on health. Fortunately, comparatively few humans have to undergo the rigors of massive epidemics, concentration or prisoner of war camps, and constant bombardment. Nevertheless, while going about our ordinary, mundane lives in a society presumably at peace, we encounter stressors of strong meaning and impact. Such events as being promoted or demoted, losing one's job, gaining a new job, getting married, getting divorced, losing someone close through death, or making a major move over a long distance, are the very stuff of modern life in America.

Can these quotidian happenings affect one's health? Well, of course everyone believes this to be so. Even the most hardened advocates of the idea that all diseases are purely mechanical events, merely the random dance of atoms operating in a physicochemical framework, do not act as if their faith in pure mechanical reductionism were total. Everyone wonders whether he or she is working too hard, or feeling too sad for personal good, and if this will not somehow help to bring on an illness. In their evaluation of disease onset, physicians must take into account the character and personality of the patient as well as the effects of the environment.

In the nineteenth century, with the rise of scientific medicine, which rested upon discoveries in the basic physical and biological sciences, there was a movement away from considering social and psychological factors in disease. However, even in Victorian times, great scientists such as Rudolph Virchow, one of the founders of modern pathology, indicated that "diseases are neither self-subsistent circumscribed autonomous organisms, nor entities which have forced their way into the body, but represent only the course of physiological phenomena under altered conditions."[4] In 1872, Daniel Tuke published his pioneering work, *The Influence of the Mind on the Body*. He described many diseases, and even instances of sudden death, which seemed to follow dramatic changes in the patient's life, accompanied by very strong emotions. More than 60 years ago, Sigmund Freud and Karl Abraham described the appearance of a specific disease, that is, depressive illness, following the death of someone whom the patient had loved.[6] Freud and Abraham thought that in order for a clinically significant depression to develop, the love had to be alloyed with some hatred. If the patient's feeling toward the deceased had not been ambivalent in character, the loss of the loved one would have been followed by normal mourning. Usual mourning resembles pathological depression in some ways, but is characterized by far less severity and persistence of symptoms. They were the first to point out clearly that, in certain susceptible individuals, the death of an individual such as a spouse or parent may regularly be followed by a specific disease, namely, a depressive illness. Clinicians soon realized that the concept of loss was a powerful one and could be generalized to include much more than the death of a spouse or a close relative. It was apparent that, for some individuals, the loss of their home, their career, their youth, or their beauty could be sufficient to precipitate a depressive episode. The concept that losses or, as they are sometimes called, "exits" from one's life can be etiologic agents in pathologic states continues to be a popular notion.

An elaboration of this idea has been put forward by Schmale and Engel, who have made explicit the concept of "giving up" as a prelude to illness.[7] Simply, this means that prior to the onset of an illness, which need not be of a psychiatric character and may include entities as diverse as ulcerative colitis or myocardial infarction, the individual is caught in the grip of malign life circumstances in which he or she is forced to "give up" some cherished part of life. This given-up thing could be the physical death of someone near, or the symbolic loss of a long-cherished dream. The individual reacts to the loss with rage, depression, and disappointment. If he or she feels incapable of rectifying the situation, and finds that alternative pathways to esteem and gratification are not available, the result is a surrender. It is at the moment of conjunction for these two processes, when there is simultaneously the giving up of a cherished thing and the loss of hope that things can ever be made right again, that illness strikes.

In studies of various individuals, Schmale and Engel found that perhaps 80 percent of the patients interviewed had had a predisease experience of actual, threatened, or symbolic loss of some highly important form of gratification. The patients had had feelings of *helplessness* which they defined as a feeling of deprivation resulting from a change about which the individual felt powerless to do anything. *Hopelessness* was defined as a feeling of despair or futility which is perceived as coming from a loss of satisfaction. The individual has the final responsibility for bringing about the loss. The hopeless feeling encompasses a sense that there could be no rectification of the situation.

The following case vignette illustrates these ideas vividly.

> The patient was a 65-year-old woman who had had 43 years of a very happy marriage. She had always been petite and doll-like, and her husband treated her with adoration and respect. She had not worked for remuneration outside the home, and had found all her satisfactions in the comfort of this particular kind of relationship. Her husband, who was a few years older, died of cardiovascular disease. Three months after his death she showed obvious weight loss and fatigue. Evident cachexia made it appear that her condition was more than ordinary mourning. She received a thorough workup at the University hospital. An exploratory procedure showed that she had an inoperable carcinoma of the pancreas. She took everything with a kind of eerie calm. She returned home, where she went steadily downhill. Throughout her last few months she seemed to be in quietly good spirits. She had a beatific smile and announced that she would soon be reunited with her beloved husband. She was able to chat quite freely and lucidly with friends and children until the day of her death. She evinced no interest in any kind of further treatment, and no wish for prolongation of her life. The course of her illness was brief and she died within a few months.

Whatever the mechanical factors in the genesis of her carcinoma, the course of the illness was clearly influenced by the husband's death and her reaction to it. The intense loss of the central figure and support in her life was followed by a sense of giving up on life itself because there was no hope of resurrecting her husband, nor, in her mind, of ever forging new relationships which would approach the satisfactions of the old one in terms of intimacy and security.

QUANTITATIVE STUDIES OF LIFE STRESS

Every practicing physician could bring forth many similar cases to buttress this point. This kind of material is anecdotal in character, and thus not scientifically persuasive. However, in the past 20 years a large body of information of a more quantitative and regularized character has appeared in the medical literature. This information helps to confirm the basic idea that life stress plays a role in the onset and course of human illnesses. The work of Holmes and Rahe has moved the emphasis from the subjective to the objective and toward the quantification of the aspects of life stresses themselves.[8] Earlier work, such as that of Engel and others, concentrated primarily on patients' subjective perceptions of life events and their inner feelings of depression, helplessness, hopelessness, and dependency. Other workers wished to introduce more precision and quantification into the whole field. In the 1950s, Hawkins and Holmes had noted the clustering of many life-change events in the 2 years preceding the onset of pulmonary tuberculosis in patients.[9] In the 1960s the systematic measurement of life-change events was largely standardized, and scaling studies were used to evaluate the relative weight or significance of these events for the average individual.[8,10] Basically, the idea was to choose a single life event, the death of a spouse, and give it an arbitrary weight of, say, 100 points, and then ask various groups of people to measure other life events against the death of the spouse in terms of the disruption of life and the amount of coping that would be necessary to adjust to them. The events included getting married, getting divorced, the birth of a child, taking on a mortgage, moving, being promoted, being demoted, trouble with the law for a minor infraction, and so forth (see Figure 9-1). Over the years the scales have been standardized with many groups in the United States and abroad. In all instances save one, there was a general convergence of opinion, even among people from widely different cultures. Items dealing with death and illness were uniformly given high scores. For example, death of a spouse was ranked first or second in all groups. On the other hand, items such as change in number of family get-togethers and taking a vacation were generally ranked rather low. However, in a recent study conducted in a Peruvian city that had been devastated by a major earthquake in 1970, no significant relationship was found between the generally accepted scale for the United States and the one in the still earthquake-blighted city of Huaraz in Peru.[11] Nevertheless, people in ordinary life generally seem to agree on the degree of significance of particular life events for the average individual. Life-change studies concentrate solely on punctate and current transitions in people's lives. They do not speak to chronic problems and prolonged stress.

After the development of the initial scale of life-change units, the investigators began studying groups of humans in terms of their life changes and their patterns of illness. The basic hypotheses was that those people who had had a high life-change score during the preceding period of, say, 1 year, because of either many life changes or a few life changes of high weight such as marital separation or personal injury, would be more likely to fall ill than would people in similar circumstances who had had a placid year with a small number of life changes. This basic hypothesis has been confirmed by literally hundreds of studies of both a retrospective and prospective character.

Even before birth, life changes may be of significance to both mother and child.[12] Those mothers who had high life-change scores in the 6 months prior to pregnancy had significantly more complications during pregnancy and parturition than did the control group of pregnant mothers. Irish mothers of newborns who developed pyloric stenosis gave a history of more problems of family illnesses, marital difficulties, fathers' unemployment, housing problems, and bereavement, than did the mothers in a comparison group.[13] Children afflicted with diabetes show more life changes in their families than did comparison groups.[14] Young male drivers of automobiles involved in serious traffic accidents have been found to have high life-change scores as compared to nonaccident controls.

Important work in the confirmation of the basic life and illness hypothesis was carried out in the United States Navy by utilizing a prospective design involv-

A *Health*

Have you experienced

1 an illness or injury?
2 a major change in eating habits?
3 a major change in sleeping habits?
4 a change in your usual type and/or amount of recreation?
5 major dental work?

B *Work*

Have you

6 changed to a new type of work?
7 changed your work hours or conditions?
8 had a change in your responsibilities at work?
9 experienced troubles at work?
10 experienced a major business readjustment?
11 retired?
12 experienced being fired or laid off from work?
13 taken courses by mail or studied at home to help you in your work?

C *Home and Family*

Have you experienced

14 a change in residence?
15 a change in family get-togethers?
16 a major change in the health or behavior of a family member (illnesses, accidents, drug or disciplinary problems, etc.)?
17 a major change in your living conditions (home improvements or a decline in your home or neighborhood)?
18 the death of a spouse?
19 the death of a child, brother or sister, parent, or other close family member?
20 the death of a close friend?
21 a change in the marital status of your parents (divorce, remarriage)?
22 marriage?
23 a change in arguments with your spouse?
24 in-law problems?
25 a separation from spouse due to work or marital problems?
26 a reconciliation with spouse?

27 a divorce?
28 a gain of a new family member (birth of a child, adoption of a child, a relative moving in with you)?
29 wife beginning or ceasing work outside the home?
30 wife becoming pregnant?
31 a child leaving home?
32 wife having a miscarriage or abortion?
33 birth of a grandchild?

D *Personal and Social*

Have you experienced

34 a major personal achievement?
35 a change in your personal habits (your dress, friends, life-style, etc.)?
36 sexual difficulties?
37 beginning or ceasing school or college?
38 a change of school or college?
39 a vacation?
40 a change in your religious beliefs?
41 a change in your social activities (clubs, movies, visiting)?
42 a minor violation of the law?
43 legal troubles resulting in your being held in jail?
44 a change in your political beliefs?
45 a new, close personal relationship?
46 an engagement to marry?
47 a "falling out" of a close personal relationship?
48 girlfriend (or boyfriend) problems?
49 a loss or damage of personal property?
50 an accident?
51 a major decision regarding your immediate future?

E *Financial*

Have you

52 taken on a moderate purchase, such as a TV, car, freezer, etc.?
53 taken on a major purchase or a mortgage loan, such as a home, business, property, etc.?
54 experienced a foreclosure on a mortgage or loan?
55 experienced a major change in finances?

Figure 9-1   Recent life changes. *(Adapted from Recent Life Changes Questionnaire, in Richard H. Rahe, "Epidemiological Studies of Life Change and Illness," Int'l. J. Psychiatry in Medicine, 6(1/2):133–146, 1975.)*

ing the crews of a number of large vessels, many thousands of subjects in all.[15] Prior to the beginning of a voyage, the members of the crew filled out life-change questionnaires which were analyzed to provide each individual with a life-change score. At the end of the 9-month cruise the health and illness history of each crew member was analyzed and compared to the recent life-change scores. The results from all the ships were the same. Those individuals with the highest life-change scores prior to departure were the greatest risks for illness and injury of all kinds, while those with the lowest scores were the least risk. Similar studies have been conducted in university populations, with the same results. This particular kind of life change and subsequent illness methodology has been utilized to study psychiatric illness as well. Investigators both in London and in Connecticut have demonstrated a life change build-up in the history of patients who became depressed or developed schizophrenia.[16,17] The life-change scores of those who became psychiatrically ill were often twice those of a healthy control group. In the case of patients who committed suicide, the life-change score was four times the level of the controls. Patients with acute cardiovascular disease have demonstrated similar phenomena, and retrospective studies of individuals who experience sudden death have shown that they, too, have a very sharp build-up of life-change events in the few months or weeks prior to the fatal event.

These studies and similar ones have unequivocally established a statistically significant relationship between the level of life-change experience, particularly in the recent past, and the subsequent development of illness of all types. Diseases of newborns, children, young adults, and the elderly frequently occur at a point in life when there has been a definite increase in life changes. It needs to be emphasized strongly, however, that all these studies involve groups of humans, and the analysis is based on mean life-change scores and mean illness data. The prediction of future illness from a life-change questionnaire score must necessarily be an actuarial rather than an absolute one. If one takes a thousand individuals with a high life-crisis score, a much larger number of those from this group will become ill in the next 6 months than would become ill from a group of a thousand people with very low life-crisis scores. However, even among people with the highest life-change scores, some will not fall sick, and even some individuals with very low scores will develop a major illness. We have already mentioned that some prisoners of war subjected to very high but submaximal stress did not develop any impairment of health. Similarly, it was obvious even in the earliest life-change studies that there were a significant number of people with high scores, say 30 percent, who did not become sick during the following year.

Dissatisfaction with the relatively low level of correlation between the sum of life-change scores and subsequent illness has led to various attempts at refining the life-change methodology. Investigators have tried to divide life events into socially desirable versus socially undesirable ones, or into events controlled by the individual versus those over which the individual has no control. In addition, there have been studies in which life-change events are simply counted rather than given a particular weight. Unfortunately, efforts at the refinement of life-change measurement have not been very successful in increasing the ability to predict illness based upon an individual's life changes. There are several reasons for this.

One is the frequency with which selected life-change events occur. One glances at the list and sees that most of the life events have low scoring weights. The high-weight events, such as death or loss of a job, are comparatively infrequent and therefore their incidence is low in the samples of individuals studied. With such a low rate of occurrence of big events, refinements of measurement for these particular events produce very little change in the predictive power of the instrument. Additionally, while obviously undesirable events may produce great demands for coping and adjustment, even events seen as desirable, such as getting a promotion, may require considerable adjustment for any given person.

On the other hand, recent studies in which the subjects scaled their own individual life changes did increase the predictive validity slightly as compared to using the standard scale. However, it does not seem as if further refinements of the life-change scale will result in any great improvement in its powers of prophesying who will become ill.

THE INDIVIDUAL'S RESPONSE TO LIFE STRESS

The life-change, or life-stress, idea is a seminal one but in itself it is not adequate to deal with the complexity of disease onset. We must add an evaluation of the person involved to any consideration of the psychosocial events in order to have a comprehensive picture of stress and illness. After all, why do some people succumb to the weight of all their life changes while others do not? What are the intermediate steps by which the changes in someone's life proceed to effect bodily changes which in turn may help result in illness?

We will begin with a few life changes and see how their effects ripple through a series of internal lenses and filters to produce a specific reaction in a given person. For example, let us take a life change: loss of one's job. The event may be perceived very differently by two different individuals. To a 55-year-old male engineer who has worked for one company for 30 years and who currently has children in college, a continued mortgage on his home, and quite apart from any financial considerations, an intense emotional attachment to his job and its meaning, being laid off would be perceived as a catastrophe. To a 19-year-old vagabond who has already gone through a number of casual jobs such as washing dishes or pumping gas in a service station, being laid off from yet another job is a matter of the most trifling concern. In addition to these obvious kinds of differences, there are other more subtle influences on the perception of the life change. For instance, the experiences of early life may have conditioned the individual's attitude about certain life-change events. The attitudes of parents toward their child, the issue of whether the individual had an intact home, or whether one or both of the parents died or deserted, religious experiences, and the financial status of the parental home, all may have a persistent influence on how a life change is viewed in adult life. An individual who was brought up during the Great Depression and experienced catastrophic financial loss in his or her parental family, may be trying to build as much security as possible, and will obviously be more devastated by the loss of a job and its attendant income than someone who was brought up in an era where money always seemed available. Positive early life influences can be termed *biographical assets* in the sense that they strengthen the individual's ability to tolerate stress in later life; conversely, negative early life experiences can be termed *biographical liabilities* because they appear to weaken the individual's ability to adjust to the vicissitudes of later life. In addition to the individual's personal perception of life change which is conditioned by his or her upbringing, the deleterious effects of the life change can be enhanced or reduced by what are called social supports.[18] In fact, studies of workers who were laid off by reason of closure of the factories in which they worked indicated that the social support that was available to the unemployed was the largest single factor in reducing the incidence of new illness in the group. Individuals who had no support from their environment found the life change far more difficult to deal with than those who had such support. For example, if an individual was laid off a job but a comprehensive retraining program was available, as well as adequate unemployment insurance, the support of a loving and concerned family, and the promise of a new position in due course, then the person would have considerable protection against the malignant effects of the life change.

The concept of social support as a method of defense against the untoward effects of life changes can be broadened to include consideration of life satisfactions or gratifications. There is a body of evidence that indicates that a sense of gratification or satisfaction about what one is doing can help minimize adverse psychophysiological responses to what outside observers see as enormous stress. To take an extreme example, among Special Forces in Vietnam those individuals who knew their job and were doing it well, even though they were in an isolated camp under siege by the enemy, were found to have normal or low adrenal arousal and no other evidence of adverse bodily reactions, even though outside observers would have felt that these soldiers were under extreme stress.[19] Similarly, there is some evidence to indicate that satisfaction at work is the best single indicator of expected longevity in men.

In another study, individuals were followed over a period of months by means of daily diaries and frequent examinations of biochemical indicators of stress.[20] Once again, at times when the individual felt a sense of high job satisfaction and gratification, the indexes of arousal in the emergency endocrine system remained low despite many life events of a stressful nature.

There is also the factor of previous exposure to life-change events. It is not yet clear from our research whether previous exposure sensitizes an individual so that the next job loss is even more traumatic than the first, or whether it tends to desensitize the individual. Obviously it is a complex issue but very likely, as in the example given in the beginning of this section, someone who has lost 20 or 30 jobs after battles with bosses is less likely to be distressed about one more job loss than the faithful employee of 25 to 40 years who loses the only job he or she ever had.

Let us now think in terms of another life event, the death of a spouse. The way the individual perceives this catastrophe will partly depend upon the elements that made up his or her early life. It is probable that the death of a parent in childhood will influence the pattern of perception when the death of someone very close occurs in adult life. The present situation and the available social supports also impinge upon the impact of the tragedy. Contrast the perception of someone who loses her husband while living in an isolated retirement community in Florida or Arizona, with the social supports available to a widow in a large extended family in a small Italian hill town. In the first instance, the bereaved wife may literally have no one close to whom she may turn. Children, if any, may live at the opposite end of the nation and, in any case, have not been directly concerned with the daily lives of the parents for years. There are casual friends and the impersonal attention of the authorities, but there is no large group of people with whom to carry out a collective mourning.

To the woman in the former circumstance, the death of a husband may seem virtually like the end of the world. The Italian widow may also be desolated, but small and close-knit societies assign a definite role to widowhood as well as to other stages of life, thus providing considerable support at a time of severe stress.

The public health and medical advances of the twentieth century have made the death of young adults in the United States rather rare. However, in previous centuries dying young was the norm. Death connected with childbirth was common, and it might very well be that a long-lived male who survived until age 70 would have had three, four, or even five wives. It is impossible to gauge after all these years whether these repetitive losses were desensitizing or sensitizing to the constantly bereaved. Fortunately, few modern Americans are thus tested.

As we move beyond the perception of a life change, we might next consider the role of the patient's characteristic psychological defenses. These may include such common ego defense mechanisms as denial, displacement, repression, isolation, or reaction formation.

Psychoanalytic theory postulates that these mechanisms develop during the course of infancy and childhood, and reside in the ego where they function to protect the person against various unconscious drives that arise from the primitive id. Although initially thought of as mechanisms to maintain the internal stability of the psyche, they also can be thought of as mechanisms by which someone deals with external reality, particularly of an unpleasant sort. Severe threats to someone's very existence can be filtered through the psychological mechanism of denial or repression, and physiological harm can be minimized. For example, patients who have suffered myocardial infarction and who are hospitalized in a coronary care unit seem to have less physiological turmoil as measured by various biochemical indexes when they deny the serious reality of their illness, as compared with fellow patients who are acutely aware of their life-threatening sickness and are extremely anxious about it.[21] In a study of the parents of children with known leukemia, those parents who used denial, repression, intellectualization, and isolation of emotion, that is, who appeared to be able to ignore the obvious lethality of the disease or who spoke about their child's illness in very detached or intellectual terms with no apparent emotion, showed no evidence of adrenal arousal. On the other hand, those parents who were acutely aware of the imminent death of their children showed extremely high levels of adrenal hormonal release.[22]

There are other mental mechanisms which can be used by various patients in response to unpleasant life events. It is common enough to project one's own anger about the blows of fate and the unfairness of life onto the outside environment and in that way maintain an internal equilibrium. There is a large repertoire of psychological mechanisms which come into play in response to a life change. These defenses are found to some degree in all humans, but each individual has his or her own particular ensemble of responses and an individual way of dealing with the vicissitudes of life.

PHYSIOLOGICAL FACTORS AND LIFE STRESS

We now will consider the physiological responses of the body to a life stress which has been filtered through a person's perceptive and psychological defense mechanisms and then modified by life supports and gratifications. Over 130 years ago, the great French experimental physiologist, Claude Bernard, put forward the concept of the internal environment or *milieu interne* which represented that inner compartment enclosed by the skin in which all sorts of physical chemical systems work.[23] For life to proceed, it is necessary that there be a constancy of the inner being. There is a vast array of interlocking physiological systems which impinge upon each other. If one system oscillates out of phase, other systems attempt to restore this constancy. In his landmark book, *The Wisdom of the Body,* Walter Cannon of Harvard conceptualized this regulation of the constancy of the internal environment into a function which he called *homeostasis.*[24] Homeostasis is the tendency of the living organism to repair the damage caused by an insult of any kind and to restore the biological status quo. Cannon also studied bodily responses to emotion and adumbrated the concept of the "fight or flight" phenomenon.[25] The phenomenon is a heritage from our primitive past, when physical action was required constantly. Emergency situations activate the sympathetic nervous system and the adrenal medulla, which prepare the body either for fleeing or for doing battle. When a human, whether in Paleolithic times or in a modern city, is confronted with a menacing situation, the heart beats faster, the blood sugar rises, pupils dilate, blood pressure rises, muscles tense, and the individual is ready for battle or swift retreat. The three concepts central to modern studies of stress effects on human health are the internal environment, homeostasis, and fight or flight.

Selye was another great pioneer of stress research. He advanced the idea of *the general adaptation syndrome* and what has come to be called *stress-Selye.*[26] He clearly demonstrated that animals subjected to physical insults such as heat, chilling, or exercise to the point of exhaustion had stereotypic physiological reactions, including adrenal activation. He also showed that the stressors did not need to be of a physical kind, since the body also reacts to noxious social influences in the animal's environment. There have now been literally thousands of studies demonstrating activation of the entire endocrine system by psychosocial stress. If we look at the studies of the most popular organ, the adrenal gland, we see that adrenal arousal occurs when a person is confronted with a new life demand about which he or she feels some uncertainty in coping. As we previously mentioned in connection with the Special Forces unit in Vietnam, even the stress of combat does not necessarily produce adrenal activation if the individual feels confident and competent to cope with the situation.

In the last 15 years, detailed anatomical and neuroendocrine research of a biochemical and physiological character has proven that the pituitary is not the autonomous master gland that the biological teaching of 30 to 40 years ago represented it to be. The pituitary, while crucial to the endocrine regulation of the body, is under control of the hypothalamus, an integral part of the brain. In turn, the hypothalamus is part of the limbic system of the brain, which deals with such basic elements of life as hunger and emotion. The hypothalamus, through its secretion of *releasing factors,* carefully modulates pituitary output. We now know that the brain itself is the master endocrine organ and that it is within the brain that the perception of life events and the psychological reactions to them are transduced into physiological or even pathophysiological states. It is now apparent that the transfer of information between cells within the brain itself follows a biochemical process similar to that of the endocrine system. In the endocrine system hormones, or chemical messengers, are carried by the blood to various parts and alter the physiology of the target cells. These targets have special receptors either on the surface or within the cell itself. There is within the cell a so-called "second messenger," cyclic AMP, which carries on the physiological process begun by the hormone. Similarly, within the substance of the nervous system, molecules are released from a portion of one cell and, after traveling a very short distance, put in motion a set of physiological responses in the responding cell. It would appear that the neurohumoral transmitters within the brain, such as dopamine, norepinephrine, or serotonin also activate a cyclic AMP system. Thus, there is a striking parallelism between the central nervous system and the endocrine system, and the influence of one upon the other is now a well-established physiological fact. Constant activation of the endocrine system can lead to adrenal exhaustion and deleterious bodily effects elsewhere from secondary processes such as elevated blood sugar. In certain subgroups of individuals who have a particular kind of renin-angiotensin system, life events that produce anger can result in blood pressure elevations which may become sustained and eventually pathological in character.[27]

Of course, it is not only the endocrine system which is affected by life events. The controlling mechanisms for regional blood flow can be affected by emotions which reverberate in the brain. The capillaries of the nasal mucosa are particularly sensitive to emotional influences, and there can be blanching or transudation of the fluid produced by mind body interactions.[28] These changes in local blood flow could predispose an individual to the outbreak of illness. Pathogenic organisms are invariably present on such body surfaces, and their penetration and growth are enhanced by ischemia or the presence of transudates.

Yet another crucial body system in the prevention of illness is the immunological one. A recent study of 26 people whose spouses had recently died showed that a critical function of their T-cells was impaired as compared to the

T-cells of controls.[29] The T-cells are an integral element of immunological competence. This is further evidence that the period of bereavement is one that is accompanied by profound physiological and even pathophysiological effects, as well as the obvious social and psychological ones.[30]

At this time, many psychophysiological responses have to be categorized as a "black box" type phenomenon because many of the intermediate mechanisms are as yet unknown. Nevertheless, after life changes have occurred and have been filtered through the perceptual mechanisms and characteristic psychological responses to these life changes, psychophysiological responses occur. These may be responses of which one is aware, such as muscle tightness, stiffness, tension, headache, and sweating. On the other hand, most of the changes are imperceptible to the individual. A life event which produces anger may produce an immediate physiological response. Blood pressure, blood sugar, and blood fats may go up without the individual's becoming aware of the changes. These physiological responses may happen immediately, or there may be a time lag before their occurrence. Some of the changes may occur in phase with each other or in a multiphasic manner. There can be interaction between certain biochemical responses to stress, and it is likely that there is never a unitary physiological response to stress. Although the changes are multiple, because of the limitations of our measurement techniques we must rely on only a few measures. There are studies which show correlations between recent life-change experience, that is, changes over a 1-week period, and levels of catecholamines such as epinephrine and norepinephrine.[31] The higher the life-change unit score, the more likely it was that the subject would have an elevated epinephrine. In studies of naval populations, we were able to demonstrate that someone's perception of stresses could be correlated with certain simple biochemical measures. For example, those volunteers in the extremely demanding Underwater Demolition Team training course who were anxious to succeed and who viewed the challenge of the course as potentially surmountable, had high uric-acid and low cholesterol levels.[32] On the other hand, those subjects who perceived training as overly burdensome, distressing, and very likely too much for them tended to have a fall in uric acid and a rise in serum cholesterol.

Life events filtered through the individual's perceptions and characteristic defenses may cause physiological responses. How does a person try to manage recognized physiological changes? Perhaps the most noticeable psychophysiological response is muscle tension. There have been various informal methods of dealing with muscle tension over the years, including attempts at self-relaxation and massage. Recent years have seen the popularity of biofeedback, meditation, and other techniques aimed at loosening up muscles. Similarly, the unpleasant feelings that go with headache, muscle tension, and dysphoric mood, may be partly ameliorated by physical exercise. This is a popular method, and more and more evidence is accumulating to show that a regular exercise program has beneficial effects.[33] Another commonly used alternative is medication of various sorts. Previous ages used wine or tincture of opium for relaxation. In our era, there are a wide variety of tranquilizing medications which are widely used. These drugs are an attempt to expunge the dysphoria and associated physical manifestations that accompany unpleasant life experiences and the characteristic reactions to them.

Another extraordinarily important technique might be labeled cognitive strategies. These represent the stricken person's intellectual attempts to find ways out of the difficulties caused by life change. The richness, complexity, and effectiveness of cognitive strategies naturally depend on the intellectual and emotional assets which the individual possesses. Such awesome events as loss of a job or the death of a spouse demand considerable use of a wide variety of thought strategies before a new and satisfactory way of life can come into being.

If we continue to follow our model of life-change effects on health, we see that after the life changes have occurred they have been perceived by the individual in a characteristic way; psychological defenses have been mobilized and various physiological events occur. With the death of a spouse, the physiological changes in the bereaved may involve not only endocrine arousal but changes in the immune system itself, as well as a mourning process which closely resembles or may even merge into a pathological depression. The person may try to manage these deleterious effects with the aid of medications such as antidepressive drugs. He or she may then utilize other techniques such as physical exercise, which can be very helpful in depressive states, various forms of meditation and muscle relaxation techniques, and cognitive strategies which call for developing new friends, new interest, and reengaging with life.

If the defensive and coping systems of the person fail to deal with the problems occasioned by adverse psychosocial events, physical or psychological symptoms may appear. The person must then make a decision whether to seek medical care, except, of course, in the most obvious emergency situations. Many humans of a stoical type can carry on for a considerable time with symptoms that are remarkably painful and disturbing. Others seek immediate help for the most trifling of complaints. There is a vast literature in sociology about illness behavior and the so-called "sick role."[34] Certain demographic characteristics, such as age, sex, race, and socioeconomic status, impinge on the individual's readiness to seek medical care. Institutional variables such as the availability of medical care and health insurance also influence whether or not the individual seeks medical care. The sick role has profound implications in most societies. In ours, if one is diagnosed by appropriate authorities as having a bona fide illness, one is given a license, as it were, to miss work and be relieved of various kinds of responsibilities of an important sort. This unloading of responsibilities may be very congenial to some people and abhorrent to others. In any case, only when the person seeks medical treatment and certification by diagnosis can we complete the process of recording the illness and the series of steps that began with the life changes.

In the case of someone who has suffered the death of a spouse and whose response-management techniques, initial medications, and cognitive strategies have all failed, the individual may develop an illness, either a psychiatric illness such as severe depression or some physical illness. The patient consults a physician and is certified as a case. Once again we see the large number of intervening steps between the life changes and the counting of someone as a case, and why it is that life changes will always be only modestly predictive of future illness at best.

We will now turn to some specific examples of the intertwining of person, events, and disease.

The patient was a physician who died at the age of 55. He was the only son of a modestly successful and highly respectable Jewish couple who lived in the lesser section of a wealthy suburb in a large Eastern city. He grew up with the values of ambition, education, and respectability deeply inculcated. He attended a fine, competitive public high school, which selected students from all over the city, and then attended the very prestigious Eastern university which his father had attended as a day student many years before. He was a brilliantly successful student and received many academic honors. The particular university he attended had always loomed large in his thinking as a boy, and association with it represented the highest and most desirable element to which he could aspire. After graduating with honors from the liberal arts college of his university, he attended Oxford University. After completing his work there, he went to another prestigious university in the United States to obtain his Ph.D. Meanwhile, World War II broke out, and after taking his Ph.D. he served in the armed services until the end of the war. He then returned, completed his premedical requirements, and attended the medical school of his initial alma mater. During all this period he had been in absolutely robust health, and he moved steadily from triumph to triumph without interruption. After completing medical school with a superb record, he took further training in internal medicine. Throughout medical school and subsequent medical training, he continued to maintain his research interests in an area that lay on the boundaries between basic science and clinical medicine. When his formal education was finally completed, he became a faculty member at his beloved university. Unfortunately, at that point in time he was only able to obtain a faculty post in one of the smaller professional schools of the university, and although he quickly reached the rank of associate professor, this particular school's financial structure was such that associate professors did not have tenure, in the sense of permanency of employment. Although his research work continued to be very successful, it was obvious that it did not completely fit into the major work of the department. The department chairman felt that the department's research effort should be of a monolithic character and ultimately he asked the subject to leave. This was an extremely severe blow, and one which he never fully dealt with emotionally. Simultaneously, at his wife's behest, he had become involved in a large business venture which necessitated the purchase of a great deal of land. As it turned out, the project was ultimately successful, but its final financial success did not occur until after his death, and during the initial years it appeared very "chancy." He had always been extremely careful and conservative in the handling of money, and had lived comfortably but parsimoniously. It was an extreme wrench for him to go heavily into debt on a business venture. Several months after his loss of professorship, and a few months after the signing of the papers which mortgaged all his property, he noticed the first appearance of a skin lesion which ultimately proved to be a manifestation of an internal malignancy. This was treated with radiation therapy and the lesions melted away. About the time of his initial treatment, he was able to secure a post on the general campus of his university in the same discipline in which his Ph.D. had been obtained.

Unfortunately, this post, too, was not of a tenured nature. On the other hand, there were many promises given to him that he would indeed be part of the permanent faculty. During this entire time he continued to receive many offers from other universities which would have been delighted to have him either as a full professor in the regular sense or as a member of a pure research service. However, he could not bring himself to leave the university with which he identified so strongly. He then had a period of remission from physical symptoms, which went along with several years of placidity and success. He helped to inaugurate several innovative educational programs which proved to be extremely successful and highly popular with the students. He also brought out several books documenting his research findings over the years. However, he was left dangling as to his future prospects. During this time he made several wide-ranging expeditions to various parts of the globe to gather data for his studies and, after one of these, he noticed a recrudescence of some of his previous symptoms and other manifestations of the disease. The exacerbation was treated and again he seemed perfectly normal. During the ensuing 18 months things began to come to a climax—the great investment was paying off slowly and his academic future was finally decided. After much deliberation and discussion, the university declined to give him a professorship on the grounds that he was now too old. His disappointment and frustration were extreme. However, he resolved to carry on in the capacity of a lecturer. About this time the disease returned in full force, with new manifestations involving the pleura, the abdominal cavity, the liver, and other viscera, and he began to go downhill rapidly with the onset of weight loss, the melting away of his musculature, edema, and other untoward signs. He continued working right up to the end of his life, and indeed on his final day he was still conscientiously seeing students up until an hour before he actually died. At the memorial service in the chapel of his university, those who eulogized him correctly pointed out a noble character which included an enormous sense of dedication, self-sacrifice, conscientiousness, and self-abnegation. It had always been difficult for him to show outward anger, and he tended to keep his anger and disappointment inside himself and not reveal his feelings in their entirety even to his family members and closest friends.

If we follow our model with this patient, we see that his major life events included losing a coveted position and an ultimate occupational failure as well as severe financial jeopardy. The patient perceived these life events as being particularly traumatic because of the special qualities of his past life which made him sensitive to the questions of prestige, status, and security which are involved with these life changes. He utilized such mental mechanisms as repression and, to some degree, denial. The pathophysiological changes which occurred are unknown to us, but it may well have been that there were changes which affected those body surveillance mechanisms which guard against cellular changes of a malignant character. His cognitive strategies were not equal to the task of coping, and the medications and radiation therapies used by his physicians were unable to deal with the biological potential of the tumor plus whatever enhancement of its growth was occasioned by troubled circumstances and homeostatic failures.

Naturally, as in all these cases, one cannot prove that the life events and environment in which he found himself had anything to do with either the genesis or the course of the disease, but to those who were able to see him from the time of his healthy and athletic youth until his last hours, it was certainly clear that both the initial appearance and the recurrences of the tumor had an eerie synchrony with great blows and losses in a life that (perhaps unwisely) had been dedicated to a romanticized and ultimately hollow ideal.

> The second patient was a 30-year-old woman of compelling beauty and vivacity. She had come from a small town in the remote rural area of a large Midwestern state, and from her early years had an ambition to move up in the world and obtain a certain kind of social position and material affluence. She had been a very successful athlete as a girl and had been an extremely popular figure in her own rural high school. She began university in another part of the state, but at age 21, with a year of college left to go, she married a man somewhat older than herself who seemed to be a "comer." He was energetic and resourceful, or so she thought, and it appeared that he would eventually be a man of means. Alas, this did not prove to be so. His early promise seemed to fade, and after 8 or 9 years of marriage it appeared that he was not going anywhere and that they would be mired in a somewhat limited existence. It was about this time that she met a man who seemed to be the embodiment of many of her youthful dreams in that, while not rich, he certainly had far more money than her husband and seemed to represent the hope of a vastly greater amount of success than either her present or future situation could afford. She quickly became attracted to this man, and it seemed possible at that point that they might each abandon their respective families for a life together. However, there were impediments on both sides—she was reluctant because of her children, who were greatly fond of their father, and she also had some religious scruples. The man had similar religious doubts and pangs of conscience. At the time when she was seriously considering fleeing her husband, she developed an attack of gouty arthritis. This was extremely painful and rendered her immobile for a period of time. Subsequently she continued to have remissions and exacerbations. What with one illness or another and other reality obstacles, the romance collapsed and she returned to urging her husband to become more successful. He had, in the interim, inherited some land from his family. He took the proceeds from the sale of the land, and instead of investing it prudently, invested the money, plus all their savings, in commodities' futures. He managed to lose virtually all the money in the process. When he summoned up the courage to disclose his recklessness and failure to his wife, she had further attacks of gout, which only remitted when she finally made definite preparations for the dissolution of her marriage. Subsequently, she remarried, this time to an older professional man of high and assured income. She moved to a more fashionable section of the city than the one in which she had previously lived. Her gout was well controlled under the new circumstances.

In this patient, life events included considerable difficulties in home life and changes in relationships with spouse and significant others. The patient perceived these life events in terms of her background, which placed a heavy emphasis on the outward trappings of success and social mobility. She used denial, repression, and displacement as psychological mechanisms, but these were not entirely successful. It was during this period of initial stress that her uric acid rose to very high levels, 15 to 16 mg percent. This high uric acid level correlated with her extreme energy, vivacity, and alertness. She then developed gouty arthritis, which has a predilection for appearing on occasions when there is a strong conflict about fleeing or staying. A subsequent life event, the loss of all family money, led to a more determined cognitive strategy, namely to remove herself from the situation. As her life stabilized, her uric acid level dropped and the amount of medication necessary to maintain her in remission fell sharply as well.

Occasionally an illness episode, traumatic as it is at the time, may actually serve a useful function in prolonging the life and happiness of the patient. For example, I know of a physician who had a heart attack at age 55. Previously he had been an extraordinarily hard-working and self-sacrificing individual who had built his practice to the point where it virtually precluded all other aspects of life. Following his heart attack, he changed his life-style drastically and, while he continued to be a contributing pediatrician, he limited his practice to allow appropriate time for ample rest, relaxation, and other nonmedical activities. He refused to reenter the frantic, overwhelming life that had preceded the infarction. He is still alive at the age of 79 and has never had another heart attack. On the other hand, the author knows of several other individuals who lived similarly overburdened lives but who returned to the old overwhelmingly hurried style of living even following a heart attack. Although they initially thought they would change, apparently they later felt that they could not live in other than a frantic way. Both these individuals had fatal myocardial infarctions 2 or 3 years after their initial attacks.

CONCLUSION

The daily demands of medical practice and the vast amounts of technological knowledge and expertise needed for the solution of patient problems make it difficult for the usual physician to approach illnesses from an ecological point of view. Yet this ecological or combined systems focus is what the work on psychosocial factors in pathogenesis of illness teaches us. Psychosocial studies of illness focus on the physical and emotional environment which surrounds the individual and illuminate the ways in which an individual construes the events of life in terms of his or her own interior templates. This all-embracing point of view adds an important dimension of understanding that can be helpful in patient care. I hope I have shown that life changes in themselves play a role in pathogenesis, but that we need to add knowledge of other systems in order to make the best prediction of future illness. It must not be thought, therefore, that the psychosocial aspect of illness is all-explanatory. Even if we knew everything about the patient and the surrounding environment from the psychosocial point of view, in many instances we would still only know a small portion of the variance that goes into becoming sick. Many illnesses have rather clear physical antecedents with little or no psychosocial input. If one eats a bowl of contaminated potato salad at a picnic, one will most likely develop enteritis regardless of one's premorbid psychological state, although psyche may well affect the course and sequelae of the illness incurred. Psychosocial stress is important and dangerous and at its most severe level, as in the concentration camp experience, it might be compared to work in a radium or asbestos factory. Fortunately, the average person is usually subjected only to episodic mild-to-moderate stress situations. Nevertheless, a physician who lacks an understanding of emotional aspects of patients' lives must necessarily be limited in his or her effectiveness as a practitioner. The psychosocial viewpoint must be added to the biological one for completeness of understanding.

REFERENCES

1 Arthur, Ransom J.: "Extreme Stress in Adult Life and Its Psychic and Psychophysiological Consequences," in *Life Stress and Illness,* Springfield: Charles C Thomas, 1974, p. 195.

2 Spicer, C. C., D. N. Stewart, and D. M. de R. Winser: "Perforated Peptic Ulcer during the Period of Heavy Air-Raids," *Lancet,* 1:14, 1944.

3 Berg, W., and M. Richlin: "Injuries and Illnesses of Vietnam War POWs," *Military Medicine,* 142(7):514–518, 1977.

4 Eisenberg, L.: "Psychiatry and Society," *New England J. Med.,* 296:903–910, April 21, 1977.

5 Tuke, D. T.: *Illustrations of the Influence of the Mind upon the Body,* London: J. & A. Churchill, 1884.

6 Freud, Sigmund: "Mourning and Melancholia," in *Collected Papers,* vol. 4, London: Ho̦arth Press, and The Institute of Psycho-Analysis, 1959, pp. 152–170.

7 S▓▓▓e, A. H., and G. Engel: "Giving Up As a Final Common Pathway to Changes in ▓▓lth," in *Psychosocial Aspects of Physical Illness: Advances in Psychosomatic Medicine,* vol. 8, New York: S. Karger, 1972, pp. 20–40.

8 Holmes, T. H., and R. H. Rahe: "The Social Readjustment Rating Scale," *J. Psychosom. Res.,* 11:213–218, 1967.

9 Hawkins, N. G., R. Davies, and T. H. Holmes: "Evidence of Psychosocial Factors in the Development of Pulmonary Tuberculosis," in *Am. Review of Tuberculosis and Pulmonary Disease,* 75:768–780, 1957.

10 Rahe, R. H. et al.: "Social Stress and Illness Onset," *J. Psychosom. Res.,* 8:35–44, 1964.

11 Janney, J. G., M. Masuda, and T. H. Holmes: "Impact of a Natural Catastrophe on Life Events," *J. Human Stress,* 3:22–34, June 1977.

12 Gorsuch, R. L., and M. D. Key: "Abnormalities of Pregnancy As a Function of Anxiety and Life Stress," *Psychosom. Med.,* 36(4):352–372, 1974.

13 Dodge, J. A.: "Psychosomatic Aspects of Infantile Pyloric Stenosis," *J. Psychosom. Res.,* 16:1–5, 1972.

14 Stein, S. P., and E. Charles: "Emotional Factors in Juvenile Diabetes Mellitus: A Study of Early Life Experience of Adolescent Diabetes," *Am. J. Psychiatry,* 128(6):56–60, 1971.

15 Rahe, R. H. et al.: "The Epidemiology of Illness in Naval Environments: I. Illness Type, Distribution, Severities, and Relationship to Life Change," *Military Medicine,* 135(6):443–452, 1970.

16 Paykel, E. S., B. A. Prusoff, and J. K. Myers: "Suicide Attempts and Recent Life Events," *Archives of General Psychiatry,* 32:327–333, 1975.

17 Brown, G. W., and J. L. T. Birley: "Crises and Life Changes and the Onset of Schizophrenia," *J. Health and Social Behavior,* 9:203–214, 1968.

18 Cobb, S.: "Social Support As a Moderator of Life Stress," *J. Psychosom. Med.,* **38**(5):300–314, 1976.

19 Bourne, P.: *Men, Stress and Vietnam,* Boston: Little, Brown, 1970.

20 Rahe, R. H., R. T. Rubin, and R. J. Arthur: "The Three Investigators Study Serum Uric Acid, Cholesterol and Cortisol Variability during the Stresses of Everyday Life," *J. Psychosom. Med.,* **36**:258–268, 1974.

21 Klein, R. F., T. F. Garrity, and J. Gelein: "Emotional Adjustment and Catecholamine Excretion during Early Recovery From MI," *J. Psychosom. Res.,* **18**:425–435, 1974.

22 Wolff, C. T. et al.: "Relationships between Psychological Defense and Mean 17-Hydroxycorticosteroid Excretion Rates: I. A Predictive Study of Parents of Children with Leukemia," *J. Psychosom. Med.,* **26**:576–591, 1964.

23 Bernard, C.: *Introduction to the Study of Experimental Medicine,* New York: Dover, 1957.

24 Cannon, W.: *The Wisdom of the Body,* New York: W. W. Norton, 1939.

25 _____: *Bodily Changes in Pain, Hunger, Fear, and Rage,* Boston: C. T. Branford, 1929.

26 Selye, H.: *The Stress of Life,* Toronto: McGraw-Hill, 1956.

27 Esler, M. et al.: "Mild High-Renin Essential Hypertension: A Neurogenic Human Hypertension?" *New England J. Med.,* **296**(8):405–411, 1977.

28 Holmes, T. H. et al.: *The Nose: An Experimental Study of Reactions within the Nose in Human Subjects during Varying Life Experiences,* Springfield: Charles C Thomas, 1950.

29 Bartrop, R. W. et al.: "Depressed Lymphocyte Function After Bereavement," *Lancet,* April 16, 1977, pp.834–836.

30 Madison, D., and A. Viola: "The Health of Widows in the Year Following Bereavement," *J. Psychosom. Res.,* **12**:297–306, 1968.

31 Theorell, T. et al.: "A Longitudinal Study of 21 Subjects with Coronary Heart Disease: Life Changes, Catecholamine Excretion and Related Biochemical Reactions," *J. Psychosom. Med.,* **34**:505–516, 1972.

32 Rahe, R. H. et al.: "Serum Uric Acid and Cholesterol Variability: A Comprehensive View of Underwater Demolition Team Training," *JAMA,* **206**:2875–2880, 1968.

33 Arthur, R. J.: "Swimming and Cardiovascular Fitness in the Older Age Group," *J. Sports Medicine,* **3**(1):35–40, 1975.

34 Mechanic, D.: *Medical Sociology,* New York: The Free Press, 1968.

Chapter 10

The Neuroses

John Donnelly, M.D.

EDITORS' INTRODUCTION

What is it like to be fearful of getting into an elevator? How does it feel to be compelled to wash one's hands repeatedly until they are raw and bleeding? How embarrassing it is when others remark about this, or about a frequent urge to check the gas jets on the stove and to make certain that the front door is locked. To "know" that nothing is wrong, yet "have" to check it. What is it like to be deeply depressed, with overwhelming feelings of inadequacy, insecurity, worthlessness, and hopelessness—what is the purpose of even seeing a physician when one's condition is hopeless?

What is it like to be a physician dealing with a person who has a germ phobia and obsessive-compulsive thoughts and rituals? What is the feeling within physicians when they take time to no avail to explain about germs and the fact that the compulsive acts really are not necessary? How does it feel to deal with an intelligent person who has a depression that the physician knows to be treatable, and yet have the patient insist that his or her condition is hopeless? What are the feelings of the physician as the patient shrugs and refuses to accept what seems so simple?

Physicians are constantly dealing with many neurotic symptoms, which are sometimes the presenting complaint, but more often serve as a concomitant condition to organic pathology. The physician may feel exasperated when the patient insists that there must be something wrong physically, that the rapid and strong heartbeat must be evidence of heart disease, or that the abdominal pain could not just be "all in the mind."

The manner in which the physician handles patients with neurotic symptomatology or overlay to organic pathology will usually determine the patient's receptivity to the possibility that the symptoms may be emotional in origin. This manner of handling patients requires extra time and great patience on the physician's part. How easy it is to brush off such patients and consider them just hypochondriacs—"crocks." However, how frustrating further involvement with the patient may be if the physician does not understand neurotic symptomatology.

Then, too, physicians are not immune to significant neurotic psychopathology; quite the contrary. Physicians have their share of neuroses. Most function very well in spite of them. A few decompensate and function inadequately. Some turn to alcoholism, which often masks a depression. Narcotics addiction may be considered an occupational hazard.

The physician who is oblivious to the prevalence of neuroses or even deep emotions is often the physician who denies the presence of these tensions within him- or herself, and too often decompensates into an incapacitated state. It is not surprising that physicians have a high suicide rate.

To the extent that the physician is open to dealing with feelings and conflicts, he or she will be able to help patients more fully.

This chapter, written by a prominent psychiatrist from a large, distinguished, private psychiatric hospital, should help physicians understand more about the etiology of neurosis, the different types of neurosis, what nonpsychiatrists can do to help, and how they can best call upon a psychiatrist when further help is indicated. It should also aid the physician in grasping a better understanding of the neurotic overlay to medical illness.

Under the category of the neuroses falls a group of conditions which cause the patient varying degrees of emotional distress but in which organic pathology that accounts for the symptoms cannot be demonstrated. These conditions have been designated as functional disorders.

In most cases, the differentiation between neuroses and psychoses is made on the basis of an overt break with reality in the patient's thinking. Psychoneurotic patients usually recognize the fact that they are suffering from an illness or incapacitating disorder. In this sense, they may be said to have insight into their illness, though not into its etiology. Those who suffer from severe symptoms that usually lead to the diagnosis of psychoneurosis, but who do not recognize the gross abnormality of their thinking or behavior, are out of contact with reality. Their illnesses fall, therefore, into the category of functional psychoses. Perhaps the best example of this occurs in some obsessive-compulsive states.

Though they may occur in children, psychoneuroses are generally phenomena of adulthood. The vulnerability of an individual to the onset of a psychoneurosis is frequently found in the patient's premorbid personality structure. The psychoneuroses are best understood as reactions to the stress that arises out of the individual's internal conflicts. The specific symptoms are primarily the compromise resolutions of the conflicts, the partially effective operations of the individual's defense mechanisms (see Chapter 2). Just as a chronic bronchitis may be the result of an inadequate resolution of an acute bronchitis, so a psychoneurosis may be the outcome of an inadequate resolution of conflicting forces within the personality.

CLASSIFICATION OF THE NEUROSES

While specific psychoneuroses have been delineated, there is no pure form; the types overlap. Since a psychoneurosis represents a pathological exaggeration of emotional experience or of behavioral phenomena occurring in all human beings, it is to be expected that psychopathology in one area of the personality will be accompanied by disturbance in other areas. Consequently, the diagnosis of a specific neurosis is made on the basis of the primary symptom affecting the patient. Marked anxiety is present in almost all psychoneuroses. In some, the patient attributes the anxiety as secondary to another symptom, while in others the anxiety is repressed. For example, the patient with a phobia about high places feels uncomfortable in high places, in contrast to a patient with a conversion reaction, who does not experience any distress despite the conversion symptom.

The conditions are classified according to the following diagnoses:

1 Anxiety neurosis
2 Phobic neurosis
3 Hysterical neurosis
4 Conversion neurosis
5 Dissociative neurosis
6 Neurosis following trauma
7 Depersonalization neurosis
8 Obsessional neurosis
9 Depressive neurosis

DEGREES OF SEVERITY

As previously noted, the psychoneuroses represent the outcome resulting from the imbalance of internal conflicting psychologic forces within the individual. Just as there can be many degrees of imbalance, so can there be degrees of severity in the manifestations of this imbalance. Thus, within the normal range of personalities, some individuals are more prone to feelings of anxiety than others, yet their level of anxiety is not incapacitating. Similarly, in a given social or cultural group, concern about cleanliness can fall within a range of normal expectations of behavior; excessive concern, on the other hand, may be evident in behavior ranging from eccentric to clearly abnormal or pathologic.

In the abnormal range seen in the psychoneuroses, there are also degrees of pathology with corresponding degrees of severity up to the totally incapacitating. Because of the variations in severity of these clinical pictures, from normal through abnormal manifestations, many people unfortunately have attributed pejorative connotations to the word "neurotic."

ANXIETY NEUROSIS

The most universally experienced emotion is that of anxiety. Far from being pathologic, the experience of anxiety is normal and essential to survival. It is the feeling that arises when there is a threat to one's well-being or welfare. While fear and anxiety feel the same subjectively, they differ objectively. When the anxious feeling results from the threat of an identifiable external danger in the environment, the term *fear* is used. Thus, fear serves a most important function in alerting the individual to prepare for protection by taking appropriate measures.

Whereas fear arises when the specific external cause of anxiety can be delineated, similar feelings can also occur in situations in which the cause in the environment is not immediately apparent. While the potential consequences when the brakes of a car fail is clearly the origin of fear in the driver, the loss of a job may arouse equally distressing feelings of anxiety in many individuals. In the case of a job loss, the threat to the physical well-being of the individuals and their families may seem to be an externally generated danger. However, the immediate cause of the anxiety is the individual's fear of being unable to provide adequately for dependents in the future, according to personal expectations. While the *threat* of the loss of a job generates fear, the *result* of the loss of a job is anxiety. The drive to avoid anxiety in most individuals is a normal motivating force.

Most individuals, at one time or another, experience the emotion of fear. This can be induced by external dangers; for example, the child may fear fire as the result of being burned. Or the fear may be the result of discipline involving either physical or psychologic punishment, such as the threat of withdrawing parental love. In an age when corporal punishment as a means of achieving conformity is so greatly deprecated, the threatened loss of maternal or paternal approval is perhaps the most effective use of fear with the child.

The converse, of course, also holds true. Providing love, approval, and other appropriate positive reinforcement gives the child the foundation for healthy personality development, which helps to avoid undue fear and anxiety in present and later years.

Anxiety occurs when the threat to the individual's well-being arises within his or her own psychological structure. This may occur as the result of forces operating at two different levels. At the first level, there are impulses or drives to behave in ways contrary to the individual's ethical standards (e.g., sexual needs which are gratifiable only in unacceptable ways, or the urge to carry out an aggressive act antagonistic to personal principles).

The second level at which anxiety may occur is related to the capacity or incapacity to live up to personal expectations. Each person, as a result of rearing or acculturation, develops a self-image, a set of ideals and aspirations that, hopefully, are achievable. These standards and aspirations vary greatly from one person to another. For some, these standards are of the greatest importance, and failure to adhere to them results in feelings of marked anxiety.

The origins of anxiety neurosis, and indeed of all the psychoneuroses, lie in large measure in the standards of personal behavior which have been incorporated into the person's self-concepts. Because humans, as distinct from other members of the animal kingdom, pass through a long stage of dependency, they are for this period of time subject to the benevolence (or otherwise) of parents or parental surrogates. Just as feelings of physical well-being (e.g., relief from hunger, thirst, cold, or pain) are derived from relationships with others, particularly parents, so are feelings of security or freedom from anxiety dependent on them. Parents, in turn, expect conformity to their expectations of appropriate behavior at the different stages of development. In this long process, the child learns to avoid immediate expression of instinctual forces, especially aggressive and sexual acts; failure to do so would automatically result in painful experiences.

In the process, the child learns and adopts parental rules of conduct, including the acts and behavior that are permitted and praiseworthy, and rejects those that are prohibited. Because these precepts are laid down by those who also relieve pain and restore feelings of well-being, they become, in large measure, the code of acceptable behavior in adulthood. Just as childhood actions contrary to this code raise fears of loss of parental approval and love, so in adulthood actions contrary to the code result in loss of self-esteem. The arousal of contrary impulses or the temptation to act them out results in feelings of anxiety.

The instinctual forces that are the most frequent sources of anxiety are those of anger, rage, and hostility, and those associated with sexual drives. The ability of the individual to deal with these forces, which are potentially destructive to the sense of well-being, appears to be determined in some part by the physical substrate of the nervous system, but most significantly by the experiences of the individual during the maturing process.

Normal Anxiety

Fear resulting from the perception of an external environmental danger is a normal emotion necessary to alert the individual to prepare for defense and ensure survival. In the same way, anxiety arising from internal impulses that are a threat to the person's sense of well-being is a normal motivating force. Anxiety becomes a pathologic condition when it is so incapacitating that the individual's normal functioning is disrupted.

Just as the anxious child often can be reassured by the parents, so can anxiety in adults often be dissipated by the reassurance of an authority figure, such as a physician in the case of physical illness or a supervisor in an occupational situation. Similarly, the achievement of a sought-after objective, such as a promotion or other accomplishment, relieves and removes anxiety generated by an individual's doubts about his or her performance.

There are a number of etiologic hypotheses about the origin of anxiety, each related to the subject area on which the author focuses.[1] Cannon's concept that fear and anxiety are alerting mechanisms to prepare for "flight or fight" is based on the theory that perception of danger produces a disturbance in the homeostatic physiologic balance of the organism.[2,3] On the basis of a broader theory, Kelman postulates that people live in a unitary system that includes the organism and its total environment.[4] The latter embraces people's societal and cultural relationships, the disturbance of which results in the feeling of anxiety. In a narrower framework, psychoanalytic theory specifies that anxiety is the emotion resulting from a conflict between the *id,* or instinctual forces, and the *superego,* or conscience. Anxiety is experienced when an instinctual drive threatens to overcome the forces opposing it.[5]

Manifestations of anxiety and fear are experienced identically by the individual, though they differ in degree and in kind from individual to individual and depend on the severity of the threat. There is a feeling of apprehension, the feeling that something bad is about to occur and that one's security is in some way about to be threatened. Bodily changes accompany this—palpitation or tachycardia, often beginning with the sensation of a missed heartbeat; hyperhidrosis of the armpits, the hands, or, indeed, of the whole body. There may be quickened or deepened breathing, or there may be disturbance of the alimentary tract, with dryness of the mouth, even nausea. The person may show pallor, while inwardly experiencing the feeling of "gooseflesh"; the pupils of the eyes may be dilated; the individual may feel restless, be unable to sit still for any length of time, may pace the floor and exhibit sudden movements, nervous mannerisms, and tremors or trembling of the hands, arms, or of the whole body. In some cases, movements may be uncoordinated, so that there is inability to walk. If the onset is sudden and the cause sufficiently distressing, there may be temporary paralysis or even temporary loss of consciousness. At night, there may be an inability to get to sleep, characteristically with marked feelings of anxiety, and the sleep may be restless, troubled by nightmares.

All these symptoms may be present either singly or in combination in the same person, depending on the severity of the threat and on the varying capacities of different individuals to withstand stress.

Pathologic Anxiety

In "pure" anxiety neurosis, the feeling of apprehension has a diffuse quality and is unrelated to a recognizable specific cause. This is free-floating anxiety.

On the other hand, an individual may cope with anxiety unconsciously by focusing attention on a particular object, a body organ, or a symptom, in which case the anxiety is said to be "fixated." Thus, a whole range of symptoms may occur without any demonstrable organic pathology. These symptoms are to be distinguished from those occurring because of psychosomatic diseases, such as peptic ulcer, asthma, or ulcerative colitis.

Pathologic anxiety may be classified as acute and chronic. Acute anxiety arises with a relatively sudden onset, usually as the sequela of a specific event, though it may not appear immediately and it may increase in severity over a short period of time. The occasions for such attacks are often easily recognizable—an accident, a divorce, a change of environment (either threatened or forced), a promotion when the individual has doubts about the ability to fulfill the responsibilities entailed. The physical concomitants may be multiple.

Depending on the capacity of the individual to cope with the sources of the stress, the symptoms may subside quickly, gradually diminish, eventually disappear, or persist.

Chronic anxiety represents a prolonged continuation of the condition and frequently results in impaired performance. The patient tends to live in a state of hyperalertness, so that acute symptomatology may be triggered easily by sudden events which would not evoke it in other people. There is insomnia, especially in falling asleep, although early awakening may also occur. There may be anorexia, but sometimes, paradoxically, weight increases because of overeating. The anxiety may be free floating or may be focused on physical symptoms.

When a chronic anxiety neurosis has developed, it tends to persist for long periods of time, though there may be fluctuations in degree, depending on the current life situation.

Differential Diagnosis

Anxiety is a general concomitant of almost all pathologic and psychopathologic conditions. Thus, physical illness is a threat to the feeling of well-being, and the more ignorant the patient is about the illness, the greater the stress.

A thorough physical examination is imperative. It is necessary to consider organic disease, in particular those conditions which may in themselves cause symptoms which also occur in anxiety states. These include thyrotoxicosis, organic brain conditions, and drug addiction and withdrawal (see Chapter 14).

A thorough mental status examination should also be performed, because anxiety frequently accompanies other psychiatric conditions—depressive states, obsessional neuroses, and phobic conditions. The presence of a phobia may sometimes be elicited only by careful questioning. It may be difficult to differentiate even moderately severe depressive syndromes in which there are hypochondriacal complaints.

Treatment

The approach to therapy depends on the level or intensity of the anxiety and on the acuteness or chronicity of the condition.

In severe, acute conditions following trauma, whether physical or psychologic, early sedation that is sufficient for effective control of the anxiety may be necessary, until the level of anxiety drops to manageable proportions.

Thereafter, the dosage is reduced progressively to a maintenance level at which the individual can reinstitute mechanisms for coping with the stress. A wide range of anxiolytic medications is available. Barbiturates are effective, but have become increasingly abandoned because of their depressive potential and because of complications such as dependence and withdrawal sequelae.

With all forms of anxiety, but especially with acute conditions, reassurance is indicated. Initially, this may require a firm but gently authoritative manner. The role of the physician in these cases should be identical to that of the strong and caring benevolent parent. When the acute stage has passed, supportive psychotherapy should be continued as long as there is improvement.

When other approaches are required, the alternatives include psychoanalytically oriented psychotherapy and orthodox psychoanalysis, in both of which there is exploration of unconscious factors accounting for the conditions. For some, group therapy may be very useful.

PHOBIC NEUROSIS

The word phobia is derived from Phobos, the Greek goddess of fear. More for descriptive purposes than for any scientific rationale, phobic conditions were named by prefixing the Greek root of the word for the phobic object; for example, agoraphobia, fear of open spaces; claustrophobia, fear of confined spaces; mysophobia, fear of dirt or germs. The list is endless.

Although phobia connotes that the source of danger lies in the external environment, this is only a partially accurate understanding. The feared object or situation has a very specific meaning to the person who is suffering from the phobia. It represents an object or situation that in the past stimulated or gave rise to an internal impulse or drive, the acting out of which would be unacceptable to the individual. The phobic object is often symbolic of a past danger.

A *phobia* may be defined, therefore, as a disorder characterized by a state of anxiety aroused by an object, animal, or place that would not arouse the same level of emotions in the ordinary person, emotions for which no reason is apparent. Moreover, the phobic individual recognizes the irrationality of the fear intellectually.

Because the phobic object is specific to the affected individual, and its power to arouse anxiety is based on personal experience, there is no rationale for a classification of phobias. Many of the phobic objects are things which would cause discomfort under certain circumstances in numbers of people, such as darkness, thunder, snakes, or being locked in a confined space, but the anxiety is much more intense in the phobic subject. Other phobias are more specific in nature, and anxiety is aroused when it would not normally occur. Such phobias are those associated with places, such as public parks, open streets, crowded shops, heights, or flying; animals, including dogs, cats, and horses; insects such as spiders; and plants and flowers. Much less frequently, specific persons may be the objects of phobias.

Origins of Phobias

Although phobias have been recognized throughout history, and had previously been studied intensively, new understanding of their origins began with the introduction of the psychoanalytic method by Freud and his disciples.[6,7,8] In the framework of this approach, a phobia represents an inadequately resolved conflict within the individual caused by impulses or drives that are unacceptable to the superego or conscience, the expression (or even the recognition or acceptance) of which would result in injury or damage to the individual's self-concept. The most frequent impulses giving rise to phobias are those of a sexual nature and those of aggression, anger, and hostility directed at other people. Another source of phobias is the drive to possess desired objects, the acquisition of which would be possible only by internally prohibited acts. Such impulses normally have been brought under firm control during the process of maturation in childhood and adolescence by the coping mechanisms of the ego. In the phobic person, the resolution of the conflict has been inadequate and the power of the ego is sufficient only to keep the impulse out of the immediate awareness of the individual.

The proximity of an object or occasion that would stimulate the memory of past danger or increase the power of a prohibited impulse in the present gives rise to anxiety. In the history of the individual, the experience of anxiety becomes associated with and fixated on that object, which must therefore be avoided at all costs.

While the phobic object is symbolic as a disguised form of a repressed, prohibited impulse, a specific object or situation may have different associations for different people. For example, acrophobia, the fear of high places, may be a clue to a self-destructive impulse in one person, a hostile or aggressive impulse in another, or loss of control in yet another. Similarly, fear of leaving home may represent avoiding temptations of sexual behavior, exhibitionism, stealing, or other impulses.

Most adults complaining of a phobia give a lengthy history of its presence, often dating from adolescence. In some patients, however, the onset may have occurred after a previously phobia-free life. In these cases, investigation will usually reveal a significant change in the living situation of the patient, representing a removal from one in which the person was secure (e.g., a change of job, a new boss, or a move to a different city). The origin of the prohibited impulse often can be identified easily and rapidly.

Comprehensive psychiatric evaluation of phobic persons almost always uncovers maladjustment in other areas of the patient's life. These include marital and sexual maladjustments of varying severity, a generally insecure, immature personality, and the presence of symptoms of other psychoneuroses. There is frequently a history of an anxious childhood. For example, school phobias most frequently represent the fear of being separated from an overprotective mother, with resultant anxiety in an insecure child. Apprehension may be aroused in children by a variety of situations—thunder, lightning, the appearance of strangers, moving to a new home or school. At birth the child is a helpless organism vulnerable to a continuing series of anxiety-provoking events. An essential element of nurturance is reassuring and assisting the child to deal with these events as they arise. In this way, the child learns to control and master impulses and emotional reactions. The relative tranquility of the home is essential as the child grows and identifies with the models that are provided by the parents. A troubled home, on the other hand, does not provide the desirable models for coping with difficulties. A constantly angry or punitive parent is the source of fear which may be transposed to all subsequent authority figures in the child's life. The child learns to control and repress the inclination to act out angry and aggressive impulses because he or she fears retaliation by physical punishment, loss of security, or the inculcation of guilt feelings. The success of the civilizing process in the child varies from individual to individual.

In adolescence, with the development of adult sexuality, the individual learns to control and repress the desire to act out sexual drives, which often can be strong. Again, the level of success varies with each person. Throughout childhood and adolescence, the individual achieves some degree of control of all impulses that are contrary to the subculture in which he or she lives.

The development of a phobia is one form of an inadequate or incomplete maturation process. The many fears and phobias of childhood and adolescence are dissipated, at least on the conscious level, with increasing experience, familiarity, and control. They may persist into adulthood in an attenuated form, such as a fear of meeting new people or going to strange places. Many adults cope in the same ways that children deal with their fears. For example, they may carry "magical" tokens, amulets, and other objects to "protect" them from the feared danger. Others find methods which permit them to overcome their apprehension; for example, the agoraphobic woman who fears the expression of an unconscious sexual drive is able to do her shopping when accompanied by a family member or close friend. The other person serves the purpose of reinforcing control over the feared impulse, much as the presence of a police officer serves to keep law-abiding those who might not be so otherwise.

The vast majority of phobic subjects manage their lives so that they will not be exposed to the phobic object or situation, or at least in such a way as to render the phobia less incapacitating for them. Others, however, seek less constructive ways of dealing with their anxieties through the excessive use of alcohol or medications. With still others, the degree of disability may completely dominate their lives.

Differential Diagnosis

When the patient complains of a specific phobia and of the incapacity resulting from it, the diagnosis may seem evident. Nevertheless, it is advisable to carry out a full physical and neurologic examination to eliminate possible conditions, especially organic cerebral changes which may contribute to the emergence or intensification of the disorder. In phobias such as cancerphobia, which focuses on a specific body organ, a firm diagnosis can be made only by exclusion of physical disease. With the exclusion, however, the patient is not relieved of the phobia, though the anxiety may be temporarily alleviated.

Phobias seldom occur in pure form, so it is necessary to evaluate the degree to which other psychoneurotic disorders are present. It may be difficult to differentiate obsessive-compulsive conditions that, on occasion, are accompanied by phobias secondary to the obsessional neurosis.

Because of the disability resulting from a phobia, many patients develop a secondary depressive state which may mask the primary condition; hence, a good psychiatric history, not only from the patient but also from a family member, is most important.

Treatment

A phobic patient seeking treatment has usually had a wealth of well-meaning but ineffectual advice from a variety of relatives and friends. Frequently, the result has been deleterious rather than therapeutic. Phobias have roots deep in the past experience of the individual. The therapeutic plan should have the purpose of deemphasizing the symptom.

Because the symptom is a manifestation of anxiety, reassurance is necessary in a good therapeutic relationship. Just as a phobia rarely emerges suddenly in a person previously without it, so it is rarely resolved in a quick or dramatic way. Most require a specific therapeutic approach over a period of time.

There are two principal forms of treatment: psychoanalytically oriented psychotherapy, including orthodox psychoanalysis; and behavior therapy based on learning theories. Both approaches require a high degree of motivation and cooperation by the patient.

With the psychotherapeutic method, the patient is encouraged to trace his or her personal history back to the early experience of the phobia and the related circumstance and to discover that what was pertinent in the past is no longer so. The method calls for a reevaluation and modification of the patient's concepts and values, and of important personal relationships, including familial and occupational. Therapy is in large measure a completion of the maturation process. By its very nature it is a long procedure.

In many cases of phobia, especially those in which it is the only symptom, behavior therapy may be effective. After completing the history and mental status evaluation, the physician organizes a list of the pertinent difficulties associated with the phobia, ranging from the least to the most severe. The patient is encouraged to think repeatedly about and confront the least severe problem until the anxiety so aroused diminishes to minimum levels. The process is repeated with each problem in the ascending order of magnitude, until eventually the patient is able to confront the object of the phobia repeatedly, with diminution and eventual elimination of anxiety. This desensitization or deconditioning approach, which takes less time than the psychotherapeutic technique, has had major success.

Many variations have been introduced to the behavior modification technique, notably that of *reciprocal inhibition*.[9,10] This is the process of associating the anxiety-provoking stimulus concurrently with an opposing emotion of sufficient quality and strength to overcome the anxiety.

One approach is that of *implosion* (or flooding in imagination), whereby the patient imagines and confronts the most intense anxiety-provoking scene until the anxiety diminishes and, over a period of time, disappears.[11]

The simultaneous use of anxiolitic medications,[12] hypnosis, or relaxation techniques has also been employed in association with the desensitization process.

Claims of high success rates (including greater effectiveness and a greatly reduced duration of therapy when compared with psychotherapy) have been made for behavior modification as the treatment of choice. The effectiveness of behavior modification appears to be limited, however, to treatment of single phobias and some anxiety states.

The use of antidepressants, sometimes combined with other medications, has been advocated, especially for those patients for whom other approaches have not been possible or effective, and who require maintenance over a period of months or even years.

HYSTERICAL NEUROSES

Hysterical neuroses conditions, which are characterized by an impairment or loss of function, are grouped in two principal categories—conversion symptoms and dissociative states.

Conversion symptoms are manifested by impairment of the voluntary nervous system, including muscular control and both general and special sensory perception. The particular symptom has a personal meaning for the patient. It represents an inadequate method of dealing with the anxiety aroused by the fear of acting out unconscious impulses or drives unacceptable to the individual. The symptoms include pareses, paralyses, ataxias, anesthesias and paresthesias of portions of the skin, anosmias, blindness, and deafness.

Dissociative states are the result of alterations in psychologic functioning under stress. In the majority of these conditions, portions of the normal consciousness of the patient are repressed so that amnesia is a common component. The amnesia may be limited to segments of time or to specific events, or it may involve the suppression of the identity of the individual.

There appear to be several common elements in the premorbid personality of these patients. They tend to be inadequate in meeting and dealing with stressful situations. There is a large degree of dependence on others. They exhibit a high degree of suggestibility, as evidenced by the ease with which they can be hypnotized.

Hysterical Personality

Sometimes called the histrionic personality disorder, the hysterical personality structure displays many of the characteristics just mentioned. It is a disorder of immature, dependent, self-centered individuals who seek approval and attention from others through a marked tendency to dramatize. They intrude on other people in order to monopolize attention. They tend to overreact, both positively and negatively, to people and events, and display emotional lability and overexcitability. They are frequently seductive, yet much of this attention-seeking behavior is not conscious. Lack of real warmth or deep attachment characterizes their personal relationships with others. They are vulnerable to the development of conversion or dissociative symptoms under the stress of severe emotional trauma.

CONVERSION NEUROSIS

A conversion reaction may be defined as an impairment of a normal physiologic function of the voluntary nervous system, or of the special senses, for which no organic cause can be demonstrated and which results from an unconscious psychologic process. The purpose of this process is to deal with internal conflicts which would otherwise give rise to anxiety. As in other psychoneurotic states, there is an unconscious impulse or drive, the acting out of which is in conflict with the need of the individual to preserve feelings of security and well-being; one example would be a soldier who is reprimanded by his sergeant and has the impulse to strike back, but when he begins to raise his hand he suddenly develops a paralysis of his arm.

Conversion reactions may occur in any of the motor areas that are under voluntary control. They range from complete paralysis through varying degrees of paresis or weakness in the limbs; they also include such disorders as aphasia and dysphonia, globus hystericus, aerophagia and dysphagia, dyspnea, vomiting, pseudocyesis, blepharospasm, tremors, and convulsions.

Other types become manifest in the sensory field, including anesthesia of areas of the skin or mucous membranes, and paralgesias such as sensations of burning, formication, or cold. Characteristic of such symptoms is the absence of correlation of the anesthetic area with the nerve distribution, so that there is often a clear demarcation by pinprick between the affected area and the nonanesthetic portion of the skin. Classical examples are the glove or stocking distribution of an affected area and sharp midline demarcation on the trunk. It is typical of the conversion symptom that the impairment is always a reflection of what is commonly believed to be anatomically correct—a feature which is significant in making a correct diagnosis.

Other conversion reactions are corneal, pharyngeal or palatal anesthesia, and loss of the gag response. Loss of associated reflexes is common in these sensory disturbances. Loss of vibration sense may also occur, and be as sharply demarcated as the overlying anesthetic area.

In the special senses, a variety of symptoms are seen. Ocular disturbances include amblyopia, which ranges up to total blindness either in one or both eyes. With bilateral blindness, the patient appears to be able to navigate accurately when alone, but has great difficulty when others are present. Partial or total deafness and loss of smell or taste tend to occur much less frequently.

Affect in Conversion Reactions

Typical of these conditions is an obvious absence of the concern that would be experienced by normal persons when suffering such severe loss or impairment of function. This lack of anxiety, named *la belle indifference* by Charcot, is characteristically associated with conversion symptoms and arises because the impairment itself serves the purpose of removing the anxiety associated with an unconscious conflict. Moreover, the symptom may serve other secondary purposes, such as avoiding situations or activities which may be unpleasant to the patient, much as phobic symptoms may do.

Pain as a Conversion Symptom

In contrast with the usual lack of concern associated with these conditions, complaints of pain that arise as a result of an unconscious conflict frequently present very serious problems in diagnosis. As with other manifestations of conversion reactions, the distribution of pain may suggest the nature of its origin. More often, the pain is diffuse. Episodes of acute abdominal pain may be reported (as in the Munchausen syndrome in which the patient undergoes repeated surgical procedures), but no cause of the pain can be found at operation.[13] Less severe forms of this syndrome appear in some of the "professional" patients who present themselves in an emergency room. Following admission, workup, and preparation for laparotomy, they discharge themselves from the hospital.

Headache as a manifestation of conversion pain is particularly difficult to differentiate from that due to physical causes. Similarly, low back pain may present a difficult diagnostic problem in many patients.

The actual experience of pain that is diagnosed as a conversion symptom may be severe in some patients, and should not be dismissed lightly as if the patient is not suffering. The willingness to undergo surgery is, in part, evidence of this suffering. The severity of the pain may be an indication of the severity of the underlying conflict.

The Symptom as Body Language

As with phobic reactions, the "selection" of the specific function that is impaired may provide a clue to the nature of the prohibited impulse. Sometimes the connection appears clear, on other occasions it is obscure. Nevertheless, whether it is paralysis of an arm, an aphonia, or an anesthetic area, to the patient the symptom has a meaning that is thought to be not consciously recognized.

Of notable interest is the still occasional appearance of hysterical epidemics in closely knit groups of individuals, as in boarding schools, military barracks, and isolated rural communities.[14,15] The particular symptom, which may be either a conversion or a dissociative one, varies, but is always one which first occurs in a member of the group who has a marked influence on the others. The original case may be a symptom occurring as the result of a genuine physical illness or upset. Such epidemics may range from fainting, tics, and crying spells to generalized convulsions or total paralysis of a limb. Noteworthy from a historical viewpoint is the epidemic of *tarantism,* or dancing sickness, which swept southern Europe in the Middle Ages.[16] Whole communities were affected and started dancing in groups—sometimes to the point of complete exhaustion and, on occasion, death.

The contagious nature of these epidemics clearly demonstrates the close association between individual suggestibility and the conversion and other hysterical disorders which occur in closely knit groups that are undergoing a common stressful experience.

Differential Diagnosis

Since the forms of conversion symptoms are protean, and the specific symptom represents the patient's understanding or misunderstanding of physiologic functions, almost any neurologic condition may be simulated. Disease of other systems must be excluded. While obvious diagnoses may be made in glove-and-stocking type anesthesias, the mere exclusion of organic disease by routine testing in other cases should not lead to hasty diagnosis of a neurotic condition. Sophisticated history taking is necessary, including an evaluation of the premorbid personality structure and adjustment. Furthermore, such conditions are not restricted to females. Evaluation of the suggestibility of the individual by the use of specific tests may be valuable. Also to be differentiated are subjective somatic symptoms, which are a frequent and prominent manifestation of depressive states and, more rarely, cases of malingering.

DISSOCIATIVE NEUROSIS

Under this rubric are gathered a number of conditions which have in common two attributes. The first is the absence of observable anxiety or other painful emotion; the second is a temporary splitting off of a part of the personality that appears separate and distinct from the ordinary character of the patient. There is no apparent conscious connection of the two portions by the patient.

In this group fall somnambulism, amnesia, fugue states, automatic behavior, and double and multiple personalities. Dreaming and *pavor nocturnus,* or night terrors, are closely related phenomena which are sometimes included, as are depersonalization and hypnotic states.

Somnambulism

Although immediately after waking, or being aroused from sleep, most people may recall some of the content of their dreams, dreams are autonomous activities. The dreamer may be physically active in the dream content, but there is no corresponding muscle activity accompanying the content. The dream is a *dissociated state,* a separation of the normally integrated mental and physical functions of the person.

With somnambulism the mental and physical functions are integrated, for it appears that the individual is carrying out purposeful, coordinated activities. Often the sleepwalker is apparently searching for something which has a special or personal meaning, or is trying to make sure that something is as it should be.

In other cases, the individual is in a highly emotional state, usually of marked anxiety. The somnambulist may be seeking to escape from some perceived danger, or may be reliving a severe traumatic experience from the past. In still other cases, there may be an absence of either purpose or emotional state, the predominant impression being one of an intense preoccupation with staring into space. In all episodes of somnambulism, the individual is out of contact with the environment and characteristically does not hear when spoken to by others.

Sleepwalking is common in children but it is rare in adults. With the latter, it may occur as single or repeated episodes, often with the same content each time; it may appear without a previously known history of sleepwalking, or it may occur after an absence of many years. As with other neurotic conditions, it emerges at times of great tension and anxiety, often when adequate means for dealing with the causes of the stress are obscure to the individual.

Pavor nocturnus, or night terrors, occur mainly in children and are probably a manifestation of delayed nervous system maturation. They are to be distinguished from nightmares or frightening dreams, which occur during normal REM sleep patterns. The individual is apparently undergoing a terrifying type of experience, accompanied by great anxiety and much vocalization. As the episode subsides, the child falls again into a calm, deep sleep. As with somnambulism, there is usually amnesia about the event. Children generally grow out of this condition over a period of years.

Amnesia

Amnesia is the term applied to loss of memory, particularly to pathologic forgetting. It may arise from a number of causes, including organic brain damage, a psychologic trauma in the absence of injury, or a combination of both. Amnesia is a manifestation of the mental mechanism of repression by which memory of painful or disturbing events is removed from awareness.

Organic amnesia may be caused by head injury, acute or chronic alcoholism, drug abuse, brain disease, and the aging process. Even when organic pathology is present, psychologic factors may operate to produce the amnesia, as revealed by the selectivity of the events forgotten. The memory loss may be complete, or may be of major or minor proportions with respect to events occurring over a period of time.

Amnesia of psychologic origin may follow an accident involving or witnessed by the patient, severely distressing news of personal significance, or an action by the person him- or herself which has damaging effects on others. Because amnesia may be claimed following the perpetration of a serious crime, differentiation from malingering must be made. This may be difficult, since both conditions have the same apparent purpose. In major cases where the diagnosis is in doubt, arousing the individual suddenly from sleep and asking specific questions about the "forgotten" events may, on occasion, be helpful in reaching a conclusion.

The memory deficit may be for events before the precipitating occurrence, that is, *retrograde amnesia;* or it may be sharply demarcated with respect to events within a specific time span, as in so-called *circumscribed amnesia*. The duration of an amnestic state may vary from relatively short periods of time, measured in hours to days, to those rare occasions when it lasts for months to years. Recovery may be sudden or may occur gradually.

Amnesias have been classified as (a) localized, (b) general, (c) systematized, and (d) continuous. With the localized form, the memory loss is confined to specific items of information which may form a cluster. In the general type, there is a complete loss of memory for events occurring over a period of time and for the individual's own identity. With systematized amnesia, the loss is for specific events that are usually significant in nature, while memory for events occurring in the same time frame is retained. Continuous amnesia refers to an ongoing process in which the forgetting involves ongoing events.

When amnesias are present, the individual is otherwise alert and in good contact with his or her surroundings. The person is usually aware of the memory deficit, but often does not exhibit the concern which might be expected. This is not surprising, since psychologic amnesia serves the purpose of repressing from awareness experiences and conflicts which would be painful.

With psychogenic amnesia, the lost memory may sometimes be recovered by placing the patient under hypnosis or by interviews conducted under the influence of intravenous sodium amobarbital. Even when successful, however, such approaches do not deal with the basic conflicts of which the amnestic episode is only a symptom. The level of psychotherapeutic intervention depends on several factors, such as the intelligence of the patient, the nature of the stress, and the degree of emotional support available to the individual in the environment.

Fugue States

A *fugue state* is a major state of dissociation or splitting off of the personality in which the identity and customary life patterns are completely repressed. In many of the cases, the individual wanders about for days, far from home, without any memory of who he or she is. In other cases, the individual appears to lead a "normal" life unconnected with his or her customary self. There is complete amnesia for the usual self, and the person is unaware of loss of memory. The patient may appear quite purposeful and seem to function well, or may be less organized than in his or her usual personality, even to the point of appearing confused.

With some fugue states, the individual may suddenly disappear from home, take up residence in a distant place, and establish a new life and identity. The pattern followed is one of avoiding local attention or prominence and engaging in a modest occupation, which is sometimes different from the previous one. These individuals experience the usual range of emotional reactions. After varying periods of time, which range from months to years, they may suddenly "wake up" in their previous identities without any recollection of what happened to them in the intervening interval. They often turn to the police, hospital emergency rooms, or physician to seek help.

Double and Multiple Personalities

These appear to be fugue state variations in which there are alternative recurrent episodes over short intervals where the "second" personality takes over for a time and then disappears. Each "personality" is significantly different, and together they appear to reflect conflicted aspects of the usual or "normal" character.

Insofar as documented cases are concerned, double and multiple personalities are rare. Public and medical attention to the syndrome was aroused by the initial report, published in 1905 by Dr. Morton Prince, about Miss Christine Beauchamp, a patient who presented three different "personalities," two of whom were unaware of the other.[17] The few other reported cases appear to be more descriptive of the behavior of histrionic personalities. The most widely known "case" of double personality is that of the fictional *Dr. Jekyll and Mr. Hyde* by Robert Louis Stevenson, published in 1886.[18] It would be interesting to know whether Miss Beauchamp had read this novel, in view of the high degree of suggestibility customarily associated with people experiencing these disorders. More recently, several more patients with this disturbance have been reported and have received much public attention.

Other examples of these multiple personalities are hypnotic states, automatic behavior, and the trances of the so-called spiritualist, or psychic. In all these cases, the common features involve loss or absence of normal control of cognitive and conative functioning. The simplest example of nonpathologic automatic behavior is the individual who when driving to work becomes so preoccupied with thoughts that suddenly he or she recognizes that a considerable distance has been traveled.

Of social, legal, and clinical significance in recent years has been the deliberate pursuit of dissociative states by a large proportion of society through the abuse of psychoactive drugs such as LSD, cannabis, peyote, and other illegal psychedelic agents. Receiving some attention medically has been the *flashback phenomenon,* in which, after a long period of abstinence, the individual suffers an acute recurrence of the dissociative state.[19] Rather than being of organic origin, as has often been proposed, these flashbacks would seem to be more likely of psychologic etiology.[20]

Differential Diagnosis of Hysterical Neuroses

As mentioned earlier, any symptom normally occurring in a conversion neurosis may be feigned by a malingerer, not only in the motor and general sensory areas, but also in the special senses. Thus, visual hallucinations may be claimed to occur, and it may be very difficult to differentiate whether or not they are hysterical in origin. Visual hallucinations may also occur in acute schizophrenic reactions. In these latter conditions, they tend to be simple in content, whereas hysterical hallucinations are usually complex in nature and are usually part of an elaborate account. With the latter, there is the notable lack of concern characteristic of hysterical disorders. With schizophrenic reactions, there is usually also evidence of a concurrent thought disorder.

Visual hallucinations also occur with toxic conditions, but there is a history involving the intake of, or exposure to, alcohol or other toxic substances, and the prominent affect is usually one of anxiety and agitation.

Both conversion and/or dissociative symptoms may be present in some schizophrenic reactions. Special diagnostic difficulty may be encountered in those cases in which there is flatness of affect.

With chronic depressions, particularly the masked variety with a predominance of hypochondriacal complaints, the demarcation is made largely on the basis of the premorbid personality, the history of onset, and the presence of depressive emotion.

Prognosis and Treatment

The prognosis and treatment of all hysterical neuroses depend on a variety of factors other than the specific symptom. The premorbid personality and the circumstances surrounding the onset of the symptom are especially important. The greater the stress in an acute onset, the better the outlook. The more stable the prior adjustment of the patient, the more favorable the prognosis. Other favorable factors include the quality of the supportive environment, especially the immediate family and, in some cases, the occupational situation.

Of unfavorable significance are a long duration of the symptom, high degree of invalidism, the degree and quality of the secondary gain derived, and the apparent lack of capacity to experience emotions.

Many hysterical syndromes, such as fugues and amnesias, subside independent of any approach. Theoretically, hypnosis should be an effective approach. However, hypnotic removal of a conversion symptom deals neither with the underlying emotional conflict nor the vulnerable personality, and is largely effective only in those cases in which the symptom is no longer necessary to the patient.

While about half the conversion symptoms disappear in about one year, the remainder tend to persist indefinitely. Patients with persistent symptoms tend to be those who have the least favorable response to treatment, irrespective of the therapeutic approach. Indicated for these patients is emotional support together with psychotherapy, including insight therapy for those individuals with the capacity to distance themselves from their symptoms and to examine the cause and onset of the symptom. In the absence of anxiety or depressive affect, chemotherapy and electroconvulsive therapy are ineffective.

NEUROSES FOLLOWING TRAUMA

Neuroses may occur following physical injury to the body, particularly to the head, or to the self-concept of the individual. In the past, these conditions were regarded as the sequelae of, or as organic damage to the brain. Today they are differentiated into two categories. The first includes symptoms which are evidence of residual brain damage, and the second includes those symptoms that result from the psychologic insult to the individual, whether or not the original injury was a physical one.

The possible manifestations of neuroses following trauma are innumerable, depending on the premorbid personality, the kind of injury, the circumstances surrounding the accident, and the unconscious conflict with which the neurosis deals. The conditions range from acute to chronic depressions, a variety of conversion symptoms, fatigue states, phobic disorders, and more rarely, obsessive-compulsive reactions and dissociative states. Hypochondriacal symptoms may be part of a depressive condition. Diminution of sexual and other normal functions often occurs. A typical characteristic is an excessive degree of impairment in comparison with the severity of the injury or with the residual organic damage, if any. Often, the psychologic response may be totally out of proportion and may occur even without the presence of physical injury to the person.

The psychologic impairment may continue in the absence of any clear-cut, demonstrable organic pathology when the individual is receiving monetary compensation while remaining away from work. Yet, such a neurosis does indicate a psychologic disorder of serious proportions. The unconscious psychopathologic patterns may be very complex, especially when the issues of so-called secondary gains complicate the clinical picture. The symptomatology has a primary significance in the personality structure of the patient. The question of secondary gains enters the picture when the original accident or injury provides the individual with the means to avoid an unpleasant situation, duty, or obligation that is unrelated to the injury itself; for example, the worker who is unhappy with his or her supervisor, or dislikes the conditions of employment, may use the original accident or injury to avoid a stressful work situation. Another example of secondary gain is the avoidance of intimate relations with a sexually demanding spouse. In many cases, the secondary gain may be as simple as the increased attention and solicitousness of a spouse, relatives, or friends.

Malingering

The term *malingering* is used when an individual deliberately simulates an illness in order to achieve a beneficial advantage. When amnesia is feigned, it is almost always for the purpose of escaping the unpleasant consequences of an act. It especially has to be considered in instances when a person has been injured on the job or in an accident and financial compensation may be a possibility. This is obvious when an individual has been identified as the perpetrator of a criminal act and the claim of amnesia is used as a defense of insanity. Amnesia is not a valid insanity defense, nor a valid basis for a claim of incompetence to stand trial. Malingering may be difficult to establish in an intelligent person. Repeated detailed questioning over a period of time, with recordkeeping of the answers, will often yield inconsistencies and contradictions. Willingness to undergo hypnosis, pentothal interviews, or lie-detector tests is not a decisive criterion of either condition and, in any case, the results of such procedures are unreliable. Questioning following sudden arousal from sleep is at times effective in making a diagnosis of malingering. Because the symptomatology is related to the patient's understanding of the physical disease and is manifested through an unconscious mechanism, differentiation from malingering presents great difficulty. Usdin has noted some guidelines in differentiating malingerers from psychoneurotics.[21] The malingerer, fearing detection, is often unwilling to undergo medical reexamination; there is no pain or disability to respond to treatment. The psychoneurotic who is having uncomfortable symptoms searches for diagnosis and treatment. The neurotic is faithful in taking medication and is eager for additional medications, physiotherapy, injections, or other treatment; the possibility of a surgical procedure may be brought up by the genuinely psychoneurotic patient. The malingerer naturally would not want any exploratory surgery or painful procedure. The psychoneurotic patient talks considerably about the accident and symptoms and often becomes markedly upset when relating details. Malingerers frequently overact the part and embroider with a luxury of words that their feelings do not reveal. Malingerers maintain capacity for pleasure in activities not concerning the alleged symptom or injured part. The psychoneurotic usually has a multiplicity of symptoms, often seemingly unrelated to the injured part. Neuroses usually invade the patient's entire personal life, causing a loss of capacity for pleasure and work, with introversion occurring frequently. Neurosis may bring with it many objective symptoms such as hyperhidrosis, hyperactive reflexes, pupillary changes, increased tension, psychomotor retardation, or any of the symptoms of anxiety or depression.

Possibly the most important evidence concerns adjustment in society. The malingerer often falls into the diagnostic category of antisocial personality (see Chapter 11).

With increased public education about psychiatric disorders, there has been an increase in the feigning of psychiatric symptoms such as hallucinations. In some cases, the individual has even sought admission to a psychiatric hospital.

The diagnosis of malingering always carries serious implications and consequences for the individual and, therefore, requires careful psychiatric observations and evaluation.

DEPERSONALIZATION NEUROSIS

Although officially classified as a specific neurosis, the depersonalization neurosis syndrome should more properly be categorized as a variety of dissociative neurosis. It is seen in two forms, depersonalization and derealization, which may be present independently or together.

In depersonalization, the individual is keenly aware that there is an absence of any feeling for or about himself. It is as though the person is looking at him- or herself from the outside, as through the eyes of a stranger. The individual recognizes that there is no other difference with regard to appearance, functioning, or identity. Although there is a feeling of being devoid of emotion, the individual may exhibit many of the signs of anxiety and agitation.

In derealization, the person feels like his or her customary self, but experiences a complete lack of feeling for even the most familiar environment and the objects in it. The individual is fully aware that there has been no physical change in the surroundings. Indeed, there is often an increased vividness of perception.

Such experiences are not uncommon at some time in life, most frequently in adolescence, but are usually of short duration, remit spontaneously, and are not of pathologic significance. They may also occur when the individual is faced with an acute situational stress, and sometimes are prodromal symptoms of a more serious psychiatric disorder, such as an acute schizophrenic or depressive illness.

OBSESSIONAL NEUROSIS

In obsessional neurosis, the individual repetitively and persistently experiences particular thoughts or is prompted to carry out certain acts. For descriptive purposes, these are divided into obsessional thoughts and compulsive acts. With the former, the same (or closely related) unwanted words, thoughts, or ideas enter the mind persistently despite efforts to suppress or avoid them. Compulsive acts are those which the individual feels compelled to perform even while recognizing that they are irrational. With attempts to resist the compulsion discomfort mounts, so that the patient can gain relief only by yielding to it. A typical example from literature is that of Samuel Johnson, who suffered from the compulsion to rap the railings of houses he passed with his walking stick.

The psychopathology of these conditions is discussed in Chapter 3. Briefly, the compulsive acts represent magic, though unconscious, rituals to ward off the anxiety that arises out of conflicts within the personality of the individual. These neurotic conditions represent an extreme form of behavior that in normal degrees can be of substantial benefit psychologically, occupationally, and socially.

Obsessive-Compulsive Character

In normal development the child must learn to control impulses, especially hostile and aggressive ones that erupt easily with frustration or anger. Some children have stronger impulses to control than others, or are exposed to more frustration and anger. Most children learn to control their behavior and to conform to the demands of their environment. The suppression or repression of their drives is carried out with varying degrees of success and, accordingly, leaves its mark in the development of the individual's character traits. Particularly common are concerns with cleanliness, punctuality, orderliness, and conventionality, all attributes that are highly valued in many societies. In a technologically advanced society, they are often very highly prized. People with obsessive-compulsive traits do have limitations in that they tend to be overly rigid and conform to minute details. In many circumstances this can be a handicap because the traits may be irritating to others. The inability to see the "forest for the trees" is perhaps an apt metaphor for many obsessional characters.

Obsessional Neurosis

Thus, obsessional defenses are effective in most individuals not only for preventing the eruption of anxiety, but also for forming personality characteristics that
may be beneficial by facilitating adjustment to society. The demarcation between
normal and neurotic is not clear-cut. The clinical picture usually appears in adults
when exposure to stress leads to a decompensation or less effective operation of
these defenses. Two types of conditions may occur, though one form is usually
more obtrusive than the other.

Obsessional thoughts or ruminations are related to personal experiences and
specific impulses that threaten to emerge into the patient's awareness. These
thoughts may range from obscene words and blasphemous phrases to hostile and
assaultive expressions. The sexual or aggressive feelings underlying these
thoughts are not consciously experienced. Rather, there are feelings of anxiety
which are attributed to the alienness of the thoughts and the inability to control
them. A not-uncommon form of obsessional neurosis is indecisiveness, the inability of a person to make up his or her mind. As a consequence, the individual is
constantly in doubt as to whether the "right" thing has been done, for example,
when locking the doors at night or turning off the lights. This condition, called
folie de doute, is also demonstrated by the person who, when faced with the
choice of several brands of the same product in the supermarket, spends a long
time making a decision and then goes on worrying whether the best selection has
been made, or even goes off without making the purchase at all.

Compulsive acts involve the acting out of obsessional thoughts, though the
connection may not always be obvious. Whereas the normal person dresses
routinely in the morning, an obsessional neurotic individual has a definite
ritualistic order in which clothes are put on. Whereas washing one's hands is ordinarily performed before meals or after gardening, the compulsive neurotic may
be so afraid of contamination that his or her hands are washed many times a
day. Many superstitions are a form of neurotic phenomena, such as the ritual of
avoiding the cracks between the stones when walking on the sidewalk, or refusing
to walk under a ladder. These rituals always have a magic component and are
usually elaborated to placate an omnipotent and punitive authority. The carrying
of magic tokens or talismans to ward off danger is another form of obsessional
behavior.

When the compulsive acts intrude so much that the individual becomes
aware of the deleterious interference with adjustment, resisting them may result
in such discomfort that it can be alleviated only by yielding to the compulsion.

When the obsessive and compulsive defenses decompensate, phobias may
emerge. Excessive concern about cleanliness and fear of contamination may
become so strong that the individual restricts and fears personal contact with such
everyday things as money, door knobs, or eating utensils. Other patients develop
fears of implements with obvious aggressive associations, such as knives or guns,
and may keep these locked up to prevent the temptation to use them.

Obsessional Neurosis and Psychosis

Decompensation of the obsessional defenses may occur as part of a schizophrenic process. The difference between a neurotic and a psychotic state is often defined in terms of the break with reality in the latter condition. An example would be the schizophrenic with severe obsessional symptoms. The neurotic patient is well aware of the inappropriateness of thoughts or acts and, when attempting to control them, experiences distress or anxiety. The psychotic patient, on the other hand, has no awareness of the irrationality of the behavior and makes no attempt to resist it. The concern about dirt or contamination acquires such delusional strength that the hands may be washed continuously until they become macerated. Similarly, ritualistic acts are performed repetitively with a complete lack of insight.

In a psychotic state, insight into the incongruity of obsessional thoughts is also absent. As a consequence, delusional ideas emerge, often in the form of paranoid beliefs that a malign force or influence is at work. Sometimes this evil influence is projected externally so that the patient may believe that the thoughts are not his or her own, but rather the work of an outside force.

Differential Diagnosis

With the obsessional neurotic patient, the diagnosis is made on the basis of the feeling of compulsion associated with repeated and irrational thoughts and acts. In a schizophrenic state with obsessional features, this insight is lacking, and the obsessional thoughts are regarded as completely valid. The compulsive actions come to dominate the behavior of the patient; the acts are of a bizarre nature, and preoccupation with them leads to complete disorganization of the individual's life.

There may be difficulty in differentiating between a phobic and an obsessional condition with compensatory phobic symptoms. In the former case, the object of the phobia is customarily specific in nature, and insight into its irrationality is present. In the latter case, a diffuseness or lack of specificity regarding the phobic object is often present.

Depressive states frequently occur in obsessive-compulsive individuals. The major distinguishing feature is the presence of the depressive affect and symptomatology. Often there is a recent history of the onset or intensification of the obsessional phenomena. The recognition of the depressive condition is important because of the availability of effective antidepressant therapeutic modalities.

Treatment

Therapy of obsessional neurosis may be extremely difficult. Psychoanalysis or psychoanalytically oriented therapy may be effective in some cases, especially where the personality structure is well-preserved. A major problem, however, is encountered in the tendency of obsessional individuals to rationalize or intellectualize as a defense against confronting their unconscious feelings and conflicts.

When the symptoms emerge as the result of the exposure to stress, treatment centered around dealing with the latter is often effective.

When associated with depression or schizophrenia, the primary treatment is directed to the psychotic condition. With the former, amelioration or reduction of the obsessional features to a nonincapacitating level is obtained as the depressive element is eliminated.

The place of psychosurgery in the treatment of obsessive-compulsive neurosis has been strongly debated. It is generally considered to be only a last resort treatment for dealing with severe obsessional states in patients with well-preserved personality structures, especially when associated with psychotic depression. It is contraindicated for any patient with schizophrenia or symptoms suggestive of it.

DEPRESSIVE NEUROSIS

The phrase, "I'm depressed," is commonly used to describe a variation from one's usual feeling state, and is sometimes expressed as being "out of sorts" with oneself. This temporary state may last from hours to a day or two, but does not interfere significantly with normal pursuits. There is a lowering of spirits, a feeling of dejection or gloominess, and a loss of spontaneity and pleasure. Such spells are very common and may or may not be triggered by some minor change in the environment, but are usually self-limited in time.

The term *depression* is used in a clinical sense to describe a more severe mood disorder which is associated with impairment of normal activities. There is a definite feeling of sadness, of being alone, or of not being close to those with whom there are usually friendly relationships. The degree of the feeling of desolation may be marked, in its most severe forms reaching feelings of utter despair.

Depressed affect may occur, therefore, on the continuum stretching from the mildest degree at one extreme to the feeling of complete futility or the uselessness of living at the other. There is no clear-cut demarcation beyond which it can be definitely stated that a clinical disorder exists. Perhaps the best criterion is the point at which the degree of disordered affect interferes with the ability of the individual to pursue normal activities.

Classifications of Depression

Depressive neurosis is "an excessive reaction of depression due to an internal conflict or to an identifiable event such as the loss of a love object or cherished possession."[22]

Prior to this century, clinical depression was called *melancholia,* a term used by Hippocrates, who postulated that it was the result of black bile. During the last hundred years, a variety of classifications of depression have been formulated, usually with emphasis on the more severe forms. Each proved unsatisfactory because of confusion or lack of specificity when the proposed criteria are applied.

The first major classification was that of Kraepelin, who divided depressions into endogenous disorders resulting from organic pathology and exogenous disorders resulting from external stress.[23] The endogenous group included manic-depressive and involutional depressions and depressions occurring without environmental stress. It became evident that this diagnostic dichotomy was unsuitable for classification because careful psychiatric evaluation revealed that many so-called endogenous depressions were actually triggered by environmental stress.

Excluding the manic-depressive and involutional illnesses, depressive disorders are reactive in origin and fall within a spectrum of increasing severity. The symptomatology varies with the intensity of the depressive affect. In the borderline between neurosis and psychosis, there may be overlapping of the symptoms that are present, making a precise differentiation difficult. This differentiation between a psychotic and a neurotic depression is based on the presence or absence of a break with reality in the mental activity, as evidenced by frank delusions or by the gross impairment of the individual's life pattern.

Symptomatology

In the great majority of neurotic depressions, stressful events in the life of the person can almost always be identified as having occurred prior to the onset of the condition. The development of the disorder is usually rapid, though there may be a period during which symptoms gradually intensify.

Almost invariably, the precipitating cause is the loss of someone or something which is highly valued. Thus, the death of, or separation from, one who is dear is a frequent cause. Similarly, rejection by a person on whom the individual is emotionally dependent or being passed over for a strongly coveted promotion are other common types of precipitating events.

The depressed affect is the result of the loss of self-esteem, triggered by the trauma of the event or occurrence. The severity of the loss of self-esteem is related to the degree of importance which the lost person or object occupied in the life of the individual. The duration of the illness is often related to the degree of significance of the loss.

The symptoms of the depressive neurosis fall into two categories. The first are those associated with the feeling state of the patient, and the second with the mental activity that is reflected in the content of the individual's verbalizations.

The affective symptoms include feelings of sadness; loss of initiative; apathy; and loss of interest in people, objects, or occupational, social, and cultural activities which previously afforded gratification. This withdrawal from involvement with matters outside the patient may reach degrees of severity to the point of almost complete personal neglect or to a state of almost complete immobility. In other patients, there may be considerable anxiety, with agitation and restlessness as prominent features.

With regard to mental activity, the patient may express loss of self-esteem in terms of a negative evaluation of self, particularly in those areas of behavior that are thought to carry the highest values. There are unduly self-critical and self-depreciatory statements regarding past performance. These expressions are all associated with feelings of failure to live up to the person's ethical or moral standards. The self-critical and self-accusatory symptoms vary from person to person, but in each case are related to the personality of the individual and may not have any obvious relationship to the precipitating traumatic experience. Expressions of worthlessness may develop in the man who has been passed over for promotion, because of the lifelong belief that devotion to work should bring recognition and the appropriate reward; or in the woman who has idealized motherhood but finds that the continuous burdens and responsibilities of child care overpower any sense of gratification.

One form of depression occurs when a longed-for success in a particular area or field has been achieved. For example, the individual may find that with the glory of advancement to a high executive position comes associated, but unforeseen, responsibilities for decision making which carry potentially adverse impact for both reputation and self-esteem.

Many self-depreciatory symptoms fall into three groups: those of health, wealth, and worth. In the last case, the individual expresses feelings of inadequacy or worthlessness with respect to ethical or occupational performance. Religious people in severe depressions may accuse themselves of having sinned, an individual who has equated personal security with the acquisition of money or material things may express the belief that he or she is poverty-stricken, and the person who has been devoted to lifelong health rituals and concerns may develop hypochondriacal symptoms.

Depression and Mourning

Ordinarily, the loss of a loved one is followed by a period of mourning. There occur feelings of sorrow, sadness, and grief. The intensity of the grief is related to how much the deceased person was loved and how important the individual was to the psychologic life of the survivor. There is a deep sense of loss with diminution in interest for daily routine activities. The individual feels that part of him or her has disappeared. The psychoanalytic studies of Abraham and Freud in the early decades of this century led to recognition of the differences between depression and mourning.[24] The latter is a normal process during which the individual learns to accept the loss and readjust patterns to the new situation. The process of mourning is self-limited, lasting usually for a year or so. As the individual adjusts to the loss, the intensity of the grief abates and eventually disappears. In mourning, there is no significant loss of self-esteem. While there may be strong feelings of regret about acts of omission or commission, there is an absence of self-accusatory ideas.

In clinical depression, however, there is an additional important component. There are negative or hostile, as well as warm, feelings toward the departed. These may not be conscious, but the loss arouses the memory of them. The depressed person associates the loss with the negative or hostile feelings, which results in feelings of guilt or remorse. The guilt feelings may be present, even though not verbalized.

The depressed individual frequently displays episodes of sudden irritability and anger, especially when pressure by others is exerted in efforts to change the preoccupation with him- or herself. This irritability is a manifestation of repressed hostile feelings which are typical of the clinical depression.

The recurrence of depression on the anniversary of the date on which the loss first happened is common. This suggests that the conflict still continues within the personality of the individual.

Because suicide is covered in Chapter 20, brief mention of it is made here only because self-destructive drives are a prominent feature in many patients suffering from moderate to severe depressive states. The risk of suicide must be evaluated in all cases of depression. By far, the highest rate of suicide is associated with depression. The open expression of self-destructive impulses ranges from the verbalization of thoughts that life is not worth living, or that others would be better off without the patient, to symbolic suicidal gestures, to successful attempts to take one's own life. Some symbolic gestures end in death because the anticipated intervention by others does not occur.

In recent years, some people have ascribed suicidal efforts to "a cry for help." While such a description may apply in some cases, it is difficult to interpret in the action of the man or woman who jumps from a 30-story building. Evaluation of the potential danger is necessary in all cases, especially when self-destructive feelings are expressed.

Physical Symptoms in Depression

The physical changes of depression range in their manifestations. There may be loss of appetite and weight, pallor, constipation, and diminution in skin temperature, especially in the extremities. Much more frequent are symptoms such as headaches, fatigue, loss of energy, insomnia, decreased sexual desire and performance, and accentuation of preexisting minor physical complaints. In severe depression, women may have amenorrhea.

In some cases, the complaints of the patient are primarily focused on somatic symptoms such as back pain or disorders of the digestive tract, so that the presence of a depressive affect is elicited only by direct and appropriate questioning. These patients illustrate a variety of the disorder called "masked depression." This should be remembered when no evidence of organic disease to account for the symptoms can be found and the symptoms persist over a long period of time.

Incidence

The incidence of depressive neurosis is difficult to establish, largely because such neuroses range so widely in degree and in their manifestations, and are part of, or overlay other illnesses. They are, however, extremely common.[25] A significant proportion of the patients attended by general practitioners exhibit depressive states, not infrequently of the masked variety. Depression is exceedingly common in the elderly, whose daily patterns and personal relationships have been severed by retirement, impairment of physical health, and the loss of the possibility of achieving cherished objectives such as occupational accomplishment or financial security. Similarly, for many elderly persons, the quality of retirement life fails to provide the long-anticipated contentment.

Chronic illness and disability are frequently accompanied by depressive states, especially in individuals, both young and elderly, who were previously active and self-sufficient. The complexities of modern life provide a nutrient medium for the development of these conditions. Along these lines, for example, the recent overemphasis by parents and society on the success to be derived from a college education may well have laid the groundwork for a future increase in the incidence of depressive states.

Premorbid Personality

In addition to environmental influences operating from an early age, there appears to be a constitutional factor involved in the individual's susceptibility to depressive reactions. The predisposition to depression is most noticeable in people who are overconscientious, perfectionistic, and overconformists to rules and regulations; they are rigid in their outlook and compulsive with regard to details. Such individuals usually have high expectations of performance and are driven to meet them by internal forces. They are very agreeable and pleasant, and tend to be compliant to the demands of others; they try to please those who occupy positions of authority over them. Although it may be far from evident on the surface, they tend to be very dependent on those in authority. They are also very sensitive to criticism. Their sense of humor is often of the dry, intellectual kind rather than of a robust nature.

People with this characterological structure are dependent for their self-esteem on the approval of others. They tend to have constricted views of life. They are self-centered in the sense that they constantly seek emotional support from others, to obtain from them what is usually attained as much by giving as by receiving.

There is often one parent who is strict and undemonstrative and who is experienced by the child as harsh and punitive. The approval of the parent is obtained only by total compliance. The hostile and angry impulses that the parent arouses in the child have to be repressed, but they remain buried within the individual throughout life. Most children pass through a stage of ambivalence toward parents at an early age, during which time the aggressive impulses are moderate in intensity, relatively infrequent, and are soon overcome by the love and affection which is demonstrated clearly. By contrast, the child of the harsh parent has impulses that are strong, frequent, and rarely dissolved, because of the absence of love and affection.

Another category of individual that is vulnerable to depressive conditions is the person with a perpetually pessimistic view of life. This so-called depressive personality is characterized by a lack of self-esteem and confidence, by passivity and lack of initiative, and by a sourness of disposition which inadequately covers a bitter attitude toward others.

The obsessional and depressive personality structures render the individual more vulnerable to the development of a clinical depression in the event of a traumatic experience, but the onset of this disorder is far from inevitable. For depression to occur, a combination of factors must be operative concurrently.

These include the importance of the psychologic insult or trauma to the person, the specific meaning of the lost person or object, and the absence of the support that is provided by others. Certain psychologic defenses often associated with these types of personality structure diminish the degree of reaction. For example, a common feature of the obsessional character is the aforementioned tendency to isolate the ego from the painful effect of trauma. This defense may be so effective that the depressive feelings are largely suppressed. With the depressive character, the individual is often able to rationalize that the loss is in keeping with "how life is," thus providing reinforcement of the embittered view of life.

Though certain types of personalities are more vulnerable, it must be emphasized that depressive neuroses frequently occur in the general population and may develop in individuals who have been regarded as mature and stable persons.

Differential Diagnosis

Differentiation must be made between the mild depressive feelings which frequently occur and are of short duration, and a clinical depression which grossly impairs the state of well-being and interferes with normal activities and relationships.

The diagnosis is made on the basis of the feeling state reported by the patient and the history of a prior significant loss. The loss may be an obvious one in the environment, such as death or desertion, or may be more subtle, as when an idealized value or ambition is found to have been unrealizable. In such cases, the distinction between a normal mourning and a clinical depression is necessary.

Differentiation between neurosis and psychosis may be difficult because of the range of severity with depressive states. The fundamental demarcation is the absence or presence of a break with reality in the thinking and behavior of the patient. The presence of firm, unshakable beliefs, such as self-accusatory or self-depreciatory delusions, is clear-cut evidence of a psychotic state. Of importance also is the degree of the patient's insight both into the relationship of the condition to the precipitating event and into the disproportion between the severity or persistence of the reaction and the loss suffered. Another diagnostic criterion is the intensity of the disruption in the ordinary life patterns of the patient.

With regard to the appropriateness of the reaction to the precipitating event, the physician, who is using subjective judgment, should be cautious about making a hasty conclusion, especially in those cases where normal mourning may be quite intense.

Depressive feelings are commonly associated with, and are often an early feature of, other psychiatric disorders, such as a schizophrenic illness. In delusional states, for example, where the delusions are largely of the self-depreciatory or self-accusatory kind, the differentiation is made on the basis of the content of the false beliefs, the prominence of the depressive affect, and a prior traumatic event.

Depressive feelings may also complicate the clinical picture in other neurotic states, such as obsessional and phobic conditions. Here the differentiation generally is based on the identification of these disorders and their presence prior to the onset of the depressive condition.

Special difficulty may arise with those patients in whom the depression is expressed primarily through somatization of the feelings, with resulting hypochondriacal symptoms. In many such patients, the presence of depression may be elicited only by careful questioning. In some cases, the patients may regard depressive feelings as secondary to a physical illness which they are convinced exists.

Secondary depressive states may be present in patients who are suffering from physical illness, especially in cases of chronic illnesses, which necessitate modification in the patient's activities and life-style.

Depressive states, which are present at various levels of severity, may be of considerable duration. Frequently the individual seeks relief from internal distress by resorting to alcohol and drugs. Many depressed patients ultimately become alcoholics and drug abusers. For all patients with alcohol problems, careful psychiatric evaluations should be carried out to establish the presence or absence of underlying depression.

There are a group of patients who present themselves primarily as patients with depressive neuroses and a history of insidious onset without any prior traumatic event. A thorough neurologic and psychologic examination may reveal evidence of organic brain changes with diminution of the individual's capabilities, a diminution of which the patient may be only vaguely aware. Such cerebral conditions include premature cerebral atrophy, premature onset of the normal aging process, and changes due to cerebrovascular disorders.

Mention should be made of *neurasthenia,* a syndrome originating in the theories of the last century that psychiatric illnesses were caused by cerebral pathology. The term, which means weakness of the nerves, was used to categorize a group of symptoms, together with complaints of chronic, severe fatigue or exhaustion. The diagnosis is rarely made today. Rather, it is recognized that in the past the category included a variety of conditions which on closer evaluation should more properly be identified as manifestations of anxiety, phobic, hysterical, and schizophrenic disorders, usually with the common feature of depression. It sometimes is, therefore, one variety of a masked depression in which withdrawal, apathy, loss of interest and initiative, and complaints of weakness are prominent.

Treatment

The identification of depressive neurosis is extremely important because effective treatment modalities are now available. These fall into two categories, psychotherapeutic and chemotherapeutic.

Because people who are suffering from depressive neuroses characteristically suffer from loss of self-esteem and are almost totally dependent for their emotional well-being on the attitudes and opinions of others, a crucial element of all treatment is the provision of emotional support and reassurance by the therapist.

Because of the role of authority which physicians occupy in society, the physician is in a unique position to provide the constant and repetitive reassurance that the patient needs. The supportive relationship between doctor and patient may enable the latter to talk about painful feelings and problems. This often enables the working-through of difficulties, while the natural process of readjustment is operating. The physician may be able to help the patient evaluate the importance of his or her reaction in the context of the overall life situation. It is, however, generally antitherapeutic to assume a too directive approach, because it may reestablish the parent-child relationship, and it is the patient who must learn to resolve the internal conflicts. Because dependency needs are greatly intensified in the depressive neurosis, a physician's failure to demonstrate a real concern for the patient is equally antitherapeutic. The demands of the patient for emotional support are repetitive and give rise to loss of patience in some physicians because there is not the expected rapid improvement. This impatience is felt by the patient to be yet one more rejection.

Psychotherapy that is aimed at helping the patient gain insight into the causes of the condition is a specialized type of treatment which should be undertaken only by those trained in this technique. With severe depressions, insight psychotherapy is often ineffective because the thought processes are slowed, the attention-span shortened, and the preoccupations overwhelming. Patients whose depression is of a significant degree and who do not soon respond to therapy should be referred for psychiatric evaluation and treatment.

With moderate degrees of depression, utilization of supportive elements in the patient's environment can often be of significant assistance. These include close relatives and friends who sometimes become impatient with the repetitive nature of the depressed person's complaints as the illness continues apparently without amelioration. Explanation of the constructive therapeutic role that they can assume may be of considerable importance in enabling them to provide a portion of the emotional support needed.

In recent years, the advent of antidepressant medications has resulted in a revolution in the treatment of depression. The preferred drugs are the tricyclic group such as imipramine and amitryptyline. It is generally better to start with lower doses, which over a period of days are increased to the maximum therapeutic dosage. The therapeutic effectiveness of antidepressant agents may not be evident immediately, and it is necessary to maintain the patient on the maximum dosage of the selected medication for at least three to four weeks before effectiveness can be evaluated. When a medication of one chemical structure is not effective, another may be found to be so.

Another group of powerful antidepressant drugs is the monoamine oxidase inhibitors (MAOI). However, the dietary restrictions and the distressing and sometimes dangerous side-effects associated with them have resulted in their prescription only for the severest forms of depression, when the tricyclics have proved ineffective.

At a time when the side-effects of all medications have become the object of legal and public preoccupation, it may seem superfluous to emphasize the importance of alerting the patient to the possible appearance of them. With antidepressants, side-effects are common reactions and the same drug may affect different physiologic systems in different patients. It may be difficult to provide the required information and yet not intensify the concerns of the patient. However, from a psychiatric viewpoint, preparation for the possible side-effects is a form of preventive medicine.

The effectiveness of these drugs frequently results in early amelioration of the depressive state to a level which renders the patient amenable to the concurrent use of psychotherapy.

With the introduction of antidepressant medications, the administration of electroshock treatment, which was once the major treatment modality for moderate to severe depressions, has become a relatively infrequent procedure. It is still extremely valuable, but is now reserved for depressions of a psychotic degree, especially those in which a significant risk of suicide is present, and for patients who fail to respond to medications and psychotherapy.

The vast majority of neurotic depressions respond to psychopharmacologic and psychotherapeutic approaches. Those that do not, usually respond to electroshock therapy. There are rare cases in which all treatment modalities fail. In such cases patients often present a clinical picture of very severe, incapacitating depression over a long period of time, frequently with a premorbid obsessional character. There may be a temporary response to one or more courses of electroshock therapy, but with a rapid relapse after each. For some of these patients, recent psychosurgical approaches—but not lobotomy—may be considered as a treatment of last resort.[26,27]

REFERENCES

1   May, R.: "Historical Roots of Modern Anxiety Theories," in P. H. Hoch, and J. Zubin (eds.), *Anxiety,* New York: Grune & Stratton, 1950.
2   Cannon, W. B.: *Bodily Changes in Pain, Hunger, Fear and Rage,* 2d ed., New York: D. Appleton, 1929.
3   Cannon, W. B.: *The Wisdom of the Body,* 2d ed., New York: W. W. Norton, 1939.
4   Kelman, H.: "A Unitary Theory of Anxiety," *Am. J. Psychoanal.,* 17:127–160, 1957.
5   Freud, A.: *The Ego and the Mechanisms of Defense,* New York: International Universities Press, 1946.
6   Freud, S.: "Obsessions and Phobias: Their Psychical Mechanism and Their Aetiology (1895)," in J. Strachey (ed.), *The Standard Edition of the Complete Psychological Works of Sigmund Freud,* vol. 3, London: The Hogarth Press, 1962.
7   Freud, S.: "Analysis of a Phobia in a Five Year Old Boy (1909)," in J. Strachey (ed.), *The Standard Edition of the Complete Psychological Works of Sigmund Freud,* vol. 10, London: The Hogarth Press, 1955.
8   Fenichel, O.: *The Psychoanalytic Theory of Neurosis,* New York: W. W. Norton, 1945.
9   Marks, I. M.: "The Current Status of Behavioral Psychotherapy: Theory and Practice," *Am. J. Psychiatry,* 133:253–261, March, 1976.
10 Wolpe, J.: *Psychotherapy by Reciprocal Inhibition,* Stanford: Stanford University Press, 1958.

11   Marks, I. M.: "Flooding (Implosion) and Allied Treatments," in W. S. Agras (ed.), *Behavior Modification, Principles and Clinical Applications,* Boston: Little, Brown, 1972.

12   Brady, J. P.: "Drugs in Behavior Therapy," in D. H. Efron (ed.), *Psychopharmacology: A Review of Progress, 1957–1967,* Washington, D. C.: P.H.S. Publ. no. 1836, 1968.

13   Asher, R.: "Munchausen's Syndrome," *Lancet,* **260**:339–341, February 10, 1951.

14   Levine, R. J.: "Epidemic Faintness and Syncope in a School Marching Band," *J.A.M.A.,* **238**:2373–2376, November 28, 1977.

15   Smith, H. C. T., and E. J. Eastham: "Outbreak of Abdominal Pain," *Lancet,* **2**:956–958, October 27, 1973.

16   Gloyne, H. F.: "Tarantism: Mass Hysterical Reaction to Spider Bite in the Middle Ages," *Am. Imago,* **7**:29–42, March, 1950.

17   Prince, M.: *The Dissociation of a Personality,* New York: Longmans, Green, 1905.

18   Stevenson, R. L.: *The Strange Case of Dr. Jekyll and Mr. Hyde,* London: Longmans, Green, 1886.

19   Brown, A., and A. Stickgold: "Marijuana Flashback Phenomena," *J. Psychedelic Drugs,* **8**:275–282, October–December, 1976.

20   Heaton, R. K.: "Subject Expectancy and Environmental Factors as Determinants of Psychedelic Flashback Experiences," *J. Nerv. Ment. Dis.,* **161**:157–165, September, 1975.

21   Usdin, G.: "Neurosis Following Trauma," in L. A. Bear (ed.), *Law, Medicine, Science—and Justice,* Springfield: Charles C Thomas, 1964, pp. 234–246.

22   American Psychiatric Association, Committee on Nomenclature and Statistics: *DSM II: Diagnostic and Statistical Manual of Mental Disorders,* 2d ed., Washington, D.C.: American Psychiatric Association, 1968.

23   Kraeprelin, Emil: *Clinical Psychiatry,* New York: William Wood and Company, 1912.

24   Freud, S.: "Mourning and Melancholia (1917)," in J. Strachey (ed.), *The Standard Edition of the Complete Psychological Works of Sigmund Freud,* vol. 14, London: The Hogarth Press, 1957.

25   Ripley, H. S.: "Depression and the Life Span—Epidemiology," in G. Usdin (ed.), *Depression: Clinical, Biological and Psychological Perspectives,* New York: Brunner/Mazel, 1977.

26   Donnelly, J.: "The Incidence of Psychosurgery in the United States, 1971–1973," *Am. J. Psychiatry,* **135**:1476–1480, December, 1978.

27   The National Commission for the Protection of Human Subjects in Biomedical and Behavioral Research: *Psychosurgery: Report and Recommendations,* Washington, D.C.: DHEW Publ. no. (OS) 77-001, 1977.

Chapter 11

Personality Disorders

Chester M. Pierce, M.D.

EDITORS' INTRODUCTION

What is it like to be schizoid—to feel more comfortable alone than with others, to focus almost entirely on what is going on within one's own world rather than in the surrounding world? How must it be to invite inattention by one's behavior and, at the same time, be very sensitive to rejection?

What is it like to be hysterical? To court attention with dramatic desperateness, and at the same time genuinely not understand the sexual advances invited by what is experienced as seductiveness only by others?

What is it like to feel that winning is the only game, that people are but pawns to be used and discarded, and that, beneath their facade, all others are just as exploitive but are only fooling themselves? How must it be to feel that rules are only made to be broken; that larceny, graft, and cheating are not wrong—indeed, that the only sin is getting caught?

What is it like for the physician to identify empathically for a few moments with the discomfort and loneliness of the schizoid patient? What conflicting feelings are aroused in the physician who feels a strong sexual response to the hysteric's seductiveness? How does it feel for the physician to realize that he or she has been charmed by a patient with an antisocial personality, and that the fee for medical services will never be paid? What is it like for the physician to recognize finally that this same patient has been obtaining codeine as a treatment for headaches from a number of physicians? What can the physician do with his or her feelings of dismay, hurt, and rage? How will having been "taken in" affect the establishment of effective relationships with subsequent patients who seem somewhat similar in their behavior?

The personality disorders are a group of psychiatric syndromes that are often unrecognized by physicians and, when recognized, are poorly understood. In mild form, they are often considered normal personality variants and pose no unusual strain on the doctor-patient relationship. In their most severe form, however, they tax the most patient and understanding physician. In this chapter, a leading psychiatrist with a special interest in behavior disorders presents a concise summary of current knowledge about these fascinating syndromes.

INTRODUCTION

Personality disorders are characterized by maladaptive behavior patterns which may be lifelong in duration and are accompanied by little, if any, obvious anxiety. Such disorders seem, therefore, to be habitual or typical ways of being, rather than a complex of symptoms added to the basic personality. "He has always been explosive" or "She has been extremely shy and withdrawn since early in her life" suggests the enduring quality which distinguishes personality disorders from psychiatric disturbances with a clear, reactive component, such as neuroses, acute psychoses, and many forms of depression.

This distinction has important implications for the clinician. First, the acknowledgment that some individuals have disordered personalities suggests that there are normal personalities. *Normal* can be defined as without pathology, as the statistical average, or as the optimal state.[1] Depending on how the concept is used, the description of normal personality will vary. Any description of normal personality, however, must take into consideration the enormous range and variability possible. Personality disorders may be of different intensity or severity, ranging from mild to moderate to severe. Mild personality disorders (often seen as personality quirks) fall close to the normal range of functioning; moderate personality disorders (often seen as eccentric personality quirks) are usually clear to the clinician and are associated with some disability; severe personality disorders (often seen as severely disturbed behavior) have major impact on the patient's life and, often, on the lives of those connected to the patient by blood, friendship, or work.

Since the very concept of personality disorder involves a consideration of the normal personality, it is important to clarify some of the current thinking and data about normality. If the concept is used to suggest an optimal level of personality functioning, the question "Optimal for what?" is immediately raised.

A variety of writers, including, for example, Freud, Menninger, and Maslow, have suggested that high levels of personality health involve the ability to love, to work, to be reasonably free from distressing symptoms, and to be able to realize a great deal of one's potential as a person.[2,3,4] It is apparent that such definitions involve value judgments about what "ought" to be. There is no way to consider the normal personality as optimal functioning without involving such value judgments. To make such judgments is perfectly appropriate as long as the core judgments are clearly stated and understood.

Optimal personality functioning does, however, necessitate strong consideration of the role of the context. One cannot assure that what is optimal in one situation or culture is also optimal in others. Some years ago, Normal Mailer suggested that this country was experiencing a change in its "preferred personality," with the more disciplined, self-controlled, task-oriented, and compulsive personality giving way to the more manipulative con artist.[5] He suggested that the latter "worked best" in a culture that needed to increase consumption constantly rather than to save for periods of deprivation, and pointed out that in certain fields (advertising, the military) manipulative ability had achieved ascendency.

Put simply, what is optimal in personality functioning for a complex, crowded, urban society might be different from what would be found in a sparsely populated pioneering society. Context, however, cuts even more deeply into the definition of normality. Within a given society and historical period, socioeconomic and ethnic factors have influence. A child growing up in an Italian-descent family with severe economic deprivation, living in a crowded, substandard tenement, with poor schools and a high crime rate, is exposed to an environment in which the socioeconomic realities and ethnic influences shape the definition of optimal profoundly. What works best in this situation is apt to be very different from that which is an optimal personality for a child growing up in an upper-middle-class suburb with a markedly different population density, school system, crime rate, and traditional white, Anglo-Saxon values.

It is in the clinician's attempt to evaluate people from one context with criteria that have evolved from another context that much damage is done. The search for a universal standard does injustice to those whose lives are spent in conditions of extreme deprivation. The fact that some truly remarkable, creative individuals emerge out of such contexts should not blind the clinician to the impact of the deprivation on the many.

In addition to the impact of context, the clinician must think in terms of a range of functioning that can be considered normal. Rollin, for example, has stated, "We can all indulge in certain minor deviations—pecadilloes if you like—and still remain well within the accepted range of normal behavior . . . we can—and who does not?—occasionally lie, occasionally cheat, occasionally get drunk, occasionally gamble, occasionally become aggressive, hurtful and spiteful, particularly towards those we love best. As far as sexual behavior or misbehavior, conscience in all probability could make cowards of us all."[6]

The attempt to apply rigid and narrow standards of normality to everyone damages and distorts the range and richness of human variability. Currently, for example, this country has witnessed a long-needed revolution in the description of gender identity. Women, in order to be considered normal, no longer need be passive, compliant, and helpless, nor men need invariably be disciplined, self-contained, and aggressive.

Within this conceptual framework there has been a growing body of research data about normal personality functioning. Vaillant's longitudinal study of college men indicates some of the enduring personality features associated with high levels of personality competence.[7] Studies of normal adolescents by Offer, Sabshin, and Marcus; Masterson; and Westley and Epstein, have helped to clarify the characteristics of effectively functioning middle- and upper-class white adolescents.[8,9,10] There is, however, a paucity of data about women, the aged, the poor, and ethnic minorities.

Patients with personality disorders, despite the relative absence of observable anxiety, have been found through psychotherapeutic and psychoanalytic investigations to be struggling with anxiety and depression that is repressed. The distorted personality characteristics have evolved, in part, as an enduring way of dealing with these unconscious feelings. Often the underlying feelings and conflicts have to do with intimacy, sexuality, or aggression. Nowadays, there are relatively abundant pathways to express sexuality. Therefore, compared to the nineteenth century, anxiety associated with conflicts about sexuality may be different in quality as well as in quantity. Recently, since sexual expression is relatively easier in present-day society, people seem, on the average, to have relatively greater difficulty in the suitable expression of aggression and the need for intimacy. For the practicing doctor, this means that a more common and complicated everyday situation will arise with patients whose personalities are distorted by the need to punch others in the mouth or to retreat from closeness with others, rather than distorted by problems concerning sexuality.

The concept of personality disorder includes a number of synonymous terms often used interchangeably in clinical discussions and reports. These include personality defect, character disorder, behavior disorder, and character neurosis. All these terms refer to a category of disorders, which contains a number of separate entities. In this chapter the syndromes to be considered as personality disorders are the following:

1. Schizoid personality
2. Cyclothymic personality
3. Paranoid personality
4. Explosive personality
5. Obsessive-compulsive personality
6. Hysterical personality
7. Passive-aggressive personality
8. Asthenic personality
9. Inadequate personality
10. Borderline personality
11. Antisocial personality

CLINICAL DESCRIPTION OF PERSONALITY DISORDERS

Often complex issues are involved in the diagnostic process when the possibility of personality disorder is being considered. Clinical practice regards as essential the establishment of a proper diagnosis, and yet often this diagnosis is established only by the exclusion of more clearly defined psychiatric syndromes. The issue is complex because the patient may be suffering from several different syndromes. For example, a man with a severe passive-aggressive personality disorder may, under stress, develop a severe phobic reaction. The clinician may see only the phobic symptoms and not appreciate the underlying personality disorder. Under stress, a patient with a paranoid personality disorder may develop a clear paranoid psychosis in which habitual suspiciousness is replaced by frank delusional thinking. Once again, the clinician may be impressed only with the obvious psychotic symptoms without recognizing that the patient's personality had been distorted by strong paranoid trends prior to the onset of psychosis. A person with a cyclothymic personality disorder may develop a clear-cut manic psychosis following a head injury. Patients with personality disorders comprise a large segment of those individuals with serious drug dependencies and addictions. Often the clinician may respond only to the substance abuse and think of the patient as an alcoholic or addict, without exploring the possibility of underlying personality disorder. In practice, therefore, differential diagnosis which considers both a personality disorder and a second psychiatric disorder is important.

Another problem involved in the process of diagnosis is the fact that personality disorders, which lack clear reactive components, do not appear to fit a model of illness which is based fundamentally on an infectious disease concept. There is often no sharp beginning, predictable course, and clear response to medication. Although a case can be made for personality disorder as chronic illness, the physician's model of illness is more apt to be of the infectious disease or acute variety.

Another complicating issue is the fact that patients with certain personality disorders tend to be involved in behavior which is antisocial and offensive to the values of the physician. The physician may quickly assign the patient a diagnosis of personality disorder that represents consignment to a waste-basket category and relieves the physician of further concern. The legal situation adds to this concept of "not sick but bad" by insisting that although psychotic patients may not be responsible for their actions, patients with personality disorders are invariably responsible for their behavior.

The importance of the often negative attitude about personality disorders lies with the jeopardy in which it places the doctor-patient relationship when treatment interventions are instituted. Many patients with certain personality disorders are difficult to treat—they can be inaccessible, irresponsible, seductive, charming, or fear-inducing. The doctor may come to feel frustrated, afraid, or angry, which in turn may lead to the patient's feeling a lack of compassion and increasing hopelessness. The caution to the clinician is to be aware of the societal and personal factors that make one assign a negative value to these disorders, which, in fact, can be looked at more profitably as the plight of the patient attempting to cope with firmly entrenched response patterns and styles of relationships.

The Nosology of Personality Disorders

1 Schizoid Personality This person is an "odd ball." The exaggerated behavior patterns that are manifested include introversion, seclusiveness, seriousness, and detachment. Characteristically the person is exceptionally shy and reticent. Such a person seems unable to socialize and have close interpersonal relationships. Often the patient avoids competition, overt aggression, and the direct expression of ordinary hostile and assertive emotions.

There is a reluctance to reveal feelings of any sort and the individual remains "shut in," frequently with a very active fantasy life but a marked preference for the inanimate world. Sometimes, under stress, the person sustains a schizophrenic psychosis.

A doctor is impressed with how uncomfortable and afraid such people seem to be when establishing human contact. The awkwardness they project can make the doctor hesitant about how to interact without either frightening the patient or showing the pity that such sequestered lives may inspire.

Outside informants reveal that such individuals have a tendency to nomadism. Their isolation and aloofness from routine interpersonal interactions often make those around them regard them as eccentrics.

Since such a person seems more an observer than a participant in life routines, others are not disturbed by their presence except for not knowing how to include them and how not to hurt them. Sometimes the schizoid individual can be present at a function and apparently comprehend everything that is happening. Perhaps days later there will be a verbalization or discovery that tells others that the schizoid individual has just "caught on" to what had happened during the function and to what everyone assumed was recognized by all at the time.

This sort of "being out of it" makes it quite difficult for the schizoid not to be thought of as being unsociable. This sets up a cycle whereby the schizoid is not able to be included, and each exclusion makes the patient more hesitant to initiate social contact. As a result, life continues in the same pattern of isolation, seclusion, and withdrawal.

Mr. B was quiet and always ill at ease around people. He felt himself to be graceless and clumsy in interpersonal skills. In a vigorous fantasy life he imagined himself as polished, smooth, and in social demand. His good work record as an engineer enabled him to earn enough money so that he could aspire to associate with the "best young people" in his community.

However, Mr. B seemed always to be tolerated rather than welcomed. He wondered why people didn't seem to like him more and "to take me in." He revealed that he was wooden and mechanical as he danced, and that he could not think of anything to say to his partner. He recognized that, at the end of the dance, she would do as other young women and thank him for the dance but walk off. Thus he thought to say to her, "Be careful and don't step on my feet." He made this statement without any levity and with the knowledge that he was the more likely to step on someone's feet while dancing. Yet this maneuver satisfied him because then, he stated, he knew what had caused the rejection he expected forthwith. Therefore, he believed that he, not his dance partner, controlled the rejection. Nevertheless he was without insight as he soberly recalled this story. He was too deficient in everyday relationship skills to recognize how destructive this pattern was for future interaction with the young lady. He merely puzzled dreamily and silently about why she didn't like him and why people didn't seem to take to him. Mr. B continues with his literal, concrete, out-of-step view of the world as his method of coping.

2   Cyclothymic Personality   This person is the "chameleon." The exaggerated behavior patterns that are manifested include fairly prolonged mood swings from depression to elation. These mood swings seem endogenous in that they appear to be without relationship to external stimuli. Sometimes, under stress, such persons may develop either a manic, depressive, or manic-depressive psychosis.

In the extroverted phase the individual works long hours and is engaged in a multitude of projects and activities. During this time the patient is warm, friendly, outgoing, and energetic. Such persons may seem ambitious and unable to stop work.

The doctor managing such a patient may feel a paradox. One side of the paradox makes the doctor appreciate the aspects of personality which are mature and productive, such as the ability to contribute at work. The other side of the paradox, however, is that the patient seems immature in such ways as being unable to relax and enjoy him- or herself.

During the introverted phase, sadness occurs. The patient exchanges action for inertia, optimism for pessimism, and outgoingness for seclusiveness. There is a gloomy focus on the futility of past gains, and the patient concentrates on his or her alleged inadequacies, failures, and lack of accomplishment.

> Ms. Z was a successful career woman. In fact, her everyday work embraced three separate career endeavors, all of which she negotiated with vitality and flair. Her infectious enthusiasm and boundless energy combined to propel her, at a young age, to the top of several career endeavors.
>
> Yet, suddenly and without any known precipitating event, she would be plunged into severe despondency. During these episodes she would remain at home mulling over her failure to have a family and minimizing the abundant material comforts she commanded. To those few to whom she talked at this time she would discount any personal achievement and obsess over her multiple, all-pervasive inferiorities, which in her opinion ranged from being an inadequate cook to not having had a satisfying adolescence.
>
> Her gynecologist mentioned that she "fascinated" him because of her prodigious accomplishments and surpassing charm. Yet, inexplicably, on some occasions she was moody, morose, demanding, critical, or apathetic.

3   Paranoid Personality   This person often is thought of as the "crank." Although such individuals often exhibit social withdrawal like those with schizoid personalities, the distinguishing characteristic is the pervasive use of the mechanism of projection. Others are constantly blamed for life's misfortunes. Paranoid persons frequently see malevolent intent in the behavior of others. Occasionally they will single out a specific person, race, or religious affiliation and ascribe to it all sorts of evil intent and influence.

Such individuals unknowingly project their own characteristics to others. This unconscious projection of their anger, guilt, or other feelings may protect them from even more serious or psychotic states. In this sense, the paranoid personality has an adaptive component, but the psychological price is high. Viewed by others as suspicious, jealous, stubborn, difficult, and even dangerous, such persons are often avoided. The wide berth given to them by most others adds fuel to the paranoid fire. They see in the response to their behavior evidence that confirms their paranoid view of the world. They are unable, however, to sense that which they provoke in those around them.

Most such individuals go through life stabilized at this level of function. Isolated and avoided, they lead solitary lives, emerging only to blame and accuse angrily. If they marry, there is a strong tendency for their paranoid stance to dominate the lives of spouse and children, and the entire family may be seen as different but often even as difficult, dangerous, or crazy. If such an individual does develop a psychosis, it is likely to be a paranoid illness with delusions and hallucinations.

Mr. C was the bane of existence for the preteenage boys on his block. He called the police frequently, beseeching their intercession to keep the boys from playing stickball or to stop them from laughing so loud or to curb their boisterousness, which he complained was a deliberate effort to keep him from being able to enjoy his television.

The boys dreaded that their tennis ball would go into the yard of Mr. C, for on more than one occasion he had confiscated the ball, cut it in half with his pocket knife and contemptuously thrown the two halves back into the street. At Halloween, following a vandalism in which garbage was spread all over his doorsteps, he accused neighborhood parents of collaboration, since no neighborhood boy was punished to his satisfaction.

His general practitioner, after hearing about Halloween, thought to herself, "Good for the parents, this old goat is always complaining and raising hell about every damn little thing." With some guilt she rushed him through his examination, knowing that somehow he didn't present "good vibes" to her. Later she told a psychiatrist colleague that in her view, neighborhood anger and indifference to Mr. C was brought about his first week there because of his angry accusations that a shop owner let his dog bark too much. The psychiatrist replied that although Mr. C was a paranoid person, he probably was not the sort of paranoid personality who did grisly things like send bombs through the mails.

4 Explosive Personality This person is the "hot head." Minimal frustrations, often unnoticed by others, lead to explosive reactions of rage. The suddenness and explosive qualities led some to suspect that there is an underlying brain disorder of the seizure variety. Some of these patients, although the minority, have been found to have a form of temporal lobe epilepsy. This is an important finding because anticonvulsive medication may help this group. For the majority, however, no such abnormality is present and emphasis is given to a psychologic etiology.

Some of these individuals are often placid, quiet, and retiring. They may seem without aggression until an explosion occurs. Other individuals, however, are tense, hyperactive, and "testy" between episodes. During the explosive episodes, the individual may be destructive to property and dangerous to others. The rage which surfaces can be of tremendous intensity, and the individual seems totally out of control. On occasion the episodes can be precipitated by alcohol or other drugs.

After an episode the individual may experience morbid and pathological resentment. Blame is usually placed on the circumstances or on others, but occasionally one sees individuals who seem truly regretful. Most frequently patients with explosive personalities have little understanding of their disturbance, although a few develop a kind of insight that at least involves seeing their behavior as a form of illness.

Living with such a person is similar to living with a bomb which has a randomly set timing mechanism. Physical abuse often occurs in such families.

Ms. J, a divorcee, worked hard to support her two children and herself. She permitted her 10-year-old son to bring his friends to their home. One day, however, when the child came in with two other boys, Ms. J flew into a tirade which included acts of throwing kitchen utensils to the floor, verbal screaming, and a cuffing for her son. Inexplicably (for the son) she demanded that the boys leave the house immediately. The boy knew that his mother was subject to temper tantrums even without provocation.

On another occasion the children sat talking to their mother about models of recent cars. The conversation drifted evenly and pleasantly until the daughter, age 12, made a mild contradiction to a statement expressed by the mother. With astonishing celerity, the daughter was slapped across the face. She never understood why such an innocent expression of difference of opinion should result in such swift and awesome retaliation.

5 Obsessive-Compulsive Personality This is the "over-conformer" or "perfectionist." Such people are characterized by a hypertrophied self-discipline. They are rigid, unbending individuals for whom punctuality, "doing things right," and control of themselves and life situations are very important. Often they are orderly and drawn to activities that require a meticulous approach to fine details.

At the level of mild personality trends, these personality characteristics are associated with competence in many fields and such people often make good employees or professionals. However, as the intensity of these personality features increases, the rigidity and stubbornness is apt to be self-defeating. At the level of the severe personality disorder such individuals are indecisive. They analyze each detail on both sides of any decision to such a degree that they cannot move in either direction. Obsessive thoughts and compulsive rituals may further incapacitate them.

Often there is a noticeable lack of openly expressed feelings in their lives. A concern with "strength" and being in control adds to the absence of normal emotional responsiveness.

These people may be strongly competitive and driven to excel in every aspect of life. They do not form close, intimate relationships, and their concern with power often makes others wary of close involvement. In their families they frequently are authoritarian and strongly dominant. Since they are often drawn in marriage to individuals who are much more expressive of feelings, dependent, and outgoing, the marital relationships frequently become distressed because the spouses feel shut out, dominated, or unloved. At severe levels, individuals with this type of personality disorder are vulnerable, because of the rigidity of their personalities, to the development of depression and/or paranoid illnesses.

> Mr. A, an undergraduate of a famous school of engineering, presented himself at the student health clinic four weeks prior to an hour examination. His fear was that he'd fail and that he wasn't preparing himself sufficiently for the test. He acknowledged that in his three years of college he had never received any grades but A and that no one else in the class was probably preparing for the test a month away. Mr. A had called home and was reassured, as he had been all his life that grades were not of extreme importance to his parents. Despite this reassurance (which he conceded to be genuine), he felt compelled to excel in academic performance. As a result he studied nearly all the time and in fact at the time of interview was relatively sleep deprived.
>
> Dr. Z was not surprised that Mr. A was not certain about what he wished from her or whether he should continue to come to see her. Nor was she surprised to hear that the crisis of an hour examination loomed large enough in Mr. A's mind that he contemplated suicide because he believed he might not get a passing grade.
>
> Depressions are frequent in people with obsessive-compulsive personalities. Dr. Z, accordingly, agonized over the real possibility that Mr. A might indeed make a suicide attempt. She felt that the issue of grades wasn't that important to most people but to a man like Mr. A the threat (real or imagined) of poor academic performance could be enough cause for an extreme resolution.

6 Hysterical Personality This person is the "attention-seeker." Dramatic, often behaving in flirtatious or seductive ways, the individual with a hysterical personality constantly seeks to be the center of attention. In this culture there are more women with this disturbance, as there are more men with obsessive-compulsive personality disorder. The reasons for this are not known, although in severe forms these two personality disorders are seen as stereotypes of a rigid gender assignment in which men must be "very strong" and women "weak and needing to be taken care of."

At the center of these disturbances is the behavioral plea to be taken care of and often what superficially appears to be an interest in sexuality is in reality the wish to be cared for, protected, or treated with great specialness. Such individuals are often seen by others as self-centered or selfish.

Mild hysterical traits in women are often seen by men as attractive. The coquettishness, appeal to the "strength" of the man, and subtle promise of a lush future, combine to add excitement and spice to such encounters. At more severe levels of the personality disorder, however, the self-centeredness and need to control others through helplessness marks these individuals frequently as persons to be avoided.

Women with this type of personality disorder often marry men with strong obsessive-compulsive features in their personalities. Although the marital "fit" may be complementary, conflict frequently develops as the woman finds the "strength" of the man is really emotional remoteness and the man finds that the woman is never satisfied with his attentions.

> Ms. U was a charming, vivacious, flamboyant woman who much enjoyed her work as a kindergarten teacher and her avocational pursuits in community theatre. She dressed in skimpy or seductive apparel and complained that she didn't know why neighbors, door-to-door salesmen, husbands of her friends, or strangers on the street seemed always to be "making passes" at her. Ms. U, according to her sister, spent much more time than most women doing her ablutions, catering to her body, and trying to enhance her appearance. Ms. U's interpersonal relations, especially with females, tended to be impetuous, turbulent, and competitive.
>
> When Ms. U went to her grocery store, the post office, or her doctor's office, she expected—and usually received—swift, gracious, and accommodating treatment. Once she flew into a rage because a bus driver didn't accord her special consideration by letting her board a half-block from the assigned bus stop.
>
> Dr. T was told by a medical student that while talking to Ms. U, the student's eyes wandered to a passerby. Garrulous Ms. U, without breaking her loquacity, said, "Don't look at other people when I'm talking to you, look at me!" Dr. T exchanged an observation that Ms. U caused furor in his office because the nurses and secretaries believed Ms. U always insisted on extra and special care, and they thought that she was so fond of herself that she couldn't have sincere, deep relationships with others. Dr. T then thought to himself that that was probably true, but nevertheless he felt annoyed if by random circumstance one of his partners got to see Ms. U on her visit to the office, instead of him.

7   Passive-Aggressive Personality   The passive-aggressive personality is the "tough baby." Aggressiveness is expressed in more indirect, legally permissible (but frustrating) ways in which the victim is hard-pressed to be able, in good social conscience, to deliver any retaliation. The aggressiveness, therefore, is passive and more covert rather than active and overt. It takes the form of pouting, stubbornness, noncompliance, procrastination, inefficiency, and obstructive resistance. Such individuals may accept designated authority but defy it by means of these passive techniques. The passive characteristics are seen, therefore, to control and manipulate the environment and, in particular, people with considerable power and authority.

Often the aggressiveness underlies a need to be dependent upon others or upon institutions. Therefore, at times the "tough baby" appears more as a "cry baby" (or some individuals appear more or less constantly as either tough or cry babies). The passive-dependent mode is characterized by helplessness, indecisiveness, tenacious clinging to others, and a practiced ability to force others and institutions to provide nurturing support.

George was a teenager whose stormy scholastic and home life led to a naval enlistment. Within the first week of boot camp it was apparent to George that he "couldn't stand the service." On the grinder during military drills, George infuriated his company commander by being totally unable to distinguish his left foot from his right foot. George's shipmates became disenchanted with him when the whole unit was penalized several times because George had not responsibly discharged duties such as cleaning the latrine, making his bed, or tidying his locker. One officer noted that of several thousand men whom he saw that year, George was the only one who got lost for over an hour in finding his way from the barracks to the staff headquarters.

Within several weeks it was obvious to peers and officers that, indeed, George was unsuitable for military service. He was sent to a neuropsychiatric unit to be evaluated for possible discharge. The corpsman complained to the medical officer that George appeared each day at sick bay with a new battery of complaints which he alleged made it impossible for him to perform even a modest detail of work. A month after entering service George was back in his home town, boasting on the street corner how he had "fooled" the Navy into letting him go. However, he had already made several trips to be certain that any veteran's benefits to which he was entitled should be forthcoming.

8 Asthenic Personality This personality is the "doleful soul." Descriptively, such individuals are lethargic, apathetic, and oversensitive to all types of stress. They seem especially vulnerable to fatigue, and they seem to have little energy. Others see them as difficult to be around because their "blue" look at the world makes them always pessimistic. Yet they seem to need and demand, because of their lack of vitality and enthusiasm, much help and support from others. They complain of being directionless and with little motivation to accomplish minimal daily routines.

Such individuals seem to be missing energy and enthusiasm, and often look to their surroundings to provide it. There are often depressive undercurrents to their personalities, and the development of clear depressive illnesses is not rare. They often are attracted to outgoing, energetic, and enthusiastic others, but the degree of their dependency on others for energy and direction often comes to be felt as a burden by spouses.

The husband of Ms. K felt confused, helpless, and exhausted. He went to his pastor for guidance because he was developing uncharitable opinions about his wife. He recited a long catalogue of woes, and indicated that they were having serious and negative impact on the entire family.

The doctors had not been able to find any health problem with Ms. K, and despite the more than comfortable existence Mr. K provided, Ms. K remained joyless, complaining that she didn't see where she was going in this life or what its purpose could be. Yet Mr. K was sure she wasn't suicidal, and he believed she enjoyed talking like this because it engaged constant attention from the entire family. But no matter what was suggested or what interpretation was placed on a life value, Ms. K rejected it as meaningless and beyond her effort. Now Mr. K revealed to his spiritual advisor that he was beginning to keep a record of those times Ms. K was too far exhausted and overwhelmed to do routine things (e.g., cook supper) but yet more than able and willing to do things she wished to do (such as to go to a movie after one of the children had cooked supper).

9   Inadequate Personality   This person is the "sad sack." Such people have no physical or mental deficiency, yet they exhibit poor responses to physical, social, intellectual, or emotional demands. The inability to respond means that they are particularly inept in new situations and that they exhibit poor judgment. Often they appear to lack physical stamina and their social relations are often based on the public acknowledgment of their incompetence. That is, others tease them, make them the butt of pranks, or disregard and minimize their opinions and presence.

Patients with inadequate personalities, because they pose no threat, may be well-liked and tolerated or even welcomed (usually to be the target of playful abuse). However, being unable to meet the demands of everyday existence, such people rarely become productive citizens.

These individuals often appear to drift through life. They may go from job to job or work for years at menial occupations. They avoid responsibility and seek relationships with powerful others. Marriages to dominant spouses may occur and in such relationships the spouse may serve as a parent figure.

> Dr. V's patient was a man in his late twenties in satisfactory health. He had graduated from grammar school and now worked on the "city roads." His foreman had to assign less taxing jobs to him because he was easily overextended and then would take time off from the job.
>
> To Dr. V's knowledge, her patient had never had a girlfriend, yet he knew lots of young women. The patient frequented the local bars in the company of other young people. However, often he was used for such roles as seeing how fast he could drink large amounts of beer, to fetch the car for one of his friends, or to regale the customers with his comical effort to dance with the neighborhood beauty.

10   Borderline Personality   These individuals present a frequently confusing array of symptoms. Basically the personality structure is fragile, and brief periods of frank psychosis are common. When not functioning at a psychotic level, such individuals may demonstrate obsessive thoughts, phobias, high levels of anxiety, and frequent brief depressive periods. This neuroticlike aspect of the clinical picture, combined with episodes of psychosis, led to an earlier designation of "pseudoneurotic schizophrenia." During the past decade, however, clinical studies have clarified an underlying and profound personality disorder.

The central aspects of the personality disorder include a basic disturbance in relationships with others, which is characterized by intense fixations during which the other individual is seen as all-good. In fact, there is a tendency for such people to respond to others as being either all-good or all-bad. Central to these personalities is a primitive fear of abandonment and, as a consequence, the need to attach themselves strongly to others. Consequently, they may be clinging, demanding, and childlike. Often, despite their attachments to others, they complain of loneliness or emptiness.

This form of personality disorder is one of the more severe types, and although there may be milder variants that do not come to the attention of clinicians, those who do are usually seen as significantly disturbed. The disturbance in relationships with others, the multiple and frequently changing neurotic symptoms, and the tendency to psychotic regression combine often to render such individuals capable only of tenuous family, social, and vocational adjustments.

Ms. R's ophthalmologist knew her well. Like many before him, he had developed a quick, easy, and strong relationship with Ms. R. The more he knew her the more surprising this attachment seemed, because in most ways Ms. R resembled a schizoid personality and Dr. W didn't think individuals with schizoid personalities were capable of such intense and lasting interrelationships. However, he realized that in many ways Ms. R kept the relationship afloat, but did so with a quality of wariness.

Ms. R's verbal content was filled with distress over fear of abandonment. Further, in a pleasant, gentle manner she would repeatedly express her anger, chagrin, and annoyance at a variety of unfortunate experiences. These included anger that her father had died a quarter of a century ago, and that everyone from her saleslady to her son was always telling her what she could do and what she was incapable of doing. She also felt that powerful personalities threatened to engulf her and thereby abbreviate her individuality, and that she was handicapped because she was so infantile that she couldn't take trips unless accompanied by a family member.

Despite many successes in her work and an obvious supportive, interested, and sustaining claque (including Dr. W), Ms. R held herself in low esteem and consciously curbed her anger that she would be abandoned, exploited, or made to seem "foolish." Thus she went through life with a depressive diathesis, feeling empty, helpless, and hopeless—and angry. She worried about her "weaknesses" and used a rigid conscience both to justify distancing from others and to verify her own unworthiness. Ms. R continues through life engaged in very active fantasy. Sometimes she appears engaged and optimistic. Other times she is down in the dumps. Frequently she is dreamy.

11 Antisocial Personality This is the "confidence" man or woman. Clinically such individuals may be referred to also as psychopaths. Such individuals typically are suave, facile, and smooth. They give a long history of repeated authority clashes and are said to be unable to profit by past experience or punishment. Such people operate as if standard and conventional ethical values are both unacceptable and incomprehensible to them, save on an insincerely verbalized basis. Hence they appear to others as unreliable, superficial, and disappointing, despite apparent high intelligence. The antisocial patient is regarded as being able to operate without a conscience, demonstrating emotional instability, poor judgment, and a dearth of moral standards. An egocentric impulsiveness combined with a lack of restraint permits such people to take risks. Frequently they seek dangerous thrills or kicks, even though realizing that such actions could result in injury to others, criminal charges against themselves, or destruction of institutions.

The bravado, insouciance, and ability to rationalize and project blame to others for their own socially disapproved behavior may make such people impressive to others. Such admiration may lead to unhappy consequences, since the antisocial personality permits the patient to exploit, with ruthless disregard, anyone who chances to believe or trust in him or her. The patient seems driven by senseless, illogical behavior which appears to provide instant gratification with emphasis on how to keep others from interfering with personal happiness.

These individuals, driven by a strong need for satisfaction and pleasure and with a massively defective conscience, often become involved in the heavy use of drugs and in crime. Many end up in prisons and, upon release, repeat the patently self-defeating behavior and are returned for longer and longer incarcerations.

As with the other personality disorders, there are various levels of severity. The milder forms of this particular disorder are characterized by manipulation of people, more subtle and skillful law breaking, and a pronounced self-centeredness. These characteristics can be associated with a degree of economic success in certain types of work that are based upon superficial charm and exploiting people. The more severe forms of antisocial personality disorder, however, frequently result in unskilled, and illegal behavior so as to bring such individuals in frequent contact with the law.

Those individuals who become attached to people with antisocial personality disorders lead lives of misery. When they are manipulated, used, and treated with little respect for their own needs, life becomes unbearable. Remaining with such a person over long periods of time may involve a pathological need to be hurt and to suffer.

> Mr. S was the son of a judge. From first grade he had been extraordinarily persuasive, often convincing others, including his teachers, that he had done things or been places, when in actuality he had not. By age 10 he had been in numerous scrapes with the local police, but his family's good standing in the community blocked any serious punitive action. When he was 14 he impregnated the grocer's 17-year-old daughter. Later she said that she thought he was 18 as he had told her, and that he had promised to marry her. At 16, following a high school football game, Mr. S, under the influence of liquor, was suspected of having grievously assaulted a crippled, mentally defective youth. Shortly afterwards he was expelled from school for a long series of infractions including gambling on the premises, selling marijuana to elementary school children, and cheating in exams.
>
> Dr. D saw Mr. S soon after he had returned from a federal reformatory. On the occasion of his son's seventeenth birthday, Judge S gave him a new automobile. That same evening Mr. S was arrested in another county in a car he had stolen. Mr. S told Dr. D that while in the reformatory he had decided to give himself a course in chemical engineering. Proudly he reported that he had commanded this material with such mastery that he had been able that week to pass himself off at a local plant as an advanced chemical engineering student from a prestigious eastern university. Dr. D listened but felt bereft of ideas about what he could do both to help this young man and to protect other people who might come in contact with him.

ETIOLOGY AND COURSE OF PERSONALITY DISORDERS

The personality disorders, like other syndromes, are not caused by a single etiologic factor but are invariably the result of the interaction of a number of variables. The major etiologic factors can be included in biologic, developmental, family, and social categories. For some patients one category seems to play a major role but for most there are clinical data to support the role of at least several categories of etiologic factors.

The evidence for the role of biologic factors is, at best, suggestive. There are, for example, basic tempermental differences among newborn infants that appear to persist at least through childhood (see Chapter 3).[11] These differences are thought to be related to genetic influences upon the integration of the central nervous system. Some infants, for example, appear to retreat from strange stimuli, cling to the mother, and overreact to noise or other sudden change. These biologic tendencies interact immediately with the surrounding environment, in particular, the personality of the mother and her specific capabilities for responding to these traits of the infant. Clinicians, however, have considered that some of these traits may represent a tendency toward, or diathesis for, poor personality formation, which in adult years would be characterized by retreat from interpersonal relationships, poor social skills, and excessive shyness.

Other infants, for example, come into life with a hyperactive tendency. They move a lot, thrash about, and seem easily excitable. Here, again, the capacity of the mother to deal with these specific traits is considered to be an important determinant of the interaction. For example, a mother who is herself very controlled may be uncomfortable with the infant's activity pattern and this may influence the subsequent development of these biologic characteristics. Some clinicians have considered these characteristics as a tendency toward a personality configuration involving a high activity level, the expression of feelings in the form of behavior (acting out) and the development of behavior disturbances.

These hypotheses grow out of clinical work with patients and do not have the firm data base that the twin and adoption studies provide for the genetic tendency to develop schizophrenia and manic-depressive illness. Other bits of evidence, however, add to the strength of clinical observations. Patients with antisocial personality disturbances have been found, as a group, to have more frequent electroencephalographic abnormalities than the general population. Unusually prolonged or difficult birth experiences have been correlated with a wide range of psychiatric syndromes, including personality disorders. Children with "soft" neurologic signs are often found to have a higher incidence of behavioral difficulty.

Although the evidence is far from conclusive, and the problems involved in doing longitudinal studies that include the interaction of many variables are tremendous, many clinicians think that biologic factors may contribute, often in significant ways, to the development of personality disorders.

There are clinical data that suggest strongly that personality disorders can be understood as arrests in the infant or child's psychologic development. If the early developmental needs of the infant are not met, or, conversely, are overgratified, the infant's personality may tend to fixate, with strong features of that developmental phase incorporated into the subsequent adult personality. The borderline personality disorder, for example, is seen as a severe disturbance because the developmental arrest occurred very early in the life of the infant, at a time when the infant was attempting to separate psychologically from the mother and experience himself or herself as a separate person. The obsessive-compulsive personality disorder is usually seen as less serious because the developmental arrest occurs later, at the time when control and self-discipline is the central developmental issue.

Those clinicians who emphasize the role of developmental arrests in the etiology of personality disorders do not exclude the role of biologic, family, or social variables. The central focus is, however, the developmental arrest. The earlier in the infant's or child's development the arrest occurs, the more profound is the adult personality disorder. In addition, as suggested by the above examples, this perspective also states that each personality disorder has, at its core, a specific developmental arrest and subsequent conflict. These concepts, which are often associated with psychoanalysis, have achieved considerable prominence and are a part of current psychodynamic practice. There is strong clinical evidence from both psychoanalytic and psychotherapeutic work with patients and the research field of child development that the basic concepts have validity. What remains to be elaborated regarding the specific area of personality disorders is the interaction of the developmental problems and the biologic, family, and social variables.

The third category of factors involves the more recent field of family systems research and family therapy. In this perspective the family is studied or treated as a system and the emphasis is to understand and intervene in those characteristics of the family system which are involved in the etiology of the individual patient's psychiatric disturbance.[12]

At this time in this relatively new field there is evidence that several family configurations can be involved in the etiology of certain individual personality disorders. The configuration is that of the dysfunctional family tightly controlled by a very dominant parent, often the father. The parent's tyrannical use of power is associated with active rebelliousness on the part of one or more children. The spouse may covertly encourage the child's rebellious behavior as part of his or her own impotent anger toward the dominant parent. The child's rebelliousness is then seen to generalize to all authority figures and the acting-out behavior becomes a part of the child's personality.

Another family process often encountered, usually in families containing one child with a personality disorder, is that of scapegoating. In these families all the problems and everything "bad" about the family is ascribed to one member. The child "selected" for this role may be physically or temperamentally different from the other children and must, at least in part, accept the role assignment. Here, again, the role of the "bad guy," the "troublemaker," or the "evil one" is incorporated into the child's developing personality and is seen in action in the outside community. The scapegoating process is seen often as a way for a family to avoid facing a deeper and potentially disruptive problem, frequently in the parental relationship.

A third configuration involves families who are grossly disturbed. The family itself encourages using others, exploiting the innocent, manipulating for individual gain, lying, cheating, and other characteristics seen in individual patients with severe antisocial personality disorders. The basic family message is that humans are all frauds, totally self-serving, and corrupt. The trick is to get ahead of, outsmart, and outmaneuver others. Needless to say, intimacy is to be avoided because it involves vulnerability.

The evidence from the fields of family research and family therapy continues to mount and does suggest that there are a variety of ways in which what goes on day after day in the life of a family may contribute to the etiology of a family member's personality disorder.

Social factors may play an important role in the genesis of personality disorders. The diagnosis, for example, of antisocial personality disturbance is made more frequently in dealing with lower socioeconomic patients than in dealing with more affluent groups. Some of this may be a reflection of middle- and upper-middle-class professionals dealing with lower socioeconomic patients and failing to understand their social reality. Some of this may also reflect the professional's disinclination to deal with behavior that includes actions offensive to middle-class value orientations.

However, there is the real impact of social deprivation to be considered. If a child grows up in circumstances where the provision of food, clothes, and shelter is always problematic and, at the same time, he or she sees on television or some blocks away a totally different life-style in which there seems to be an easy affluence, ostentatiousness, and gross material wastage, this is bound to have its impact. Certainly some youngsters exposed to this discrepancy may work hard to change their life circumstances. Others, however, will fall into a gang of peers in which stealing and other crime is accepted. Under circumstances of deprivation, the family may have a more difficult time offering children the strength and cohesiveness necessary for personality development. It is not surprising, therefore, that there may be an increased number of people who are judged to have antisocial personality disorders and who come from environments of social deprivation.

This brief overview of some of the factors thought to be important in the etiology of personality disorders is not inclusive or exhaustive. Rather it is meant to demonstrate that the physician must recognize that multiple factors are invariably present in the causation of such disturbances. The clinician must evaluate, as best as possible, the role of each etiologic variable in the individual patient in order to plan treatment effectively.

Little, unfortunately, is known about the natural history of untreated patients with various personality disorders. Some continue to function in society, others periodically regress and are hospitalized. Many are in prisons; some experience a violent death. Robins suggests something of the outcome for some of these patients.[13] She was able to contact a group in their forties who had been seen as children in a guidance clinic. When compared with matched controls from the same neighborhood, those who as children were diagnosed as having personality or behavior disorder had very poor outcomes as adults. More of them were dead, hospitalized, in prisons, on drugs, or on some type of government subsidy than those in the control group. This suggests that, at least for some personality disorders, life continues to be a losing struggle.

TREATMENT OF THE PERSONALITY DISORDERS

The treatment of patients with personality disorders taxes the acumen of competent clinicians. As in all excellent treatment, the first step is to make a precise diagnosis. Knowledge of the differential diagnostic possibilities, plus a grasp of the multiple etiologic factors involved, will permit the doctor to proceed with treatment interventions.

Such patients come to medical attention often because of secondary symptoms. Alcoholism, drug abuse, or traumatic wounds are common. Often physicians come to know such patients during treatment for a medical illness, and after finding the patient "odd" or difficult, may come to recognize the presence of a personality disturbance. It is frequently important to obtain historical information from other family members because the patient may be grossly inadequate in providing historical data.

A thorough history, physical and neurological examinations, and, on occasions, psychological testing are necessary. Once the diagnosis is established, the next question concerns the degree of disability and destructive impact upon others. Patients with mild personality disturbances may need help, and patients with severe personality disorders usually need help desperately.

The problem is that frequently the patient is not uncomfortable; the disturbance does not result in enough personal anxiety or depression to push the patient to do something about himself or herself. Often, in antisocial personalities, for example, apparent motivation appears only when the patient is facing a trial or is in other trouble with authorities. The family may wish to have "something done about the patient," but the patient seems little interested.

The physician's most potent therapy is to form an alliance of trust and respect with the patient, taking into account that many patients with severe personality disorders have difficulty with interpersonal relationships. However, the doctor's warmth and interest may play a crucial role in effecting a treatment alliance.

Often these patients are referred to a psychiatrist for treatment. The psychiatrist, following evaluation studies, will make recommendations to the patient and often the family. The psychiatrist will base treatment recommendations on the following guidelines.

1   Most such patients are not benefited by psychopharmacologic approaches, except for periods of crises. Further, this group of patients includes many individuals who have a propensity to misuse or become dependent upon drugs.

2   Although crisis intervention or brief psychotherapeutic treatment is

helpful during crises, often such patients are inaccessible to or are uninterested in psychotherapy aimed at examining and changing the basic personality disturbances.

3 Some such patients are accessible to intensive psychotherapy, and often a trial of such treatment is necessary in order to know whether the individual patient can be helped.

4 Group psychotherapy has been helpful as either an adjunct to individual psychotherapy or as the primary treatment effort.

5 Marital or family therapy has been useful if the personality disorder is mild or moderate, and if both patient and spouse wish to preserve the relationship.

6 Biologic treatments such as electroshock are of no use in the treatment of personality disorders.

7 Patients with severe personality disorders may be helped by psychiatric hospitalization in a facility where an intensive, confronting, interpretive milieu is combined with intensive individual and group psychotherapy. Under these circumstances, hospitalization may have to be continued for a year or more in order to produce basic personality change.

In summary, these patients are often difficult to treat, and some appear impossible to help with any form of current therapy. However, treatability cannot be generalized to all such patients, for many are accessible and derive much gain from a variety of psychotherapeutic techniques. It does require, however, a therapist with an appreciation of the often deep-seated nature of the patient's difficulty, and the patience and skill to involve the patient in the psychotherapeutic adventure.

PREVENTION

Because of the lack of solid data about etiology, natural history, and treatment, few studies have been done on preventing the development of personality disorders. Such research, as with other longitudinal studies, requires prodigious effort.

Some have focused on the social factors often involved in the etiology of these disturbances and have suggested that efforts at alleviating the plight of the socially deprived would reduce the prevalence of some personality disorders. Others with an interest in family education have suggested that the family is the obvious focus of preventive efforts. Still others would point to educational programs directed at early infant development and increasing the important maternal skills.

The truth appears to be that medicine and psychiatry are a long way from having the skills and proven techniques to prevent personality disorders or any other major psychiatric disturbance. The widespread prevalence of personality disorders, however, ensures that most physicians will be requested to care for such patients. The more the physician understands this group of patients, the better he or she will be able to provide help to them and to their families.

REFERENCES

1 Offer, D., and M. Sabshin, *Normality,* New York: Basic Books, 1966.

2 Strachey, J.: *Collected Papers of Sigmund Freud,* New York: Basic Books, 1959.

3 Menninger, K., M. Mayman, and P. Pruyser: *The Vital Balance: The Life Process in Mental Health and Illness,* New York: Viking Press, 1963.

4 Maslow, A. H.: *The Farther Reaches of Human Nature,* New York: Viking Press, 1971.

5 Mailer, N.: "The White Negro," in G. Sykes (ed.), *Alienation, The Cultural Climate of Our Time,* vol. I, New York: George Braziller, 1964, pp. 171–189.

6 Rollin, H. R.: "Personality Disorders," *Brit. Med. J.,* **1**:655–667, 1975.

7 Vaillant, G. D.: *Adaptation to Life,* Boston: Little, Brown, 1977.

8 Offer, D., M. Sabshin, and D. Marcus: "Clinical Evaluations of 'Normal' Adolescents," *Am. J. Psychiat.,* **9**:864–872, 1965.

9 Masterson, J. F.: *The Psychiatric Dilemma of Adolescence,* Boston: Little, Brown, 1967.

10 Westley, W. A., and N. B. Epstein: *The Silent Majority,* San Francisco: Jossey-Bass, 1969.

11 Thomas, A., and S. Chess: *Temperament and Development,* New York: Brunner/Mazel, 1977.

12 Lewis, J. M. et al.: *No Single Thread: Psychological Health in Family Systems,* New York: Brunner/Mazel, 1977.

13 Robins, L. N.: *Deviant Children Grow Up,* Baltimore: Williams and Wilkins, 1966.

Chapter 12

The Functional Psychoses

John S. Strauss, M.D.

EDITORS' INTRODUCTION

What does one do with a patient who is "crazy," out of contact with reality, belligerent, and unable to understand why the physician and the rest of the world cannot see things precisely as he or she does? All physicians face this problem, and it may be a most exasperating, frustrating experience. The physician may urge the patient to settle back, be rational, and recognize the need for help—often to no avail. The physician may encourage the patient, again to no avail, to see a colleague—a psychiatrist, for example—or go to a hospital.

At other times, a physician may feel helpless when the family phones to say that Aunt Helen or young John is hearing and responding to voices, yet the family insists that there is nothing wrong and that, certainly, there is no need to see a doctor.

The physician may also feel helpless when recognizing the civil rights and liberties of the patient, who may or may not be dangerous to self or others. Perhaps the best way out is to contact a psychiatric colleague to see if the psychiatrist will take over the management and treatment of the patient.

On the other hand, how exasperating it is for the psychotic patient when no one seems to understand, to appreciate the perils or the importance of something which is so real to the patient. What is wrong with everybody and what makes them think there is something wrong with you? Why do others not recognize that the television announcer is talking directly to you? The physician who understands the basic structure and different varieties of psychosis, recognizes how real the events are to the disturbed patient, and does not react in a cavalier manner may be in the best position to direct the ill person toward treatment.

The physician can offer more than chemical relief. The physician may offer the patient his or her own presence—a sense that someone is "with" the patient in at least some of what the patient is experiencing. Often, however, this does not happen, and frequently it is because the physician does not understand the underlying structure of the acute psychosis and retreats from what appears to be a chaotic situation.

There are, however, many parts of the psychosis that may be understood from the vantage point of the physician's personal experience. Most individuals have experienced periods of impasse—occasions where life seemed bogged down, goals appeared unattainable, and the urge to retreat was strong. Peak experiences, although not common, have been experienced by many; for some, these occurred in a religious context, and for others they may have been drug-related. Some individuals have experienced such periods during a deeply intimate encounter with a loved one, others with Bach or a mountain sunset. At such times, there may be heightened perception, a sense that one is close to a new level of meaning.

Perhaps only a few physicians have experienced some loss of the sense of self. One can, however, experience something of this state when awakening from deep sleep, during early phases of anesthesia, or even after long periods of being entirely alone.

There is, of course, much in the content of the acute psychosis that is idiosyncratic and emerges out of the individual's experiences, conflicts, and defenses. If the physician can reach beyond this highly personal content to the structure of the acute psychosis, he or she will find much that can be understood from the viewpoint of the physician's own life experiences. It is with this kind of orienting view that the reader should approach this chapter by a renowned authority in the field of the functional psychoses.

INTRODUCTION

In considering the functional psychoses, it would be a mistake to jump immediately into issues of diagnosis, etiology, treatment, and prognosis. Although important, these issues far too often obscure another major consideration—the feeling, or even worse, the absence of feeling when the clinician is faced with a psychotic person. The statement by Euripides, "Those whom the gods would destroy, they first drive mad," gives a hint of the horror with which mankind through the ages has viewed the losing of one's mind. Certainly references commonly made to "the nuthouse" or to a person who does something unusual, "he belongs in _____ (the psychiatric hospital serving the area)," are evidence of the continuing contempt and fear people have about going crazy. These feelings are reflected also by ignorance about schizophrenia even among highly educated people. Schizophrenia is often viewed by such people as a disease characterized by a "split personality," while among less educated people the schizophrenic has the image of someone wearing a Napoleon hat, standing with his hand inside his shirt. The degree of feeling and misinformation produced by these images is something that the physician cannot avoid when confronting a psychotic patient, at least not successfully. These feelings must be confronted as they exist in the "treater," the "treated," and society in general.

Often the inexperienced physician, or even an experienced physician who is meeting a psychotic patient for the first time, deals with some of the anxiety and uncertainty in working with such persons by becoming extremely objective or distant. This tendency may not be entirely bad, since the other extreme, allowing the patient's disorganization and misperception of reality to dominate the clinical interaction, would of course be even more unfortunate. But the polarity between becoming detached on the one hand, and overwhelmed on the other is not satisfactory. The physician dealing with a psychotic patient must attempt as much as possible to establish a clinical relationship, to establish the necessary controls with the patient (depending on the patient's condition), to carry out an adequate evaluation for the purposes of diagnosis and treatment, and still empathize with the patient's distress. Sometimes the psychotic patient expresses this distress openly, as in a fear of inner confusion or of what might happen. Often, however, this distress is more implicit, and expressed as delusional fear of others or as an absolute certainty about a view of reality shared by no one else.

In any of these instances, besides the usual work of evaluation, diagnosis, and treatment, the physician must attempt to comprehend what it must be like to be experiencing what the psychotic patient describes. The isolation, the alienation, the hearing of strange voices, the belief in powerful forces not accepted by others, the unpredictable agitation and hyperactivity, or severe depression and retardation—all have a serious impact on the patient's sense of self and of the world, life, occupation, and relationships. Even in those cases where the psychotic patient does not or will not acknowledge intense feelings, the physician must attempt to the utmost to comprehend what it would be like to be so out of step without, however, reacting to it. The understanding that comes with such empathy is not just a luxury for the physician or the patient. A major part of the psychosis is the alienation it causes and reflects; to help the patient deal with this experience requires as much understanding as can be generated.

Naturally, such understanding does not need to be maudlin pity. Even during the initial interview, the physician can increase his or her grasp of the problem and help the patient relate by asking the patient direct questions about how the experience feels, such as, "Do other people hear these voices?" or "Is something unusual happening to you?'' These inquiries will help considerably in developing a relationship between the physician and the psychotic person.

If the physician has trouble relating to the psychotic patient, the patient frequently has extreme difficulty in relating to the physician, for after all, the physician is the person who will give the final judgment whether or not this patient is mad. The feeling that this message conveys, perhaps that the patient is not competent and has lost his or her mind, is not something that a person takes lightly. The uncertainty about craziness in the future, the implications of madness regarding the patient's family, life, and hopes, obviously have a major impact.

And yet most psychotic patients want to be helped, and see the physician as a major resource, perhaps a final resource, for such assistance. The mixture of feelings this conflicting situation stirs up in the individual who wants help to overcome uncertainties and fears, and yet is struggling perhaps even to a delusional degree to maintain self-respect, is considerable. The physician working with such patients must recognize both the hopes and the fears the patient has, and then attempt to deal with them.

A further aid to understanding these experiences can be obtained by reading first-person accounts of someone who has been psychotic. But the reader should be aware that often the best publicized accounts are not either the most accurate or the most representative. Particularly well-documented descriptions of being psychotic are to be found in Kaplan[1] and in Sechehaye.[2]

After it has been recognized that dealing with psychosis may be strange and/or frightening for both physician and patient, the process of evaluation can begin. At the very beginning of the evaluation—even before attempting to reach a diagnosis—three questions should run through the physician's mind: Is the patient likely (1) to be dangerous, (2) to act impulsively, or (3) to be alienated easily? You simply do not know in the first minute or two what the patient is like, even when psychotic. The patient may be neither dangerous nor impulsive, and may be willing and eager to enter into a sustained treatment relationship without being readily alienated.

If the physician feels that the answer to any of the three questions is in the affirmative, however, appropriate steps must be taken. If there is some reason to believe that the patient may be dangerous, security for both the physician and the patient should be ensured. Such measures as the physician's sitting near the open door during an interview taking place in an emergency room, and being accompanied by one or two strong assistants, or other such measures, are perfectly legitimate approaches to potentially dangerous patients. It is often possible to be direct with the patient about such fears: "Until I can understand things better, I prefer to have Mr. X, our hospital aide, with me." "What's the matter, doctor, are you afraid of me?" "Well, I'm not sure yet." Of course, sometimes these judgments are difficult; however, it is often better to err on the side of caution, an approach which then leaves the physician freer than otherwise to ask the necessary questions in order to find out more about the patient's problems.

Another frequent difficulty at the beginning of evaluating psychotic patients is that the physician accepts hearsay from other people about the patient too readily, or assumes some predigested view about what psychosis is all about. The patient often knows and can communicate much crucial information that can be all too easily cut off by physicians who think they know more about the patient than they really do. Even the patient who responds to the question, "What brought you here?" with the answer, "They think I'm crazy," can give much helpful information if the physician pursues this lead by asking more about what they think, and also more about how the patient feels. These principles are basic, of course, to psychiatry and to medicine in general. However, they are sometimes ignored or forgotten in dealing with psychotic patients, as though somehow with such patients all the basic rules for a clinical relationship no longer hold true.

Besides these issues, important from the start, there are certain general principles for dealing with psychotic patients that need to be maintained throughout the entire evaluation and treatment. The first of these is candor. It may seem unnecessary to note the importance of this quality in the physician, but once again, one sees a separate set of rules used in dealing with psychotic patients so often that it is essential to reaffirm the importance of even these basic principles. Frequently when a psychotic patient asks the physician, "Do you think I'm crazy?" the response is likely to be a quick "no." Such a misleading response is rarely indicated. An answer that avoids being brutal on the one hand, and lying on the other, is almost always possible. For example, one might respond, "That word means so many things to different people, I won't use it with patients. You are having serious problems, however, and one of them appears to be hearing things that other people don't hear." Even if answers do not come to mind rapidly, it is still possible to respond by leaving time to reflect on an answer, saying something like, "I think words like that are very misleading, but I do want to give you my opinion of the problems you are having after we have a chance to talk further." Such a perfectly legitimate delay allows the clinician time to get more information that may be needed, and to think of a way of responding that will be candid without endangering the interview and treatment. Naturally, an answer must be given if one has been promised, and it is usually too mysterious and alienating to avoid the issue, attempt to make an interpretation, or leave such questions unanswered.

The second basic principle of the evaluation interview is structure. While being candid and empathic, the clinician has a task to accomplish, and the structure needed to achieve that task is not only practical, but can be reassuring for both physician and patient. The structure of the psychiatric evaluation, especially with psychotic patients, can sometimes be made particularly explicit and thus give extra help to both the patient and the physician. For example, the physician can say at the beginning of the interview, "First, I would like to talk with you for about half an hour to get some idea of the problems you've been having and what kind of treatment you have had for them." A comment like this at the beginning of the evaluation can serve to calm any fears the psychotic patient might have about the mysterious, powerful physician, and help to establish a clear task for the evaluation session.

But what structure should the evaluation interview use? To some extent, this will depend upon the particular orientation of the clinician. Nevertheless, the newly developed multiaxial diagnostic systems in psychiatry provide a helpful framework for collecting clinical information. These systems, which will be described in more detail later, generate not merely a single diagnostic label, such as "schizophrenia," but classify a patient in terms of several characteristics or axes. For example, one such system that has been recommended includes five axes focusing on the individual: symptomatology, duration and course of symptoms, associated (or precipitating) events, social relations functioning, and work functioning. These five headings provide an outline for information collection which will give the clinician the data he or she needs to evaluate the nature of the disorder, its prior course, possible etiological factors, and the strengths and disabilities of the patient in dealing with the world.[3] A more comprehensive addition to this multiaxial diagnostic system has been suggested. This would include four axes beyond the basic five. Two of the additional axes deal with family characteristics (type of psychiatric disorder in first-degree relatives, and family living situation and interaction patterns), and two axes cover general social conditions, social class, and a description of the patient's social network.

Clearly, these nine axes are mostly cross-sectional. They do not focus on the patient's early childhood and other background. Such background information is also important, but often it can best be collected and understood in terms of the basic axes.

Now that these general principles for the initial orientation to the psychotic patient have been stated, it would be possible to describe the classical functional psychoses: schizophrenia, manic-depressive (or bipolar affective) psychoses, psychotic depression (or unipolar affective psychosis), and schizoaffective schizophrenia (or schizoaffective psychosis). Description of these diagnostic types will again be postponed, however, since they are still being redefined and reconceptualized, and because of these uncertainties it may be better to describe some basic psychotic characteristics first before trying to fit them into diagnostic categories that have important shortcomings as well as values. In the following sections, therefore, we shall describe the evaluation of patient characteristics for each of the nine diagnostic axes before proceeding to discuss diagnostic categories.

Evaluating Symptoms and Signs

It is obvious, though sometimes neglected in practice, that the best way to find out about the patient's symptoms is to ask. Although asking an individual about hearing voices, for example, might seem likely to destroy rapport, almost all patients answer if they are asked, especially when such questions are posed with helping phrases such as, "Some people (e.g., hear voices); have you had any experiences like that?" Many times, however, physicians merely fail to ask, which often results in misdiagnosis and poorly focused treatment.

Since hallucinations, delusions, thinking disorders, and bizarre behavior are considered the major criteria of psychosis, it is generally wise to inquire routinely about these when evaluating possible psychotic conditions. The first two of these, hallucinations and delusions, are usually relatively easy to elicit and evaluate. The last two, however, are frequently judged present on dubious grounds. Often, for example, communication errors attributable to the patient's agitation or uncertainty during the initial interview will be considered as reflecting loose associations or other signs of considerable diagnostic importance, when in fact they are well within the range of normal deviation. The same may be true in judging appropriateness of behavior. It is important in evaluating these characteristics not to have too idealized a view of what nonpathologic behaviors are. Sometimes, to avoid this error, it is valuable to note the range of communication styles and aberrations that is present in persons who are clearly nonpsychotic. Especially in patients from subcultural groups and social classes different from those of the interviewer, patterns of communication and behavior can be misinterpreted as psychotic, when in fact they are within the normal realm for those subgroups.

Evaluating Precipitating Events

It is often difficult to be sure which factors cause a disorder in medicine generally, and this is especially true for psychiatric disorders. Events that appear stressful and are temporally related to the onset of a disorder may or may not reflect etiological contributions to the manifest pathology. Nevertheless, it is important to investigate routinely the occurrence of such possible precipitants. The most common stressors preceding psychiatric disorders appear to be losses in relationships or occupational functioning, the occurrence of severe illness, or success.

There is evidence to suggest that for neurotic disorders precipitants of these kinds are indeed important. For psychotic disorders, however, these usual "stressful events" have not been clearly demonstrated as playing a causal role. Although it has been suggested that this is evidence that stressful events do not appear to contribute to psychotic episodes, another answer seems more likely. Events related to psychotic episodes may have a relatively idiosyncratic impact on the individual vulnerable to psychosis and may not be one of the more commonly noted stressful situations. For example, the second year in college has been suggested as being particularly stressful to many individuals because for them it marks a considerable increment in their commitment to leaving the parental family. That event is not recorded in any of the common life-event scales. For these reasons, in evaluating possible precipitants in psychosis, it can be useful to pay special attention to the existence of such idiosyncratic precipitants to help untangle the types of causal factors that might be operating.

Evaluating the Course of the Disorder

This characteristic is especially important in evaluating psychotic patients. For one thing, it has been suggested by several schools of psychiatry that a major diagnostic criterion for differentiating schizophrenia from the affective psychoses is whether the disorder is continuous (schizophrenia) or remitting (affective psychosis). Besides its diagnostic implications, the course of the disorder is also important prognostically; the longer the patient has been symptomatic in the past, the more likely he or she is to be symptomatic in the future. Understanding the course of the disorder is also important in providing further information to the physician regarding what the patient and those around the patient are experiencing. There is, for example, evidence to show that patients who have been hospitalized three or more times tend to be given up by family members, who search for alternative relationships. Such facts are important to recognize because they influence the context in which treatment will be given.

Information on a Patient's Social Relations Functioning

Data on this topic, although perhaps seeming far afield from a narrow version of the medical model, is valuable prognostically as well as for treatment planning. There is considerable evidence to show that patients with poor premorbid social functioning have poor prognoses and may need more help in social skills training and dealing with social situations than other patients do. It is important in assessing these factors to judge the patient's isolation and the depth, number, and constancy of relationships.

Occupational Function

Occupational function is another characteristic which may seem somewhat distant from a narrow medical model yet has important prognostic and treatment implications. Besides being one of the better prognostic indicators, occupational functioning is a major sign of a patient's abilities and disabilities in relating to the environment. A satisfying job often provides considerable support for individuals going through stressful situations, including periods of psychiatric symptomatology. Patients with major difficulties in the occupational area may need vocational rehabilitation, or other types of training, to help them deal with job situations more successfully and thus provide them with a major source of self-respect and material security.

Family

Two family characteristics are particularly important. First, it is valuable to determine whether any first-degree relatives of the patient (parents, children, and full siblings) have had a diagnosable psychiatric disorder, and if so, what that diagnosis was. Both the affective psychoses and schizophrenia have a genetic tendency to run in families.

The second family characteristic is environmental. It is important to determine with whom the patient lives and the nature of their relationships. Hostile and intrusive family situations can render a patient's prognosis more guarded and may require active intervention.

Social Conditions

Social class (based on evaluation of occupation and education) appears to be an important characteristic in the etiology and treatment of psychiatric disorders. Individuals from the lower class (for example, unskilled laborers or unemployed individuals with only elementary school education) appear to be particularly vulnerable to schizophrenia. Besides this, social class to some extent determines the subject's expectations and ways of dealing with the treatment situation. Although it is wise not to assume prematurely that a person from a particular social class will have those norms, it is also wise to consider that he or she is likely to, and that this should be considered in treatment planning. For example, physicians sometimes underestimate the reality problems of patients in lower social classes in terms of the difficulties encountered in dealing with welfare agencies, violence, and substandard housing conditions.

TRADITIONAL DIAGNOSTIC CATEGORIES OF THE FUNCTIONAL PSYCHOSES

Although the multiaxial system, including the types of axes described above, is recommended for classifying and evaluating psychotic patients, it is also important to discuss the more traditional diagnostic categories of functional psychoses. There are two main types of such psychoses: schizophrenia and the affective psychoses. The latter include manic-depressive psychosis (also called bipolar affective psychosis) and the psychotic depressions (often called unipolar affective psychoses). Even recently, it appeared that these different disorders could be differentiated rather clearly based on the principles defined by Kraepelin and others at the beginning of this century. However, there have also been continued controversies about this division, and some changes in classification are continuing to take place. In spite of these changes, the basic split in the classification of functional psychoses between schizophrenia and the affective psychoses is likely to be maintained. Another classification, schizoaffective psychosis, which represents descriptively a mid-point between the two other psychotic types, has been identified. Although schizoaffective psychosis was originally considered a subtype of schizophrenia, there is increasing evidence to suggest that it may be more similar to the classical conception of the affective disorders since it may have the heredity pattern, prognosis, remitting course, and perhaps even treatment response generally considered to be characteristic of the affective psychoses. In the following sections, each of these three disorders, schizophrenia, affective psychosis, and schizoaffective psychosis will be discussed.

Schizophrenia

Description   Classically, schizophrenia (originally called dementia praecox) was considered to be a disorder with a chronic deteriorating course usually beginning in adolescence or early adulthood. The deteriorating course first described is less common today, apparently to some extent having been a result of the kind of institutional care given to such patients in the past. The age of onset is still commonly in adolescence and young adulthood, although both younger and older patients are often diagnosed as schizophrenic.

The clinical picture considered most characteristic of schizophrenia consists of delusions of passivity (being controlled by an outside force) and other psychotic phenomena, such as auditory hallucinations or other delusions, in the absence of either marked elation or depression. Social isolation and flat or incongruous affect have also been considered characteristic of schizophrenia. Several subtypes of the disorder have been defined. Those most commonly agreed upon are the following:

1   Catatonic—the major signs are motor abnormalities, either excessive activity (catatonic excitement) or inactivity, including muteness and immobility
2   Paranoid—the predominant symptomatology is delusions, especially delusions of reference or persecution which may provoke the compensatory mechanism of grandiosity
3   Hebephrenic—marked by deterioration as shown by a childlike manner and inappropriate affect, such as giggling or disorganized or ritualistic behaviors
4   Simple—most marked by withdrawal and flat affect and occasional bizarre or inappropriate behavior

Strangely, these traditional subtypes are much less often seen in most clinical settings today than in the past. Perhaps the disorder itself has changed. Perhaps newer treatment techniques, with active intervention and attempts to combat institutionalism, have minimized clinical pictures which in many instances may have been treatment artifacts. Whatever the reason, the smaller number of the classical types has added to the disagreement about who should be considered schizophrenic. Clearly those patients who fit the traditional descriptions should be. But what about those who have auditory hallucinations and various delusions but without flat affect or social isolation, and who have a brief course with complete recovery? These types of patients and others are the center of much diagnostic controversy. However, a major recent advance in psychiatry is the systematic use of operational descriptions. The American Psychiatric Association's new diagnostic manual (DSM III) will have these descriptions for each diagnostic category. Whether the categories defined are diseases or even true disorders is open to question, but they provide descriptive clarity, so that in terms of symptoms at least, physicians using the categories will understand the type of patient being described.

Epidemiology   Schizophrenia is the most common of the functional psychoses. Incidence and prevalence figures vary considerably, especially in relation to diagnostic criteria, but a common figure given for incidence (new cases per year) is 1/1000, and for prevalence (number of people affected during a 1-year period) is 4/1000, with a lifetime prevalence (percentage of people affected during their lifetime) of about 1 percent.

Etiology   Although there continues to be a vigorous search for "*the*" cause of schizophrenia, the more information that is obtained, the more it appears that there is no single cause. As each clue to etiology is pursued, it is found to be either not related to schizophrenia at all, or quite definitely related, but only accounting for a certain fraction of the causal process. Thus, with the considerable advances in genetic research for example, there is increasingly solid evidence for a genetic contribution to schizophrenia. However, where many years ago some investigators considered that schizophrenia was a "genetic disease," it is clear now that genetic factors play an important but nevertheless small role in determining whether an individual will become schizophrenic. Genetic research has been perhaps the most successful in studying the etiology of schizophrenia.

Specific biochemical and psychophysiological factors have also been suggested as causes of schizophrenia. One of these suggested as a possible mechanism is the hyperresponsiveness of certain neurotransmitter systems. It has been suggested that since certain types of drugs, e.g., amphetamines, cause schizophrenialike states, and since the antipsychotic drugs operate almost without exception by inhibiting specific types of neurotransmission, the abnormalities in these biological systems may be one of the causes of schizophrenia. The specific mechanism or definitive proof of such a process has been elusive, but increasing evidence suggests that these neurotransmitter systems play an important role in contributing at least partly to schizophrenic symptomatology. Even recent evidence on long-acting effects of abnormal inputs into these systems has provided theories about the etiology of chronic schizophrenia based on unusual patterns of habituation that have been demonstrated to amphetamine-related drugs.[4] A new focus of biochemical research in schizophrenia involves evaluating the role of polypeptides, many of which serve as types of neurotransmitters never before considered. This research, too, may provide a clue to abnormalities found in schizophrenia.

As with the biochemical studies, research on psychophysiological contributors to schizophrenia has also produced important information that is not yet conclusive. Various studies of reaction times in schizophrenia, cerebral cortex responses to stimuli, and measures of skin conductance have suggested the pervasiveness and importance of unusual patterns of arousal and recovery. It is argued that if schizophrenics have abnormal nervous system response patterns, they may be ineffective in warding off excessive stimuli and focusing attention. These defects in turn may produce aberrations of thought and perception, such as delusions, hallucinations, and the characteristic patterns of thought disorder.

The problem of schizophrenia has provided a major stimulus to biological research on the nature of brain function and its relation to perception and cognition. Although some of the biological theories of schizophrenia are becoming less plausible, such as the belief in an etiological role of monoamine oxidase (MAO), the work in this area appears to be providing important information about the nature of brain function, and some theories may be getting progressively closer to key biological factors in the functional psychoses.

Does the evidence for genetic, psychophysiological, and biological factors in schizophrenia mean that psychosocial factors in this disorder are negligible? Although the pattern in the past has often been for polarizations to develop between those who believe in biological causes and those who believe in psychosocial causes, an increasing number of investigators and clinicians believe that both factors are truly important, and even more, are able to consider seriously both psychosocial and biological characteristics in trying to discover the causes of schizophrenia and then work out treatment programs. This development is mirrored in what has happened recently to the age-old split between nature and nurture theorists. First, one group argued against the other, then one group pursued its own directions while more or less peripherally acknowledging the existence of the other, and now there are increasing attempts to relate the genetic and psychosocial elements in a serious fashion. Thus, for example, Kinney and Jacobsen[5] have described ways for studying how genetic predispositions might interact with certain environmental stresses to cause psychotic episodes. Others have suggested a scheme by which a variety of premorbid characteristics (biological, psychosocial, and developmental), may combine to predispose persons toward schizophrenia.

What psychosocial characteristics might be important in the etiology of schizophrenia? Many have been suggested, but all are controversial. The importance of disruptions in early childhood, disruptions caused by parental loss or bizarre family life, has been suggested for many years. Surprisingly, however, there is little evidence that these factors are causal elements in schizophrenia. One body of psychosocial research suggesting another possible etiology is the work of Wynne and Singer, who found that parents of schizophrenics often have an abnormality in their communication patterns which may not be immediately apparent clinically, and is not necessarily associated with parent symptomatology, but which nevertheless may be related to impairments in developing offsprings' abilities to deal with reality issues.[6] This impairment may render these individuals vulnerable to more serious cognitive or perceptual disruption at times of stress.

Do stressful events contribute to the cause of schizophrenia? Strangely, as with the early childhood trauma theories, there is very little evidence to show that stressful events precede the onset of schizophrenic psychoses. One suggestion has been that this failure is because these disorders are almost entirely biological in nature. Another suggestion, noted earlier, has been that the methods for measuring stressful events have been inappropriate for reflecting the more idiosyncratic situations that might be particularly important in setting off a schizophrenic episode.

One other factor that appears to be important in the cause of schizophrenia is the subject's social class. Schizophrenia is found more frequently in individuals from the lowest class. Some of this finding is apparently attributable to "social drift," the phenomenon by which individuals who are not very competent drift into the lowest class. In many instances, however, the findings of more schizophrenia in lower-class persons appear to be related more basically to social-class structure itself. Lower-class individuals from the largest cities especially are commonly diagnosed as schizophrenic, suggesting that there may be greater isolation of these individuals than of their counterparts in smaller towns, or from middle- and upper-class life-styles, and that this isolation may make people particularly vulnerable to schizophrenia.

Although one day there may be a discovery of the cause of schizophrenia, the best evidence now suggests that all the factors described above, and perhaps others still unknown, may interact in such a way that they cause a person to become schizophrenic. No single variable, biological or psychosocial, appears to be necessary or sufficient to make someone schizophrenic. When one considers that there may also be many types of schizophrenia, that schizophrenia may be a syndrome somewhat like dropsy with many specific causes, treatments, and prognoses, the complexity of the problem becomes clearer. Perhaps this should come as no surprise. In other types of disorder, including renal disease, blood dyscrasias, and pulmonary disorders, increasing knowledge has also tended not to simplify, but to reveal the complexities of the problems involved. Yet clearly the complexities need not be overwhelming. In fact, to the degree they are understood rather than oversimplified, they provide the physician as well as the investigator with increasingly realistic methods for dealing with patients who have the disorder.

Treatment   Treatment, like the processes of evaluation or diagnosis, should involve attention to several components of the patient's functioning. In the history of treatment, once again too narrow a view has been a major problem. Thus, when psychoanalysis first came to be used with schizophrenics, many thought that it would be the definitive treatment. That did not prove to be the case, although psychoanalytically oriented therapy can have an important part in the treatment program.

The era of antipsychotic medications then began, and many felt such medications would be the definitive treatment for schizophrenia. Recent evidence suggests that this, too, may not be the case. Although antipsychotic drugs often play an important role in reducing the symptoms and perhaps in helping with other aspects of the disorder as well, it appears that these medications are in many instances not of appreciable value in helping patients recover or develop their abilities to relate socially and to work.

In treating schizophrenics, the first concern besides establishing a relationship, as described earlier, is to attend to the "first-aid" measures necessary for any disorder. Schizophrenic patients may (or may not) be impulsively violent or suicidal. Many of their symptoms may alienate them from their families, friends, and employers, causing the patients more psychological hurt and rendering reentry into the community extremely difficult. Obtaining relevant history from the patient and relatives, and dealing with interpersonal processes like alienation and mystification in the evaluation interview itself, must be focused to determine the extent to which problems such as violence and alienation pose major difficulties. Again, it is important to remember that the patient—if asked—may provide the best information about these kinds of problems. This suggestion runs counter to the commonly held belief that schizophrenic patients do not have any insight into their problem and do not know that they need treatment. That belief is simply not accurate; in fact, a large percentage of schizophrenic patients will know when they need help and participate actively, especially if they have a feeling of trust for the physician who is working with them.

Clearly, if a definite risk of violence or suicide is present, hospitalization or some similar kind of care will be necessary to ensure the patient's safety and the safety of those nearby. For problems of social alienation, reaching a decision about hospitalization is sometimes more difficult. It must also be remembered, however, that some schizophrenic patients will not need hospitalization.

Treating Symptoms   The symptoms and signs of schizophrenia, such as delusions, hallucinations, and bizarre behavior, can be treated in several ways. Sometimes hospitalization itself, with its structure and supportive environment, will alter the course of symptoms that previously had worsened progressively, perhaps under the pressure of environmental stresses. Another factor is that, especially with patients whose symptoms are of recent onset, the natural history of the disorder is often for these symptoms to remit relatively spontaneously.

Antipsychotic medication can also be helpful in treating symptoms. There is, however, a tendency sometimes, in working with schizophrenic patients to start medication immediately, before the evaluation is completed, even when there is no urgency to do so. It is important to avoid this practice, and whenever possible to talk with the patient and the family long enough to clarify the nature of the symptoms, their duration, the kinds of living problems that they are causing, and possible specific stresses that may have helped to generate the psychosis.

Once the clinician has assessed the patient and the situation fully, he or she can then begin to consider treatment alternatives—and there are alternatives. For the physician who only rarely treats schizophrenics, it is perhaps best to refer such patients to a psychiatrist when you can. If this is not possible, it is probably better to use conservative management, including such things as talks with the patient and the family to clarify living problems they might be having, and the use of antipsychotic medication. In more difficult situations, hospitalization for a period of evaluation can be helpful. Following discharge the patient, and where indicated, the family members, can be seen periodically to discuss problems they may be having or, where medication is required, to adjust dosage. For those clinicians who have more extensive experience working with schizophrenics, still more flexibility in using psychosocial treatment approaches is possible and advisable.

For physicians working with schizophrenics, as with any other kind of patient, it is important to recall that no matter how severe the disorder, it is essential, with few exceptions, that some expectations for the patient's functioning be maintained. As with other disorders, some balance needs to be reached between the amount of responsibility that the clinician takes, the amount given to family members, and the amount expected of the patients themselves. When the responsibility is taken away from the patient, especially for extended periods, the result can be a progressive deterioration of the ability to function and a tendency to lean on symptoms excessively in order to avoid difficult situations. Establishing reasonable expectations for the patient's self-care and relationships to others can help prevent such an outcome.

Psychosocial approaches to working with schizophrenics can involve individual treatment and/or family treatment. In working with the patient as an individual, it is usually most helpful to begin by focusing on problems in daily living. These include the effects that symptoms have on patients and their environment, ways patients have found for alleviating symptoms, factors that make them worse, and all the usual things one asks about in a medical history.

The physician should attempt to titrate the detail with which he or she delves into family, competence, and other interpersonal issues at a level that may cause some anxiety, but not the disorganizing kind. This approach should not be viewed as merely supportive treatment. It can be the essence of psychotherapy if it helps the patient to understand how the symptoms appear to operate in the way he or she handles daily life, the types of stress that may make the symptoms worse, and things to do that may help. This kind of interaction with a patient can also generate more trust and lay the groundwork, if it seems useful, to investigate possible sources of symptoms in the patient's intimate family, social relationships, and occupational experiences and background.

Medication is especially helpful for states of agitation or when psychotic symptoms become particularly disturbing (see Chapter 26 for full details). Once the dosage range has been established, medication can be switched to a single bedtime dose. This can help with any sleep disturbances there might be, and will also minimize drowsiness during the day. Phenothiazines should not be used primarily as sedatives, however, since they have a much greater incidence of side effects than the usual sedative preparations.

Since the four classes of antipsychotic drugs currently used all have generally the same therapeutic effects, it is most useful to select one or two types and use them with most patients who require such treatment. In that way it is possible for the physician to become familiar with the preparation and the dosages required by various patients. The most justifiable reason for changing medications is not so much to afford a change in therapeutic effects, since these are minimally different, but to overcome certain side effects, since patients developing severe side effects with one medication may not have any such reactions to another.

The only preparations that are distinctively different from the others in their therapeutic action are the long-acting injectable medications. Fluphenazine has the advantage of ensuring "compliance," but the corresponding disadvantage of rendering the patient more passive in the treatment program, a feature that may have ramifications for the way he or she is treated by the family and for all attempts at taking more responsibility for personal functioning. An additional danger is that if side effects occur, they may be more severe and/or last longer because of the long-term action of the drug.

The antipsychotic drugs have the potential for a wide range of side effects. Some of these side effects, such as certain types of abnormal muscle tone, can be controlled by using an anti-Parkinsonian agent like trihexyphenydil. Acute, severe reactions can be treated with intramuscular antihistamines. Routine use of anti-Parkinsonian agents is not recommended. In fact, the goal of reducing side effects can often be obtained merely by lowering the dosage of the antipsychotic drug itself.

It is no longer generally considered optimal to treat patients with antipsychotic drugs for extremely long periods unless absolutely necessary. The occurrence of tardive dyskinesia—abnormal movements whose occurrence may be irreversible—is a serious effect whose considerable prevalence has become apparent. Depending on the course of the disorder and previous history regarding the likelihood that a patient's psychosis will recur, courses of medication might be continued for up to 1 month, 6 months, or a year. Some patients will need to be treated longer, but the clinician ought to be careful to justify the continuing need for such medication.

Treating Precipitants and the Course of the Disorder   In the process of the initial evaluation, possible precipitating factors that may become apparent should provide a focus for continuing investigation and evaluation of the ways in which the patient can deal with precipitating situations more effectively, or if absolutely necessary, avoid them. Pursuing this information and helping the patient deal with stresses more adequately can provide a basis for psychotherapy, as noted earlier. It is surprising how often clinicians ignore the existence of such possible precipitants, when in fact patients frequently request some help with them.

The course of the disorder, too, needs to be treated. It is important to discuss the history of the disorder with the patient and the family, to learn their feelings about it and to help them with the experience. Especially with chronic or recurring disorders, the tendency toward isolation, frustration, and surrender must be explored, and optimal ways of handling these feelings and the realities of the disorder need to be considered.

Treatment of Social Relations and Work Functioning.   In working with schizophrenics, it is important for the clinician to evaluate, and when necessary help to improve, the patient's social relations and occupational functioning. Social and occupational skills programs, especially when given by those who are familiar with the needs of schizophrenic patients, are often extremely important for the patient trying to establish a personal life in a role other than that of patient.

Treatment also ought to involve explicit attention to the family and the social matrix in which the schizophrenic lives. Gaining some understanding of the patient's environmental context and the problems being faced can guide the clinician to the kind of interventions required, whether it is obtaining help with a welfare problem, talking with the family together, or making a home visit to ameliorate difficult situations that the patient's disorder may have caused or that may exist independently of the patient's schizophrenia.

Family interviews can often help in the process of clarifying many issues, such as fears, expectations, frustrations, and ways family members have of dealing with each other. In such encounters, it is important to try to deal with all members, including the patient, as people with legitimate questions and needs. It is also important to avoid a frequent tendency either to join certain family members in treating the patient as though he or she were defective in some way, or, on the contrary, to blame the family members for possible contributions to the patient's problems.

Finally, with schizophrenics, as with many others, a balance must be found between the removal of the patient from stressful situations and the encouragement to take on responsibilities. An extreme at either pole appears to generate unfortunate consequences. For this reason, a gradual pacing of increased responsibility is generally most helpful, while the physician is monitoring the degree to which the patient is able to take on the responsibilities and helping him or her through stressful situations.

Prognosis   Schizophrenia originally was considered as having a deteriorating course almost invariably, thus accounting for the original name, dementia praecox. More recent research, however, demonstrates that, depending on the specific diagnostic criteria used, deterioration is by no means a constant or even a frequent outcome. Often patients have some residual dysfunction or symptomatology, although some recover completely. The best way to predict the outcome is by considering three major factors: previous duration of the patient's symptoms, previous level of social functioning, and previous level of occupational functioning. These three characteristics together provide the maximum amount of predictive power for speculating about the patient's outcome. And the word "speculating" here is an appropriate one. Even using the best-known indicators of prognosis, the clinician is able to predict the likelihood of a particular outcome in less than half the cases. Because of this, prognostic measures can provide rough guidelines but leave much room for individual variation, the sources of which are not understood.

The Affective Psychoses

In discussing the affective psychoses there are two choices: to consider them as having discrete disorders, or to describe the numerous controversies about the boundaries and nature of the syndromes generally included in this category. For the sake of simplicity, the first alternative would seem preferable; for the sake of accuracy, the second is more appropriate. But for general clinical use, it is perhaps most important to discuss some of both.

In general, the affective psychoses include those psychiatric disorders in which the predominant symptomatology involves high or low mood, concomitant thought disorder, and sometimes perceptual disorder as well. Psychotic depression is marked by severe depression, psychomotor retardation, sleep disturbance, and constipation. Many authorities believe that the label *psychotic depression* should only be employed when the usual symptoms of psychosis are present, namely, delusions, hallucinations, bizarre behavior, and thought disorder. Others use the term as a synonym for severe depression. In this discussion, the first of these two alternatives will be followed.

Classically, the psychotically depressed person is severely depressed, and often experiences depressive delusions, including belief in his or her own guilt or worthlessness (not just because of ineffective functioning, but also at a delusional level, with the patient believing, for example, that he or she has squandered the family fortune or has killed off relatives). The patient may have auditory hallucinations with a depressive content, such as voices saying how worthless he or she is. Psychomotor retardation and diminished speech can be so severe that it is difficult to distinguish these patients from mute, retarded, catatonic schizophrenics. It is generally agreed that the latter diagnosis should not be used when depressive affect is present. The diagnosis of catatonic schizophrenia is more suitable with patients who have bizarre motor behaviors, or are disorganized in their thinking. There may actually be several types of psychotic depressive disorder, but these will not be described here.

Mania represents the opposite pole. Classically, the manic patient is elated and hyperactive, has pressure of speech, and delusions of grandeur (knowing everything, having just made a fortune and invented exciting new machines). The patient may stay awake all night for several days, believing he or she has connections with important people, and carrying out extravagant acts, such as buying two or three cars in a few days or developing an elaborate plan for world peace. Manics can also be litigious and often feel that efforts to limit their effusiveness are persecutory. These characteristics can make it difficult to determine whether paranoid schizophrenia might be a more appropriate diagnosis in some instances. Often the schizophrenic diagnosis is considered more reasonable when cognitive disorganization is present and the affective component is less predominant.

Interestingly, patients with manic states and those with psychotic depressive states are notable for the amount of antagonism they can generate in people who deal with them. Manics are notorious for the infectiousness of their wit, but they often have an exhausting ability to find and work on the most sensitive topics of psychiatric staff members as well. Many inpatient units find it extremely difficult to deal with more than one or two florid manic patients at a time.

Psychotic depressed patients are also extremely frustrating to those around them, mixing as they do a tragic sense of anguish and pain with what appears to be a tenacious resolve to think only of themselves and not lift a finger to help themselves or those around them. This mixture of pain and apparent stubbornness often leaves those who treat such patients with strong feelings that may interfere with treatment efforts.

Patients who have had both manic and psychotic depressive episodes, either cycling from one to the other and back—or just one episode of each at some time, are considered to have bipolar affective disease (or the equivalent label, manic-depressive psychosis, circular type). In some classical descriptions of manic-depressive psychosis, the patient goes repeatedly from one of these states to the other and back again. However, such patients are the exception rather than the rule, and it is common to have an episode of one state resolved, to be followed after some time by another such episode or by the opposite state. It is also possible for patients to have hypomanic conditions and to cycle between subpsychotic depressive states. Finally, it is also possible for a person to have only manic episodes, although such patients are rare.

As with schizophrenia, there is currently much controversy about the nature and delineation of the affective disorders. Fortunately, this controversy is not limited to idle speculation and verbal struggles between various schools of thought, but reflects the emerging pictures of a psychiatric disorder that can be generated by increasingly sophisticated research efforts. In spite of the progress that has been made, however, there are many questions still to be resolved. Should all affective disorders be grouped together, or should they be separated depending upon whether they are primarily characterized by manic or depressive states or both? Should affective psychoses be separated from affective neuroses as distinctive types of disorder? These and many other questions remain to be answered.

The practicing physician should be aware that these controversies exist, but some structure is needed for thinking about and caring for patients coming for treatment. For this purpose, a descriptive orientation may be the most useful. This involves assessing the degree and type of affective abnormalities and the presence or absence of other symptoms.

Evaluation   For evaluating patients with possible affective psychoses, it is useful to determine first whether the patient is depressed, elated, or has had episodes of both. Once this has been clarified, the question of whether psychotic symptoms (hallucinations, delusions, thought disorder, or bizarre behavior) are present can be pursued. If psychosis is present, and there is both limited or absent disorganization and predominant manic and/or depressive affect, the diagnosis of affective psychosis is justified.

Within this very general category, the particular nature of the symptoms and their course will determine the specific diagnostic title given. These titles will be changing when the new diagnostic manual is published; since it is still in draft stage, however, it may be best to assume that two general categories will be used, bipolar affective disorder (previously called manic-depressive psychosis, circular type), and unipolar affective psychosis, either manic or depressed type (previously called psychotic depression).

Although conventionally the focus is primarily on using symptomatology to define the traditional diagnostic categories, it is recommended that the nine axes be evaluated as with other psychiatric disorders. There is a tendency, especially now that psychopharmacologic agents that help to alleviate and often prevent symptoms of the affective psychoses have been found, to consider other characteristics of the patient as irrelevant to evaluation or treatment. Such conclusions, however, are not justified at this time.

Epidemiology   As might be expected, figures for the incidence and prevalence of the affective psychoses depend heavily on the diagnostic criteria used. Given the relatively narrow criteria suggested here, an incidence of slightly over 4/1000 is sometimes given. This figure is similar to that given for schizophrenia, which is difficult to reconcile with the clinical impression in many centers that schizophrenia appears to be far more common. Some of this impression may be a result of the greater chronicity of schizophrenia, so that patients who have it spend a longer period of time in treatment. In any case, epidemiologic data are extremely dependent on the diagnostic criteria used, with some centers viewing schizophrenia as a rare disorder and affective psychoses as common, others viewing affective psychoses as rare and schizophrenia as common.

Etiology of the Affective Psychoses It would be nice to describe a simple etiology for these disorders, but perhaps by now the reader has noted that any claim of a single etiology or absolute knowledge of what the etiologies are for the functional psychoses should be viewed with considerable suspicion.

As with schizophrenia, there is evidence of a genetic contribution to the affective disorders, especially for bipolar affective psychoses. There is also some evidence of unipolar disorders subtypes that have specific genetic components.

As with schizophrenia, this does not mean that these are "genetic disorders." It is possible, almost certain, that other etiological factors are also important. These might include such characteristics as precipitating stresses, patterns of family interaction, and early childhood traumas. Unfortunately and interestingly, there is little solid information about the possible contribution of these factors to the affective psychoses, and the basis for considering their role rests primarily on general clinical theory, anecdotal evidence, and the limitations of the ability to predict the occurrence of these disorders from genetic data alone.

There is also some evidence to suggest that biochemical etiologies may be important in the affective psychoses. Two major theories accompanied by some supporting evidence have hypothesized that a disturbance in the metabolism of either catecholamine or sodium is involved. Currently much research is being carried out to pursue these hypotheses.

Finally, there is some evidence that social class might have an impact on the genesis of affective psychoses, since it appears relatively well established that, in contrast to schizophrenia, these disorders are found proportionately more often in upper-class individuals. It has been suggested that the reason for mania being found proportionately more often in upper-class persons is the fact that such individuals have had the experience of accomplishment in their daily lives.

Treatment In treating patients with affective psychoses, the most urgent concern is for those in depressive states. Psychotically depressed patients are high suicide risks. This risk is great during all symptom phases of the disorder, and seems to be especially high during the phase in which the patient is recovering from the psychotic episode. Although some patients in manic states are violent, far more frequently, the problem is their considerable power to disrupt and to alienate. Wastefully spending large amounts of money, disrupting efforts in which they are participating at work or at home, they can make the lives of others miserable with grandiosity, hyperactivity, and hyperassurance. Family, friends, and employers all suffer frequently. The suicide risk of the psychotic depressive and the manic's power to alienate and disrupt are two major reasons why these patients are hospitalized frequently.

The treatment most widely recommended for the affective psychoses is lithium. For the bipolar disorders especially, the advent of lithium treatment has made a major impact on the control of the symptomatic states. Some have claimed that it is also useful for unipolar psychotic depression, although its value in this disorder is more questionable. Lithium does have potentially serious toxicity as well as side effects, and its administration needs to be monitored. However, its value for those patients on whom it does work is so considerable that it is often worth trying lithium treatment, even in somewhat questionable cases. A common starting dosage is 300 mg three times a day. The main determinants of dosage are both plasma levels (.8–1.6 mEq. per liter) and the absence of such side effects as tremor, diarrhea, and ataxia. Since lithium often needs 1 or 2 weeks to take effect, it is sometimes necessary with manic patients to prescribe phenothiazines for the first week or two, during which time the lithium levels are building up.

For psychotic depressed states, the antidepressants that are now available appear to be a particularly effective treatment. Imipramine and amytriptyline at the commonly recommended dose of 150–250 mg/day are two preparations that have proved to be particularly valuable. These too have side effects, primarily based on their anticholinergic properties, and they especially need to be monitored in patients with glaucoma and tendencies to urinary retention.

Electroconvulsive shock treatment (ECT) is often used, especially for psychotic depression, and is somewhat more controversial than medication. Some claim that electric shock is the best treatment for psychotic depression. In other centers, electric shock is used only as a last resort after a full trial of medication, and possibly psychotherapy as well, has been attempted. Although ECT often does appear to have a significant effect in lifting depression, it causes short-term memory impairment, and some patients (as well as physicians) have extremely strong feelings against this treatment. Some individuals with jobs requiring major intellectual activity have complained that their memories were impaired in important ways for many years following shock treatments. In spite of these anecdotal reports, clear evidence of such long-term memory loss is minimal.

Medication and shock treatment often have a major effect in ameliorating symptoms. In many centers it is felt that these modalities also treat the basic disorder and that no other care is either useful or required.

Although there is scant evidence regarding this specific issue, many clinicians believe that individuals who develop these kinds of symptomatology also have serious psychological problems (especially difficulties in dealing with anger) that somatic treatments do not help. For this reason it is wise to consider psychotherapeutic approaches to dealing with these problems. Because of the possibility that a basic part of these disorders is a malfunction in dealing with affects and relationships, some clinicians believe that psychotherapeutic approaches are in fact the mainstay of treatment. Even with the demonstrated effectiveness of somatic treatments, the definitive resolution of this controversy awaits clearer evidence regarding the nature of the underlying pathological processes involved.

Treatment of both the possible precipitants and the course of the disorder is often overshadowed by the efficacy of medications in controlling symptoms and is therefore not pursued intensively. It is not clear presently whether or not this overshadowing is justified, but it appears that frequently situational factors set off affective psychotic episodes. Possible precipitants, as well as the patient's and family's response to the course of the disorder, must be considered routinely in working with such patients. One important thing the clinician can do for patients with affective psychoses and those around them is to carry out some educational activity and help the people involved to be sympathetic, yet not allow the patient to dominate their lives totally.

In the more severe or long-standing instances of the affective psychoses, family members will often begin to distance themselves from patients, and employers may give up on them. In some families, for example, a member with a long-standing psychotic depressive disorder may come to be treated almost as subhuman. It is important not to attempt to focus blame on the patient or the family for this, but to work with both regarding reasonable expectations and demands, and ways in which family members can take care of their own lives while still continuing to relate to the patient. At the same time, many patients with these disorders need help in dealing with relatives and employers, especially in expressing anger and in making their needs known.

Social Relations and Work Functioning   Perhaps depending on the specific type of disorder, problems in social competence may or may not be apparent in these patients. Medications may be useful for treating symptoms, but psychosocial care is required to help improve the commonly found dysfunction in social relations and occupational function. Some patients with affective psychoses, when healthy, often demonstrate considerable social competence. This may be partly because they tend to come from upper classes, and have received considerable help in these areas. It may be because they have reached higher developmental stages, or may arise from other causes not yet determined. Although these people are often highly competent in at least general ways, the problems many have in dealing with specific aspects of competence, such as handling anger or assertiveness when not in an episode of illness, need to be explored. Because individuals with these disorders appear to be so competent, it is often especially difficult to engage them in psychological treatment. Nevertheless, some form of psychotherapy is often indicated and should be seriously considered.

Prognosis   There long has been an implication that schizophrenia is a deteriorating disorder where the affective psychoses are not. This simple rule appears to have some justification, but as with most such rules in psychiatry, is overly simple. As more systematic research on prognosis of the functional psychoses has been carried out, it is clear that a sizeable number (about 13 percent) of patients with affective psychoses remain chronically ill. This is not as many (depending on diagnostic criteria) as is usually found in schizophrenia, but is still a sizeable number. Although the classical cyclical or recurring course of the affective psychoses is found occasionally, it is also common for there to be only one episode of disorder. Because of this considerable variability, it is not possible to make a specific prediction of how patients with these disorders will fare over time. Especially with the medications now available, prognosis appears to be better than it was before those treatments were discovered.

Schizoaffective Disorder

The third group of functional psychoses is of special interest and is also especially controversial. This is the group known as schizoaffective disorder (it has been called by many other diagnostic titles as well). The clinical picture of this diagnostic category can be considered either as a type of schizophrenia with many affective symptoms, or a type of affective psychosis with schizophrenic symptoms. Some believe it is a subtype of schizophrenia, others that it is a subtype of affective psychosis, and still others that it is neither. The final solution of this controversy will have many important theoretical implications regarding the relative importance and incidence of the two (or three) major types of functional psychosis and the pathological processes involved. Nevertheless, for practical purposes, the physician need not be overwhelmed by the uncertainty that exists in this area. Treatment of schizoaffective disorder is generally similar to treatment of schizophrenia, with one possible important exception. Especially when there is a manic component to schizoaffective disorder, a trial of lithium might be warranted. Although some hold the opinion that lithium is specifically for manic psychoses or manic-depressive psychoses, this may well not be the case. There is some evidence, in fact, to show that the elation that occurs in certain schizophrenic pictures may also be helped by this medication.

Differentiation of the Functional Psychoses
from the Organic Disorders

It is sometimes extremely difficult to differentiate schizophrenia and the affective psychoses from organic disorders on the basis of symptomatology alone. Many investigators have noted that amphetamine psychosis, for example, often mimics very closely the symptomatology of schizophrenia. The same is true for toxicity from "angel dust" (Sernyl, PCP). The hyperactivity of the manic state can be mimicked by agitated states produced, for example, by amphetamines. More rarely, even other organic CNS pathology such as tumors or temporal lobe epilepsy can produce symptoms similar to schizophrenia, and less often, similar to the affective psychoses. The presence of confusion or the history of drug ingestion can help to provide clues to organic etiology, but careful physical examination with special focus on neurological abnormalities and laboratory analyses to detect drug ingestion are especially important.

CONCLUSIONS

The functional psychoses present a serious challenge to the practicing physician. Their symptoms and the degree of disorganization they often reflect can be frightening to the doctor as well as to the patient. In the light of such severe symptomatology, it is important for the physician to find some path between excessive rigidity and detachment on the one hand or overinvolvement and amorphousness on the other. As hard as it sometimes is, a balanced empathy, structure, and interest in understanding what the patient is communicating appears to be the best approach to working with these patients and their social systems. Approaches to patient evaluation certainly require this balance, but the same is true for diagnosis and treatment. Diagnostically, rigidly forcing patients into diagnostic categories that do not fit can be useful for some purposes, but should be accompanied by the same reservations one would have with excessively rigid evaluation procedures. The patient needs to be diagnosed, but at the same time also to be seen as an individual and not as a stereotype, particularly if the model does not fit. The new multiaxial diagnostic systems ought to improve to some degree the fit between the real individual patient and the diagnostic categories.

In treatment, too, a balance between extremes of structure and amorphousness is essential. The use of psychosocial treatment approaches and/or medication and other somatic treatments requires a clear goal orientation and specificity. The concepts for treating schizophrenia or manic-depressive psychosis are just too crude an approximation to permit the specific tailoring of treatment to the needs of real patients. Yet there are enough general principles that apply to these disorders so that the likelihood that a given modality might be useful can at least be signalled by the diagnostic labels.

Finally, prognosis too can be seen as a balance between the too vague and the too dogmatic. Prognoses are likelihoods, not definitive predictions. They provide guidelines regarding what can be anticipated, but no certainty that the course of disorder will not be much worse, or much better. And like evaluation, diagnosis, and treatment, prognosis is complex. The functional psychoses are not simple disorders, but progress in understanding them over the years has done away with some of the total confusion—and oversimplification—of the past.

REFERENCES

1 Kaplan, B.: *The Inner World of Mental Illness,* Harper & Row, New York, 1964.
2 Sechehaye, M.: *Autobiography of a Schizophrenic Girl,* New York: New American Library, 1970.
3 Strauss, J. S.: "A Comprehensive Approach to Psychiatric Diagnosis," *Am. J. of Psych.,* **132**(11):1193–1197, 1975.
4 Segal, D. S.: "Behavioral and Neurochemical Correlates of Repeated D-amphetamine Administration," in A. J. Mandell (ed.), *Neurobiological Mechanisms of Adaptation and Behavior,* New York: Raven Press, 1976.
5 Kinney, D., and B. Jacobsen: "Environmental Factors in Schizophrenia: New Adoption Study Evidence and Its Implications for Genetic and Environmental Research," in L. C. Wynne, R. L. Cromwell, and S. Matthysse (eds.), *Nature of Schizophrenia: New Findings and Future Strategies,* New York: Wiley, in press.
6 Wynne, L., and M. Singer: "Thought Disorder and Family Relations of Schizophrenia: II A Classification of Forms of Thinking," *Arch. of Gen. Psych.,* vol. 9, p. 199, 1963.

Part Four

Special Areas

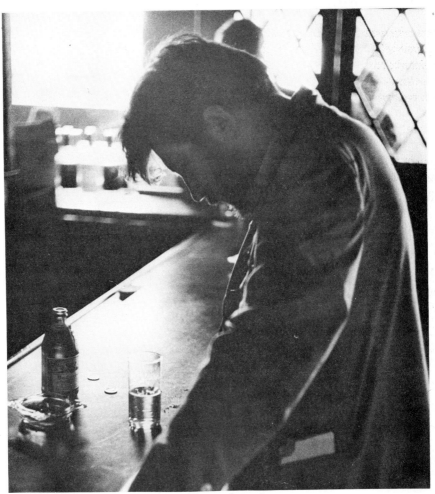

Courtesy of David Krasnor/Photo Researchers, Inc., NYC.

Chapter 13

Alcohol and Drug Dependence

E. Mansell Pattison, M.D.
Edward Kaufman, M.D.

EDITORS' INTRODUCTION

What is it like to be unable to take an alcoholic drink without taking another, and still another, and yet another? What is it like to feel so completely different from others when spouse, friend, or physician tells you that you must not drink? How does it feel to have to ask for plain soda at a party? What is it like to come home worried that your mate will smell alcohol on your breath? How does it feel to be sitting at home, dreading the arrival of your spouse because he or she may realize that you have been nipping at the bottle during the day?

What is it like to find yourself smoking a joint each morning before work, another during the lunch hour, and a third during a late afternoon coffee break? How does it feel to realize gradually that you no longer see friends who are not into grass? What is it like to feel that you cannot go to the supermarket, prepare for a party, or have sex without taking a drink or a pill?

What is it like to be husband, wife, parent, child, or close friend of a person who is moving toward dependence on alcohol or drugs—to see the gradual change in personality, life-style, and physical appearance? What must it be like to try to intervene, and come to feel increasingly helpless?

Physicians, too, are no strangers to feelings of helplessness. How do physicians feel when, despite their efforts, they recognize that a patient has a growing drug dependence? What is it like to be called at inconvenient times because Joe or Mary is drunk or on a bad trip again?

Alcoholism and drug dependence are problems that affect people as individuals, but they are also social problems of staggering proportions. Recent estimates place the number of alcoholics in the United States close to 10 million. The number of women who are afflicted by alcoholism appears to be growing rapidly, the economic impact of alcoholism and drug dependence is huge, and there is no way to estimate accurately the damage done to families and friends.

The physician faces such problems on a daily basis. These problems may take many forms: the alcoholic patient who experiences severe physical consequences (for example, cirrhosis, peripheral neuropathy, brain injuries, fractures, and postoperative deliria, to mention but a few), the concerned and depressed spouse, the parent struggling to understand the adolescent's use of drugs, the addict "conning" for a prescription, the patient's insistent demands that there "must be something I can take to feel better."

Often there are no simple answers. Rather, the physician must evaluate each patient's dilemma and then keep in mind a wide range of treatment possibilities. Office psychotherapy, referral to Alcoholics Anonymous or an alcoholism clinic, use of disulfiram, referral to a psychiatrist, use of marital or family therapy, hospitalization—all these treatments and others may be useful. At the heart of the matter, however, is the physician's willingness to be involved rather than to join those who have retreated into professional apathy in the face of these problems.

Perhaps one of the most tragic problems is the physician who personally has a dependence problem. How easy it is for physicians to rationalize that they know all about the dangers of narcotics, that if they take codeine now for that severe tension headache they will know better than to take two or three grains later when the headache no longer responds to the smaller dose. How easy it is to rationalize about the need, about the lack of necessity for bothering a fellow physician, and about the simplicity of self-medication. Securing the drugs constitutes no major problem—at first. Later, the physician, like other addicts, uses illegal means to obtain drugs. This is one of the occupational hazards of medical practice; the sick physician constitutes a major problem to the medical profession itself and to the patients whom this physician treats.

This chapter, which was written by two leading investigators and authorities in the field, presents the reader with an overview of current knowledge. The physician will find useful information for evaluating and treating patients. The resulting improved treatment is beneficial not only to the patients who are treated and to their friends, but also to the physician, with all his or her personal tensions and vulnerabilities.

INTRODUCTION

Use, misuse, and abuse of alcohol and drugs is a major health problem in the United States today. Alcoholism is the third most prevalent public health problem in our society. Alcohol and drug use are more than just health problems; they also lead invariably to personal, familial, social, and legal problems.

Ours is an "overmedicated society" in which various psychoactive substances are viewed by some people as being desirable. Alcohol and drugs are positively desired as "change agents" in the lives of perhaps the majority of the population, and the use of these agents is supported by legal, personal, professional, social, and cultural sanctions.

Alcohol and psychoactive drugs are no respecters of age, sex, ethnicity, geography, or legality. The physician will encounter problematic use of alcohol and drugs routinely in clinical practice. The patient who is clearly "addicted" to alcohol or drugs is but a small part of the problem. This chapter stresses the multiple forms of alcohol and drug dependence as encountered in medical practice.

DEFINITIONS OF ALCOHOL AND DRUG DEPENDENCE

Because the use of alcohol and drugs is interwoven with contradictory personal, social, and cultural attitudes and values, there is no unanimous agreement about when use is to be considered misuse or abuse. Often, alcohol and drug abusers are labeled as "sick" and "addicted." Although there is ample social justification for labeling problematic human behavior as an "illness" that requires health care, this simplistic approach distorts the meaning of the label "disease" and the diagnostic use we make of that label. As Engel has pointed out, the medical model of disease incorporates biological, psychological, and social parameters of health behavior.[1] Different health problems will present a different mix of biological, psychological, and social factors. So it is with alcohol and drug dependence, where different patterns of psychoactive drug use will involve different mixtures of these factors. Consequently, Engel proposes a "bio-psycho-social" concept of illness.

From this perspective, alcohol and drug dependence may be considered a "health syndrome." A set of propositions can be set forth that any person can develop some degree of alcohol or drug dependency; that this dependence can be manifested in a variety of combinations of biological, psychological, and social symptoms; that the degree of severity of the syndrome can range from minimal to severe; and that the clinical course can vary widely from highly contained to progressively severe.

There is no specific entity of alcohol and drug dependence. Rather, there are degrees of alcohol and drug use that have adverse biological, psychological, and social consequences, which may be labeled as misuse or abuse. These consequences may be virtually absent (except for legal consequences, as in the use of marijuana), or may range along a continuum from mild, to modest, to severe dysfunction.

As a health syndrome, alcohol and drug abuse may be defined as any degree (mild, moderate, severe) of psychoactive drug use that results in physical, emotional, interpersonal, or vocational dysfunction; or psychoactive drug use whose purpose is to maintain or improve function.

To use this definition properly requires taking a careful history of the patient's use of a psychoactive drug. The frequency, quantity, and circumstances in which the patient uses a psychoactive drug should be detailed. This history should explore three specific items: (1) Does the person feel different or experience himself or herself differently when drinking, smoking, or ingesting the drug? (2) Does the person's behavior change when he or she is under the influence of the drug? (3) Does the person demonstrate any adverse consequences of drug use in terms of physical, emotional, interpersonal, or vocational function? The person who uses a psychoactive drug in a moderate, low-risk fashion will answer negatively to these items, except perhaps under the most controlled of social circumstances. When there is a degree of positive response, it must be assumed at least that the person is engaging in high-risk psychoactive drug use. Then the physician must explore in more detail the evidence for minimal, moderate, or severe consequences.

Use, Misuse, and Abuse

The *use* of certain psychoactive drugs may be problematic for various reasons. In France it was long the custom to give young schoolchildren diluted wine with their meals. Consequently, many young French children developed cirrhosis. The use of psychotomimetic drugs may trigger untoward psychological reactions in certain vulnerable people. The use of marijuana may bring with it legal problems. Thus, the use of certain psychoactive drugs may in itself produce adverse consequences that are quite apart from any drug dependence.

The *misuse* of psychoactive drugs can likewise be considered as a separate issue from alcohol and drug dependence. For example, many people misuse alcohol at parties and on other social occasions. This may result in arguments, fights, displays of inappropriate behavior, sexual misconduct, and accidents. Yet persons who misuse alcohol may never become alcohol-dependent. In like fashion, the use of psychotomimetic drugs has led to mental illness, unfortunate accidents, suicides, and destructive behavior.

The *abuse* of psychoactive drugs occurs when a person uses such drugs in a chronic fashion, some degree of dependence on the drug is established, and chronic adverse consequences accrue. Such abuse can be relatively acceptable socially, as with heavy chronic tobacco smoking or with the socially marginal alcoholic.

Addiction, Habituation, and Dependence

Various terms have been used to denote drug dependence. In the first half of the century, many efforts were made to define a specific disease or state of addiction that was thought to be different from more moderate states of dependence, and was variously termed as drug habituation, drug dependence, drug misuse, or problematic drug usage. These "levels" are ambiguous and clinically meaningless, for the syndrome of drug dependence varies widely in symptomatology and severity. Such labels could well be discarded.

It is more appropriate clinically to discuss the syndrome of psychic dependence and physical dependence. The differences are clearly stated in the World Health Organization Bulletin of 1965.[2]

> Drug dependence is a state of psychic or physical dependence, or both, on a drug, arising in a person following administration of that drug on a periodic or continuous basis . . . . All these drugs have one effect in common: they are capable of creating, in certain individuals, a particular state of mind that is termed "psychic dependence" . . . this mental state may be the only factor involved, even in the case of the most intense craving and perpetuation of compulsive abuse . . . psychic dependence can and does develop . . . without any evidence of physical dependence . . . . Physical dependence, too, can be induced without notable psychic dependence, indeed, physical dependence is an inevitable result of the pharmacological action of some drugs with sufficient amount and time of administration. Psychic dependence, while also related to pharmacological action, is more particularly a manifestation of the individual's reaction to the effects of a specific drug and varies with the individual as well as the drug.

The phenomenon of *psychic dependence* results from the fact that all drugs that produce dependence are *psychoactive.* They change the conscious state of the consumer in one way or another. It does not matter much what change in consciousness is produced. The drug-dependent person relies upon a change in consciousness to cope more effectively with self and to experience reality. Thus, drug-dependent people commonly switch from one type of drug to another, depending upon what drug is available, is most desirable socially, or is personally appealing. The drug-dependent person has a psychological reliance on the psychic effect of the drug to produce an altered state of consciousness.

As noted above, physical dependence is not necessary for a person to acquire psychological dependence. Anyone can be made physically dependent on almost any psychoactive drug, without necessarily acquiring a psychic dependence. For example, after surgery a person may develop a mild physical dependence on morphine if it is administered regularly and in large amounts.

The development of physical dependence lies in the pharmacological properties of certain drugs, which allow them to become incorporated into the metabolic cycles of cellular physiology. This is the pharmacological "addictive property." As a result of this metabolic incorporation, two clinical features emerge. The first is the development of tolerance. That is, the body can tolerate more of the drug biologically without manifesting the pharmacological effects of the drug. As a result, one must consume more of the drug to produce a consciousness-changing effect. The second clinical feature is the production of withdrawal symptoms when the drug is withheld. Withdrawal is a manifestation of altered organ function as a result of deprivation of the acquired drug as an essential metabolite. Some common properties of psychoactive drugs of abuse are shown in Table 13-1.

Table 13-1 Some Pharmacologic Properties of Psychoactive Drugs

Properties	Alcohol	Barbiturates, sedatives, major tran- quilizers	Opiates, heroin	Stimulants, amphetamines	Cocaine	Marijuana	Hallucinogens
Central nervous system							
Effect							
Low dose	Disinhibit	Disinhibit	Depressant	Excitatory	Excitatory	Disinhibit	Hallucinatory
Moderate dose	Disinhibit	Disinhibit	Depressant	Excitatory	Excitatory	Hallucinatory	Hallucinatory
High dose (toxic)	Depressant	Depressant	Depressant	Excitatory	Excitatory	Hallucinatory	Hallucinatory
Ratio:							
Toxic dose/Effective dose	High	High	Low	Moderate	Low	Moderate	Low
Organic brain damage	High	Low	Low	Moderate	Low	Low	Low?
Systemic organ damage	High	Low	Low	Low	Low	Low	Low
Physical dependence	Moderate	Moderate	High	Moderate	Low	Low	None
Psychological dependence	Variable	Variable	High	Variable	High	Variable	Low
Withdrawal syndrome severity	Variable	Moderate	High	Moderate	Moderate	Low	None

Modified and adopted from data in B. Kissin, "Alcoholism as It Compares to Other Addictive Substances" in W. Keup (ed.), *Drug Abuse: Current Concepts and Research*, Charles C Thomas, Springfield, Ill.: 1972, pp. 251–262; and S. Cohen, "Pharmacology of Drugs of Abuse," *Drug Abuse and Addictive Newsletter*, **5**(6), 1976.

Tolerance and Cross-Tolerance

Tolerance occurs when greater doses of a drug are required for the same or lessening effects. The lethal dose of drugs is variable, and is dependent on tolerance. As tolerance builds up, the range between the lethal dose and the intoxication dose narrows. Therefore, the risk of lethal overdose with psychoactive drugs is quite high. *Cross-tolerance* results when use of one drug leads an individual to require greater than normal doses of another drug or drugs. Cross-tolerance exists among all the sedative hypnotics, minor tranquilizers, barbiturates, and alcohol. This cross-tolerance does not affect the lethal dose. Thus, when these drugs are taken simultaneously by individuals who are dependent on one or more of them, they may act additively and produce toxic or fatal reactions. For example, diazepam is almost never fatal by itself but is frequently found as a contributing factor in deaths from multiple drug ingestion.

Because of the pharmacological similarities among all the above sedating drugs and alcohol, these substances are frequently mixed together or substituted for one another, which results in polydrug abuse.

Types of Polydrug or Multiple Drug Use, Misuse, and Abuse

The term *polydrug abuse* was originally introduced to describe the trend that evolved early in the 1970s toward using more than one drug. However, the term came to be defined as what the National Institute of Drug Abuse (NIDA) considered polydrug abuse, that is, a dependence on psychoactive drugs where the primary drug dependence was not heroin, methadone or alcohol.[3]

A recent study of emergency room drug-abuse incidents noted 5,755 two-drug combinations.[4] The total number of possible combinations of abuse drugs is in the billions. However, four predominant patterns of multiple drug abuse emerge as critical. They are:

1　Narcotic abuse, with the abuse of other psychoactive drugs and alcohol
2　Methadone maintenance, with the abuse of other drugs and alcohol
3　Alcohol abuse, with the abuse of other drugs
4　The abuse of more than one nonnarcotic drug

Drugs as Magical Solutions

"Better things for better living through chemistry" has become a byword for the seeking of the instant relief of emotional or physical pain through a magical pill or substance. Physicians have responded by providing prescriptions for magical relief. This applies not only to psychotropic drugs, but also to the public's demand for penicillin for a cold, a potent analgesic for a headache, or codeine for a cough. It takes only a few seconds to write a prescription, but it can require far more time to determine what the real problem is. The public's response to the media's prodding by multiple ingestion of over-the-counter (OTC) drugs and vitamins also perpetuates the magic of the pill. Too frequently, it does not matter what the substance is as long as it is in a form that can be taken into the body. The potent placebo effects of these substances are well known.

Psychoactive Drugs as Coping Mechanisms

Drugs are used to facilitate, or obliterate concern with, sexual performance, communication, or assertion; to have a thrill; to seek oblivion; and/or to relieve anxiety and depression. In more disturbed individuals, drugs may provide a psychological homeostasis. There are common myths that such drugs as methaqualone, cocaine, and amphetamine augment and improve sexual performance. Actually, they may relax tense persons or activate passive persons, thus enabling them to overcome sexual inhibitions. Heroin has a reputation for dampening sexual drives. However, many heroin abusers find that initially heroin aids sexual performance through promoting mental relaxation or physiologic retardation of ejaculation. Many heroin users take their first dose with friends before a dance or party to deal with anxieties about social contacts. Most sedatives, including heroin, alcohol, and minor tranquilizers are used to diminish anxieties about self-assertion in vocational performance and social contact. These drugs are also used to obliterate anger and avoid hostile confrontation. Unfortunately, when individuals become intoxicated by means of sedatives or alcohol, rage is frequently released in ways that are out of control and destructive.

Drugs and alcohol have become a readily available and sanctioned means for dealing with minimal amounts of anxiety or depression.

Drugs and Hypochondriacs

The hypochondriac may present with multiple diffuse somatic complaints and a history of doctor "shopping." He or she may also use many over-the-counter drugs as self-treatment, and the extent of such use must be carefully documented. Family and friends frequently become impatient with the hypochondriac's constant complaints, and encourage further medical care or self-treatment. The physician must be cautious in prescribing for such patients, in order to avoid perpetuating misuse of drugs.

Iatrogenic Drug Dependence

Many patients are initiated into drug dependence by the physician. Sedative hypnotics for insomnia must be used with caution, and their danger must be weighed against the genuine problems caused by insomnia (see Chapter 18). Most patients are better off struggling with the problem of minimal insomnia, rather than using drugs for relief. Drug-free solutions, such as interdictions against napping, moderate exercise, and relaxation techniques, should be tried first. The underlying problems that lead to the insomnia can be explored and hopefully ameliorated. When depression is the root of insomnia, this can be treated by support, psychotherapy, or nonhabituating antidepressants. When the decision is made to treat sleeplessness with medication, nonhabituating drugs like antihistamines should be tried first, followed by drugs that are relatively noneuphoric, such as flurazepam hydrochloride, which does not depress REM sleep as most hypnotics do. If more potent sedatives are indicated, they should be used only for a few nights at a time, to avoid tolerance while reestablishing a normal sleep cycle.

Similarly, habituating flurazepam should be avoided for pain relief, particularly for low-level or chronic pain. Many patients become dependent on analgesics such as pentazocine hydrochloride, propoxyphine hydrochloride, codeine, or oxycodone when they are prescribed casually for extended periods (see Chapter 15).

Alcohol Switching

The number of alcoholics who also abuse prescription sedatives and minor tranquilizers has been increasing rapidly over the past few years. Careful history taking reveals that at least half of the alcoholics who present for treatment are ingesting high levels of these drugs as well. The younger the alcoholic and the greater the intake of alcohol, the more likely there is to be concomitant drug abuse. The physician who prescribes these drugs for individuals who are struggling with problematic consumption of alcohol is only compounding the problem. Any detoxification of an alcoholic must evaluate the intake of these drugs, since the drugs may lead to a prolonged and dangerous withdrawal.

Polydrug Abuse and Dependence

In 1974, the National Institute on Drug Abuse estimated that there were two million polydrug users in the country. Drug abusers no longer limit themselves to one drug or to one category of drugs. The five top-selling pharmaceuticals in the United States include four drugs that are a vital part of the polydrug abuse problem: diazepam, chlordiazepoxide, propoxyphene hydrochloride, and codeine.[5] In 1972, 7 percent of adults used proprietary psychoactive drugs, 4 percent used ethical sedatives, 5 percent used ethical stimulants, and 4.6 percent used hallucinogens.[6] Another study showed that one in ten adults used diazepam at least once in 1973.[7] There is no reason to believe that the use of these drugs has not increased. Given the fact that so many individuals use these drugs, the percentage of those who become dependent is rather low. However, the overall numbers are quite high. After alcohol, diazepam is the leading cause of drug emergencies in our society. Although every few years we see society's attention focus on a new drug of abuse, the problem of the abuse of multiple drugs, and particularly of the nonnarcotic "polydrugs," has been our primary drug problem for at least 5 years.

Mixed Methadone Dependence

Methadone maintenance is a method of treatment for heroin dependence. With motivated, selected patients, it has a high rate of retention in treatment, reduces criminal behavior, and increases employment. A fairly accurate estimate of drug abuse in this group can be determined since urinalyses are performed regularly. One problem has been that there is little testing for many drugs of abuse. Frequently, when new tests are instituted for drug abuse, the percentage of abusers is surprisingly high. When abusers become aware that a drug is being tested for, the abuse of that drug lessens. An accepted estimate of abuse in long-term methadone patients is drug abuse with 10 percent of the patients, and alcohol abuse with another 10 percent.[8] Chambers found that in a 1-month period in 1970, 97.5 percent of methadone maintenance patients abused other drugs.[9] These included heroin (92.3 percent), barbiturates (43.6 percent), amphetamines (69.2 percent), and cocaine (43.6 percent). Other widely abused drugs for which there were no tests until recently include diazepam and tricyclic antidepressants. Patients who are on methadone treatment are desperately seeking supplementary drugs to provide the euphoria and oblivion that they do not experience from methadone. Some claim that methadone increases their tolerance for alcohol. Whatever the reason, patients on methadone maintenance who drink seem to develop severe cirrhosis much more rapidly than alcoholics who are not on methadone.[10] A serious problem with abusers of methadone and other drugs is their high mortality rate. In 1973 in New York City there were 181 deaths from methadone poisoning, and 98 of these were attributable to heroin.[11] However, most "methadone deaths" are a result of supplementary alcohol and drug abuse. A review of 21 deaths from methadone in a 6-month period in Washington, D. C. reported that 15 had ingested ethanol recently, 1 had ingested barbiturates and amphetamine, and 6 had ingested quinine or morphine.[12]

MECHANISMS OF DRUG DEPENDENCE

No one factor produces or maintains drug dependence on any psychoactive drug. Rather, drug dependence is the final common outcome of biological, psychological, social, and cultural variables. People vary in their vulnerability to drug dependence, and that vulnerability may vary so much with time and circumstance that the vulnerability shifts back and forth.

There is no such thing as an "addictive personality"; some people are more vulnerable psychologically than others and therefore more likely to become drug dependent given the right circumstances. Neither is addiction genetically determined, in terms of biological disposition to drug dependence. Although with alcoholics there is some evidence of increased statistical probability of developing alcoholism along genetic lines, such evidence is equivocal. More likely is the probability that genetic differences may influence rates of drug metabolism and drug response, which in turn may influence the degree of pharmacological response to a drug. In itself, however, that does not produce drug dependence.

Although many people may derive some psychic pleasure and other psychological rewards from psychoactive drug use, most people observe control and limits over psychoactive drug use. Such controls and limits include legal constraints, moral and religious constraints, social expectations and sanctions about drug use, cultural norms, and personal values about the relative merits and costs of psychoactive drug use. As a result, most people establish a personal cost-benefit limit on how much they are willing to pay in a legal, social, fiscal, and personal sense in exchange for the psychic rewards of psychoactive drug use. Most people are able to live within these personal cost-benefit limits.

On the other hand, under certain psychological conditions a person may be unable to set such limits, may be unable to behave in accordance with personal limits, may believe that the benefits outweigh the costs, or may develop distorted perspectives in which they believe that they are paying much less than they actually are to maintain a pattern of drug dependence. In all these different circumstances, the development of drug dependence may be seen.

Table 13-2 outlines a variety of patterns of development of drug dependence that will be discussed briefly.

Persons who might otherwise be highly vulnerable to developing drug dependence may avoid such a possibility through total avoidance of drug use. This drug avoidance may be for legal, moral, religious, psychological, or social reasons. Former alcoholics and drug addicts learn that for the most part a drug-free existence is a major and necessary step to maintain a life-style that is devoid of dependence on drugs.

The *drug experimenter* typically does not start out seeking or expecting to develop drug dependence.

1 If the drug experience is not rewarding, or if it produces adverse effects, the person may then become a non-drug user and drug avoider.

2 Some people will experience nothing or will experience adverse drug effects, but will use psychoactive drugs occasionally as they participate in socially desirable or expected behavior. This use includes the social uses of tobacco, caffeine, and alcohol in reasonable amounts in solely social situations.

3 Some, including a large number of average people, experience some positive, rewarding effects and engage in occasional legal use of psychoactive drugs without any adverse effects. This use includes caffeine, tobacco, and alcohol. Here the frequency and amount are well controlled, and there are no adverse consequences.

4 A small number of people, who experience positive effects but who are not susceptible psychologically, will engage in more frequent use of psychoactive drugs in larger amounts. They may not experience loss of control over drug usage, or develop any sense of psychic dependence, yet the amount of drug use may produce adverse effects physically, psychologically, or socially. This pattern includes chronic smoking and heavy alcohol use.

5 There are those who are vulnerable psychologically and who engage in heavy drug use in a socially acceptable manner. They have a significant degree of drug dependence. This category would include neurotic smokers, hypochondriacal and neurotic OTC drug users, and moderate alcoholics.

The *prescribed-drug users* present yet another developmental pattern.

1 Patients with primarily neurotic symptoms, such as anxiety, depression, or hypochondriasis, may find that the psychoactive drug has symptom-relieving effects. Such patients may become dependent on the drug to allay their symptoms, and they may develop a primary psychological and physical dependence on the drug after their initial symptoms have vanished. This is a common pattern.

2 An uncommon pattern, but one that is nevertheless seen occasionally, is that of psychologically vulnerable patients who have some significant medical

Table 13-2 Patterns of Psychoactive Drug Use

Drug use category	Experience	Pattern	Consequence
Non-drug user	No drug experience	Drug avoidance	No adverse experience
	Unrewarding or adverse experience	Non-drug user	No adverse experience
Drug experimenter	Unrewarding or adverse experience	Occasional legal drug use in social context	
	Positive or rewarding experience (low vulnerable population)	Occasional legal drug use—well controlled	
	Positive or rewarding experience (moderate vulnerable population)	Frequent legal drug use	Possible legal, social, physical, personal abuse consequences
	Positive or rewarding experience (high vulnerable population)	Drug-dependent abuse pattern	Significant adverse consequences
	(Illegal drugs) Variable experience (all populations)	Variable use	Legal consequences
Prescribed drug user	Unrewarding or adverse experience	Non-drug user	
	Rewarding or positive experience and symptom relief	Drug-dependent abuse pattern	Significant adverse consequences
	Variable experience and major symptom relief	Secondary dependence on drug to minimize symptom relief	Variable adverse consequences
Drug seeker	Unrewarding or adverse experience	Drug switching	
	Variable experience and symptom relief	Drug dependence	Major adverse consequences
	Variable experience and major life-style relief	Drug dependence	Major adverse consequences

problem for which psychoactive drugs are prescribed (for example, acute pain from an injury). When introduced to the psychic effects of a psychoactive drug, such patients rapidly develop a primary drug dependence.

3 Occurring with intermediate frequency is the pattern of patients with chronic pain, a chronic illness, or a fatal deteriorating illness. Here the primary dependence on a psychoactive drug may realistically be seen to be for relief of pain and misery. A secondary psychic and physical dependence may ensue. For the dying patient such a situation may realistically be accepted. However, with chronic disease and pain problems, the complications of drug dependence usually outweigh the palliative value.

Finally, there is the group of *drug seekers*. This can be divided into the self-medication group and the life-style group. Those in the *self-medication group* typically face a life crisis, and turn to some type of psychoactive drug deliberately to provide symptom relief. Anxious and depressed persons may turn to alcohol, stimulants, and depressants deliberately to assuage their psychic state. In a sense, they do not care about becoming drug-dependent because they seek relief at any cost. Another category is that of psychotic patients, who may find that alcohol or opiates cause their psychosis to remit. Such persons are usually very resistant to initial treatment, because the drugs are already their treatment.

The *life-style group* represents those who start out in life with major maladjustments. They typically turn to alcohol and narcotics early in life deliberately to escape from their unhappy existence. The rewards of living in an altered state of consciousness outweigh all the costs of a destructive, drug-dependent life-style. For these people, a drug-free existence is no existence at all. Therefore, the development of a new life-style is critical to any rehabilitation program.

In brief, there are many roads to drug dependence. An individual may start down the road to drug dependence from many points in life. The progression and maintenance of drug dependence have different meanings in these different patterns of drug dependence. In turn, treatment interventions will have to take into account major differences in drug-dependent patterns.

RECOGNITION AND IDENTIFICATION

The identification of the drug-dependent person is an important aspect of medical practice in virtually every clinical setting, for the physician will encounter all the many patterns of drug dependence that we have outlined. Therefore we shall briefly describe some of the typical settings and clinical situations in which drug dependence is encountered.

The Medication-Prone Person

Any patient who is a firm believer that any symptom can be magically relieved by the appropriate drug is a potential abuser. The patient who immediately treats most minor aches or pains with an OTC remedy is more likely to misuse medication than the patient who tolerates an occasional headache, gastrointestinal upset, or cold without resorting to drugs. This assessment provides a measure of a patient's frustration level as well as a general measure of his or her pain threshold. The attitude toward relief of pain in the home where the patient was raised is also crucial, as is parental use and abuse of drugs and alcohol, which are almost directly proportional to the incidence of substance abuse in offspring.

Most Americans presently view medical care as a right rather than as a privilege. This right frequently includes freedom from discomforts, including those related to the stresses and strains of contemporary life. Thus, the average patient often expects and demands relief from the emotional pain that is associated with such stress. It is tempting, simple, and quick to provide the patient with *the* pill that will provide instant relief. The patient who experiences immediate relief may be just the one who is getting started on the path to drug dependence.

Some patients feel that they are entitled to the drug of their choice for what they consider to be recreational use. Even the word "recreational" is destructive when applied to drug use, since it perpetuates the myth of chemical solutions to personal problems and discourages the development of more meaningful forms of recreation. Furthermore, many recreational drug users do become drug abusers and addicts.

The Drug-Abusing and Drug-Dependent Person

Individuals may progress from controlled and moderate drug use in the early stages, to heavy abuse in later stages. As this occurs, there are reports of progressively more accidents, injuries, and rebound depressions or "hangovers." Regular usage and expenditures for drugs tend to be rationalized as non-drug expenditures, and responsibilities become neglected. The patient or family will report neglect of work or school, termination of friendships, acute anxiety attacks or panics, intermittent alienation of the family, and financial difficulties. Prior medical history may include abrupt onset of seizures, treatment for overdoses, detoxification, suicide attempts, or a history of "doctor shopping." An excess of special social problems, such as divorce, bankruptcy, and a history of delinquency or driving offenses, is also suspect.

The language of hardcore drug users and teenagers is pervaded by idioms of the drug culture, which shift rapidly as these terms are taken over by "normal" teenagers and by the mass communications media. Friends are limited to those who use drugs, and the individual may become seclusive and furtive to hide drug use.

A crucial aspect of the drug abuser's office visit is the physician's determination of the extent of the problem. The physician must make a consistent effort to obtain specific historical material. This should include the types of drugs (and alcohol) used, the amounts, and the duration and pattern of usage. Questions used to determine this should be nonjudgmental and matter-of-fact. Pejorative or idiomatic terms such as abuse, "strung out," or "hooked" should be avoided.

All drugs of abuse have nicknames, which are determined either by the color of the drug, by the name of the manufacturer, or by the real or imagined effect of the drug ("red"—secobarbital; "Cibas"—glutethimide; "ups"—amphetamines;

"smack"—heroin, etc.). The physician should be alerted to the potential for abuse in any individual who refers to the drug by its "street" name. Likewise, any patient who asks for a specific drug or combination of drugs, or hints heavily about receiving certain types of drugs, is suspect.

Drug abusers have little concept of time, except when an appointment will result in obtaining drugs. Even then they are often late; they think they can get their drug. Drug abusers become deceitful, conniving, and resentful of authority. They become accustomed to lying, until they no longer know what is and is not true. Many drug abusers are obstreperous, challenging, angry, or violent when they do not get what they want or when they are on stimulants, sedatives, or in withdrawal. Although some individuals can maintain jobs even while regularly using heroin, sedatives, or stimulants, most serious drug abusers neglect work or school. This is in contrast to the situation with alcoholics, who frequently maintain employment. Old friends tend to be lost, and they become targets of manipulation and hostility. Associations become limited only to other individuals who will share in drug-taking or procurement. A history of sudden personality change frequently accompanies drug intake. There may be a history of acute anxiety attacks or panics, particularly from cocaine, stimulants, and hallucinogens. Drug abusers are very unreliable with money and pay bills late, if at all, as more and more of their funds are devoted to their drugs. Frequently, the family will relate a history of money and small articles being missing from the home. This situation can progress to theft of many family valuables and possessions.

Children of drug abusers are subjected to a great deal of abuse and neglect, and a history of child abuse should alert the clinician to the possibility of parental drug and alcohol abuse.

Certain behavior in the office should alert the physician that the patient is a potential drug abuser. Any patient who returns to the office for a prescription renewal of an abuse-prone drug before the prescription should have been used up is suspect. Such patients may be very skilled at making up excuses for why they have run out prematurely. Some examples include "My friend's mother died and I gave him some" and "I lost the prescription" and "The pharmacist only gave me half because he didn't have more in stock." In fact, many drug abusers share and trade drugs with their friends, and frequently sell such drugs at highly inflated prices.

Evidence from a pharmacist that a prescription has been altered is definitive evidence of a drug abuser. Any patient who can tolerate therapeutic or large doses of a drug without experiencing the expected psychological or physiological effects is probably tolerant, and therefore is dependent on that drug or on a chemically related drug. These patients are particularly skillful at asking for their drug of choice. They invariably give a history of allergic and hypersensitivity reactions to phenothiazines. Although in some cases these histories are valid, in general they are fabricated to avoid phenothiazines because they do not cause euphoria, and because the drug abuser has a low psychological tolerance for the side effects of these drugs. The more mentally disturbed or desperate drug abusers will try to obtain any drug that will alter their mental state, and they will even settle for phenothiazines when no other drug is available.

An "accidental overdose" is a common sign that an individual is abusing or is dependent on a drug or combination of drugs. Likewise, a definitive suicide attempt is a frequent symptom of the desperation of drug abusers. It is a "cry for help" to the individual's family and to the physician, and an indication of serious problems that require a multiplicity of solutions. Even with chronically drug-dependent patients, there are brief attempts at abstinence, which are used as rationalizations to "prove" that the individual is not "hooked." However, there is evidence of impairment even between episodes of dependence and intoxication. There is apathy, fatigue, decreased productivity, depression, and anxiety. Even when the patient is not intoxicated, there is memory loss, impaired judgment, and inability to make decisions. In this phase, even abusers of prescription drugs spend over $1,000 yearly through medical and illicit channels, and combined with their decreased work performance, this leads to heavy debt and bankruptcy. Heroin addicts spend from $20 to over $200 daily, and cocaine users can "snort" $100 worth in an hour, so that their lives become totally preoccupied with obtaining drugs and the money to pay for them.

The manipulative drug abuser may find and exploit the weak points in the physician's personality. Thus the doctor will be flattered or coerced, or guilt will be induced. Flattery may take the form of "You really understand me" or "You really are knowledgeable about drug use" or "I know you truly trust me because you prescribe X." Coercion may include "You hooked me, so you must continue to help me" or "You prescribed X for my friend, so why not do it for me" or "Prescribe X again or I will report you." Guilt induction includes "Prescribe the drug legally or I will have to steal to buy it" or "Prescribe X or I will have seizures" or "Prescribe X or I will kill myself." Regrettably, for a few physicians economic gains influence clinical practice.

A family interview is frequently indicated with drug abusers. This is important for evaluating the extent of the problem and its effect on the individual and on those close to him or her. The family can also be an invaluable ally in motivating the drug abuser to seek treatment.

Signs and Symptoms of Drug Abuse and Dependence

The signs and symptoms of drug abuse are directly related to the specific drug or drugs being abused and to whether the patient is stabilized, intoxicated, or in withdrawal. Nevertheless, certain findings are common enough to warrant discussion.

One of the first of the areas that are neglected by the chronic drug abuser is that of personal appearance and dress. The individual may dress poorly or inappropriately, or may assume the garb of drug-using peers. Sunglasses may be worn at inappropriate times to hide conjunctival injection (marijuana), constricted pupils (narcotic use), or dilated pupils (withdrawal). Eye contact is usually avoided.

Vital signs may reveal a rapid pulse, blood pressure fluctuations, or elevated temperature in sedative or narcotic withdrawal, in the absence of other physical causes. Halitosis is common. Many serious drug abusers have a characteristic pallor or grayness to their faces, particularly around the eyes and mouth. At other times, they may appear flushed, with heavy perspiration and warm or clammy skin. Dental care is often overlooked, and inflamed mucous membranes, pyorrhea, receding gums, neglected caries, and missing teeth are common. Often food and nutrition are neglected. There may be progressive weight loss, with symptoms of vitamin and other nutritional deficiencies. Examination of the skin commonly reveals abrasions, bruises, old abscesses, and scars, particularly around the ankles, head, and face. Heroin addicts and other intravenous drug abusers have needle marks and scarified tracks over veins. Multiple tattoos are common manifestations of the drug abuser's identity.

Thrombophlebitis, tuberculosis, upper respiratory infections, pneumonia, septicemia, pulmonary infarcts, subacute bacterial endocarditis, hepatitis, and toxic nephropathy are commonly seen in drug abusers, depending on the drug, on its route of administration, and on the patient's life-style. Individuals who are ingesting high doses of amphetamines may present with symptoms of hypertension, cerebral hemorrhage, or endarteritis. As in states of withdrawal from CNS depressants, patients who abuse amphetamines, hallucinogens, and especially phencyclidine (PCP) may present with acute or chronic psychosis.

Individuals who are intoxicated by any sedative or narcotic drug usually experience a dissociated, sublime contentment. They may repeatedly fall into a light sleep for a few seconds ("nodding"), from which they readily waken only to believe that they have not slept. They may be subdued, unreachable, and withdrawn, or unusually talkative. Those who are intoxicated with heroin, persistently, often with evident enjoyment, scratch themselves, particularly around the face.

Although these findings are seen mainly with hard-core addicts, such patients are being seen more and more in general practice as they attempt to relieve withdrawal symptoms with depressants or boost the effects of progressively weakened and expensive heroin.

TYPICAL OFFICE SYNDROMES

Several specific types of patients will present to the physician with incipient or overt drug abuse. These include children and adolescents, neurotics, "bored housewifes," executives, and the aged.

Children

Inhalants have been widely abused by children for the past 20 years. The average age of an inhalant abuser is 13, with abuse frequently beginning at age 8. Solvents commonly used include airplane glue (polystyrene cements containing toluene), paint thinner, varnish remover, nail polish remover, spray can aerosols, lighter fluid, cleaning fluids, and gasoline.

The technique of administraton for liquid solvents is to saturate a rag and hold it over the mouth and nose. Glue is placed in a plastic bag, which may be placed over the head or over the mouth and nose. The immediate effects are similar to those from drinking an alcoholic beverage. There is a euphoria that is almost immediate and lasts 30 to 45 minutes. There is also incoordination, restlessness, excitement, confusion, disorientation, ataxia, and delirium, which may progress to coma that may last for a few hours to several days. Individuals under the influence of inhalants may be glassy-eyed, with pupils showing little reaction to light; they will smell strongly of solvent. They may show irrational, antisocial, or violent behavior. Inhalants lead to a delirium, and chronic exposure may lead to liver, kidney, bone marrow, and brain damage.

Prescription drug abuse in this age group is also increasing rapidly. The nonmedical use of prescription psychotherapeutic drugs by 12- and 13-year-olds was found to increase from 1 percent to 6 percent in the 2 years from 1974 to 1976.[13]

More recently, latency-age children have increasingly abused prescription drugs, marijuana, alcohol, and hallucinogens. This trend is also reflected in the increased use of all these substances by adolescents.

The Adolescent

During the latter part of the 1960s, the terms "adolescence" and "drug abuse" became almost synonymous. Behavior that would be considered aberrant or even pathological during other developmental stages occurs as part of the normal spectrum of adolescent behavior. The internal and external challenges to sexual and personal identity that are experienced daily by the adolescent are often extreme, as is much of the behavior elicited by these challenges. Mood swings are especially rapid and often inexplicable. The most minor comment or event may precipitate psychic turmoil and difficult, obnoxious, acting-out. Drug abuse provides a maladaptive, potentially hazardous fulfillment of many of the adolescent's psychological and social needs, but inhibits the required completion of many maturational tasks.

The rebelliousness and impulsiveness that are so often a part of adolescence, combined with the punitive responses that such behavior frequently elicits, make the adolescent vulnerable to the abuse of drugs.

The Neurotic

The most common neurotic symptoms that lead to the search for pharmacologic relief are depressions and anxiety. Frequently, one may precede or mask the other. (For a full discussion of depression and anxiety, consult Chapter 10.) Quick relief for anxiety may be provided by anxiolytic agents, but vulnerability to potential drug dependence must be evaluated before such agents are prescribed.

In prescribing medication for a depressed patient, the physician must take into account the potential for self-punitive and dependent behavior, since such behavior may lead to drug abuse, dependence, and in some severe cases to possible suicide. Tricyclic antidepressants have little potential for being abused, and can frequently provide relief of depression as well as of secondary anxiety.

The Bored Housewife Syndrome

The housewife who chronically overuses or abuses drugs constitutes a major social and medical problem. In a study of drug use in New York State, the incidence of unemployed housewives who were found to use nonbarbiturate sedative/hypnotics, antidepressants, diet pills, and relaxants/minor tranquilizers was significantly in excess of that recorded for the general population.[14]

The housewife who is not employed or engaged in some demanding, rewarding avocation may suffer from diminished self-esteem and a negative self-image. She may feel isolated. Everyday tasks and problem solving are often regarded as unimportant, unfulfilling, and dull. Financial, social, and familial obligation stresses often go unshared, and the resulting tension may be manifested as anxiety, depression, or hypochondriasis. Self-treatment may begin with alcohol; with diet pills that are legitimately prescribed for weight loss; or with a sedative, antidepressant, or minor tranquilizer that is prescribed initially for insomnia. When prescribing for such a patient, the physician should bear in mind the potential for misuse of any drug with psychoactive properties, and the possibility of dependence.

The Executive Abuser

An analog of the pressured executive alcoholic, this patient utilizes drugs to help cope with professional, financial, and familial stress. Presenting complaints may be insomnia, anxiety, or diminished performance caused by fatigue. Somatic symptoms such as headache or backache are common. Frequently, in the course of a regular physical examination, the executive will ask directly for medication to help sleep or to increase energy. While in a majority of cases drug use will probably not progress to misuse or habituation, the physician should not prescribe such medication without first making an assessment of the psychological status of the patient. Depression, hypochondriasis, passive-dependence that is masked by an "aggressive" affect, and alcoholism are factors that should be considered. When possible, information about other family members should be obtained to avoid the hazard of making drugs available not only to the patient, but to other potential abusers in the home as well.

The Aged

Family conflicts, retirement, bereavement, isolation, and diminished independence are major stresses of old age, and may precipitate severe decompensation, especially when they are complicated by loneliness, chronic pain, disability, or anticipation of an undignified death. The hypochondriasis, anxiety, and depression that can accompany such decompensation may be implicated in the prevalence of drug dependence among the elderly. Habituation to sleeping pills, insistence on sedatives for chronic pain, the abuse of many OTC drugs, and the overuse of tonics for their alcoholic content are common. The simple reassurance that sleep requirements are lessened in the aged may be sufficient to avoid sleeping medication.

Evaluation of the geriatric patient involves both a physical and psychological assessment. Psychopathology that may predispose to drug abuse and functional CNS impairment that can lead to accidental misuse of medication should be regarded as crucial determinants in prescribing. Since the elderly frequently present with multiple complaints, many are likely to be taking a variety of medications. This, in addition to the fact that some physicians may prescribe drugs too freely for their older patients, poses a hazard of toxic drug interactions. In addition, advanced age, decreased body mass, and impaired kidney, heart, liver, and CNS functions all can contribute to diminished drug tolerance and to the danger of intoxication. While caution especially should be exercised in the pharmacologic treatment of psychiatric disorders in the elderly, undertreatment and delayed treatment can be dangerous as well, and should be avoided. Drugs, when administered appropriately and monitored diligently, have an important role in the care of the elderly.

Familial Patterns of Drug Abusers

The psychopathology in the families of drug abusers is best seen as quantitative rather than qualitative. That is, it is not the specific behavior or interaction, but rather the *degree* to which it is carried that seems to foster abuse. Communication in such homes is negative, and life often may be described as dull, deadened, lifeless, shallow, or having an affectless quality. Remarks like "It's as if we live in a hotel and not in a home" or "We each go our separate ways—as if we lived in different boxes," are very common.[15] These homes may be scenes of overwhelming criticism on the one hand, and unrealistically high expectations on the other. Destructive or deviant behavior may be reinforced when the family rallies to a crisis that is precipitated by one of its members, thereby breaking the routine of isolation and inattentiveness. Parents and grandparents often do not set consistent limits on the behavior of their children. At times inappropriate behavior will be rewarded, and at times it will be punished or ignored.

The drug-abusing child in such a family situation may be crying out for love, affecton, help, and attention, and may be escaping through intoxication. Parental ambivalence in responding to the child's drug abuse may also stem from personal guilt about drug-taking or drinking behavior. In one survey, it was found that the children of mothers who used tranquilizers were three times more likely to use marijuana or LSD; six times more likely to use opiates; five times more likely to use stimulants, other hallucinogens, and amphetamines; and seven times more likely to use tranquilizers and barbiturates than the children of mothers who did not use tranquilizers.[16]

Anger frequently is utilized pathologically by family members, because the open expression of positive emotion is regarded as threatening. Enraged by a sense of deprivation of love, warmth, and attention, and terrified by his or her own anger, the child may turn to drug abuse as an act of revenge. Self-destructive behavior allows the child to punish his or her parents and to punish himself or herself for hostile-aggressive impulses. Unfortunately, the parents are likely to deny that a problem exists, even in extreme situations, and the child may go farther and farther to gain the negative recognition that is sought.

Drug abusers frequently are linked symbiotically to the parent of the opposite sex in a way that perpetuates both their drug abuse and the parent's need to keep them as a child. This situation tends to disengage the same-sex parent, who will react with brutality, alcoholism, emotional distance, or divorce. Sensitivity to these patterns in families should alert the physician to the possibility of drug abuse in offspring.

Identification of the Alcoholic in the Medical System

The physician in the medical care system usually does not treat the alcoholic for a primary complaint of alcoholism. The alcoholic typically enters the medical system with nonalcoholic complaints, illnesses, and symptoms. The alcoholic may seek medical care for major complications of alcohol abuse, such as hepatic, cardiac, dermatologic, or peripheral neurologic complaints. Such persons often do not consciously link their medical illness with their alcohol abuse. A second group presents in medical settings with severe consequences of alcoholism, such as fractures and head trauma that are caused by falls, burns, or peripheral palsies (which occurred while intoxicated), or a variety of acute or chronic brain syndromes. Such patients may recognize that their medical problems are linked directly to their drinking, but they are not likely to complain of their alcoholism. A third group may recognize and seek medical help for their alcoholism, but may complain principally of insomnia, nervousness, tremors, anxiety, anorexia, or dyspepsia.

Many physicians first meet alcoholics while the physicians are working as interns and residents in large public hospitals, where the alcoholic patient may well have been the prototype skid row bum. This is a misleading stereotype. Only 5 percent of all alcoholics are on skid row, and only 5 percent of the people on skid row are alcoholic.[17] Thus, the skid row alcoholic is atypical. The more typical alcoholic is likely to be employed; married; a church, lodge, and club member; and a respectable member of the community. Since the alcoholic patient does not look or act like the stereotyped alcoholic, the condition is likely to be overlooked.

These respectable "community alcoholics" appear in the everyday case load of the physician. In a survey of 3,376 internists, Jones and Helrich found that only 3 percent saw no alcoholics, whereas 16 percent saw over 20 alcoholics during a 1-month period.[18] Significantly, half of the alcoholics were women. This finding highlights the importance of the "hidden housewife" syndrome of alcoholism.[19,20] Dunn and Clay reported that 10 percent of general physicians' and internists' patients are alcoholics.[21]

The incidence of alcoholics in hospital populations is even higher. The type of hospital, however, is a critical variable. Edwards and his associates studied four different hospitals and found that each hospital was actually admitting different types of alcoholics, ranging from skid row alcoholics to working class individuals to professional people.[22] Thus, the incidence and type of alcoholic population will vary with the hospital. The proportion of hospitalized patients who have been identified as having moderate to severe alcoholism problems ranges from 27 to 60 percent.[23],[24],[25]

MANAGEMENT OF ALCOHOL PROBLEMS

Often the physician is not in a position to provide complete rehabilitation programs for alcoholics. However, there are several specific services that the physician in office practice can provide.

1   The physician can maintain regular contact with patients who are not yet willing to accept treatment. Over time, the physician may be able to guide the patient by virtue of a positive doctor-patient relationship into a rehabilitation program.

2   The physician can be an effective diagnostic and triage agent.

3   The physician can safely manage acute intoxication syndromes as well as mild withdrawal syndromes, and can use this contact to guide the patient into rehabilitation.

4   The physician can provide a regular contact program of disulfiram maintenance with motivated patients who need to maintain abstinence, but who do not desire or require other avenues of rehabilitation.

5   The physician is in an excellent position to involve the spouse and family members in the process of rehabilitation. The alcoholic behavior patterns have a direct impact on spouse and family. Conversely, the spouse and family are likely either to exacerbate and play into the perpetuation of the alcoholic behavior, or to contribute signally to changes and effective rehabilitation.[26],[27] Therefore, effective management of the alcoholic and effective involvement in treatment are highly likely to be directly related to the degree of effective family involvement.

6   All of these services do require that the physician become acquainted with local community resources. The physician should learn what types of Alcoholics Anonymous groups are available, so that the willing patient can be referred to a group that is most like the patient. The physician should be able to hospitalize and manage effectively alcoholic patients who require inpatient care. The physician should have personal information about the facilities, admission requirements, fees, and suitability of different community rehabilitation programs, so that he or she can counsel the alcoholic in terms of the program that is best suited to the patient.[28],[29]

7   The physician can effectively promote increased awareness and acceptance of the importance of evaluating alcohol use carefully among patients.

8   The physician who is knowledgeable about alcoholism may serve as a resource for public education and may be available for discussions and talks (including the media).

Management of Medical Complications

The major problem of medical management in the hospital is overmanagement. Finer has detailed the excessive use of medications, diagnostic procedures, and unduly prolonged hospitalization for uncomplicated medical problems that are associated with alcoholism.[30] The physician must be wary lest good medical treatment of the complications from alcoholism obscure the treatment of the alcoholism itself. Treating the physical complications without dealing with the underlying condition itself is simply not good medical care.

Specific criteria for hospitalization should be employed.[31,32] An alcoholic should be admitted to a psychiatric hospital or to a general hospital psychiatric unit when the individual is psychotic, depressed, or behaviorally disordered enough to require hospitalization. There are some alcoholics who cannot stay off alcohol unless they are hospitalized with a rigidly regulated, "protected" environment where alcohol cannot be gotten.

Freed believes that psychiatric hospitalization should be used only when the patient has a severe, acute psychiatric problem other than alcoholism.[33] It must be noted that almost all acutely ill alcoholics will demonstrate some degree of depression, thought disorganization, and behavioral disorder. But these transient disturbances must be differentiated from an essentially psychotic, rather than drunk, demeanor. One exception is the so-called 24-hour-schizophrenia syndrome. Patients with this syndrome present with what appear to be classic schizophrenic symptoms while they are intoxicated. After a 24-hour sobering up period, the psychotic manifestations vanish. It is virtually impossible to make this differential diagnosis, except after the fact.

A general hospital admission is indicated when the patient is:

1 Unconscious, or has evidence of a head injury
2 Seriously hemorrhaging
3 Suffering from actual or impending delirium tremens
4 Suffering from a severe or persistent disulfiram-alcohol reaction
5 Jaundiced, or shows other signs of liver disease
6 Convulsing
7 Dehydrated, or shows signs of significant malnutrition and vitamin deficiency
8 Evidencing any medical pathology that is judged serious enough for general hospital care.

Put simply, acute general hospital admission is necessary for any medical disorder, other than the alcoholism itself, that is serious enough to require admission. Specialized hospitals or units for alcoholic patients may be helpful in initiating the alcoholic into treatment.

Differential Diagnosis and Management of Acute Alcoholism Syndromes

Acute alcoholism syndromes are a confusing diagnostic melange. They can be separated into three groups: simple intoxication, acute withdrawal, and psychotic states.

The psychotic group includes alcoholic paranoia, alcoholic hallucinosis, alcoholic schizophreniform psychosis, and delirium tremens. In this group the paranoid and schizophreniform symptoms usually appear during the period of

**Table 13-3   Differences Between Intoxication
and Major Withdrawal in the Alcoholic Patient**

Factors	Intoxication	Major withdrawal
Frequency	Common	Less common
Onset	Immediately after drinking	24 to 72 hours after cessation of drinking
Duration	Hours	Days
Symptoms and signs	Slurred speech, staggering gait, stupor	Tremor, hallucinations, delirium, seizures
Blood alcohol level	Elevated	Not elevated
Response to alcohol	Aggravates the symptoms	Decreases the symptoms
Mortality	Rare	10 percent with severe delirium tremens

actual intoxication and disappear when the individual sobers up; clouding of sensorium, hallucinations, and motoric-seizure symptoms usually appear after the individual sobers up. Yet this dichotomy is not neat and clean, for Gross et al. found an overlap of about 50 percent of the symptoms in these clinical categories.[34]

There is similar overlap in the symptoms of intoxication and of withdrawal states. Mild withdrawal is characterized by insomnia, irritability, and tremor; major withdrawal, in addition, includes anxiety, agitation, diaphoresis, and disorientation. Acute intoxication can trigger seizures in vulnerable persons. Seizures are rare in mild withdrawal states. Major withdrawal states may progress, if untreated, to delirium tremens with associated seizures and hallucinations. The major differences are shown in Table 13-3.

The physician must not neglect considering other causes for delirium and psychotic symptoms, despite the fact that the patient has been drinking or is even intoxicated (see Table 13-4).

The intensity and severity of the symptoms for intoxication and for withdrawal vary with the prior exposure to alcohol. Mild reactions to withdrawal appear during the sobering-up period, and usually dissipate within 48 hours. In severe withdrawal reactions, the symptoms begin to exacerbate as the blood alcohol level is falling, and become most manifest in 48 to 60 hours. Delirium tremens occurs in fewer than 5 percent of hospitalized patients with major withdrawal. Delirium tremens can be fatal, but the mortality rate has been dropping because of improved supportive treatment.

Most acutely intoxicated alcoholics are not withdrawal risks. In the past, expensive hospital detoxification units were provided for the management of withdrawal. Such units are relatively unnecessary, because only a small group of

Table 13-4   Common Nonalcoholic Causes for Delirium

MEDICAL	DRUG INGESTION
Infection (particularly pneumonia)	Bromides
Thyrotoxicosis	Steroids
Hypoparathyroidism	Stimulants
Congestive heart failure	Atropine
	Psychedelics
SURGICAL	
Head trauma	DRUG WITHDRAWAL
Postanesthesia confusional states	Barbiturates
Brain tumor	Tranquilizers
Fat embolus	Opiates
Pancreatitis	
METABOLIC	
Hypoxia	
Uremia	
Hypoglycemia	
Hepatic encephalopathy	
Water intoxication	

alcoholics requires hospitalization for acute symptomatology, or management of withdrawal, or both. The alternative is outpatient detoxification programs.[35]

The medical management of withdrawal states has been summarized clearly by Sellers and Kalant.[36] Multivitamin preparations are commonly given, but their value is unproved. Sixth cranial nerve paresis responds to thiamine (2 mg) intravenously, or 50 to 100 mg by injection. Hydration may be required, but in mild withdrawal, overhydration is more typical. Specific pharmacotherapy has been bewildering over the past 25 years, with over 135 drugs being recommended and used. The administration of alcohol will reduce the initial symptoms, but it is undesirable psychologically, has a short duration of action, and perpetuates the metabolic disturbances. Antihistamines, barbiturates, chloral hydrate, antipsychotic agents, and paraldehyde have been used, and are effective to some extent. However, the most effective and safe class of drugs is the benzodiazepines, including chlordiazepoxide, diazepam, oxazepam, flurazepam, and clorazepate. Doses in the range of 100 to 400 mg on the first day, followed by a tapering of 25 percent of the initial dose for each subsequent day, is the typical procedure. The evidence for the preventive value of oral anticonvulsants is contradictory. The patient who is hospitalized with a severe withdrawal state also requires careful, supportive medical management.

In many parts of the United States the need for detoxification triage and a simultaneous entry into rehabilitation programs has given rise to "social detoxification" centers. Management in such centers is similar to the outpatient regimen described above, and the centers provide a 24-hour-care capacity to interrupt the drinking and initiate intensive therapeutic encounter when patients are not likely to enter and remain in an outpatient program.[37,38]

Use and Abuse of Drugs in Treatment of the Alcoholic

A major problem in the physician's management of alcoholic patients is the overuse of drugs. In their survey of 3,376 internists, Jones and Helrich report that 90 percent primarily prescribed drugs.[18] The chief drugs were chlordiazepoxide, phenothiazines, diazepam, antidepressants, and disulfiram.

The judicious use of benzodiazepines in the short-term management of acute withdrawal symptoms has been acknowledged as being justified. Thereafter, there is rare justification for the use of any medications in the management of alcoholism. There have been many attempts to find the magic drug that will cure alcoholism. Both Freed and Mottin have documented these many futile attempts.[39,40] Popular fad drugs that have proved to have no better than a placebo response include antitrichomonads, although they may have a mild disulfiramlike reaction,[41,42] and lysergic acid diethylamide (LSD).[43] Perhaps the most cogent demonstration of the futility of drug therapies was a review by Viamontes of 89 alcoholism drug studies, which found that 94.5 percent of uncontrolled studies reported positive results, whereas only 5.8 percent of controlled studies showed positive results.[44] The issue has been stated so clearly by one internist, Bissell, that her observations are worth quoting:

> Arguments are still advanced at times that, if one does not prescribe sedatives for a highly manipulative patient, he will simply get his drugs from another doctor and fall into hands less expert than ours. The same reasoning could be applied whenever one is asked to give penicillin for a viral pharyngitis, but that does not justify our doing so. It is also agreed that giving drugs makes the patient more likely to keep coming back to us. Many a street-corner drug pusher would agree.
>
> I do think we need to give our patients a substitute for alcohol, but I don't think that substitute can be another sedative. I think it has to be our concern, our time, our caring, and ourselves.[45]

One drug that is useful in the physician's armamentarium is disulfiram. This drug has been used in the United States for nearly 30 years.[46] Early enthusiasm for the drug waned when widespread use did not produce uniformly positive results. There have been many misunderstandings about the mechanism of action of disulfiram. Quite simply, disulfiram is a psychological assist to the alcoholic's determination not to drink. The patient who is taking disulfiram daily cannot drink alcohol without a severe physiological reaction, not only for that day but for 3 to 7 days following ingestion of the last dose of disulfiram. The taking of the drug is voluntary, and hopefully the patient will scrupulously take the disulfiram daily, so that the "insurance policy" against impulsive drinking is kept fully in effect for the 3-to-7 day period.

Research evidence emphasizes the conclusion that the best results occur when the patient has a positive motivation, that is, when disulfiram is helping the patient to maintain a desired sobriety.[47,48] Other positive disulfiram responders include alcoholics who have a stable social and vocational history, are personally motivated to maintain abstinence, and most importantly, have a regular, ongoing positive relationship with the physician who is prescribing the drug. In a word, the drug itself produces no physiologic effect in the successful patient. Rather, the taking of the drug reinforces the daily motivation to maintain abstinence.[49]

In the early days of disulfiram's use, a "challenge" dose of alcohol was given to the patient after the patient had been taking disulfiram for several days. The concept was to have patients experience a severe reaction so that they would know what would occur if they drank alcohol. Also, alcohol would be associated with exceedingly unpleasant sensations. We do not favor this challenge dose technique, but other authorities in the field do.[46,50]

Finally, the physician should be aware of the interactions of alcohol with other classes of drugs that are commonly used in medical practice. Alcohol will aggravate possible gastrointestinal bleeding from salicylates. It potentiates the central depressant effects of the narcotic analgesics and antihistamines. Occasionally, rare disulfiramlike reactions occur with alcohol in combination with certain antibiotics: sulfonamides, chloramphenicol, and nitrofurans. Of major significance is the potential severity and unpredictability of alcohol interactions with hypoglycemic agents. Finally, alcohol may potentiate the depressant effects of antipsychotic drugs, sedatives, and hypnotics. There have been some cases of psychosis occurring with disulfiram alone, but the mechanism remains unclear. Indirect effects on drug actions are produced by alcohol-induced impairment of hepatic, renal, and antigenic systems that may secondarily influence the metabolism and activity of the above array of drug classes.

MANAGEMENT OF DRUG-ABUSE PATIENTS

It is important to differentiate which patients should have medication. Many individuals who have abused drugs in the past develop real problems that require relief of pain, of anxiety, or of depression. The former narcotic addict who has a surgical procedure requires narcotics, and generally in larger doses than normal because of prolonged tolerance effects. The patient can take narcotics postsurgically to deal with real physical pain, without becoming readdicted. There is obviously some risk of iatrogenic readdiction here, but not if the medication is stopped as soon as it is no longer clinically indicated. It is unfortunate to overreact to the possibility of iatrogenic drug dependence to such an extent that we do not give adequate pain relief to the dying patient. Likewise, patients who self-medicate to relieve tension should not be deprived of needed nonpsychoactive drugs. Patients who misuse or abuse drugs may also have real physical problems that require appropriate medication.

Psychoactive drug abusers frequently present to the physician with medical problems that may be a direct or indirect result of their abuse patterns. Such problems as broken limbs, head trauma, hepatitis, or delirium can be treated in a short hospital stay. However, to treat only these physical problems is to do the patient a gross injustice. When the drug-dependent individual presents with these problems, they provide an excellent opportunity for the physician to interrupt the cycle of dependence.

The medical consequences of intoxication, dependence, and withdrawal are definitive syndromes that can be diagnosed easily. Symptoms of acute intoxication range from depression to euphoria to true delirium. Alcohol, barbiturates, and other sedatives may initially produce behavioral excitation, stimulation, and lack of inhibition prior to sedation. The "high" from these drugs is a disinhibition euphoria, which depends on personality, setting, and expectation. The user may become happy, pleasant, euphoric, or "mellow" on the one hand; or hostile, suspicious, aggressive, and violent on the other. Barbiturates are frequently implicated in aggravated assault charges. Low-dose effects are erratic, while moderate to high doses slow reaction time; impair mental function; and produce a lessening of inhibition, a reduction in emotional control, and impairment of coordination. The minor tranquilizers produce a similar reaction. Normal doses usually provide relaxation and a sense of well-being. With excessive doses of depressant drugs, there may be disorientation, confusion, memory impairment, nystagmus, slurred speech, ataxia, double vision, personality alterations, rage reactions, and other symptoms resembling those of drunkenness.

Overdose from narcotics may present with the classic triad of coma, pinpoint pupils, and depressed respiration. However, meperidine causes mydriasis rather than miosis. Also, when death is imminent, pupils may dilate. Narcotic addicts in withdrawal evidence dilated pupils, rhinorrhea, lacrimation, yawning, and perspiration. This progresses to nausea, vomiting, diarrhea, turkey flesh (hence, cold turkey), muscle jerks (hence, the term "kicking the habit"), increased pulse, and high blood pressure.

In withdrawal from the CNS depressants, there is first anxiety, insomnia, and restlessness, which progresses to grand mal seizures, mental confusion, and delirium. The higher the dosage, the longer the period of drug use, and the shorter-acting the drug, the more likely there is to be an intense withdrawal. Multiple-depressant drug abuse results in more intense withdrawal, including the possibility of a two-stage withdrawal. Patients who withdraw from amphetamines and cocaine are depressed, agitated, restless, irritable, and paranoid.

The treatment of drug dependence will not be described in detail in this chapter. However, it is important to state that the general physician should *not* treat drug dependence anywhere but in hospital settings. Even hospitals are not always ideal—these patients do not do well in the wards of a general hospital or even in most psychiatric units. Their withdrawal is best managed in specialized treatment settings that are equipped to handle the manipulations and special needs of such patients.

To initiate detoxification, a baseline dose of sedation should first be determined, and the patient should then be detoxified by a reduction of 10 percent a day, or in seizure-prone individuals, by one sedative dose daily over a 2-to-3-week period. Detoxification, by itself, is relatively valueless unless it is accompanied by rigorous and prolonged aftercare that is tailored to the individual needs of the patient.

THE PHYSICIAN, HIS OR HER SPOUSE, AND FAMILY

Physicians and their families represent a vulnerable and high-risk population for the development of psychoactive drug use, misuse, and abuse. Because of their intimate association with illness and with bodily function, the physician, spouse, and family are likely to have a higher degree of awareness and even preoccupation with bodily function, which can generate subtle degrees of hypochondria. High levels of stress, tension, responsibility, as well as heavy work loads, tend to make physicians more susceptible to positive and rewarding personal response experiences with psychoactive drugs. The spouse and family are likely to experience more isolation, loneliness, and noninvolvement with the spouse-parent who is a physician. In turn, these conditions can be the psychological seed-beds for turning to psychoactive drug relief and escape. Finally, the physician has ready access to prescriptions, drug samples, and stocks of drugs, which can be self-dispensed or given to spouse or family members. Thus it is not surprising that physicians, spouses, and families have a high incidence of alcoholism and psychoactive drug misuse and abuse.

CONCLUSION

In conclusion, alcoholism will remain a major health problem. Its effects are ubiquitous, and involve not only the patient but all those around the alcoholic, including family, employers, employees, friends, and physicians. From an interpersonal or social perspective, its effects are ruinous. From an economic or work viewpoint, its effects may be destructive. From a physical health viewpoint, its effects may be disastrous. From an emotional health viewpoint, its effects may be deadly. One of the prime instruments of intervention in this progressive, destructive script may be the physician who is willing.

Finally, if the physician, spouse, or family members begin to misuse or abuse any psychoactive drugs, including alcohol, do not treat yourself or them. Seek reliable and competent advice, evaluation, and treatment from a professional who is skilled in the area of alcohol and drug dependence.

Physicians, their spouses, and their families often receive inadequate, inappropriate, and inept treatment for alcohol and drug problems. As physicians, we must first develop healthy attitudes toward alcohol and toward psychoactive drug use ourselves. Drugs especially must be considered an occupational hazard. If we fail to examine and monitor our own attitudes and use of alcohol and drugs carefully, we may place ourselves and our families in jeopardy, and may likewise fail to offer effective treatment to our patients.

REFERENCES

1   Engel, G.: "The Need for a New Medical Model: A Challenge for Biomedicine," *Science,* **196**:129–135, 1977.

2   World Health Organization Expert Committee on Drugs: "Drug Dependence: Its Significance and Characteristics," *Bull. WHO,* **32**:721–733, 1965.

3   Kaufman, E.: "Polydrug Abuse or Multidrug Misuse: It's Here to Stay," *Brit. J. Addict.,* **72**:339–374, 1977.

4   Gropper, B. A., and M. I. Burke: "Characteristics of Multidrug Abuse Incidents and Abuser Populations," *North American Congress on Alcohol and Drug Problems,* San Francisco, California, December 12–18, 1974.

5   Fox, V.: "Recognizing Multiple Simultaneous Drug Withdrawal Symptoms, NCA/MSA Medical-Scientific Conference," Washington, D. C., May 6–8, 1976.

6   "Reported Experience with Drug Use for Recreational and Non-Medical Purposes by American Youth and Adults," in *The New York Times,* Jan. 14, 1973, p. 47.

7   Greenblatt, D. G., and R. I. Shader: "Drug Therapy: Benzodiazepines," *N. E. J. Med.,* **291**:1239–1243, 1974.

8   Gearing, F. R.: "Methadone Maintenance Treatment Five Years Later—Where Are They Now?," *Am. J. Publ. Health Suppl.,* **64**:44–50, 1974.

9   Chambers, C. D., and W. J. R. Taylor: "Patterns of 'Cheating' Among Methadone Patients," in W. Keup (ed.), *Drug Abuse, Current Concepts and Research,* Springfield, Ill.: Charles C Thomas, 1972.

10 Bihari, B.: "Alcoholism and Methadone Maintenance," *Am. J. Drug Alc. Abuse,* **1**:79–87, 1974.

11 Boden, M.: "Methadone Deaths," *New York Post,* August 16, 1974, p.10, column 1.

12 Chabalko, J. et al.: "Death of Methadone Users in the District of Columbia," *Inter. J. Addict.,* **8**:897–908, 1973.

13 Wilson, C., and J. Orford: "Children of Alcoholics," *J. Stud. Alc.,* **39**:121–142, 1978.

14 Chambers, C. D.: *Differential Drug Use Within the New York State Labor Force,* Narcotic Addiction Control Commission, Mamaroneck, N.Y., July 1971.

15 Reilly, D. M.: "Family Factors in the Etiology and Treatment of Youthful Drug Abuse," *Fam. Ther.,* **2**:149–171, 1975.

16 Smart, R. G., and D. Fejer: "Relationships Between Parental and Adolescent Drug Use," in W. Keup (ed.) *Drug Abuse, Current Concepts and Research,* Springfield, Ill.: Charles C Thomas, 1972.

17 Plaut, T. F.: *Alcohol Problems: A Report to the Nation,* New York: Oxford, 1967.

18 Jones, R. W., and A. R. Helrich: "Treatment of Alcoholism by Physicians in Private Practice: A National Survey," *Quart. J. Stud. Alc.,* **33**:117–131, 1972.

19 Beckman, L. J.: "Woman Alcoholics: A Review of Social and Psychological Studies," *J. Stud. Alc.,* **36**:797–824, 1975.

20 Lindbeck, V. L.: "The Woman Alcoholic: A Review of the Literature," *Inter. J. Addict.,* **7**:567–580, 1972.

21 Dunn, J. H., and M. L. Clay: "Physicians Look at a General Hospital Alcoholism Service," *Quart. J. Stud. Alc.,* **32**:162–167, 1971.

22 Edwards, G. et al.: "Alcoholics Admitted to Four Hospitals in England," *Quart. J. Stud. Alc.,* **35**:499–522, 1974.

23 Barcha, R. et al.: "The Prevalence of Alcoholism Among General Hospital Ward Patients," *Am. J. Psychiat.,* **225**:681–684, 1968.

24 Gomberg, E. S.: "Prevalence of Alcoholism Among Ward Patients in a Veterans Administration Hospital," *J. Stud. Alc., 36*:1456–1467, 1975.

25 Kearney, T. R.: "Alcohol and General Hospital Patients," *Am. J. Psychiat., 125*:681–684, 1968.

26 McCusker, J. et al.: "Prevalence of Alcoholism in General Municipal Hospital Population," *NYS J. Med., 71*:751–756, 1971.

27 Steinglass, P.: "Experimenting with Family Treatment Approaches to Alcoholism, 1950–1975: A Review," *Fam. Process, 15*:97–123, 1976.

28 Cross, J. N.: *Guide to the Community Control of Alcoholism,* New York: American Public Health Association, 1968.

29 Pattison, E. M.: "Rehabilitation of the Chronic Alcoholic," in B. Kissin and H. Begleiter (eds.), *The Biology of Alcoholism, vol. 3, Clinical Pathology,* New York: Plenum Press, 1974.

30 Finer, M. J.: "Overmanagement of the Alcoholic Patient," *JAMA, 219*:622, 1972.

31 American Medical Association: "Guidelines for Admission of Alcoholic-Dependent Patients to General Hospitals," *JAMA, 210*:121, 1969.

32 Twerski, A. J.: "When to Hospitalize the Alcoholic," *Hosp. Prog., 4*:47–55, 1969.

33 Freed, E. X.: "The Dilemma of the Alcoholic Patient in a Psychiatric Hospital," *J. Psychiat. Nurs., 7*:113–116, 1969.

34 Gross, M. M. et al.: "Classification of Alcohol Withdrawal Syndromes," *Quart. J. Stud. Alc., 33*:400–407, 1972.

35 Feldman, D. J. et al.: "Outpatient Alcohol Detoxification: Initial Findings on 564 Patients," *Am. J. Psychiat., 132*:407–412, 1975.

36 Sellers, E. M., and H. Kalant: "Alcohol Intoxication and Withdrawal," *New Eng. J. Med., 294*:757–762, 1976.

37 O'Briant, R. G. et al.: *Recovery from Alcoholism: A Social Treatment Model,* Springfield, Ill.: Charles C Thomas, 1973.

38 Seigel, H. H.: *Alcohol Detoxification Programs,* Springfield, Ill.: Charles C Thomas, 1973.

39 Freed, E. X.: "Drug Abuse by Alcoholics: A Review," *Inter. J. Addict., 8*:451–473, 1973.

40 Mottin, J. L.: "Drug-Induced Attentuation of Alcohol Consumption: A Review and Evaluation of Claimed, Potential, or Current Therapies," *Quart. J. Stud. Alc., 34*:444–472, 1973.

41 Goodwin, D. W., and J. Reinhart: "Disulfiramlike Effects of Trichomonacidal Drugs: A Review and Double-Blind Study," *Quart. J. Stud. Alc., 33*:734–740, 1972.

42 Kaplan, R. et al.: "Phenytoin, Metronidazole, and Multivitamins in the Treatment of Alcoholism," *Quart. J. Stud. Alc., 33*:97–104, 1972.

43 Ludwig, A. M. et al.: *LSD and Alcoholism: A Clinical Study of Treatment Efficacy,* Springfield, Ill.: Charles C Thomas, 1970.

44 Viamontes, J. A.: "Review of Drug Effectiveness in the Treatment of Alcoholism," *Am. J. Psychiat., 128*:1570–1571, 1972.

45 Bissell, L.: "The Treatment of Alcoholism: What Do We Do About Long-Term Sedatives?" *Ann. N. Y. Acad. Sci., 252*:396–399, 1975.

46 Usdin, G. L.: "Antabuse in the Therapy of Chronic Alcoholism," *Cinn. J. Med, 32*:288–291, 1951.

47 Baekeland, F. et al.: "Methods for the Treatment of Chronic Alcoholism: A Critical Appraisal," in R. J. Gibbins (ed.), *Research Advances in Alcohol and Drug Problems,* vol. 2, New York: Wiley, 1975.

48 Lubetkin, B. S. et al.: "Difficulties of Disulfiram Therapy with Alcoholics," *Quart. J. Stud. Alc.,* **32**:168–171, 1971.

49 Billet, S. L.: "The Use of Antabuse: An Approach that Minimizes Fear," *Med. Ann. Dist. Col.,* **33**:612–615, 1974.

50 van Praag, H. M.: *Psychotropic Drugs,* New York: Brunner/Mazel, 1978.

BIBLIOGRAPHY

Green, H. I., and M. H. Levy: *Drug Use . . . Human Abuse,* New York: Dekker, 1976.

Kaufman, E., and P. Kaufmann: *Family Therapy of Drug and Alcohol Abuse,* New York: Gardner, 1978.

Kissin, B., and H. Begleiter (eds.): *The Biology of Alcoholism,* 5 vols., New York: Plenum Press, 1970–1977.

Pattison, E. M. et al.: *Emerging Concepts of Alcohol Dependence,* New York: Springer, 1977.

Smith, D. E., and D. R. Wesson: *Uppers and Downers,* Englewood Cliffs, N.J.: Prentice-Hall, 1973.

Westermeyer, J.: *A Primer on Chemical Dependency,* Baltimore: Williams and Wilkins, 1976.

Chapter 14

Physical Disease Manifesting As Psychiatric Disorders

M. J. Martin, M.D.

EDITORS' INTRODUCTION

What is it like to think you are losing your mind, only to learn that you have a subdural hematoma that can be removed surgically, or that you have myxedema that should respond to thyroid medication? How does a patient feel after having been treated for 6 months with the newer antidepressant drugs because of fatigue and depression (as well as a sore tongue and tingling in the lower extremities), before being told one had pernicious anemia that will respond promptly to a vitamin of the B complex? Many patients are misdiagnosed and treated for psychiatric disorders, while organic disease is overlooked and goes untreated. Many patients are diagnosed as having a physical disease and are treated with vitamins, diets, and thyroid, hormone, and drugs when psychotherapy and psychotropic drugs are indicated.

Patients expect accurate diagnoses and the best possible medical treatment. The physician needs to consider all diagnostic possibilities, psychiatric and nonpsychiatric. Physicians have many reasons to do this—the wish to help the patient, to maintain a good professional reputation, and to avoid malpractice litigation, among others. All physicians make mistakes in diagnosis and treatment. The amount of discomfort experienced varies from physician to physician. How disturbing it is to know that a patient has not benefited as much as he or she should, because of an incorrect diagnosis and treatment. How must a physician feel when "that alcoholic" dies of a subdural hematoma? What goes on within the physician when a colleague tells the patient that the antianxiety medication formerly prescribed will not help the patient because the patient has hyperthyroidism? What about the clinician who treats the apathetic, despondent, anorectic patient with antidepressants for months, and then has the patient bring to the clinician's attention the fact that the patient's eyes seem a little yellow—should the clinician now consider cancer of the pancreas?

The task of the physician would be much easier if the issue was clearly "either-or." Of course it is not, and many patients present with both physical disease and psychiatric disorder, which exist independently of each other. The hypochondriacal patient who has had years of diffuse physical complaints and whose newest symptom reflects a recently evolved physical disease is a common example. The neurotic man who develops a brain tumor, the hysterical patient with a recently acquired collagen disease, and the poststroke elderly patient whose convalescence is complicated by the emergence of neurotic symptoms are but other examples of patients who tax the diagnostic skills of the physician.

This chapter, which was written by a psychiatrist, who is also an internist and who now heads the psychiatric department of a major medical clinic, discusses many of the physical diseases that may manifest themselves as psychiatric disorders. Familiarity with this material will assist the physician to minimize mistakes in diagnosis and treatment.

Essentially all patients with physical disease have emotional components associated with their illnesses. Usually the emotional manifestations involve the way the individual feels about and reacts to being ill. The person who has been injured in an accident involving the automobile of an uninsured person may worry about job security and welfare of his or her family. In some instances, the associated anxiety and depression may affect recovery adversely. This is quite a different situation from that of the soldier who is injured in battle and evacuated from the source of danger. He may feel happy and relaxed to be away from the front lines. The more-or-less inevitable consequences of being ill may manifest themselves in a multitude of ways. Not all uremic patients become confused, few patients with a seizure disorder have a personality change, and the mood alterations associated with steroid treatment are quite variable. These somatopsychic manifestations of disease are of great consequence in the care of patients. All health care workers should be cognizant of the importance of the way patients feel about, and react to, their diseases. There are a number of conditions that are thought to be produced, or at least precipitated, by emotional conditions. This psychosomatic explanation for illness is discussed by Schwab in Chapter 16.

Here we shall be concerned with various physical diseases that masquerade as psychiatric disorders. The clinician must be ever-alert to the possibility that hidden organic disease may be present in the face of overt psychiatric symptoms. Proper therapy cannot be instituted unless the correct diagnosis is made. The importance of proper interviewing skills was emphasized in Chapter 1 by Lewis and

Usdin. Nowhere in the practice of medicine is an accurate and detailed history more important than it is with patients whose organic disease is hidden by a facade of emotional symptoms.

There are a wide variety of disease states that have been known to produce emotional symptoms as a part of their symptomatology. On many occasions, these diseases present with the emotional aspect of the syndrome as the most prominent feature. The physician may be distracted by the chief complaint of anxiety, depression, or personality change, and fail to pursue the possibility of underlying physical illness. This is especially true if the patient has had a history of psychiatric problems. Sometimes clinicians do not maintain their objectivity when they are making evaluations of patients who have a prior history of depression, neurotic reactions, or psychosis.

Attempts have been made to list and classify these conditions.[1,2] Since the disease processes may involve almost every organ system and are quite dissimilar, the logical classification and outline that are possible with most organic illnesses are difficult with these. An organ-system approach is probably better than a symptom classification. Because of the great variability of disease and of people who develop disease, which makes an all-inclusive listing impossible, no review is complete.

ENDOCRINE PROBLEMS

The role of the endocrine glands in maintaining metabolic homeostasis in humans is well known. These glands secrete hormones that regulate the metabolism of food and minerals. The interrelated systems are complex, with primary control coming from the influence of the anterior pituitary gland, which in turn is influenced by hypothalamic and higher cortical functions in the brain. The function of various levels of the brain is influenced in turn by the metabolic or chemical status induced by the endocrine gland functions. These alterations may affect mood states or cognitive function, and may induce anxiety. Either diminished function or hyperactivity of the endocrine glands may produce such indirect effects on cerebral function, with subsequent symptoms that appear to be primarily psychiatric in origin.

Table 14-1 shows endocrine problems that may masquerade as psychiatric illnesses.

Thyroid Gland

Hypothyroidism (Myxedema) Failure of the thyroid gland to secrete thyroid hormone may result from a failure of the anterior pituitary gland to stimulate the thyroid gland, either because of inadequate production of thyrotrophin, or because of a disease within the thyroid gland that curtails its functions. Either situation may result in the clinical state of *hypothyroidism*. Regardless of the etiology of the failure of the thyroid gland, the clinical condition most often affects middle-aged females. The onset is usually insidious and may be associated with fatigue, lethargy, and feelings of depression,

Table 14-1   Endocrine Problems

Problem		Common symptoms	Misleading signs	May be misdiagnosed as
Thyroid				
Hypo-thyroidism (myxedema)	Mild	Fatigue, apathy, cold	Dry, puffy skin	Depression
	Moderate	Intolerance, coarse voice	Depressed affect	Depression
	Severe	Irritability, delusions, paranoid thinking	Clear sensorium	Schizophrenia
Hyperthyroidism		Fine tremor, heat intolerance	Loss of strength, weight loss	Anxiety state
Parathyroid				
Hypoparathyroidism		Muscle spasms, tetany, hyperreflexia	Irritability if onset is rapid, apathy if insidious	Anxiety state Depression
Hyperparathyroidism		Renal calculi, polyuria, abdominal pain	Weakness, irritability, anorexia, fatigue	Either anxiety or depression
Adrenal				
Hypoadrenalism (Addison's disease)		Weight loss, hypotension, skin pigmentation	Negativism, apathy, suspiciousness	Depression
Hyperadrenalism (Cushing's syndrome)		Weight gain, fat face, and cervical hump, ecchymoses	Easy fatigue, emotional lability, somatic delusions	Schizophrenia
Pancreas				
Adenoma of islet of Langerhans (hyperinsulinism)		Episodic tremor, sweating, hunger, weakness	Fearfulness, confusion	Anxiety attacks, hysterical attacks, acute alcoholism, organic brain syndrome

with anergy and a loss of interest in the social environment. Classically associated with it are dry, cool skin with a puffy face; thinning hair; coarse voice; and an intolerance to cold. A weight gain may occur, but significant obesity is rare. Many patients become irritable, short-tempered, and anxious. In severe cases, a "myxedema madness" as described by Asher may occur.[3] This condition is associated with delusional thinking that is often of a paranoid type, with somatic delusions and hallucinations. This state may mimic schizophrenia. The mental status is clear but slowed, even during the most disturbed, belligerent behavior.

Since the course is slow and early symptoms may indicate depression, the physician must be alert to the possibility of hypothyroidism when middle-aged patients complain of lethargy, fatigue, and depression. The proper diagnosis is essential, since thyroid replacement therapy should not be given indiscriminately.

> A 48-year-old housewife noted progressive anergy and fatigue. She blamed her fatigue and irritability on menopausal changes, but her menstrual periods were regular. Her physician felt she was depressed and prescribed a tricyclic antidepressant. This drug had no effect. Another physician noted pale, puffy facies and a slowed return phase of the deep tendon reflexes of the ankles. Laboratory studies revealed markedly diminished total and free thyroxin levels. The patient's symptoms subsided after thyroid extract therapy was begun.

Hyperthyroidism   Hyperactivity of the thyroid, with the development of increased metabolic levels, is the syndrome of *hyperthyroidism* (Graves's disease). This condition of uncertain etiology most frequently affects females in their middle years. If the condition has a rapid onset, it is manifest by a fine tremor, weight loss, heat intolerance, and anxiety. Occasional hyperactive and grandiose behavior may occur. While hyperthyroidism is most often mistaken for an anxiety state, those cases that have an insidious onset may resemble depression, with weight loss and restlessness. When increased psychomotor behavior occurs, the mood is usually not elated, but the hypomanic phase of bipolar depression must be excluded. Uncontrolled hyperthyroidism may result in a "thyroid storm" with delirium, excitement, delusional state, and marked restlessness with insomnia.

> A 26-year-old resident physician's wife noted a rather sudden onset of anxiety, associated with tremulousness, sweating, and insomnia. She was treated with minor tranquilizers by her husband, and became more excited. She became obsessed with the idea that she was mentally ill, and was admitted to a psychiatric unit. Psychiatric evaluation failed to reveal significant emotional conflicts. Tachycardia, dry skin, and evidence of weight loss were noted at the time of the physical examination. The presumptive diagnosis of hyperthyroidism was confirmed with appropriate laboratory studies. Treatment with radioactive iodine controlled the symptoms.

Parathyroid Gland

Hypoparathyroidism   The loss of function of the parathyroid glands most commonly follows thyroidectomy or other radical neck surgery, but may be idiopathic. The associated defect in calcium metabolism produces hyperreflexia, muscle spasms, and tetany. Anxiety manifest by irritability and hyperactivity is usually associated with hypocalcemia; however, if the onset is insidious, a progressive apathy and social withdrawal, with associated depressed mood, is seen. Occasionally with severe *hypoparathyroidism,* a toxic delirious state may occur. This is manifest by confusion, disorientation, and a clouded sensorium. A syndrome of this severity is unusual, but the clinician must be alert for such a problem, which may be mistaken for depression or acute organic brain syndrome of uncertain etiology. Hypoparathyroidism should be suspected in those patients who become apathetic or confused following thyroid or other neck surgery.

Hyperparathyroidism   Renal calculi are the most common harbingers of *hyperparathyroidism.* This condition is caused by adenomatous hypertrophy of one or more of the parathyroid glands. Altered calcium metabolism with hypercalcemia and diminished blood phosphorus produces not only osseous lesions and renal calculi, but also affects the central nervous system. Anxiety, depression, and irritability are commonly seen. Occasionally a toxic psychosis can be produced by rapidly increasing calcemia. Usually the disease has a gradual onset, and the absence of clear-cut diagnostic signs frequently leads to misdiagnosis.[4]

A 68-year-old widow complained of intermittent upper abdominal pain of 4 years' duration. She also felt apathetic, weak, and depressed, but blamed her mood disturbance on loneliness. Her internist noted a duodenal ulcer during radiological examination of the upper gastrointestinal tract. A psychiatric consultation was obtained, and depression of a moderate degree was noted. Before therapy was instituted, blood studies revealed a calcium level of 12 mg per 100 ml. Subsequent studies confirmed the diagnosis of hyperparathyroidism, and a parathyroid adenoma was removed surgically. The patient's duodenal ulcer healed promptly, and her lethargy and depression lifted without specific treatment.

Duodenal ulcer is often asociated with hyperparathyroidism.

Adrenal Cortex

Adrenocortical Insufficiency (Addison's Disease)   This condition usually develops gradually, and is associated with progressive weakness, weight loss, and hyperpigmentation of the skin. It occurs in adults of both sexes, and often produces hypotension and a craving for salt. Severe depression with marked apathy and negativism is frequent with Addison's disease. Some patients become suspicious and paranoid. The syndrome resembles primary unipolar depression, and is sometimes of psychotic proportions.

Hyperadrenalism (Cushing's Syndrome)   Hypertrophy of the adrenal cortices, or a functional cortical tumor of an adrenal cortex with increased production of adrenocortical hormones, produces a syndrome similar to the familiar hyperadrenalism associated with the administration of exogenous corticosteroid drugs. A wide variety of psychological symptoms may occur, but anxiety or retarded depression predominates in endogenous Cushing's syndrome. Weight gain occurs, along with the characteristic "moon" facies and cervical hump. Patients develop fatigue easily, often become depressed, and experience emotional lability. Occasionally bizarre somatic delusions develop as the result of bodily changes, and some patients with Cushing's syndrome have been diagnosed initially as schizophrenic. The behavioral problems and mood disturbance may require symptomatic treatment, before and during appropriate surgical treatment of the adrenocortical pathology. Complete recovery may take several months.

The most frequent cause of Cushing's syndrome is the administration of corticosteroid drugs for a variety of diseases, such as asthma, rheumatoid arthritis, systemic lupus erythematosus, chronic hepatitis, and other autoimmune disorders. The psychological effects of these drugs depend upon the previous personality organization of the individual, as well as the rate of change of bodily functions secondary to the metabolic shift induced by the drugs.[5] An increase in joviality and optimism is the most frequent response to exogenous corticosteroids. This may mimic hypomania, and may be associated with emotional lability and a short temper. Some patients become severely depressed. A wide variety of psychologic and motor disturbances may occur. However, confusion, disorientation, and sensorial disturbances characteristic of toxic psychosis are unusual.

In general, the type of mental disturbance produced by corticosteroid therapy seems to be determined by the basic pattern of the patient's personality. If the patient has a tendency to be depressed, the drug may worsen the depression. Spontaneous recovery occurs upon discontinuation of the drug, but the medical condition for which the steroids were prescribed may preclude stopping the drug. In that instance, the dose may be tapered and neuroleptic drugs can be used as adjunctive therapy to help control the mental symptoms. The development of a psychiatric disturbance with the use of corticosteroids does not prevent their use at a later date. Such side effects may not occur again. The drug effects are not clearly dose related.

Pancreas

Adenoma of Islet of Langerhans (Hyperinsulinism) Hypoglycemia from any cause can produce symptoms of anxiety, with tremulousness, sweating, fatigue, and dizziness. Unfortunately, many patients with reactive or transient functional hypoglycemia and associated hypochondriacal symptoms are misdiagnosed as having true hypoglycemia. Many emotional and physical symptoms have been "explained" by inconsequential lowering of blood sugar. A cult of hypoglycemia believers has developed. Believers prescribe treatment with bizarre dietary regimes. True hypoglycemia, with blood glucose levels below 20 mg per 100 ml, is caused by excessive insulin, either from an islet cell adenoma or from exogenous administration of insulin, as with an overdose in diabetic patients or with insulin injection as a form of factitial illness.

Hypoglycemia as a result of an islet cell adenoma frequently presents with mental symptoms including episodes of anxiety, irritability, anger, apathy, depression, delusions, and hallucinations, and rarely may progress to convulsions and coma. Repeated episodes of severe hypoglycemia may produce brain damage, with personality changes and dementia. Initially the episodes may produce mild symptoms, and are infrequent. Misdiagnosis is common. Attacks of hypoglycemia then become more frequent, and obesity may develop, because ingestion of food at frequent intervals is based on the patient's increased effort to prevent the attacks, which both fasting and excessive exercise tend to bring on. Surgical removal of the insulin-producing adenoma is the treatment of choice. This is often technically difficult, and identification of the tumor by the surgical pathologist is necessary to confirm adequate surgical excision. Hypoglycemia secondary to islet cell tumors is frequently misdiagnosed as anxiety, hysteria, psychotic states, or acute alcoholism. This is especially true early in the course of the disease, when the attacks are infrequent. Later the illness may be confused with a seizure disorder, an organic brain syndrome, or even a brain tumor. Few diseases offer a greater challenge to the diagnostician.

METABOLIC ABNORMALITIES OF UNKNOWN CAUSE

Acute Porphyria

Many patients with acute intermittent porphyria have been misdiagnosed as having neurotic or psychotic illness. It is felt King George III probably had acute intermittent porphyria. The illness affects females more frequently than males, and may be associated with severe, colicky abdominal pain, paresthesias associated with peripheral neuropathy, and weakness. It is inherited as an autosomal dominant trait. The syndrome may be precipitated by the use of barbiturates, alcohol, and oral contraceptives. Associated anxiety is often severe and of acute onset. The patient's mood may be quite labile, with vacillations between relative euphoria and depression within hours. Emotional outbursts, with uncontrolled anger and destructiveness, sometimes occur. Many patients develop neurotic lifestyles, which are perhaps secondary to the intermittent, unpredictable, and often misdiagnosed aspects of their illness. Many patients with porphyria seem to live in fear of a recurrent attack. The urine of patients with acute porphyria turns to port wine color when exposed to sunlight, and porphobilinogen and uroporphyrin is found in the urine of patients with this metabolic defect.

Pernicious Anemia (Vitamin B$_{12}$ Deficiency)

This chronic disease is characterized by an insidious onset, gastric achlorhydria, with the absence of "intrinsic factor" and the development of macrocytic anemia. It primarily affects members of the white race, and usually occurs after age 40. Although initial symptoms may include weakness, sore tongue, and paresthesias of the extremities, other somatic symptoms occur frequently. Many patients with pernicious anemia are depressed. When the depression is associated

Table 14-2 Metabolic Abnormalities of Unknown Cause

Abnormality	Common symptoms	Misleading signs	May be misdiagnosed as
Acute porphyria	Colicky abdominal pain, peripheral paresthesias, weakness	Marked emotional lability, sudden onset of anxiety	Anxiety state, conversion reaction
Pernicious anemia (vitamin B₁₂ deficiency)	Weakness, sore tongue, paresthesias of extremities	Depression, fatigue, lethargy	Depression
Hepatolenticular degeneration (Wilson's disease)	Tremor, choreo-athetoid movements, hepatic failure	Aggressive behavior, mood swings, intellectual impairment	Adolescent turmoil

with the fatigue, weakness, and lethargy of the anemia, the depression may be quite intense, with feelings of guilt and worthlessness. Some patients have irritability, paranoid ideation, lack of concentration, and headache. Short-term memory defects are also seen frequently and may be related to vitamin B_{12} deficiency.[6] Sensory disturbances are common, along with difficulty in walking and impotence. The syndrome is easily mistaken for an involutional type of depression. The depression associated with pernicious anemia may progress to delusional and sometimes confused states. In the years before effective treatment of pernicious anemia, it was emphasized that mental disturbances could be the first manifestation of the disease, and often progressed to become a serious problem.[7] In recent decades, treatment with vitamin B_{12} has resulted in few such complications, but an awareness of the possible *initial* psychiatric manifestations of pernicious anemia is important.

Hepatolenticular Degeneration (Wilson's Disease)

In accordance with the name, this genetically determined inborn error of metabolism produces cirrhosis of the liver and degeneration of the lenticular nuclei of the brain. There is a disturbance of copper metabolism, with high urinary excretion of copper. The characteristic brownish Kayser-Fleischer rings in the periphery of the corneas were present in 97 percent of a recent series of patients.[8] The relative lack of available copper in the brain affects enzymes (monoamine oxidase and dopamine β hydroxylase) involved in the function of the brain. Mental symptoms in this disease frequently resemble schizophrenia, a "functional" psychosis that also is manifest by abnormal function of brain enzymes. Neurologic signs are usually prominent, with tremors or choreo-athetoid movements. The disease classically begins in adolescence, and has a chronic course terminating with dementia. If untreated, it is universally fatal. Mild alterations in personality may be present in early stages, along with irritability, silliness, aggressive behavior, difficulty in concentration, and emotional lability. Memory and intellectual impairment develop later, as do more obvious psychiatric symptoms such as paranoid episodes, uncontrolled hyperactivity, and hallucinations. Treatment with penicillamine, a chelating agent that promotes a reduction of total body copper and a marked increase in the urinary excretion of copper, is a fairly effective treatment. Since the disease often has its onset in adolescence, the personality changes may be confused with adolescent incorrigibility.

NEOPLASTIC CONDITIONS

Intracranial Tumors

Brain tumors are highly varied, both morphologically and with regard to specific symptoms. However, since the cranial cavity is a closed space, tumor growth and subsequent increase in intracranial pressure produce certain similar characteristics. Many brain tumors are of metastatic origin, but may produce symptoms like those of a primary lesion in the brain. A subdural hematoma that occurs subsequent to a blow to the head may also have similar characteristics. It should be emphasized that head injury can produce personality changes that may be either acute or chronic and may be quite variable. Delirium, memory deficits, posttraumatic personality disorders, posttraumatic anxiety and depression, or other neurotic symptoms, and a chronic brain syndrome with dementia all may be seen following head injury.[9] Posttraumatic psychosis, except for psychotic symptoms secondary to dementia, is unusual following head injury. The structural lesion that is associated with head injury and that most often manifests as a

Table 14-3   Neoplastic Conditions

Condition	Common symptoms	Misleading signs	May be misdiagnosed as
Intracranial tumor	Headache, vomiting, seizure	Personality change, depression, localized neurologic signs	Depression, senility
Pancreatic carcinoma	Abdominal pain, weight loss, jaundice	Apathy, despondency	Depression
Pheochromocytoma	Anxiety, perspiration, headache, tremor	Episodic attacks of anxiety	Anxiety state

psychiatric disorder is a *chronic subdural hematoma.* This condition begins with the tearing of small veins in the subdural space. This causes bleeding and subsequent clot formation. The injury may be relatively minor, and the patient may not recall the event in subsequent weeks or months as symptoms develop. The clinical picture is progressive, with the gradual onset of irritability, lethargy, memory difficulty, and headache. The course may proceed to a confusional state, with a variable state of consciousness. Subdural hematoma should be suspected, even with no history of head injury, if the patient complains of headache, progressive drowsiness, and becomes confused and stuporous over a period of several weeks. The diagnosis of a subdural hematoma depends upon a high level of suspicion. Focal neurological signs, roentgenologic or echoencephalographic evidence of a shift of the brain in the cranial cavity, and computerized axial tomography of the head will confirm the diagnosis and lead to appropriate neurosurgical treatment.

While the initial symptom of an intracranial tumor may occur as headache, vomiting, a seizure, or other localized neurologic sign, nonspecific symptoms such as agnosia, apraxia, memory loss, difficulty in concentration, depression, and personality changes with inappropriate behavior may occur. Early diagnosis based on such vague symptoms is often difficult. Some patients are treated by psychiatrists before more specific sensory and motor manifestations lead to studies that confirm the proper diagnosis. Psychiatric symptoms are often the earliest and occasionally the only symptoms of an intracranial tumor. The behavioral changes resulting from a brain tumor are due to insidious but relentless alteration of cerebral function and the patient's responses to these changes. The symptoms are never the result of a single cause; rather, they reflect the interplay of many forces. The rate of the tumor growth, and to some degree the location of the tumor influence the type of symptoms. For example, temporal lobe tumors may cause olfactory or gustatory hallucinations. Frontal lobe tumors often produce distinct personality change and flatness of affect, with superficial euphoria. Occipital lobe lesions frequently are associated with unformed visual hallucinatory experiences consisting of flashes of light. Patients with parietal lobe tumors sometimes have sensory or agnostic disturbances, with a lack of awareness that may appear as denial (anosognosia).[10] Fluctuating symptoms, especially behavioral changes, may be affected by variations in edema around the tumor, and may vary from hour to hour. On the other hand, slow-growing lesions such as meningiomas induce a loss of brain function so gradually that the patient can adapt more or less satisfactorily at first. The patient usually reacts to the reduction in adaptive capacity with their premorbid defense mechanisms.[11]

A 52-year-old shoe store owner became irritable and irascible. He was argumentative with his family and employees, and summarily dismissed two of his sales clerks because they did not place bills in the cash register with faces looking to the left. His wife insisted that he consult his physician. He did so reluctantly. He was examined briefly and received a diagnosis of "male climacteric" syndrome. He was referred to a local mental health center, but did not keep his appointment. His erratic, impulsive behavior continued for several more weeks. He then developed a severe headache and had a grand mal seizure. He was placed in the hospital, where computerized axial tomography of the head revealed a large mass in the left frontal lobe of the brain. Despite cobalt therapy, the patient's condition deteriorated, and he died 6 months after the diagnosis. An autopsy revealed a large grade 3 astrocytoma of the left frontal lobe, with invasion of the corpus callosum.

When the onset of psychiatric symptoms is unrelated to situational factors and the course is progressive, the physician should weigh the possibility of a brain tumor. This, coupled with a detailed neurological history and examination including a funduscopic examination, is essential. A high level of awareness is most important.

Pancreatic Carcinoma

This cancer occurs in males three times as often as in females. It usually occurs between ages 50 and 70. Early symptoms may be upper abdominal pain that radiates to the back, jaundice if the lesion is in the head of the pancreas, weight loss, and weakness. However, these symptoms may be preceded by severe depression, with feelings of imminent doom. The incidence of depression with carcinoma of the pancreas is much higher than that of the depression that sometimes occurs with other types of cancer.[12] The reason for this high occurrence of depression is unknown. Since this disease occurs in an age group that has a high incidence of depression, the physician must be especially wary of a carcinoma of the pancreas in older men who become depressed. Although the depressive symptoms are severe, there is usually little associated guilt, and a premorbid psychiatric history is most often free of specific symptoms.

Pheochromocytoma

This is usually a benign tumor of the adrenal medulla, although it is a carcinoma in about 10 percent of the cases. The tumor secretes increased quantities of epinephrine. Sustained or paroxysmal hypertension occurs. When the secretion of epinephrine is paroxysmal (in about half of the cases), the syndrome produced is characterized by severe anxiety, sweating, pallor, and a severe, throbbing generalized headache. The patient is usually unable to function during an attack, and many cases are misconstrued as an acute anxiety state. Normal physical findings between paroxysms and the erroneous development of "psychodynamics" to explain the etiology of an anxiety state often discourage further studies. Appropriate treatment is the surgical removal of the tumor. This is curative, unless the tumor is malignant and metastatic spread has occurred.

NEUROLOGIC DISEASES

There are a number of neurologic conditions that occasionally may be confused with psychiatric syndromes (see Table 14-4). Early symptoms of *myasthenia gravis,* with easy fatigability, listlessness, and irritability may be considered as

Table 14-4 Neurologic Diseases

Disease	Common symptoms	Misleading signs	May be misdiagnosed as
Myasthenia gravis	Muscle weakness, fatigability	Listlessness, irritability	Depression
Peripheral neuropathy	Paresthesias, numbness	Vague history	Hypochondriasis
Chronic organic brain syndrome	Insidious personality change, social withdrawal	Fatigue, weight loss	Depression
Normal pressure hydrocephalus	Confusion, memory loss, ataxia	Depressive affect	Depression
Multiple sclerosis	Motor and sensory loss, speech and visual symptoms	Euphoria, labile mood	Hysteria

being of neurotic or depressive origin. *Peripheral neuropathies,* with vague paresthesias and nonspecific history, may also be considered neurotic. A common diagnostic mistake involves the various *chronic organic brain syndromes.* Many forms of dementia present with vague personality changes that can mislead the clinician. Many patients who suffer from progressive and gradual loss of brain function will be depressed; consequently, the early diagnosis of depression is often made before the underlying organic brain disease is noted. Sometimes treatment for depression is initiated, and accentuates the symptoms of dementia.

A 62-year-old podiatrist was seen in psychiatric consultation, with the chief complaint of progressive depression of about 1 year's duration. He had felt sad and lethargic, and had lost interest in his work and avocations. His wife reported that he ate poorly and had lost weight. He had been impotent for several months. During examination, he appeared depressed, spoke little, and moved slowly. He was admitted to the psychiatric unit for observation. It was noted that he refused involvement with unit activities and slept much of the time. The mental status examination and psychometric studies revealed deficiencies that were felt to be compatible with retarded depression. Electroconvulsive therapy was begun. The patient became inordinately confused after five treatments, and they were discontinued. Although he improved gradually in subsequent weeks, it became apparent that the primary problem was dementia. Computerized axial tomography of the head revealed a dilated ventricular system compatible with a loss of brain tissue. The patient was transferred to a nursing home for continued supportive care.

Normal Pressure Hydrocephalus

Adams et al. reported this treatable type of dementia in 1965.[13] Patients with this problem have enlarged ventricles of the brain, and normal cerebrospinal fluid pressure. The syndrome is characterized by progressive dementia not unlike the course of senile dementia. It occurs in middle or late life, and is often associated with and treated as depression. It is thought to be secondary to an obstruction to the absorbtion of spinal fluid. Although unusual, the condition should be suspected in cases of early dementia and depression. Neurosurgical shunting of the cerebrospinal fluid from the ventricular space to either the atrium or peritoneal space has been successful in alleviating signs of this illness.

Multiple Sclerosis

This disease of unknown etiology has a lower incidence in warmer climates. The age distribution of the disease follows a normal distribution, with a mean between 20 and 35 years. The disease is characterized by remissions and exacerbations, with diffuse or spotty demyelinization of white matter in the central nervous system. There is no classic form of the disease. Early symptoms may be minor, and may involve any portion of nervous system function. About half of the patients with multiple sclerosis have mental disturbances. Feelings of euphoria and instability of mood are often reported. These changes may be secondary to the plaques of demyelinization commonly found in the white matter surrounding the laternal ventricles in the frontal lobe of the brain. Anxiety is often present, and when neurological symptoms affect gait, vision, and speech, a secondary depression may become prominent. Rarely, a form of dementia may occur early in the course of illness. The diagnosis is often difficult. There are no specific diagnostic tests for the illness. Observation for months or even years may be necessary to be certain of the diagnosis. The fleeting nature of the symptoms, and the bizarre aspect of some of the neurological findings, particularly in young adults, make the differential diagnosis from conversion reaction most difficult early in the course of the disease. The euphoria that is often noted may be taken for the *la belle indifference* of hysteria.

CONNECTIVE TISSUE DISEASE

Lupus Erythematosus

This condition primarily affects young women and involves multiple organ systems. Cardiovascular, genitourinary, and central nervous system involvement contributes to a panoply of symptoms. The illness occasionally begins with a confusional state that may be mistaken for a thought disorder. The toxic psychosis associated with the disease may occur at any stage of the illness, and produces a variable psychiatric picture. Usually the patient is disoriented and excited, but emotional lability and desultory thinking may be present. This syndrome highlights the necessity for a high level of awareness by the diagnostician. A careful assessment of organ systems other than the central nervous system usually leads to a correct diagnosis. Corticosteroid therapy is the treatment of choice for the disease.

SUMMARY

In these diseases, the underlying physical disease is disguised or hidden by emotional symptoms. Fortunately, most of these conditions are uncommon, but in all instances a correct diagnosis is essential for appropriate therapy. The physician must be especially wary of the possible existence of such primary physical disease when evaluating patients who at first appear to have primarily psychiatric symptoms. Medical evaluation is important in all instances. Awareness should extend to all patients who are seen in evaluation, consultation, or in liaison psychiatry. There may be clues to alert an astute examiner that the basic problem is physical, but a high level of suspicion is essential in order to avoid a diagnostic pitfall.

REFERENCES

1 Peterson, Herbert W., Jr., and Maurice J. Martin: "Organic Disease Presenting as a Psychiatric Syndrome," *Postgrad. Med.,* **54**:78–84, August 1973.

2 Szyrynski, Victor: "Some Psychiatric Syndromes in Internal Medicine," *Psychosomatics,* **2**:1–4, March–April 1961.

3 Asher, R.: "Myxoedematous Madness," *Brit. Med. J.,* **2**:555–562, September 10, 1949.

4 Reilly, Edward L., and William P. Wilson: "Mental Symptoms in Hyperparathyroidism," *Dis. Nerv. Syst.,* **26**:361–363, June 1965.

5 Kolb, Lawrence C.: *Modern Clinical Psychiatry,* Philadelphia: W. B. Saunders, 1977, p. 338.

6 Shulman, Ralph: "Psychiatric Aspects of Pernicious Anemia: A Prospective Controlled Investigation," *Brit. Med. J.,* **3**:266–270, July 29, 1967.

7 Preu, Paul W., and Arthur J. Geiger: "Symptomatic Psychoses in Pernicious Anemia," *Ann. Int. Med.,* **9**:766–778, December 1935.

8 Wiebers, David O. et al.: "The Ophthalmologic Manifestations of Wilson's Disease," *Mayo Clinic Proceedings,* **52**:409–416, July 1977.

9 Mersky, H., and J. M. Woodforde: "Psychiatric Sequelae of Minor Head Injury," *Brain,* **95**:521–528, 1972.

10 Horton, Paul C.: "Personality Disorder and Parietal Lobe Dysfunction," *Am. J. Psychiat.,* **133**:782–785, July 1976.

11 Mulder, Donald W.: "Organic Brain Syndromes Associated with Intracranial Neoplasms," in Alfred M. Freedman et al. (eds.), *Comprehensive Textbook of Psychiatry II,* Baltimore: Williams and Wilkins, 1975, p. 1135.

12 Fras, Ivan et al.: "Mental Symptoms as an Aid in the Early Diagnosis of Carcinoma of the Pancreas," *Gastroenterology,* **55**:191–198, August 1968.

13 Adams, R. D. et al.: "Symptomatic Occult Hydrocephalus with Normal Cerebrospinal-Fluid Pressure: A Treatable Syndrome," *N. Eng. J. Med.,* **273**:117–126, July 15, 1965.

Chapter 15

Chronic Pain
and Its Management

Wilbert E. Fordyce, Ph.D.
Jo Ann Brockway, Ph.D.

EDITORS' INTRODUCTION

What is it like to have chronic abdominal pain for which no physical cause
can be found and no further treatment suggested? What concerns, worries,
and fantasies does this situation precipitate? How does the feeling of
helplessness, coupled with no hope for relief of the pain, affect one's mood,
job performance, relationships within the family, and hope for the future?
Do these feelings cloud joyful moments? What is it like to have chronic
sacroiliac pain, which flairs up whenever one plays tennis, and have to accept that playing tennis is probably a thing of the past and that one will
have to do what the physician said—"Just adjust to it and take long walks
instead." To be told that there is no physical reason for the pain often offers
little, if any, solace Patients may feel that there must be something wrong
and that it has to be serious since the physician cannot find a cause; or,
worse yet, that perhaps the physician knows and is unwilling to disclose
that the disease is so serious.

The physician's role, too, is indeed difficult. How frustrated many
physicians feel when patients persistently demand that the physician do

something about their chronic pain, for which no specific etiology can be found, and for which no treatment seems to suffice. The authenticity of medicine as a profession may seem to be in question, no less than the physician's ability to cure.

Regretfully, too many physicians have feelings bordering on omnipotence and omniscience, and the frustration of being unable to deal successfully with chronic pain may be disturbing to them as well as destructive to the patient. Physicians may have their alternatives, their "outs"—they may label the patient a "crock" or hypochondriac or use a stigmatizing psychiatric term. Because of such concerns, the physician may retreat from the doctor-patient relationship, and however subtly this is done, such a change in the physician is perceived at some level by the patient, who may then become more anxious, frightened, or demanding. The discord in the physician-patient relationship may thus escalate and the relationship may terminate with mutual anger and blame.

Most experienced clinicians will have been called upon to deal with chronic pain; the future physician will have to learn to deal with it. But both the physician and the physician-to-be might do well to reexamine how they react to difficult conditions that have no easy solution. They might reflect on how the patient with chronic pain feels when he or she is told that there is no basis for the pain and that nothing further can be done. What is it like to know that one has cervical degeneration which is progressive and which, for some reason, has not been "cured" by two laminectomies? How does it feel to have intractable pain that is related to a terminal illness, and especially, to feel alone with this pain when the physician is conservative about the use of analgesics? The physician should always be a student who treats the patient empathically, humanely, and wisely.

It is hoped that this chapter will enable physicians to look at pain in a broader perspective, and thus help the patient better, with resulting gratification for the physician. This chapter by Fordyce and Brockway, two authorities from one of the pioneer pain clinics in the world, provides a basic philosophy and a clear picture of the treatment of chronic pain today.

INTRODUCTION

Pain is a multifaceted phenomenon that has been approached from many different points of view. To the neurophysiologist, it may be seen as the firing of a particular kind of nerve ending in response to stimulation, or the transmission of specific spatial patterns of nerve impulses. To the biochemist, pain may represent metabolic changes in the cell membranes, while the experimental psychologist may view pain as a threshold of sensation. The medical practitioner may see it as an indication of tissue damage or as a nagging and difficult problem. To the patient, pain may be an unpleasant physical sensation, an anxiety-evoking event, or a cause for despair.

What then is pain? Numerous authors have made reference to the puzzling complexities of pain and the difficulties in defining it.[1,2] Most definitions refer to some physiological component of pain, yet pain is more than a physiological stimulus. Weisenberg wrote of pain: "In some respects it is a sensation, and in other respects it is an emotional-motivational phenomenon that leads to escape and avoidance behavior."[1] Any definition of pain, particularly of clinical pain, must also include some reference to emotional or behavioral aspects of pain. Sternbach has stated, "The word 'pain' is an abstraction we use to refer to different feelings which have little in common except the quality of physical hurt . . . the injured or affected locus, i.e., the apparent source of the pain, . . . a class of behaviors which operate to protect the organism from harm or to enlist aid in effecting relief."[3] (pp. 1-2) While this definition takes note of sensory, physiological, and behavioral aspects of pain, it still does not begin to reflect the complexities of the pain experience. Nor does any other definition.

Most authors [4,5,6] believe that there is no dependable relationship between the extent of physical injury and the pain experience. Pain is influenced by situational stimuli and prior experience. Beecher's report comparing requests for narcotics for pain relief for wounds suffered on the battlefield with similar requests for narcotics for comparable surgical wounds in a hospital illustrates this point clearly. He found that only 25 percent of the men who had been wounded on the battlefield requested narcotics, while over 80 percent of the hospital patients wanted such medication. He attributed the difference to the significance of the wound. While the injured person was in the hospital in civilian life, the wound was threatening; on the battlefield it meant a ticket to safety.[4]

Pain is related to emotional state. It increases with anxiety and may also be influenced by expectancy. Beecher[7] reported that clinical pain can be decreased with placebo in about 35 percent of the cases. Cognitive variables such as instruction and advance patient preparation have resulted in patients' making fewer requests for postoperative narcotics.[8]

Numerous other variables have been reported to influence pain perception. This chapter will not delve in detail into the many variables that may contribute to the pain experience. The reader wishing to pursue this may begin with the reviews of Weisenberg[1] or Clark et al.[9] This chapter will focus on pain as experienced by patients with chronic pain problems, and on the management of such pain. Pain will be discussed from a behavioral perspective, i.e., as behavior which is influenced by situational stimuli and the prior experience of the individual, as well as by physiological stimulation. The process of acquiring chronic pain will be presented from a learning model point of view, including the contribution of the health-care system to the acquisition of chronic pain problems. Finally, techniques for the management of pain will be discussed.

PAIN AS BEHAVIOR

Pain can be conceptualized as behavior. In order for patients to communicate that they are in pain, they must behave in a certain way. Except in rare circumstances, the neurophysiological or biochemical events that may be part of the pain experience cannot be seen. While one may be able to view tissue damage, it is the total verbal, emotional, and psychomotor behavior of the patient that communicates to the environment, intentionally or not, the presence of pain.

The patient may signal the experience of pain verbally by describing the location, intensity, or quality of the pain, or by moaning or sighing. The patient may also communicate pain by nonverbal means such as limping, grimacing, or massaging the painful body part. The behavior serves simultaneously as a signal to the environment that the patient is in pain, and a stimulus that elicits some action from the environment. Behavior may elicit medication from the physician, indicate to the spouse that sex is out of the question tonight, or communicate to the boss that the patient cannot perform the job effectively. Without the behavior, there would be no pain problem clinically, but only a private and personal sensation with no outward sign.

Pain as behavior is subject to the laws of learning and conditioning, as are other behaviors. A brief discussion of learning principles will be provided here. More thorough treatments of the learning principles can be found elsewhere.[10,11,12]

Learning

Learning occurs when the conditions are right, that is, when systematic behavior-consequence sequences occur. It is important to differentiate between operant and respondent behavior. *Respondent behavior* occurs in response to specific stimulus situations; that is, a respondent behavior occurs automatically when the stimulus is adequate, or the behavior *responds* to the stimulus. Respondent pain behavior can, therefore, be said to be controlled by antecedent nociceptive stimuli. *Operant behaviors,* too, can be elicited by specific stimuli, but are influenced additionally by their outcomes. An operant that is systematically positively reinforced, that is, is systematically followed by a positive outcome, is likely to occur more frequently in the future. An operant that is systematically followed by a neutral or negative consequence, that is, extinguished or punished, respectively, is likely to occur less frequently in the future. Operant pain behavior, then, can be said to have come under the control of environmental contingencies. More importantly, this process occurs automatically when there are contingent relationships between behavior and reinforcement.

Examples of operant and respondent pain behaviors should serve to illustrate these points. A child puts one hand on a hot stove and quickly draws it away. The removal of the hand from the stove is respondent behavior; it is controlled by the nociceptive stimulus of the hot stove's burning the hand. In contrast to this example, consider what happens when the same child has fallen on the sidewalk and skinned one knee. The child begins to cry and immediately his or her parent, who has been busy and not paying attention, is at the child's side and giving him or her a hug. Later the child falls on the grass and does not skin a knee. Nevertheless, crying is begun and is rewarded by the parent's attention. The crying in this case is an operant, in that it was followed by positive consequences (was positively reinforced), and came to occur again without the original nociceptive stimulus.

ACUTE VERSUS CHRONIC PAIN

It is important to differentiate acute from chronic pain. Pain of an acute nature, perhaps from a sprained ankle, a broken arm, a burn, or a toothache, is most often the result of actual or impending tissue damage. Generally with such a pain problem, the person with the problem seeks professional advice and follows it, and the pain is relieved. Chronic pain usually begins with an acute episode, such as an illness or injury. Typically professional advice is sought, evaluation procedures are performed, and treatment is instituted. Such action is intended to lead to a resolution of the problem; however, the pain persists.

The Experience of Chronic Pain

The experience of chronic pain is different from that of acute pain. The patient with acute pain experiences increasing anxiety as pain intensity increases. Sternbach[3] describes the experience as follows. First, there may be some uncomfortable feelings or twinges that may barely be noted. As the pain increases and the individual becomes aware of it, he or she is likely to experience mild anxiety. The individual then imposes a cognitive structure on the pain, a label such as "I've probably strained a muscle." With such an understanding of the pain, the anxiety decreases. If the pain becomes still more intense, the individual may become more alarmed. The patient fears that something is very wrong, and also that the pain will reach an intolerable level.

With chronic pain the experience is different. Anxiety is replaced by despair. The patient feels worn down by what is perceived as nearly constant pain, and insomnia night after night. Hopelessness and frustration are felt, and suffering is seen as endless. Examination after examination and treatment after treatment have yielded no relief. The patient may often be angry because a physician or family member has suggested that the pain is "not real." He or she may experience the despair expressed by one patient who said tearfully, "How much should one person have to take?"

Notwithstanding the above discussion, it is important to recognize that what the patient feels is *pain*. Whether the chronic pain is respondent to the initial stimulus or has become primarily a problem of operant pain, the patient feels it as pain.

The Effects of Chronicity

Chronicity is important in that it provides the opportunity for changes in behavior sequences, that is, changes in habit patterns, to occur around the patient's pain problem. This is inevitable with chronicity. While acute pain problems may cause temporary disruption in the daily activities of the patient and family, with chronicity these disruptions become systematic changes in behavior. For example, a person with influenza does not go to work for a few days, but the laborer with chronic back pain may have to search for a new source of livelihood. Similarly, the family of the person with a broken arm may take over some of the household responsibilities for several weeks, while the family of the patient with chronic pain may have to assume those household responsibilities for months or years.

With chronicity, certain skills may be diminished. The individual who has restricted social activity as a result of pain may become ill at ease socially when attempting to reestablish social interactions. Also, after months or years of a narrow existence focused on pain, he or she may have few topics of conversation other than pain. The patient who has had chronic pain may find difficulty in obtaining employment, because employers are wary of hiring someone who has been unemployed for a long period of time, especially one who has a history of a chronic pain problem.

There is another aspect of chronicity alluded to above which needs to be recognized. Most people think of pain as a warning signal. When pain is experienced, the prudent action to take is essentially protective, to remove oneself from the noxious stimulus or to minimize its effects by stopping the activity that elicited the pain. When an ankle is sprained, one attempts to walk on it gingerly, but stops if there is a sharp increase in pain. The warning function of pain is nearly always an accurate and useful one during the early stages in the life of a pain problem. Several months and even years later, however, when the pain problem has persisted into chronicity, it often appears that the experience of pain no longer has that warning function. The healing process usually takes only a few weeks, or a few months at most. The exceptions are few. When the pain persists and is increased by activity, it does not necessarily mean that continuation of an activity will either do further tissue damage or worsen the pain problem. But the patient does not know that. He or she makes the mistake of thinking that the pain signal means to stop, because to fail to do so will make the problem worse. Thus, the patient is likely to stop activity when pain is experienced, which often results in less and less activity as time goes on. This has the ultimate effect of a physical deconditioning process, so that the patient experiences discomfort even with very little exertion.

The effect of the conditioning process is illustrated by the observation that many chronic pain patients do not show the full flower of autonomic signs that typically accompany expression of pain behaviors in acute pain problems. The recently injured patient perspires, has tachycardia, rapid breathing, etc., particularly when being examined and put through body motions that are likely to increase the pain.

In contrast, often the chronic pain patient is found to display only vestiges of those autonomic responses when put through examination procedures that are likely to increase pain. The facial grimaces, the guarded motions, the verbalizations (all operants) remain much as they have through the life of the pain problem. But the flushing or blanching of the skin, the tachycardia, rapid breathing, increased perspiration, etc., now occur only very slightly or not at all. Thus, there is a separation of autonomic responses from pain-related behavior.

The reason for this appears to be that autonomically mediated pain behaviors are less readily conditioned, that is, are less likely to come under control of contingent environmental reinforcement than are striated muscle mediated motor actions (verbal and nonverbal), which make up the rest of the pain behavior repertoire. With chronicity there is a differential conditioning effect favoring voluntary muscle mediated behaviors.

Similarly, verbal behavior and nonverbal behavior are separate and may be differentially reinforced so that what the patient says about the pain, and what the patient does, may be quite different. The patient may, for example, claim to be incapable of sitting for more than 20 minutes at a time, yet may sit watching a televised sports event for several hours without standing up. Similarly, the patient may state that he or she rarely takes medication; "I put off taking it as long as I can," or "I wait until the pain becomes unbearable before I take a pill," yet the patient may be asking repeatedly for additional medication. These inconsistencies between verbal report and patient behavior may lead the physician and often the patient's family to consider the patient dishonest, a malingerer, or "a crock." This is unfortunate, since these feelings are likely to be communicated to the patient.

The physician is faced with the decision as to whether the patient with chronic pain is suffering primarily from chronic operant pain, chronic respondent pain, or a combination of both. If the patient's pain is understood as primarily respondent, the principles to be described for the management of operant pain may still be used to great advantage. The pain and its associated disability may be diminished by treatment that is based on the physician's understanding of the pain behavior-consequence sequences.

In the management of the patient for whom chronic pain is clearly respondent to underlying, severe disease, other treatment modalities are useful. The importance of a trusting and collaborative doctor-patient relationship may be crucial. As a result of this relationship, which is essentially one of a supportive psychotherapeutic nature, the patient may come to feel less alone and despairing. The knowledge that the physician understands what the patient is experiencing is frequently what offers the patient much-needed hope.

The skillful use of analgesics is important. They should be prescribed on a time-contingent basis rather than at the patient's request. As Cassell points out (Chapter 30) in regard to the management of the dying patient, it is important for the patient to feel that symptoms are controllable. Many physicians, even in dealing with patients with severe disease or impending death, are reluctant to precribe adequate analgesics. It is as if suffering pain that is clearly related to underlying disease is preferable to becoming dependent upon analgesics, even in situations where life expectancy is short.

Patients with chronic respondent pain may be helped by other treatment techniques. Biofeedback approaches, which aim at increasing the patient's voluntary control over circumscribed muscle spasm or blood flow, are helpful to some.

Hypnosis may offer some patients significant relief. The essential issue is that physicians dealing with patients who have severe, chronic respondent pain can be pluralistic in their approach to treatment. The principles to be described for the management of operant pain often have applicability, and the physician should keep in mind the importance of his or her relationship with the patient, the appropriate use of analgesics, and such special procedures as biofeedback and hypnosis.

In order to consider all available treatment options, the physician must examine whether his or her model of pain does not preclude the use of some helpful techniques.

DISEASE MODEL OF PAIN

Traditionally, the medical model concept of disease has been applied to problems of pain. From the perspective of the *disease model* (Figure 15-1) discussed by Fordyce[13] and by Fordyce et al.,[14,15] the symptoms that the patient exhibits arise from an underlying pathological condition. Treatment then is aimed at eradicating the underlying pathological condition. The symptoms *per se* are not treated directly; the notion is that when one is rid of the pathology, the symptoms will disappear. In the case of a pain problem, the medical practitioner evaluates the patient's symptoms and makes a diagnosis identifying the underlying cause. Treatment, whether it be medications, bed rest, or surgery, is aimed at eradicating this etiological factor in order to eliminate the pain. A problem arises, however, when either the diagnostic process fails to identify an etiologic agent to account for the symptom of pain, or when, as sometimes occurs, the treatment or series of treatments designed to eliminate the underlying pathology fails to be effective in relieving the pain. Under those circumstances, particularly after a number of practitioners and treatments have been tried with little success, the patient is often referred to another treatment system, which is also based tradi-

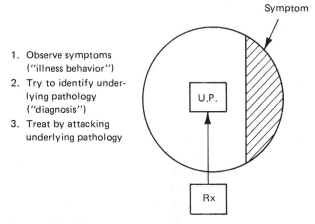

1. Observe symptoms ("illness behavior")
2. Try to identify underlying pathology ("diagnosis")
3. Treat by attacking underlying pathology

Symptom

U.P.

Rx

Figure 15-1   Disease model

tionally on the disease model. In this conceptual framework, the symptoms of the patient are referred to as psychogenic, hysterical, or psychosomatic. Here the etiologic factor causing the pain problem is considered to be not an organic pathology, but rather a personality, motivational, or emotional disorder. The conceptual model is still the same, however, for it holds that if one could treat the underlying emotional disturbance, via psychotherapy for example, pain symptoms would be eliminated.

Limitations of the Disease Model

Although the disease model continues to be a valuable perspective for the evaluation and treatment of illness, and works well for acute pain problems, it has many limitations with respect to chronic operant pain; and the longer the pain problem has persisted, the less likely it is that the disease model perspective will suffice. The first limitation relates to the notion that symptoms are controlled by underlying pathology. Earlier it was noted that symptoms, or pain behaviors, are influenced by any number of situational stimuli and prior experiences, as well as by conditioning and learning. Thus, in patients with a chronic pain problem, the behaviors or symptoms on which the physician bases diagnoses, and presumably the treatment, are not directly controlled by an etiologic factor, but have been modified to an unknown extent by the patient's environment. Thus, the expression of certain symptoms may or may not reflect a particular pathogenic problem. For the physician, the decision regarding the extent to which the chronic pain has been modified by the responses of the patient's environment is crucial for determining the nature of the treatment program.

A second limitation of the disease model relates to the concept of psychogenic pain, and the use of psychotherapy as a treatment. The effectiveness of treatment that is based on the disease model concept of psychogenic pain will not be argued here. It is certainly not denied that many pain patients do have significant emotional or personality difficulties relating closely to their pain problems. The main point to be made here is that referring the patient with chronic, operant pain for psychotherapy may not be useful. To begin with, some patients will not follow through with the referral. Of those who do, many drop out early in the process, while many others continue "because my doctor told me to," and do not invest themselves in the treatment. And of those who do persist diligently, psychotherapy may not prove, by itself, to be sufficient to bring about resolution of the problem and a reduction of pain-related symptoms.

A third related problem, when one is committed to looking for an underlying pathology to explain the pain and guide treatment, appears when the physician takes the position that pain is either "real" (that is, underlying organic pathology) or "imaginary" (that is, psychogenic conversion reactions, which are often based on the absence of convincing physical findings rather than on the presence of something). A referral for psychotherapy may communicate to some patients that the physician feels that their pain is not "real." This suggestion is resented by the patient, and is seen as a challenge to the authenticity of the pain. The patient is forced, as he or she sees it, to prove the hurt is real, and is likely to increase efforts to authenticate the extent of the pain problem by increased displays of pain, more demand for medication, or yet another treatment event. That puts the patient at additional risk that someone will attempt surgery for a problem that may be essentially operant in nature, or will prescribe pain medications too freely. Another unfortunate consequence of this problem is that the patient often becomes embittered toward physicians, thereby making it increasingly difficult to elicit cooperation and active participation in treatment.

A fourth limitation of the disease model as a sole approach to chronic pain is that it obscures other perspectives that might lead to effective methods of managing problems. When the patient continues to hurt after resolution of the acute problem, something is wrong. It is not helpful at this point to ask "Is the pain real?" Ask, rather, "What is causing the pain problem to continue?" The answer is likely to be some mixture of residual noxious stimulation, plus reinforcement of pain behavior by the environment. Looking for an underlying pathology, whether it be organic or a personality disorder, minimizes the importance of the patient's environment in interacting with the patient and the pain problem. Often chronic pain can be accounted for and understood in terms of relationships between the patient's behavior and the environmental contingencies. Such a point of view, the *learning model approach* to pain, leads to systematic methods for managing the problems of chronic pain.

LEARNING MODEL OF PAIN

The learning model approach to pain is illustrated in Figure 15-2. From the perspective of a learning model approach, one observes symptoms, or pain behaviors, that indicate to the observer that the patient has a pain problem. The necessary step then is to identify the circumstances under which pain behaviors occur, and their consequences. The assumption is that contingency arrangements between the patient's pain behaviors and the environment, whether it be family, work, or health-care system, can maintain and aggravate pain problems and may be doing so now.

1. Observe "illness behavior" (symptom)
2. Identify "illness behavior" — consequence relationships
3. Change behavior by principles of learning

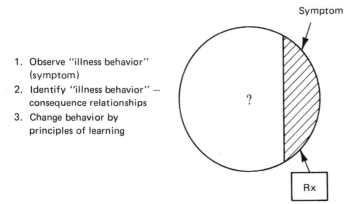

Figure 15-2   Learning model

Whereas from the disease model perspective the symptoms are seen as signs of the pain problem, from a learning model point of view they are seen as the problem itself, and as such are treated directly. Treatment involves the use of learning principles to rearrange the contingencies between the patient's behavior and the environment, so that the patient decreases the frequency with which symptoms, or pain behaviors, are exhibited, and increases the frequency with which healthy or well behaviors are shown.

DEPRESSION AND PAIN

A discussion of depression and pain seems appropriate at this point. A number of authors, such as Merskey and Spear,[16] have noted the frequent association of depression and pain in patients. Depressed patients frequently complain of pain problems, and most chronic pain patients are depressed. It is often quite difficult to distinguish whether pain or depression is the primary problem. Depression is often mislabelled as pain by the patient, spouse, or family doctor.

A psychologic or psychiatric evaluation might help to resolve the issue. If depression is the major problem, it should be treated appropriately. Treatment should include increasing activity levels and encouraging pursuits which engage the patient's attention.

The depression seen in chronic pain patients may also be attributable to the lack of reinforcers. Patients with chronic pain tend to do little, and accordingly they receive few positive reinforcers and tend to engage in few activities that become positively reinforcing in themselves. When this is the case, increasing the patient's level of activity and widening the patient's range of activities may provide sufficient reinforcements to alleviate the depression.

Depression, which is a sequela of chronic pain, is usually a self-resolving problem. It would be a mistake to assume that one must first alleviate the depression before undertaking treatment that is designed to diminish pain behaviors and increase activity and well behaviors. The operant-based strategies for increasing activities and well behaviors are part of the treatment of the depression and may be augmented by other treatment modalities.

ACQUISITION OF OPERANT PAIN

The acquisition of operant pain requires only that pain behaviors be reinforced systematically by the environment. Given the right reinforcements, such conditioning occurs automatically, without any attempt on the part of the patient to prolong the pain problem. The pain behavior occurs, signals to the environment that the patient hurts, and is reinforced by the patient's environment, family, friends, coworkers, and the health-care system.

Direct Reinforcers

Pain behaviors are often reinforced directly by the environment. The family may be particularly solicitous of a patient with an acute pain problem. The spouse, for example, may be especially attentive. The spouse might massage the patient's leg when the patient complains of leg pain, or perhaps give up outside activities to stay home more often. As chronicity occurs, there is ample time for the systematic pain-behavior reinforcement sequences to occur, for example, sequences of complaint of pain followed by an attentive response. A frequently occurring example is the female patient whose husband rarely displays overt affection or praises her activities, yet may rub her back when it hurts, or makes her comfortable on the couch and stand by attentively.

Rest may be a reinforcer for pain behavior. The patient with pain may find that activity leads to discomfort, and rest eases that discomfort. Thus, lying down or resting leads to increased comfort; or stated another way, the increase in comfort positively reinforces lying down or resting behavior, thereby assuring that it will occur more frequently in the future.

The examples represent sequences wherein activity is replaced by inactivity, and well-intentioned measures paradoxically increase pain.

Indirect Reinforcers

Pain behaviors are frequently reinforced indirectly by enabling the patient to avoid or have "time out" from difficult, stressful, or physically tiring situations. A complaint of pain may be followed by time out from disciplining children, going to work, engaging in sexual intercourse, arguing over the budget, or washing the windows.

This is frequently seen in either male or female patients who have, prior to injury, experienced some change in their vocational situation, such as a promotion or a move to another plant, which has resulted in increased stress for the patient. Avoidance of the stressful work situation may be a potent reinforcer of pain behavior. A similar situation is often seen in the older patients who have suffered a stroke or other cerebral dysfunction, and who are no longer able to function as well intellectually. Pain may provide time out from activities, such as bridge or conversation, which may be quite taxing and which threaten to reveal intellectual deficits.

Similarly, the development of certain pain behaviors, such as a limp or an unusual body posture, may be reinforced indirectly by the avoidance of discomfort. Initially, the patient may limp or assume the unusual posture as a protective mechanism that allows walking, standing, or sitting without discomfort. As chronicity occurs, the behavior may continue long after the original noxious stimulus has been resolved.

Punishment of Well Behavior

The systematic punishment of well behavior, as well as the reinforcement of pain behavior, leads to the acquisition of operant pain. The patient who has done little, but momentarily "feels better" and attempts to "do something useful," may find that pain follows the effort at activity, possibly because the patient has attempted to work for too long a time, or has attempted work that was too strenuous, considering the preceding extended period of inactivity.

Family and friends may do their part to punish well behavior. They may insist upon limitations to activity, and may sharply admonish the patient who attempts to perform beyond these limits. The spouse may tell the patient to rest when he or she attempts to help with the dishes. At the least, the spouse may simply ignore or respond neutrally to well behavior, thereby promoting extinction of the behavior.

The Health-Care System and Chronic Pain

The nature of the health-care system contributes to the development and maintenance of chronic operant pain problems. Traditional medical management is largely illness-contingent and, as such, often provides systematic reinforcement for pain behavior. Physician attention can be a powerful reinforcer, and it is most often contingent upon patient displays of pain or illness. Physician attention is a potent reinforcer in several ways. First, the physician may provide the concern for, understanding of, or interest in the patient that is not provided by the patient's family or friends. A second way relates to the long-standing pain problem. At some point, someone is likely to have suggested to the patient that the pain problem is "psychogenic," or some variation thereof, thus challenging the authenticity of the patient's pain. Continued contact with a physician may represent validation of the pain problem to the patient.

There are other ways in which the physician may unwillingly punish, or at least not reinforce, well behavior. During the examination, the physician is not only likely to focus on pain complaints, but may be neutral or nonresponsive to patient statements about engaging in activity. Should the patient feel quite well, the physician is likely to discharge that individual from care, and suggest that since the patient is doing so well, there is no need for further contact unless the patient develops some other problem.

Medication may be a direct reinforcer of pain behavior, the management of which may contribute to the maintenance of the pain problem. Many patients with chronic pain problems are habituated or addicted to pain medications. Medications are often prescribed *prn*, or on a "take only as needed" basis. The effects of the medication, be it pain reduction, anxiety alleviation, or whatever, are then made contingent on the patient's display of pain. As a patient becomes habituated or addicted, pain behaviors will continue to be displayed, even though the original noxious stimulus has been resolved.

Prescriptions for activity and rest may also serve to maintain pain behavior beyond the resolution of the original stimulus. The physician is likely to tell the patient, "Take it easy until the pain is gone," or "Do what you can, and if it hurts, stop and rest." Taking it "easy" may serve as a physician-prescribed time out from unpleasant activity and, as such, reinforce the pain behavior. The "do what you can" or work-to-tolerance prescription allows the punishment of well behavior as well as the reinforcement of pain behavior. Activity is followed by discomfort (punishment), and rest is followed by decreased pain (positive reinforcement).

PAIN MANAGEMENT

The difficulties that the physician may experience in attempting to manage patients with chronic operant pain are well recognized. Patients with such pain are often difficult to deal with. One often finds the suspicious and embittered attitudes previously described emanating from the failure of the health-care system to accept that the patient has a "real problem." Another factor is that the physician may find that there are few alternative approaches toward pain and its management. Additionally, the physician knows that if he or she fails to respond to the patient's pain, the patient may go elsewhere, perhaps to someone with less wisdom who may perform hazardous procedures or prescribe greater quantities of medication.

For management of the patient with chronic pain, one cannot overestimate the importance of sensitivity in the early contacts to help the patient understand that you are not challenging the authenticity of the problem, but are instead bent on determining how you can be of help. Additionally, the physician who recognizes the operant nature of pain behavior should examine all interactions with the patient in terms of pain behavior-consequence sequences, and modify management of the patient appropriately to minimize reinforcement of pain behavior and to maximize reinforcement of well behavior.

Medication Management

Learning model methods have been developed for medication management.[13,17] For problems of chronic pain, except for those in which there is ample evidence of an ongoing, currently active body-damage factor (for example, the active stage of arthritis or metastatic cancer), there is no justification for, and there are objections to, continued use of injectable medication. The conditioning effects are far more potent, both pharmacologically and psychologically, for injectable medication than they are for orally-administered medication.

The physician should prescribe medication on a time-contingent, rather than pain-contingent, basis. The shift to time-contingent medications breaks the association between hurting and requesting/taking medications, thereby permitting deconditioning of the medication-related cluster of pain behaviors. It eliminates the need for pain behavior to occur in order for medication to be forthcoming. If narcotics are used, they should be prescribed for a preset, limited time. An added deconditioning advantage can be gained by incorporating the various pain medications into a single mix (known as the pain cocktail,[13,17] which then is delivered in enough masking agent (for example, cherry syrup) to total 10cc of volume for each dose.

When medication is already a serious problem, that is, when the patient is habituated or addicted to pain medication, an inpatient hospitalization is needed to deal adequately with the medication issue. The patient on injectable medication should be shifted to oral intake medication. The patient should then be observed for 2 to 3 days on a *prn* regimen to identify what medication is taken, how much, and at what time intervals. After having obtained that baseline of medication consumption, the patient can then be shifted to a time-contingent regimen. The time intervals between medication doses should not exceed those that the patient displayed during the observation period, except when the physician substitutes long-acting for fast-acting narcotics, which is usually a highly advantageous shift.

The medication is then delivered via the pain cocktail described above. The total amount of medication taken in 24 hours is the same as that observed during the baseline period. With this regimen, significant reductions in medication consumption can usually be achieved simply by reducing the active ingredients by approximately 10 percent, each week to 10 days. The patient should be informed of this regimen, except for the dates of reduction in active ingredients, prior to beginning it.

Activity and Rest

Most chronic pain patients have reduced and restricted activity levels. That is one of the more important pain behaviors and functional limitations to be addressed in treatment. For most chronic pain patients, the restricted and reduced activity level stems from anticipating that movement which produces pain will also, if continued, produce additional pain and body damage, as we discussed before. There are several simple steps which can be taken to help remedy this problem.

First of all, exercises that are selected to be appropriate to the patient's general medical status should be prescribed. The very act of prescribing the exercise program is a way of informing the patient and family it is all right to move. Next, exercise baselines should be obtained. The patient goes through the exercise program several times, with instructions to "Do as many of (this exercise) as you can before pain, weakness, or fatigue causes you to want to stop. You decide when to stop." The amounts completed are recorded for each exercise, and those numbers are then examined by the physician and therapist. Quotas are then set for each exercise, so that the patient begins by doing less than he or she was able to do during baselines, and increases the amount done of each exercise each day. This arrangement breaks up the relationship between activity and pain, so that activity is not punished by the occurrence of pain. Additionally, it ensures that pain is not reinforced by rest. Instead, rest becomes work-contingent; that is, it becomes available when a fixed amount of work or exercise has been completed. Exercise ceilings should also be determined, and when they are reached, exercises stabilize at that point. Finally, quotas are both floors and ceilings. That is, the exercise effort should not end until the quota is reached, but the quota should never be exceeded, however good the patient may feel.

Physician Attention

There are several additional ways in which the physician can maximize the reinforcement of well behavior and minimize the reinforcement of pain behavior.

First, the physician can include members of the patient's family along with the patient in a discussion of findings and recommendations for treatment. Such discussions promote patient and family understanding of, and adherence to, a graded exercise program, time-contingent medication, nonreinforcement of pain behavior, and positive reinforcement of well behavior.

In addition, the physician should focus some attention on the patient's well behavior, for example, by asking what activities the patient is engaging in, and by suggesting social reinforcement for appropriate activity. The physician might also schedule several brief follow-up visits with the patient, on a time-contingent basis. As a result of using this method, physician contact is not contingent on patient expressions of pain behavior.

The Well-Behavior Problem

One of the most important implications of viewing chronic illness and chronic pain from a learning model perspective is that the reduction of illness behaviors does not necessarily lead to a corresponding increase in well behaviors. To cite a simple example, a pain patient who reclines much of the time may have reclining reduced through treatment, but unless treatment is systematic about it, that reclining may be replaced by sitting and not by standing/walking/working. As discussed earlier, people with chronic illnesses have long been on the sidelines, and may have lost much of their ability to be effectively well. Moreover, in the case of chronic pain, it may be that pain behaviors have proven to be so reinforcing for a given patient because that patient had many problems for which pain provided effective avoidance. If, then, treatment addresses itself only to reduction of pain behaviors, and does not examine what it is the patient is going to do following treatment, there will be many short-lived treatment successes that are followed by early return to the illness role. It should be noted that this is true whether one is using behavioral methods for treatment or some other approach.

Evaluation for treatment, then, should include careful review with the patient of what it is the patient is expecting to do following treatment. These target behaviors need to be studied to ensure that the patient is able to perform them with sufficient capability and confidence to achieve the reinforcement necessary to maintain performance. If there are gaps in the patient's well-behavior repertoire, treatment should strive to remedy those. This may not be the province of the physician, but may best be done in conjunction with professionals who are trained in this area.

REFERENCES

1 Weisenberg, Matisyohu: "Pain and Pain Control," *Psychological Bulletin,* **84**:1008–1044, September 1977.
2 Melzack, Ronald: *The Puzzle of Pain,* New York: Basic Books, 1973.
3 Sternbach, Richard A.: *Pain Patients: Traits and Treatment,* New York: Academic Press, 1974.

 4 Beecher, Henry K.: "Relationship of Significance of Wound to Pain Experienced,"
    JAMA, **161**:1609–1613, August 25, 1956.

 5 Sternbach, Richard A.: *Pain: A Psychophysiological Analysis,* New York: Academic
    Press, 1968.

 6 McGlashan, Thomas H. et al.: "The Nature of Hypnotic Analgesia and Placebo
    Response to Experimental Pain," *Psychosom. Med.,* **31**:227–246, May–June 1969.

 7 Beecher, Henry K.: "The Placebo Effect as a Non-specific Force Surrounding Disease
    and the Treatment of Disease," in Rudolf Janzen et al. (eds.), *Pain: Basic Prin-
    ciples—Pharmacology—Therapy,* Baltimore: Williams and Wilkins, 1972.

 8 Egbert, Lawrence D. et al.: "Reduction of Postoperative Pain by Encouragement and
    Instruction of Patients," *New England J. Med.,* **270**:825–827, April 16, 1964.

 9 Clark, W. Crawford, and Howard F. Hunt: "Pain," in John A. Downey, and Robert
    C. Darling (eds.), *Physiological Basis of Rehabilitation Medicine,* Philadelphia:
    W. B. Saunders, 1971, pp. 373–401.

10 Skinner, B. F.: *Science and Human Behavior,* New York: Macmillan, 1953.

11 Miller, Neal: "Learning of Visceral and Glandular Responses," *Science,*
    163:434–445, January 31, 1969.

12 Krasner, Leonard, and Leonard P. Ullman: *Research in Behavior Modification,* New
    York: Holt, Rinehart and Winston, 1966.

13 Fordyce, Wilbert E.: *Behavioral Methods for Chronic Pain and Illness,* St. Louis,
    Missouri: C. V. Mosby, 1976.

14 Fordyce, Wilbert E. et al.: "Some Implications of Learning in Problems of Chronic
    Pain," *J. Chronic Dis.,* **21**:179–190, June 1968.

15 Fordyce, Wilbert E. et al.: "Operant Conditioning in the Treatment of Chronic
    Clinical Pain, *Arch. Phys. Med. and Rehabil.,* **54**:399–408, September 1973.

16 Merskey, Harold, and F. G. Spear: *Pain: Psychological and Psychiatric Aspects,*
    Baltimore: Williams and Wilkins, 1967.

17 Halpern, Lawrence M.: "Analgesics and Other Drugs for Relief of Pain," *Postgrad.
    Med.,* **53**:91–100, May 1973.

Chapter 16

Psychosomatic Disturbances

John J. Schwab, M.D.

EDITORS' INTRODUCTION

What is is like to be told that you have an ulcer in your duodenum, and according to the physician, it is mainly the result of tension? What is it like to be told that you have hypertension, though you do not feel ill, and to have your doctor tell you that if you do not change your life-style you may have a stroke? How does it feel to have severe headaches, and to be told that they are due to emotions? How must it be to have a definite physical disease, and yet be told that emotions, tension, or life-style may be an important cause? The fear and anxiety about what may happen as the result of the ulcer, hypertension, or other disease may, in turn, make the condition worse. It is easy to understand why many patients may minimize or deny their disease completely. To take the prescribed medications, to follow the physician's suggestions may only keep the whole thing on one's mind. It is easier to forget, to keep the whole thing out of one's thoughts, and perhaps find another doctor.

The physician, in turn, often leads a busy and tense life. He or she may wonder whether the instructions to patients would not seem hollow if such patients knew the details of the physician's own life. How can the physician with an ulcer or hypertension talk to a patient with a similar condition?

Even for the physician who has a life that is in better balance, many patients with psychosomatic disturbances are difficult to treat. Often the very emotions that need to be explored seem inaccessible to the patient. Often the patient seems remote and very controlled. It may be hard to understand how emotions can play a role, since they are so little in evidence. The patient's inability or unwillingness to cooperate may bother the physician. On other occasions, the physician may not feel that he or she has the time to talk at length with such patients. Referral to a psychiatrist might offend the patient and strain the doctor-patient relationship.

In the following chapter Schwab, who is both an internist and a psychiatrist, emphasizes the interworking of mind and body, elaborates theory and mechanisms, and provides useful suggestions for treatment. It is hoped that, in reading this chapter, the student or physician may become intrigued by the relationship of mind and body, and come to appreciate the pleasure and gratification that can be found in treating patients with psychosomatic disturbances.

INTRODUCTION

"Each civilization makes its own diseases. But it has many ways of doing so."[1] So said the great medical historian, Henry Sigerest. The modern American way of disease is psychosomatic. More patients seek general medical care for psychosomatic and psychophysiological disorders than for all other kinds of illnesses. About one-third of all patients complain primarily of bodily pains and dysfunctions that are intertwined with various admixtures of psychic, interpersonal, and social distress.[2] In an editorial in the *Annals of Internal Medicine,* Huth emphasizes the therapeutic challenge presented by this massive group of patients, and deplores internists' relative disinterest in psychophysiologic disorders.[3]

DEFINITIONS

What are the disturbances we label *psychosomatic* or *psychophysiologic?* In the 1930s, psychosomatic medicine developed as a field concerned mainly with seven diseases that were believed to be produced in large part by personality problems and intrapsychic conflicts. These "classic" diseases are: bronchial asthma, rheumatoid arthritis, ulcerative colitis, essential hypertension, neurodermatitis, thyrotoxicosis, and duodenal peptic ulcer. Although they are the traditional psychosomatic disorders, in reality they encompass only a small fraction of the total number of psychosomatic disturbances. Today, psychosomatic medicine must also be concerned with a broad array of psychophysiologic symptoms and conditions, including tension headaches, ill-defined chest pains, a wide number and variety of gastrointestinal dysfunctions (nervous stomach, diarrhea, constipation, etc.), backaches, and pains and other symptoms in the extremities.

About 30 years ago, James L. Halliday emphasized that broad sociocultural factors that influence child-rearing practices determine the quality of human beings' interactions with the environment, and thus are responsible for psychosocial illnesses. He developed the concept of a "psychosomatic affection" as a bodily illness produced by multiple etiological factors—a "synergy of causes."[4] The synergistic factors include: (1) assortative, not random, mating (the tendency to marry within the same social class), which results in either increasing or decreasing the size of groups with hereditary predisposition to disease, particularly coronary heart disease; (2) child-rearing practices that involve approval and disapproval during critical stages of development, precipitating the utilization of defenses and adaptations that become patterns of psychobiologic reactivity and are related to health and illness in adult life; (3) broader social forces that, for example, may account for more or less stressful employment and dietary habits associated with coronary heart disease and gastrointestinal disturbances; and (4) social mobility, with its tensions and demands for alertness that are conducive to psychophysiologic dysfunctions.

In recent years the term *psychosomatic* has fallen into disfavor. (In this chapter, the word *psychosomatic* does not refer strictly to the classic seven diseases, but instead is used in its more popular sense to cover a wide variety of bodily disorders in which social and psychologic factors are considered to have special etiologic significance.) In the *Diagnostic and Statistical Manual of Mental Disorders, Second Edition (DSM II)*, which was prepared by the American Psychiatric Association in 1968, it was replaced by the term *psychophysiological disorders,* which embraced a large number and variety of disorders "characterized by physical symptoms that are caused by emotional factors and involve a single organ system, usually under autonomic nervous system innervation. The physiological changes involved are those that normally accompany certain emotional states, but in these disorders the changes are more intense and sustained. The individual may not be consciously aware of his emotional state."[5] In the newly drafted *DSM III, psychophysiological disorders* have been redefined and categorized as *psychic factors in physical condition.* This is a classification system that, in reality, is not a diagnosis, but instead can be used to indicate the extent to which ". . . psychological factors are judged to be contributory, for a particular patient, in the initiation, exacerbation, or perpetuation of a nonmental medical disorder."[6] Also, appropriate diagnoses for this category are obesity, headache, asthma, duodenal ulcer, etc.

EPIDEMIOLOGY

Epidemiologic studies show that a staggering number of people complain of psychophysiologic symptoms. The Stirling County Study reported that 59 percent of a random sample of about 1,000 adults had psychophysiologic symptom patterns.[7] The Midtown Manhattan Study, which was conducted in the 1950s, rated about 60 percent of the 1,660 respondents as having psychophysiologic symptomatology.[8] The Florida Health Study of an entire county, which was conducted in the early 1970s, indicated that *either currently or during the preceding year* about 40 percent of the respondents reported having weight difficulties or problems with headaches, 25 to 30 percent reported various gastrointestinal symptoms (indigestion, stomach ache, or constipation); 15 percent reported asthma; and 2.4 percent reported peptic ulcer.[9]

Moreover, Tringo has found that psychosomatic disturbances are considered by Americans to be "acceptable." A random sample of respondents gave diseases such as peptic ulcer, arthritis, and asthma much more favorable acceptability ratings than diseases such as tuberculosis, carcinoma, and mental illness.[10]

WHO ARE THE ILL? THEIR SOCIODEMOGRAPHIC CHARACTERISTICS

Age-Sex-Race

Older studies showed that the frequency of psychophysiologic disorders increased steadily with advancing age. However, recent research indicates that persistent complaints of headaches, nervous stomach, and diarrhea are more common in younger than in older age groups.[9] Also, more children with bronchial asthma, ulcerative colitis, diabetes mellitus, etc., are now being brought to the attention of the medical profession, which leads to the belief that these illnesses are increasing in frequency in younger age groups. The increase may be more apparent than real: it may be the result of greater awareness and improved medical care. Let us hope so, for if the increase is real, it forbodes a general increase in the occurrence of these diseases in the future. One of the maxims of epidemiology is that an increase in the frequency of any chronic or recurring illness in younger age groups—a shifting of the age base toward younger people—heralds a greater frequency of that illness in the general population in the next few decades.

Traditionally, certain psychosomatic disorders have been significantly sex-related. Migraine and fainting were considered "women's diseases." In contrast, diabetes and coronary heart disease typically occurred much more often in males. But in recent years we have been observing changes in the sex ratio for some diseases. The male-female ratio for peptic ulcer has fallen during the last 20 years from at least 4:1 to about 2.5:1.[11] From Great Britain, Shepherd and Cooper report Halliday's finding that there has been a marked increase in the frequency of diabetes among females, and that the male-female ratio for deaths attributable to diabetes has reversed—from 2:1 to 0.5:1.[12] Such changes in the sex ratios indicate that the tensions of social change are not exerting a uniform influence on both sexes simultaneously. One possible explanation may be that as women participate more actively in the occupational and social arenas, they are exposed to added stressors that, in conjunction with role conflict, can result in a psychosomatic disturbance.

Unfortunately, we do not have adequate data to gauge changes in the frequency of psychosomatic illnesses in different races over time. Rowntree's 1945 evaluation of 13 million Selective Service registrants showed a "marked increase in the incidence of psychosomatic disease in the Negro, who in peacetime appears to be relatively immune."[13] Research carried out in the 1960s showed that an alarming number of black females had hypertension, and that they are the high-risk race-sex group for death caused by hypertensive disease.[14] It appears that in the past psychosomatic conditions were underreported in certain minority or ethnic groups.

Social Class Distinctions

For many years it was believed that the seven classic diseases were mainly afflictions of the upper and middle classes—the price of success. The typical peptic ulcer patient was portrayed as a harrassed, prosperous business person, whose ulcers were evidence of striving and dedication at the expense of emotional well-being. It was also thought that among blacks, illnesses such as peptic ulcer occurred only among those who had adopted white middle-class values, and were attempting to achieve middle-class status.[15] But in the 1950s and 1960s, studies of large patient groups and extensive community surveys showed that psychosomatic and psychophysiologic disturbances generally were more common in the lower than in the middle or upper socioeconomic groups. The myth that psychosomatic illness is a middle-class affliction has been exploded.

THE THEORETICAL BACKGROUND

The Mind-Body Problem

Our scientific understanding of psychosomatic disorders has been plagued by an age-old handicap, the mind-body problem. No one questions the influence of life events on emotions, and in turn, the influence of emotions on the development of psychosomatic disturbances. But the basic issue, the one for which no resolution appears to be in sight, pivots on the major question: How do stressful events, such as a death in the family, produce bodily dysfunctions and disease processes? Advances in research are providing greater understanding of the mechanisms by which the brain regulates bodily functions. But how the intangible mind influences the brain, which is a bodily organ, baffles us. Philosophers and scientists have advanced two theses—dualism and monism. The *dualist* concept was proposed by Plato, codified by Descartes, and espoused by Sherrington. It holds that the mind and body are independent systems—different forms of reality—that interact at times in unknown ways. This dualistic thesis is consonant with those religious doctrines that emphasize the immortality of the soul. In contrast, the *monistic* viewpoint is materialistic; the mind is the function of the mortal brain.

Theoretical scientists have proposed tentative solutions that reconcile the opposing dualistic and monistic viewpoints. For example, Sir James Jeans postulates that all matter exists in two forms—particle and wave—and that the brain may be the particle form, and the mind the wave form.

Current concepts of psychosomatic medicine take for granted that understanding interactions between the mind and body—the mind at the abstract level and the central nervous system at a demonstrable psychologic level—requires different conceptualizations, languages, and scientific approaches. Because of these difficulties, many studies of psychosomatic disorders are limited to searches for correlations between stressful environmental events and circumstances on the one hand, and the occurrence of disease or illness on the other. "Disease is a process that produces physiological and psychological disorder. Illness is a state of distress expressed as symptoms. . . . Thus, a person may have a disease, yet not be ill, or a person may be ill although no disease process can be identified."[16] Most concepts of psychosomatic illness focus on the psychophysiological mechanisms involved, and dismiss the mind-body linkage as exceeding our present capabilities for understanding.

Concepts of Psychosomatic Illness

Conventionally, major concepts of psychosomatic disease are divided into two categories, the specific and the nonspecific.

The Specific Concepts An example of a specific concept is Flanders Dunbar's work in the 1930s, in which she delineated specific personality profiles she thought had diagnostic and prognostic significance for various psychosomatic disorders. She outlined the characteristics of the coronary-prone personality, the arthritic personality, and others.[17] Other workers in this field, however, were unable to replicate her findings, especially the correlation between a specific personality pattern and the occurrence of a particular psychosomatic disease. For example, some persons with rheumatoid personalities had peptic ulcers, not rheumatoid arthritis. Consequently, for years her theory has been regarded as passé. But Rosenman's recent work on the Type A and B personalities has revived interest in Dunbar's concept. He has shown that the Type A personality, which is characterized by excessive ambition, striving, impatience, punctuality, etc., is at much higher risk for coronary heart disease than the Type B personality.[18] In the last few years, Bahnson and Bahnson have described a cancer-prone personality, which is characterized by overdenial, failure to use projection efficiently, and inability to recover from depression following loss.[19]

Another specific concept that achieved popularity, especially during the 1940s and 1950s, was Alexander's psychodynamic conflict hypothesis. For example, he postulated that the psychodynamic conflict—dependence versus independence—was specific for the development of peptic ulcer. For essential hypertension, the conflict centered on the inadequate, semifrustrated expression of aggressive tendencies.[20] The relationship between a specific psychodynamic conflict and a certain psychosomatic disorder has been challenged and, in large part, repudiated. However, French and Pollock have continued Alexander's work; they now believe that they can "differentiate between the seven specific diseases on the basis of the psychological patterns associated with each of them."[21] Personality constellations and specific intrapsychic conflicts cannot be separated completely. There is some overlap between Dunbar's and Alexander's hypotheses, although Alexander emphasized the significance of intrapsychic conflict much more than Dunbar did.

The third major specific concept theory is that of psychologic and physiologic regression, a theory developed by Margolin and Kubie, who hypothesized that stressors impaired the individual's customary adaptive mechanisms, which resulted in an altered ego state, characterized first by psychological regression and later by physiological regression that appears as homeostatic fragility. For example, it was postulated that in a state of physiologic regression a person's autonomic and endocrine functions would undergo wide swings that resembed those normal in infancy and childhood, but abnormal in adulthood.[22] Thus, a person with a psychosomatic disorder would be considered to have sustained first a breakdown of normal mental defense mechanisms, and eventually *somatization*—the breakdown of the second line of defense. This is an imaginative concept that appears to have some clinical validity, but is tremendously difficult to demonstrate scientifically.

The Nonspecific Concepts   During the last 10 to 15 years, in accord with the current emphasis on general systems theory and ecologic concepts of health and disease, nonspecific concepts of psychosomatic disease have been evolving. These hold that psychosomatic disorders are the result of interactions among the following: broad social processes, environmental factors (especially stressful events), familial influences, a constitutional predisposition that is genetically determined, and inadequacy of verbal and other symbolic types of communication. Lower social-class status, with its exposure to numerous stressors and a relative lack of resources for coping, is an example of a broad social process. Adverse life events require social readjustments and have been shown by Holmes, Rahe, and others to produce stress, with its associated neuroendocrine activity that leads to psychosomatic illness.[23,24,25] By identification with a family member, a child may learn or adopt various characteristic symptoms. During childhood and adolescence a person can develop patterned responses, such as nausea and vomiting, as a reaction to conflict. Genetic defects and/or incompletely understood constitutional factors can predispose to such diseases as peptic ulcer, or contribute to "organ inferiority"—the special susceptibility of an organ. The work of Nemiah and Sifneos has shown that many psychosomatic patients are alexithymic—unable to express feelings verbally—and therefore react somatically to stressors and conflicts.[26]

At this time, most psychosomaticists subscribe to the nonspecific theory of psychosomatic illness. The fundamental principles are: a general systems theory of human behavior; a holistic view of the human being that encompasses stressful social, psychological, and biological factors; an emphasis on multifactorial etiology that recognizes a "synergy of causes"; and an appreciation of the interrelationship between the human being and the environment.

Stress

The concept of stress is integral to an understanding of psychosomatic disturbances. In the 1940s, Selye developed a nonspecific stress model to explain mental and physical reactions to stressors, and also to explain certain "diseases of adaptation," such as essential hypertension. Animals that had been exposed to a variety of stressors, for example, cold, radiation, or pneumococci, responded in a characteristic physiological way. Immediately after being stressed, the alarm reaction occurred; the animal went into a shocklike state that was followed by a rebound (countershock). Repeated exposure to the stressful stimuli led to the stage of resistance that was eventually succeeded by the stage of exhaustion. The physiological mechanisms in this *general adaptation syndrome* involve neuroendocrine responses, primarily, activation of the pituitary-adrenal axis. For example, during the resistance stage, the animal's adrenal cortices were hypertrophied; when exhaustion ensued, the adrenal cortices were depleted. Selye first visualized stress as the "wear and tear within the body," but after he saw that stress was a "dynamic protective," as well as a destructive process, and since it was difficult to distinguish precisely between damage and repair, he defined stress as the ". . . state manifested by a specific syndrome which consists of all the nonspecifically induced changes."[27] He emphasized that both stressors and stress could be measured only by the resulting psychophysiologic responses.

A useful clinical frame of reference for understanding the relationship between stress and psychosomatic disturbance has been offered by the Dutch investigator, Groen, who views such disturbances as substitutive reactions.[28] From this perspective, we can conceptualize an individual as a psychobiosocial organism who is capable of reacting to stressful psychosocial events and circumstances in only a certain number of ways. A person can: (1) sustain a breakdown of ego mechanisms and develop a psychosis; (2) employ maladaptive mental mechanisms to counteract or diminish anxiety, and thus develop a neurosis that is characterized by anxiety and the psychic defenses against it, such as phobias, obsessions, and compulsions; (3) "act out" to diminish anxiety by transforming it into some type of deviant behavior, such as alcoholism, addiction, or promiscuity, that we might term *sociopathic;* or (4) continue to internalize the stress, and thus develop psychosomatic illness. Usually the development of one type of reaction seems to protect, to a limited extent, against the development of another.

This conceptualization accounts for some clinical facts that have been observed repeatedly. For example, illnesses such as asthma and rheumatoid arthritis are seen rarely in chronic mental hospital patients. On occasion, however, when one of these patients improves and is discharged from the hospital, the person may develop a full-blown psychosomatic illness, such as asthma or peptic ulcer. Or the individual may suffer alternatively from clear-cut mental illness at one moment, such as paranoid schizophrenia, and at another time from a psychosomatic illness, such as asthma. This ping-ponging is known as *syndrome shift.*

PSYCHOPHYSIOLOGIC MECHANISMS

Flight-Fight

Our scientific understanding of the pathway from symbolic stimulus → stress → neurophysiologic processes → somatic dysfunction was developed in part by the work of Cannon. He was the first to hypothesize that stimuli were perceived by the sensory apparatus, transmitted to the thalamus, and then sent in two directions simultaneously: (1) to the cerebral cortex, where they were assessed for "danger," and (2) to the viscera and skeletal musculature, via the autonomic and endocrine systems.[29] Later, Bard's work on the hypothalamus led to a revision of this schema, so that the hypothalamus occupied an important role as the part of the central nervous system that was intimately connected with the pituitary gland, and that mediated neuroendocrine mechanisms.[30]

The stimulation of the autonomic nervous system, and the release of epinephrine and norepinephrine, prepares the subject for either flight or fight, but when the subject can do neither, the mobilization of the emergency mechanisms leads to bodily dysfunctions, especially when that mobilization is sustained. After a period of time, these dysfunctions produce lesions.

Conservation-Withdrawal

The second major psychophysiological mechanism is the "conservation-withdrawal" hypothesis developed by Engel and his associates.[31,32] They showed that object loss (real, threatened, or symbolic) produces affective and other disturbances that precede the onset of medical and psychiatric disorders. They based their concept on the observation that losses are usually adverse and stressful, and thus require social, psychological, and physiological adjustments that may be either adaptive or maladaptive. The conservation-withdrawal reaction to loss is characterized by a turning inward of the emotions that is analogous to the depressed state, which conserves energy but enhances the organism's susceptibility to psychophysiologic and other illnesses.

Support for the significance of loss in the genesis of illness is supplied by Parkes' well-designed studies of the psychosomatic effects of bereavement.[33] His work showed that in a bereaved group, both morbidity and mortality rates were significantly higher during the first year following a spouse's death, than were the rates for an age-controlled group that was not experiencing bereavement.

The Psychophysical Circuit

Hess's Nobel-Prize-winning work on the ergotropic and trophotropic systems demonstrated that subcortical centers regulate psychic, autonomic, and somatic processes via the reciprocally balanced ergotropic and trophotropic systems.[34] Kiely's recent review article summarizes:

> The ergotropic system integrates functions that prepare the individual for positive action. It is characterized by alerting, arousal, excitement, increased skeletal muscle tone and sympathetic nervous activity, and the release of catabolic hormonal products. The trophotropic system, on the other hand, integrates systems that promote withdrawal and conservation of energy: raising of the stimulus barrier to perceptual input, decreased skeletal muscle tone, increased parasympathetic nervous function, and the circulation of anabolic hormones. A developing body of data indicates that the biogenic amines, norepinephrine (NE) and dopamine (D), are the neurotransmitters

for the ergotropic system, while 5-hydroxytryptamine (5HT), or serotonin, and acetylcholine (ACh) play similar roles for the trophotropic system. . . .[35]

Certain neurophysiological mechanisms are reasonably well established, particularly the ones that mediate between the symbolic stimulus, the alerting response in the reticular activating system, the functions of the visceral brain (the limbic cortex and the hippocampus, which is responsible for memory), the cerebral cortex, and the hypothalamus, with its central role in activating and regulating autonomic and endocrine functions. This formulation provides a scientific underpinning for both the flight-fight and conservation-withdrawal hypotheses—tentative explanations of the psychophysiological basis of psychosomatic disorder.

PSYCHOSOMATIC-SOMATOPSYCHIC RELATIONSHIPS

The term *psychosomatic* implies a unidirectional path from the symbolic stimulus to the lesion in the tissue. But to understand patients' psychosomatic disturbances, we need to recognize the influence of reciprocal psychosomatic-somatopsychic processes. A person responds to the onset of a psychosomatic illness with mixtures of anxiety, denial, and depression. As a consequence, some degree of regression, or at least a limitation of activity and a preoccupation with self, is added to the existing psychologic difficulties that were etiologically significant. Regression usually involves increased dependency on others and changes in familial and interpersonal relationships. Regressed patients are often narcissistic as well as dependent, and may obtain so much secondary gain from their illness that helpless dependency persists.

In addition to the stressful effects of illness and fears about possible medical or surgical procedures or even recovery, interpersonal difficulties can ensue. Thus, psychosomatic and somatopsychic processes merge into a vicious cycle, in which one process reinforces the other. The result is a complicated illness, with a possible retardation of convalescence. A dramatic example of this is found in the patient who has had a vagotomy and a partial gastric resection for a duodenal ulcer, and then develops the "dumping" syndrome. The patient's attention is focused on gastrointestinal functioning, diet, probable weight loss, and abdominal distress. The anxiety, depression, and self-preoccupation disturb family members, who in turn respond inconsistently and often antitherapeutically to the patient's distress. The end result can be a miserable series of surgical procedures, further impairment of functioning, other failures in role performance, distortion of family relationships and, too often, invalidism. Such entangled psychosomatic and somatopsychic processes must be evaluated by the doctor who is working with patients suffering from psychosomatic disturbances.

In summary, the conceptual bases for psychosomatic disturbances have been built on a psychobiosocial view of the human being whose encounters with adverse life events and other stressors require psychic, somatic, and social readjustments. When the individual has inadequate mechanisms for coping with stressors, has deficient social support systems, and has a genetic or learned predisposition to bodily illness, the stressful state produces bodily dysfunctions, and sooner or later the lesions characteristic of a psychosomatic disturbance. As a consequence of the disease process, the individual's capabilities for problem solving and adaptation diminish, familial and other interpersonal complications develop, and the reciprocal influence of psychosomatic and somatopsychic forces eventuate in chronic illness that is characterized by bodily symptoms, interpersonal difficulties, and mixtures of psychic and social distress.

MAJOR TYPES OF PSYCHOSOMATIC DISTURBANCES

The major types of psychosomatic disturbances can be divided arbitrarily into two categories: (1) the classic seven considered to be psychosomatic disease entities for more than 30 years; and (2) the numerous and varied psychophysiologic disturbances, the most common of which are tension headaches, chest pains, abdominal distress, backache, and complaints of pain, numbness, and/or tingling in the extremities. In addition to the varied clinical pictures these groups of illnesses present, they also have differentiating psychological features.

Psychosomatic and Psychophysiologic Disorders

Patients suffering from classic psychosomatic diseases are more apt to pinpoint stressful events precisely (and these events are more likely to have a symbolic quality), than are patients with psychophysiologic syndromes. The latter generally appear to have been suffering from an ill-defined anxiety state for a prolonged time, their interpersonal and other conflicts are diffuse and entangled, and there is an arid quality to their life-style. Many patients in both these groups are also alexithymic. They tend to overuse denial and repression, and tend toward somatizing rather than symbolizing. Blackwell characterizes them behaviorally as demanding, threatening, helpless, compliant, and interpersonally manipulative.[36] Many are passive-aggressive and depressive. Thus, in the first encounter with them, the doctor can expect to contend with denial, rationalization, and alexithymia.

Differential Diagnosis

Psychosomatic disorders must be diagnosed precisely and must be distinguished from hypochondriasis and conversion reactions. *Hypochondriasis* is a distinct syndrome characterized by the chronicity and rigidity of the patient's bodily complaints, and the staunch conviction that a medical illness is present. Historically, some of the complaints involve abdominal distress, but the syndrome generally includes other bodily symptoms.

Characteristically, hypochondriacal patients engage in long symptom recitals, demand treatment (in a not-too-veiled fashion), appear to be barely controlling a great deal of anger, have tenuous interpersonal relationships, and are critical of doctors and medical science, even though they frequently return for medical care.

In contrast, the patient with a conversion state usually has a history of a sudden onset of the condition, little recognition of even obvious precipitating stressors, and an affective disturbance that betrays a true lack of concern about the possible seriousness of the physical condition, for example, paralysis of a limb. Evaluation of the conversion patient generally reveals that the symptoms symbolize both the conflict and the defense. This is illustrated by the case history of an 18-year-old female college student who was participating in a "wild" fraternity party. Her boyfriend brought her to the emergency room "paralyzed from the waist down."

As was pointed out by Ziegler and his colleagues in their articles on contemporary conversion reactions, conversion symptoms are seldom so dramatic and so clear-cut.[37] Because the general public's knowledge of medicine is increasing, many conversion patients tend to present with sophisticated symptomatology. Consequently, they are admitted to neurologic and neurosurgical services for diagnostic evaluations for such diseases as multiple sclerosis or brain tumor. Generally, doctors should hesitate to make a diagnosis of conversion reaction unless the following criteria are met: (1) a negative neurological or other thorough diagnostic examination; (2) evidence of being in an acutely stressful situation; (3) a history of a previous attack; (4) presence of some type of preexisting personality disorder; (5) an affective disturbance that at least borders on *la belle indifference;* (6) some indication of secondary gain; and (7) coherence of the preceding criteria.

EXPERIENCING PSYCHOSOMATIC ILLNESS

Although almost any type of illness induces anxiety, requires changes from the daily routine, and generates existential questions about the quality of life, possible invalidism and death, being psychosomatically ill has some added special features. In addition to anxiety about the illness and the future, the psychosomatic patient usually is plagued by doubt, shame, and guilt. The patient is beset with disquieting self-questioning that is related to blame and inadequacy. Almost all psychosomatic patients feel that they are responsible for their illnesses, that they have done something wrong—in reality or in fantasy—or that the illness is proof of inadequacy, even though they may know the probable cause, for example, excessive demands placed upon them at work. Nevertheless, blame, guilt, and doubt persist, and the illness is perceived as tangible evidence of a flaw for which one is responsible. Consequently, many of these patients attempt to conceal their inner turmoil, the facts of the illness, and even the treatment regimen. For example, many ulcer patients take their antacid tablets furtively when they are at work. The treatment regimen can include special diets that may be difficult to obtain at work or may necessitate changes in the family's mealtime schedule or choice of foods. Or, the asthmatic or hypertensive patient may no longer be able to do accustomed chores at work or at home. Thus, psychosomatic illness involves changes in routine and some degree of disruption in accustomed family activities, which in turn can be stressful for other family members. This both complicates the illness and reinforces the patient's self-blame and sense of inferiority.

Furthermore, psychosomatic illness is mysterious. Most patients think that psychosomatic illnesses tend to be chronic and certainly recurrent. The blame, sense of inadequacy, the treatment regimen's restrictions on activities, changes in the family routine, disturbed interpersonal relations, and the air of mystery about the illness conjoin to heighten fears of being unable to live healthfully and happily. When doctors tell patients that the diagnosis is a psychosomatic illness, and outline the treatment program, they must be empathic and think: "What is this going to mean for my patient? What changes in living will be required? What will it do to the family and to others? How can I help the patient (and the others) to cope?" and perhaps most importantly, "What would it be like if I were the patient?"

CLASSIFICATION AND DESCRIPTION ACCORDING TO ORGANS AND SYSTEMS

A classification of the psychosomatic and psychophysiologic disorders according to the various bodily systems can provide a useful clinical approach to diagnosis and treatment.

Cardiovascular System

Psychophysiologically, the heart is a target organ. Popularly, it is associated with emotions, heroism, chronic disease, and sudden death. The ancient Greeks, who were cognizant of the changes in the pulse and sensations in the chest, associated the heart with fear and anger, and also considered it to be responsible for courage. Our sentiments of love rhapsodize about the heart's affections, and our everyday language (for example, stouthearted) discloses this link with the past. But heart disease is also known to be the leading cause of death in the United States, and ischemic heart disease kills more than 500,000 persons annually.

Syndromes and Psychodynamics Since *effort syndrome* was first described as a condition common in frightened Civil War soldiers, it has been applied to symptoms of chest pains, shortness of breath, a sense of tightness in the thorax, faintness, and weakness. Synonomous terms are *neurocirculatory asthenia* and *cardiac neurosis*. Many patients with these syndromes are rushed to emergency rooms displaying obvious fear of the dreaded "possible heart attack." Most of them state that the attack came on suddenly—"nothing was bothering" them until suddenly they felt weak, had to gasp for air, and had pains and tightness in the chest. The first thought was of a heart attack. After they have been assured that their EKGs are normal, and are calmed by a sedative, they still maintain: "It just happened—I didn't know what to do—I thought I was dying."

Many of these symptoms are attributable to hyperventilation; the patient recovers quickly but the syndrome is likely to be recurrent, and a fixed cardiac neurosis can develop. Too often, the patient is given only reassurance and a tranquilizer. But this is inadequate treatment, because the first attack traumatizes the patient and focuses subsequent attention on any chest sensations. As one "attack" succeeds another, the cardiac neurosis develops; the patient becomes more and more apprehensive, and less able to carry out life's customary routines. Some elements of secondary gain appear as the patient avoids exertion, pleads fatigue, and obtains sympathy from others. Repeated medical examinations not only fail to relieve the anxiety, but serve instead to concentrate thoughts and worries on the heart, the pulse, the blood pressure, respiration, etc. A vicious psychosomatic-somatopsychic cycle is established.

These cases are psychiatric emergencies that require immediate psychotherapeutic intervention. One approach involves cutting through the patient's denial and repression and asking direct questions about the circumstances under which the "attack" occurred. "When did it occur? Where were you? Who was with you? What were you thinking beforehand? What fantasies did you conjure up? What occurred earlier in the day?" However, each patient must be individualized; questions that elicit cooperation from one patient and enable that patient to achieve some degree of insight, may increase resistance in others.

Two general types of situations epitomize these cases. Often the patient has identified with a family member, friend, or colleague who has recently had a fatal myocardial infarction. A typical case vignette is that of a 40-year-old machinist whose first attack occurred at about 4 p.m. one afternoon, shortly after he had started work. The rapid, probing history obtained by the resident who was on call in the emergency room disclosed that:

> One of the patient's coworkers had had a myocardial infarction and had died about a week earlier. While at work in the machine shop, the patient had been thinking about his friend. Prompt reassurance, pointing out the identification, and eliciting the patient's grief and fear, were successful therapeutic measures. The patient was referred to the psychiatric outpatient clinic for brief psychotherapy; he was told that it was important for him to talk about his anxiety with a professional in order to prevent recurrences.

Another general type is illustrated by the case of a 36-year-old housewife who had had three "attacks" in 1 month.

> During her second visit, the cardiologist ascertained that all the "attacks" had occurred early in the afternoon, while she was shopping at a center near her suburban home. The patient denied knowing anyone who had had serious heart trouble, and could not supply information about stressful events or anxiety-provoking situations. Consequently, after she had had two thorough cardiovascular workups, she was referred for psychiatric evaluation. The resident delved quickly into her personal history. She had been divorced 5 years earlier, and after a few years of "the single's life," she had remarried a few months prior to her first "attack." Between marriages, she had had a serious love affair with a man who wanted to marry her, but because

she feared that he was a potential alcoholic, she had ended the affair ambivalently. A few days before her first "attack," while leaving the drug store, she had run into him and had talked for a few minutes. Her first "attack" occurred only a few days later, as she was leaving the same drug store. When asked about her fantasies, she began talking eagerly about her pent-up feelings for her former lover, and her fears that she might acquiesce to a proposition! With the help of the psychiatrist, she gained rapid insight into the cause of her "heart attacks" and the potential for an anxiety neurosis with severe phobic as well as somatic symptoms.

Essential Hypertension Although essential hypertension has been considered one of the "classic" seven psychosomatic disorders, psychiatric therapies have not generally been regarded as adequate or successful treatment. Psychosomatic theories characterize the hypertensive personality as perfectionistic, agreeable, and striving to excel. It is postulated that people with this type of personality handle their aggressive drives poorly, either by expressing aggression at inappropriate times and then reproaching themselves, or by manifesting a "contain and suppress" attitude. In order to avoid jeopardizing interpersonal relationships, many of these patients will state that they seldom get angry. It "does no good to express anger and make an enemy." Or they feel furious but do not know how, where, or when to express these feelings, even though they equate them with their rising blood pressure. One of the major clinical problems with the hypertensive patient is that once the patient learns about the elevated blood pressure, concerns are focused on the level of the blood pressure, which then becomes a source of anxiety in itself. Often mild antianxiety agents are beneficial, and superficial psychotherapy can help the individual to live more comfortably, avoid stressful situations, and feel better, even though there is little or no proof that the hypertension (usually labile) is improved.

Coronary Heart Disease An increasing scientific body of evidence points to the psychosomatic component in coronary heart disease. Risk factors that have been identified in major collaborative studies are: high serum cholesterol, elevated systolic blood pressure, cigarette smoking, and the Type A personality pattern described by Rosenman et al.[18] (See the section "The Specific Concepts" in this chapter.) The Western Collaborative Group Study has shown that the risk for coronary heart disease in males is about twice as high in Type A as in Type B men. Furthermore, attempts to convert the Type A to the Type B personality, usually through intensive group therapy, are being conducted scientifically; statistical projections indicate that over an 8.5-year period, there would be a 31 percent reduction in coronary heart disease if all men had Type B personalties.

Gastrointestinal System

Since the gastrointestinal tract is associated with the symbolic expression of emotion throughout life, starting with nursing in infancy and proceeding to toilet training that is a model for socialization, it is the most common focus for psychophysiologic disorders. Two classic psychosomatic disturbances, peptic ulcer and ulcerative colitis, epitomize the fundamental emotional conflicts: for ulcer, dependence-independence, and for colitis, a distorted, very close relationship with the mother, excessive vulnerability to loss or separation, and an internalizing of hostility. But these distinct disease syndromes, both of which can be serious, life-endangering medical illnesses, constitute only a small fraction of the gastrointestinal complaints presented by patients with psychophysiologic disorders. Indigestion, nausea, vague abdominal pains, intermittent nervous diarrhea, and chronic constipation are taken for granted, as symptoms of emotional distress and the inevitable consequences of being human. Burkitt thinks that many of these conditions are diseases of civilization that are attributable not only to the stresses and strains of life in a modern industrialized society, but also to technological changes in the preparation of foods. For example, appendicitis, constipation, and many other gastrointestinal conditions were considered rare in Great Britain until about 100 years ago. Burkitt believes that the refining of natural foods, particularly grains, and the consequent loss of roughage, such as bran, is responsible for gastrointestinal dysfunctions that result in illnesses such as diverticulitis.[39]

Although most patients with gastrointestinal dysfunctions and symptoms can obtain relief by a change in the daily routine and diet, and the avoidance of stress, the *anniversary reaction* often appears as a GI disease and can usually be alleviated through brief psychotherapy. One case vignette is illustrative.

> A 40-year-old white married woman was referred for psychotherapy because of persistent right upper quadrant pain. Complete diagnostic evaluations revealed moderate obesity and sluggish emptying of the gall bladder. The personal history taken by the psychiatrist disclosed that the patient's mother had died of a carcinoma of the liver, almost exactly 2 years before. When questioned about her reactions to her mother's death, she stated that she had scarcely grieved. Her husband, who was a legislator, disdained the open expression of feelings, and had admonished her not to make a "public spectacle" of herself at the funeral, because it might be politically injurious if a large crowd of friends saw her break down. Encouraging the patient to grieve, and pointing out the similarity between her symptoms and those of her mother, was beneficial. Her symptoms disappeared almost completely, and her relationship with her husband improved; she dieted voluntarily, lost 20 pounds in 6 months, experienced a boost in her self-esteem, and was able to assert herself more vigorously. Her husband was relieved of fears that she would be a menopausal invalid, and was gratified by her more attractive appearance and outgoing personality, which he regarded as substantial evidence of an improvement in their relationship.

In working with patients with psychosomatic disturbances, the doctor should always look for anniversary reactions and unresolved grief. When they are found to correlate with the onset or exacerbation of symptoms, the doctor should encourage the patient to ventilate pent-up feelings and accept the accompanying ambivalences. The patient should be assured that ambivalent feelings are normal, and are not a cause for guilt or shame. These cases are especially gratifying; a doctor usually can observe improvement in the patient after just a few sessions.

Peptic Ulcer Many fundamental psychosomatic concepts can be observed in patients with peptic ulcers. Although Franz Alexander's dependence-independence conflict can be demonstrated in only a minority of these patients, problems with dependency are usually on the surface. The work of Mirsky et al. shows the significance of multifactorial etiology—the synergy of causes.[40] Their study involved two groups of Army recruits who were about to begin basic training. Those who were high pepsinogen secretors, and those with low pepsinogen levels, were evaluated by means of standard projective tests for psychologic vulnerability. All procedures were blinded. Thus, this quasi-experimental design involved life stressors (basic training), genetic predisposition (serum pepsinogen levels), and psychologic vulnerability. The groups were followed. All of the nine who developed peptic ulcers demonstrated high pepsinogen and high psychologic vulnerability.

Advances in the medical and surgical treatment of peptic ulcers have been remarkably successful. Consequently, fewer of these patients are referred for psychiatric evaluation and psychotherapy than in the past. A high-risk group for peptic ulcer are hysterectomized women in their thirties and forties. Since it is likely that women who are developing ulcers after hysterectomy are having major problems with living and multiple physical illnesses, they should receive a psychiatric evaluation.

Ulcerative Colitis Fortunately, ulcerative colitis is a rare disease, but its occurrence in children and adolescents is a matter of grave concern. The disease begins with abdominal pain and bouts of bloody mucoid diarrhea. Within a few months, the mucosa of the colon appears as a shaggy, bleeding, friable, ulcerative membrane; the patient sustains weight loss, becomes anemic, and both looks and is febrile and toxic. The principal etiologic factors are unknown; there may be a genetic defect, or the illness may be produced by unidentified microorganisms. However, it is not contagious. Psychological factors are thought to be important; these patients exhibit immaturity, have had tenuous relationships with their mothers, are covertly demanding, and are especially vulnerable to disappointments and separations (real or threatened). It has been hypothesized that the ravaged mucosa and the diarrhea symbolize the distorted expression of aggressive impulses.

Supportive psychotherapy is generally beneficial. Many of these patients have exceedingly serious psychopathology that is analogous to "malignant" schizoid syndromes; consequently in-depth psychotherapy and confrontation should be undertaken only by experienced therapists. Some of these patients require colectomies and continued supportive psychotherapy.

Respiratory System

The common cold, allergic rhinitis, and many cases of pharyngytis are thought to have a psychosomatic etiology. Bronchial asthma is the most serious psychosomatic disorder of this system. Psychophysiologic mechanisms involving the hypothalamus and the autonomic nervous system have been demonstrated, but there is little doubt that allergic and infectious factors are also influential. Psychodynamically, the patients, especially the young ones, are critically and often ambivalently involved with their mothers; the asthmatic wheeze has been described as "a cry for mother."[41] Some of these patients recognize that stressful events are conducive to the development of the asthmatic attack, and that intrafamilial conflict can sustain an attack that was originally precipitated by an upper respiratory infection.

Treatment includes regular medical management, the prevention of infections, desensitization or other procedures that reduce the influence of allergens, and a psychotherapeutic approach that emphasizes support during the acute attack and more dynamically oriented psychotherapy when the patient is in remission. Family therapy can be especially effective.

PRINCIPLES OF THERAPY

The fundamentals of treatment for patients with psychosomatic conditions are to: (1) provide the best medical care available, by utilizing diagnostic evaluations when needed but not relying on x-rays or the laboratory either to solve the patients' problems or avoid coming to grips with the anxieties and interpersonal difficulties; (2) make sure that one doctor has the basic responsibility for the patient; (3) prescribe medications according to a rational plan that includes full knowledge of their use and abuse, as well as of their pharmacologic activity, especially interactions and side effects; (4) work psychotherapeutically with the patient (the following section briefly describes some psychiatric approaches, especially individual psychotherapy, that can be employed by the physician); (5) be aware that some environmental manipulation is usually mandatory, that the doctor may have to see and work with others to ensure the treatment's success; and (6) marshal social support systems for these patients. In looking back at his more than three decades of work with doctors, nurses, clergy, and others, Gerald Caplan has recently concluded that support systems are the most significant factors in "maintaining the psychological and physical integrity of the individual over time."[42]

Individual Therapy

A number of fundamental principles are applicable to the treatment of patients with psychosomatic disturbances. The first requires that the doctor manifest a warm personal stance. Since most of these patients have already sought a number of physician's services, they tend to interpret excessive objectivity as a lack of understanding and interest. Furthermore, many of them are frightened, particularly when the illness has been diagnosed as psychosomatic. Their anxieties spring from three main sources: (1) an impression that psychosomatic illnesses are poorly understood scientifically, (2) the fact that technological medicine has little to offer therapeutically, and (3) the assumption of personal responsibility for their psychosomatic condition, which creates feelings of guilt, shame, and inadequacy. Therefore, a completely objective, impersonal manner may confirm their thinking that something has been wrong with their personal life. On the other hand, an overly sympathetic style may give the patient the feeling that the physician is substituting concern for knowledge and skill.

The second principle is awareness that the patient's anxieties are often concealed by some degree of aloofness and skepticism. Most psychosomatic patients do not express their feelings verbally; instead, they somatize. Thus, their responses to questions about feelings are often monosyllabic and taciturn. Therefore, the doctor must start teaching them to begin *talking* about their feelings, and encourage them to do so even during the initial interview. The doctor should do more than collect facts about present and prior illnesses, family relationships, work, etc. Expressions of emotional reactions that are related to events in the life history should be elicited. This can be done with such questions as: "How did you feel about that? What were your inner feelings: Anxiety? Fear? Resentment? Anger? Disappointment? A sense of being misunderstood, rejected, ignored, put down?" This may appear tedious and time-consuming (it often is), but it is critically necessary in order to enable the patient to correct an essential defect—that of being unaccustomed to regarding one's feelings as worthwhile. Later the patient will have to learn to let feelings surface (when it is appropriate), first in the office and eventually in everyday life.

The third fundamental principle of therapy is linked to the preceding one. It involves fantasizing. Most of these patients seldom admit to fantasies, or when they do, their fantasies are arid and almost unbelievably simplistic. For example, in response to a question about fantasies regarding a difficult work situation, in which most people would feel some anger and at least fantasize that they could express their resentment, the psychosomatic patient will tend to reply: "I didn't feel very much—I just wished it hadn't happened or that it was time to go home." These patients have to be encouraged to feel free to fantasize and be comfortable about doing so. Generally, this requires that the doctor interrupt or follow up the patient's statements with direct questions: "What were your fantasies when X happened? What was in your imagination?" Simultaneously, one has to be supportive, by reassuring the patient that all of us have fantasies that allow us to work out trial solutions to problems, or minimally, to release some of our feelings and thoughts in our imagination.

Even during the first interview, I often mention a fantasy of my own. For example, after the patient has talked about a family or work problem or described an illness, I ask directly: "What were your fantasies about that?" When the patient responds: "I didn't think much about it," or "I don't know what you mean," I reply, "Well, just now, as you were telling me about your experience, I had a fantasy. Momentarily, I fantasized that you would tell me that you hoped the other person would say, 'I'm sorry, let me make it up to you.'" Also, sometimes I quote Harvey Cox, who is a well-known Harvard theologian: "Fantasy is the frontier of thought."[43]

Mentioning one's own fantasy—when appropriate to the situation—can be a valuable technique that enables the patient to understand and utilize fantasies, as well as feel that it is normal and proper to do so. However, the doctor should be careful to limit remarks about personal fantasies. The goal is to label and define the word "fantasy," and to encourage patients to talk about their fantasies, not to display one's own fantasy life as a model.

The fourth fundamental principle is that the doctor's style must be both *supportive and collaborative.* This involves reassurance—evincing warmth and understanding—as the patient traverses relatively unexplored life events and conditions, and their singular personal meaning. I tend to question psychosomatic patients more actively than I do patients with neurotic disorders or characterologic disturbances. It is important to lead them with questions about their own views of the impact of interpersonal problems, and their reactions to stressful events and circumstances that are tinged with conflict. To accomplish this, often it is helpful to ask the patient to give an account of a typical day, beginning with time of awakening, breakfast, the daily routine, chores, leisure time, what happened in the evening, bedtime, and dreams. I interrupt to ask for details about interactions with family members, colleagues, and friends—who, when, what was said and done, and always, "How did you feel? What did it mean to you? What did you fantasize?" Spending some time discussing a typical day gives the doctor an intimate view of the patient's life-style, and also supplies information that can be used therapeutically. In addition, it is vital to reiterate that psychotherapy is a joint effort, that the physician and the patient are collaborating in a project that requires attention and work. Thus, success depends upon sometimes employing the principles of supportive therapy, often encouraging the patient, and always insisting that this is a shared endeavor.

The fifth and critically important principle is that these patients should be receiving adequate medical care for their physical complaints and illnesses. Ideally, this requires periodic, thorough diagnostic evaluations. Also, these patients should maintain a conventional ongoing relationship with their other physicians, by continuing prescribed medications and returning for scheduled appointments. Obviously, the patient's physician or surgeon needs to be in frequent contact. It is best for the patient when the various doctors taking care of him or her know each other and respect each other's efforts.

Pitfalls

Somatization The first pitfall involves permitting the patient to dominate office visits with long recitals of complaints, enumerations of disappointments in previous treatment regimens, and repeatedly posed queries about the efficacy of current medications or procedures. As Peter Knapp explains: "The psychotherapist must avoid . . . [making] the symptoms a battleground. His best tack is openly to focus on psychological issues inviting the patient to share the gamble that if difficulties in new spheres can be helped, the physiologic process may also change."[44] Initial acceptance of the "gamble" by the patient is not enough. Somatization has become a way of life. Attention is focused on the symptoms, which have somatopsychic as well as psychosomatic complications—

the psychosomatic disturbance is a raison d'être. Therefore, the doctor should expect physical symptoms to be emphasized, not just when therapy is being started, but later, when the patient is attempting to make changes that involve personal reactions to life situations and different behaviors. When customary mental mechanisms are inadequate, or when the patient is unsure of how to handle feelings (particularly in interpersonal situations), accustomed attitudes and behavior patterns will reappear, even though experience has shown that these are ineffective and self-defeating. When somatization threatens to eclipse psychological, interpersonal, and social issues, the doctor should express understanding, point out nonpejoratively what is occurring and why, and guide the patient toward fuller comprehension and a recognition of the desirability of breaking established patterns that are deleterious.

Medications   The second pitfall, which is often entangled closely with the first, concerns medications. Many psychosomatic patients are taking, or have access to, a variety of medications. Often they will question the doctor about the efficacy of medications that others have prescribed, or seek advice and/or approval of their use. Not too covertly, they may request new ones. Psychosomatic patients tend to rely increasingly on the sick role, especially when it is reinforced by such traditional medical practices as repeated diagnostic evaluations and the overuse of medications. The doctor has to ascertain what medications the patient is taking and, in cooperation with the patient's other physicians, set forth a regimen that is rational, humane, and does not lead to abuse.

Manipulating the Physician   Manipulation of physicians—turning the family doctor against the internist or vice versa—is the third, and often the most serious, pitfall. Consciously or unwittingly, the psychosomatic patient will try to play one doctor against another, thus creating inconsistencies in care and continuing along a self-defeating, symptomatic path. A working alliance among the physicians, and adherence by them to agreed-upon plans for medications and procedures, is the only effective strategy. This alliance among the doctors should be known to the patient, who should be receiving periodic medical checkups, and should not just turn to a specialist when symptoms become severe.

Other Therapies

In addition to individual psychotherapy, newer therapeutic approaches are being used with psychosomatic patients. These are mainly family and group therapies, use of conditioning and biofeedback, and/or intensive hospitalization in a special psychosomatic unit for about a month.

Family or Group Therapy   Family therapy can be a valuable adjunct to the medical and individual psychotherapeutic approach. Sometimes it is the preferred treatment modality. In family therapy, interpersonal conflicts can be brought to light, and role behaviors can be clarified and modified. Group therapy is particularly helpful for psychosomatic patients who lack interpersonal and other supportive networks. In the group session, the patient becomes aware that there are few truly unique situations. The patient's overuse of denial and repression often becomes a focal topic that is explored and questioned by others.

There are few absolute indications or contraindications for family and/or group therapy. When marital and other familial conflicts persist, family therapy can be beneficial. Group therapy can augment individual psychotherapy. It is seldom contraindicated. Some authorities think it is particularly useful for their psychosomatic patients who seem to lack "psychological awareness." But this criterion should not be accepted at face value as an indication for group therapy, since many of these patients are alexithymic. Therefore, the doctor's warm, supportive approach, which is felt more personally in individual psychotherapy, often better enables patients to express their feelings appropriately.

Behavior Therapy   Behavior therapy focuses explicitly on the present. The root causes of maladaptive behavior are less significant than in more traditional insight-oriented dynamic psychotherapy. The emphasis is on how the patient acts and reacts in everyday life, and/or modifying behaviors associated with psychosomatic symptoms. Behavior therapy appears to be a useful approach to certain types of problems, for example, obesity. The rationale is that obesity is the result of unhealthy eating habits. The therapeutic objective is dietary control that can be achieved by counting calories, maintaining a daily weight record, having the patient look at him- or herself in a full-length mirror for 5 minutes, three times each day, and not sanctioning the use of various wardrobes—one for "fat" and one for "thin." Instead the patient should be urged to stay with one wardrobe and to wear it, even though it does not fit well.

Biofeedback Therapy   The principle underlying biofeedback therapy—learned cognitive control of the musculature and even regulation of cortical and autonomic processes—has been demonstrated and is a significant addition to knowledge about psychophysiologic mechanisms. This type of therapy is used in some psychiatric centers to treat such disorders as migraine headache, certain cardiac arrhythmias, hypertension, Raynaud's disease, and poorly controlled epilepsy. The results of biofeedback therapies, however, have not yet been evaluated systematically. Furthermore, indiscriminate use of these therapies is potentially dangerous, especially when the patient has inadequate insight into the social and psychological processes influencing illness.

Intensive Hospitalization   A number of medical centers have developed special psychosomatic units in which selected patients are hospitalized for an agreed-upon time, which is usually 4 weeks. The unit is designed to provide a therapeutic milieu wherein patients receive intensive family and/or group therapy, behavior therapies that often make use of rewards or a token economy, and a concentrated multistaff approach that discourages talking about symptoms. Many patients benefit from an intensive regimen of this type.

CONCLUSIONS

Finally, psychotherapeutic work with psychosomatically ill patients is both desperately needed and rewarding. Because of the paucity of personnel and facilities to make the needed therapy available, the frequent failure to recognize the need, or the general attitude toward psychotherapy on the part of many technical medical practitioners, large numbers of these patients never receive the assistance that can enable them to change established illness-producing living patterns. Doctors have been criticized frequently for poor results with psychosomatic patients. However, when the doctor works intensively with these people, some degree of success is often achieved. Whatever the degree, that success not only benefits the patients by sparing them repeated diagnostic examinations and other procedures, but is also especially meaningful to the physician, who is working against odds. As Huth has insisted, medicine needs new approaches that embrace ecologic concepts, attend to patients' problems in living, and pay more than lip service to "holistic" care for them.[3]

REFERENCES

1 Morris, J. N.: *The Uses of Epidemiology,* 2d ed., Baltimore: Williams and Wilkins, 1964, p. 14.

2 Gardner, E.: "Emotional Disorders in Medical Practice," *Ann. Intern. Med.,* **73**(4):651-653, 1970.

3 Huth, E. J.: "Stale, Soft, or Chronic," *Ann. Intern. Med.,* **70**:1272-1275, 1969.

4 Halliday, J. L.: *Psychosocial Medicine: A Study of the Sick Society,* New York: W. W. Norton, 1948.

5 The Committee on Nomenclature and Statistics of the American Psychiatric Association: *DSM-II, Diagnostic and Statistical Manual of Mental Disorders,* 2d ed., Washington, D.C.: American Psychiatric Association, 1968, pp. 46-47.

6 The American Psychiatric Association Task Force on Nomenclature and Statistics: *DSM-III: Operational Criteria Draft,* Washington, D.C.: American Psychiatric Association, April 15, 1977, pp. 140-141.

7 Leighton, D. C. et al.: *The Character of Danger,* vol. 3, *The Stirling County Study,* New York: Basic Books, 1963.

8 Langner, T. S., and S. T. Michael: *Life Stress and Mental Health,* vol. 2, Thomas A. C. Rennie Series in Social Psychiatry, The Midtown Manhattan Study, New York: The Free Press, 1963.

9 Schwab, J. J. et al.: "The Epidemiology of Psychosomatic Disorders," *Psychosomatics,* **15**:88-93, 1974.

10 Tringo, J. L.: "The Heirarchy of Preference toward Disability Groups," *J. Spec. Educ.,* **4**:295-306, 1970.

11 Department of Health, Education and Welfare: "Health Statistics from the U.S.," *National Health Survey,* Series B., no. 17, Washington, D.C.: USGPO, 1960.

12 Shepherd, M., and B. Cooper: "Epidemiology and Mental Disorders: A Review," *J. Neurol. Neurosurg. Psychiat.,* **27**:277-290, 1964.

13 Rowntree, L. G.: "Psychosomatic Disorders as Revealed by 13,000,000 Selective Service Registrants," *Psychosom. Med.,* **7**:27-30, 1945.

14   Stamler, J. et al.: "Epidemiologic Studies on Cardiovascular Renal Diseases: Analysis of Mortality by Age-Race-Sex-Occupation," *J. Chron. Dis.,* **12**:440–445, 1960.

15   Kardiner, A., and L. Ovesey: *The Mark of Oppression,* New York: World Publishing, 1962.

16   Schwab, J. J., and M. E. Schwab: *Sociocultural Roots of Mental Illness: An Epidemiologic Survey,* New York: Plenum, 1978, p. 118.

17   Dunbar, F.: *Emotions and Bodily Changes,* 3d ed., New York: Columbia University Press, 1946.

18   Rosenman, R. H.: "Assessing the Risk Associated with Behavior Patterns," *J. Med. Assoc. Ga.,* **60**:31–34, 1971.

19   Bahnson, M. B., and C. B. Bahnson: "Ego Defenses in Cancer Patients," *Ann. N.Y. Acad. Sci.,* **164**:546–559, October 14, 1969.

20   Alexander, F.: *Psychosomatic Medicine: Its Principles and Applications,* New York: Norton, 1950.

21   Alexander, F. et al. (eds.): *Psychosomatic Specificity, vol. 1, Experimental Study and Results,* Chicago: Univ. of Chicago Press, 1968.

22   Margolin, S. G.: "Etiology and Pathogenesis in Psychosomatic Medicine," *J. Ark. Med. Soc.,* **60**:175–180, 1963.

23   Holmes, T. H., and R. H. Rahe: "The Social Readjustment Rating Scale," *J. Psychosom. Res.,* **11**:213–218, 1967.

24   ———, and M. Masuda: "Life Change and Illness Susceptibility," in B. S. Dohrenwend, and B. P. Dohrenwend (eds.), *Stressful Life Events: Their Nature and Effects,* New York: Wiley, 1974, pp. 45–72.

25   Paykel, E. S.: "Life Stress and Psychiatric Disorder," in B. S. Dohrenwend and B. P. Dohrenwend (eds.), *Stressful Life Events: Their Nature and Effects,* New York: Wiley, 1974, pp. 135–149.

26   Nemiah, J. C., and P. E. Sifneos: "Affect and Fantasy in Patients with Psychosomatic Disorders," in O. Hill (ed.), *Modern Trends in Psychosomatic Medicine,* London: Butterworth, 1970.

27   Selye, H.: *The Stress of Life,* New York: McGraw-Hill, 1956, p. 54.

28   Groen, J. J.: "Methodology of Psychosomatic Research," *Fortschar Psychosom. Med.,* **1**:45–56, 1960.

29   Cannon, W. B.: *Bodily Changes in Pain, Hunger, Fear and Rage,* 2d ed., New York: Appleton, 1929.

30   Bard, P., and V. B. Mountcastle: "Some Forebrain Mechanisms Involved in the Expression of Rage with Special Reference to Suppression of Angry Behavior," *A. Res. Nerv. & Ment. Dis., Proc.,* **27**:362, 1947.

31   Engel, G. L.: "Selection of Clinical Material in Psychosomatic Medicine: The Need for a New Physiology," *Psychosom. Med.,* **16**:368, 1954.

32   Schmale, A. H.: "Relationship of Separation and Depression to Disease: A Report on a Hospitalized Medical Population," *Psychosom. Med.,* **20**:4, 1958.

33   Parkes, C. M.: "Effects of Bereavement on Physical and Mental Health: A Study of the Medical Records of Widows," *Brit. Med. J.,* **2**:274, 1964.

34   Hess, W. F.: "Uber die Wechselbeziehungen Zwischen Psychischen und Vegetativen Funktionen," *Schweiz. Arch. Neurol. Psychiat.,* **15**:260–264, 1924.

35   Kiely, W. F.: "From the Symbolic Stimulus to the Pathophysiological Response: Neurophysiological Mechanisms," in Z. J. Lipowski et al. (eds.), *Psychosomatic Medicine,* New York: Oxford Univ. Press, 1977, pp. 206–218.

36 Blackwell, B.: *Paper Presented at the Annual Meeting of the Kentucky Psychiatric Assoc.,* Louisville, Ky.: September 1975.
37 Ziegler, J. J. et al.: "Contemporary Conversion Reactions: A Clinical Study, *Amer. J. Psychiat.,* **116**:901, 1960.
38 Brand, R. et al.: "Multivariate Prediction of Coronary Heart Disease in the Western Collaborative Group Study Compared to the Findings of the Framingham Study," *Circulation,* **53**:348–355, 1976.
39 Burkitt, D. P.: "Some Diseases Characteristic of Modern Western Civilization," *Brit. Med. J.,* **1**:274–278, 1973.
40 Mirsky, I. A. et al.: "Studies on the Physiological, Psychological and Social Determinants in the Etiology of Duodenal Ulcer," *Psychosom. Med.,* **23**:514, 1956.
41 Weiss, E.: "Psychoanalyse eines Falles von Nervösen Asthma," *Int. Z. Psychoanal.,* **8**:440–445, 1922.
42 Caplan, G.: *Support Systems and Community Mental Health: Lectures on Concept Development,* New York: Behavioral Publications, 1974, p. 7.
43 Cox, H.: *The Feast of Fools: A Theological Essay on Festivity and Fantasy,* New York: Harper & Row, 1969.
44 Knapp, P. H.: "Psychosomatic Medicine: An Interpretation," *Psychiat. Ann.,* **2**(8):36–61, 1972.

BIBLIOGRAPHY

Halliday, J. L.: *Psychosocial Medicine: A Study of the Sick Society,* New York: Norton, 1948.
Lipowski, Z. J. et al. (eds.): *Psychosomatic Medicine: Current Trends and Clinical Applications,* New York: Oxford Univ. Press, 1977.
Wittkower, E. D., and H. Warnes (eds.), *Psychosomatic Medicine: Its Clinical Applications,* New York: Harper & Row, 1977.

Chapter 17

The Geriatric Patient

Robert N. Butler, M.D.

EDITORS' INTRODUCTION

What is it like to be nearing the biblical "threescore and 10" and to be told by your physician that your various aches and pains are "just your age and you will have to learn to live with them"? How does it feel to look in the mirror and see not just more lines in the skin, more sagging muscles, and even changes in the face's bone contour, but an aged face? What feelings are aroused in the patient who recognizes that a cane really does make for a steadier gait and that somehow others are concerned about your tripping and falling? What is it like when you have retired, or been retired, and hear some people argue against a compulsory retirement age and others argue for it? Does an *emeritus* status really mean *emeritus*? Or does it mean you are no longer the capable, active, vital professor you have always been?

When you are in your doctor's office, and the nurse reminds you to be careful, then puts her hand on your elbow to steady you—would you rather she did not? Then, too, how difficult it is to have to find a new doctor because your friend and physician of many years retired or died. Will the new doctor understand you? Can he or she ever take the place of your former physician?

How do physicians feel about older people? Would they rather see a young, attractive individual who is actively involved in business, politics, or civic affairs? Will the patient cause the physician to reflect on his or her own aged parents, or may the aging physician see a reflection of self in the patient who is waning physically and intellectually? Will the physician start playing the "numbers game," in which he or she knows that a feeble 72-year-old patient is only 8 years the physician's senior? What feelings about self and about aging are evoked in the physician? Some physicians can handle this dilemma comfortably and empathically. Some can see the beauty and dignity of aging. Many cannot. For so long, the aged have not received the attention they merit. This disregard subjects them to a type of indignity. It becomes very important for the caring doctor to sense each older patient's specific anxieties and find ways, however subtle, to help the patient deal with them.

The provision of quality medical care requires both of the skills central to the good physician: detachment and empathy. Detachment is necessary in order to make the objective observations upon which accurate diagnosis is based. Empathy is required in order to know the patients and their dilemmas at a different level and in order for the patients to feel understood. "My doctor cares about me" is the feeling of the patient who has an empathic physician. This feeling is at the heart of good medicine. Sometimes, however, the older patient provokes in the physician strong reactions that have little to do with the characteristics of the specific patient, and that may interfere with the physician's capacity for empathy. Under these circumstances, the physician is only detached with the patient, and the patient may interpret this as a failure to care.

In this chapter, the Director of the National Institute on Aging, who is a distinguished psychiatrist, presents an overview of the mental health problems of the aged. He makes an urgent plea for the care the aged deserve, expressing an optimistic viewpoint about what must and should be accomplished.

We really do not know what aging is. Much of what was once thought to be aging, that is, inevitable decline, is actually disease. Physicians who are engaged in treating the older patient are reporting impressive therapeutic results. Researchers have demonstrated the usefulness of many levels of psychotherapy as well as varied approaches to physical treatments.[1,2,3]

New research has demonstrated that brain deterioration and mental confusion are far from inevitable and that old age can be a time of vigor and wisdom. New sensitivity to the illnesses of old age, particularly those conditions that bring reversible brain syndromes, will save many from chronic brain syndromes. Although older people were once thought to be inflexible and unresponsive, we now know that, in spite of the odds our society places against them, they are quite adaptive and able to benefit from individual and group psychotherapy as well as from pharmacotherapy. Indeed, psychotherapy may coincide with the natural process of life-review that occurs in the later years and may be particularly helpful.

There is an excitement in learning to treat the entire sweep of life and value for the physician who is learning to assist patients even to their dying days. There are demands as well. The complexities of later life demand complex therapies. The physical, social, cultural, and economic aspects are intricately woven into the psychological well-being of the elderly.

Humanism demands attention to this, and the numbers command respect. There are now some 23 million older Americans. In about 50 years, with new research achievements and improved health care, there will be a doubling of these figures, and probably one in five Americans will be over 65. The children of the post-World-War-II baby boom that "greened" America in the 1960s will be the generation that "grays" America in the next century.

OVERVIEW

Losses, grief, and efforts toward restitution characterize later life, a period laden with crises. Both intrinsic and extrinsic factors influence a person's adjustment. High among the extrinsic factors are the inevitable deaths, not only of the marital partner, but often of children and friends as well. Retirement, with its losses of status, income, and activity, is another extrinsic factor. In recent years, those living on retirement pensions and savings have been struck another blow by virulent inflation. A sense of helplessness, uselessness, and apathy often develops.

How easy it is for a person to become depressed, and yet how strong his or her zest for living is, even in a time of great sadness. The following vignette encompasses many of the problems:

> I'm a 73-year-old man who just lost my wife. That's against the usual, natural order of things. I feel quite helpless. I've never learned to cook or sew buttons on my shirts. I feel quite helpless and lonely. I understand it's more difficult for a man to adjust than a woman in the later years. It's true from my experience. I can't seem to shake the experience of loneliness. I feel quite angry. I'm surprised at myself at how angry I am at my wife for dying on me, leaving me. I'm depressed. I'm angry and anxious, and now I'm told by my doctor that I have some evidence of blood in my stool and I have to be investigated—have an unpleasant proctoscopic examination and a barium enema, and who knows what the outcome will be. If it's not something this time, it will be the next time. It's not just death. It will be the dying and the pain and the being alone. The kids are living across on the other side of the United States. I have friends, but they have their problems, or are sick or even dying. Despite this, I also have things I very much want to do. I still enjoy concerts and have a lot of things that I want to complete. I don't know whether I'm a coward or not, but I'm not looking forward to some of the tougher tests of my mettle. But I still like to travel, go to the theater, work in my workshop and, as far as I was concerned, if I hadn't been required to retire, I would have kept right on working.

The way a person has lived life and one's style—and personality—play a role in determining the quality of later years. Each of us brings the weight of our past decisions and regrets into old age. Moreover, as the Romans noted, *mens sana in corpore sano:* it is all easier if you are well. Physical disabilities deplete the older person, and some disorders are particularly threatening. Perceptual problems, particularly hearing losses, may lead to depression, the appearance of confusion, or even to paranoia. Diminished sexual desire and capacity may distress the older person, but there is reason to hope that sexuality may enhance the later years.

Organic brain disease restricts the important adaptive mechanism of intelligence. With arteriosclerotic brain disease, the damage tends to be spotty and erratic rather than complete and, as people retain the insight and judgment to understand their plight, a marked depression may result—a very important differential diagnostic point.

There are the obscure but implacable factors we still believe are part of aging: the slowing of psychomotor responses and other integrative processes. There is the subjective awareness of aging, of body losses, and the awareness of the passage of time. Some older people react to the idea of death with fear, others with denial; most face the approach of death with equanimity. Nearly all tend to review their lives.

Physical Changes

Although we tend to think that bodily changes come with age alone, this is not so. The folk saying, "You are only as old as you feel" is especially apt. There is more variance of physiological measures among older persons of a given age than there is among younger ones. It appears to be illness or health that makes the difference, not age alone. Certainly there are obvious changes: graying of hair; loss of hair and teeth; elongation of ears and nose; subcutaneous fat losses, particularly around the face; skin wrinkles; fading of eyesight and hearing; postural changes; and other manifestations of time. Resistance to disease diminishes, with those over 65 having only 10 percent of the immune capacity of adolescents.[4] Animal studies suggest that this immune response can be boosted, and this area is most promising for research with regard to the elderly. The body's other responses to disease change, too. For instance, an older person with a heart attack may experience no pain, another with pneumonia may not have the characteristic elevated white cell count, and another with appendicitis may not have the usual signs that accompany it.

Senility, which is really a wastebasket term, is not an inevitable condition, but appears rather to be a cerebrovascular disease involving destruction of central nervous system cells or an emotional state such as severe depression. Circulatory problems are not solely age connected, but are the result of vascular disease. One study showed that cerebral blood flow and oxygen consumption were essentially the same in healthy, normal, older men as they were in young men.[5] Research may bring the prevention of atherosclerosis; if that seems too optimistic, remember that once people dying of cancer were said to be "dying of old age."

It is important to be aware of the intricate connections between mind and body in the elderly; the slowing of perceptual, associative, and psychomotor functions, often thought to be caused by a lowering of the subliminal cortical excitation, may also be caused by depression. Similarly, behavioral changes may

also be the first clue to physical illnesses, dehydration, or electrolyte disturbances. As more research with healthy older persons is conducted, misconceptions, on which years of work with the ill and institutionalized were based, may
fall away.

There are unpleasant facts to be considered. Older people suffer more severe
illnesses and remain ill almost twice as long as younger people. About 86 percent
have one or more chronic ailments, although these problems may be treatable.
About 30 percent suffer hearing losses. Until mental hospitals began to refuse to
admit the elderly, they accounted for almost 25 percent of admissions. Today,
many older people who have been lifelong residents of mental hospitals have been
transferred to the community, where their days are spent in poorly supervised
programs or lonely rooms. Five years ago, of the 21 million Americans over 65,
3.4 million were profoundly poor and living below the official poverty level of
$2,100 for a single person or $2,650 for a couple. Some, particularly minority-
group members and women, are extremely poor. Almost half of older black
women live on incomes well under $1,000 a year. It is estimated that about 40 per-
cent of single older citizens have total assets of less than $1,000.[6] It is no surprise
that so many suffer from poor nutrition or malnutrition and hesitate to spend
money on "luxuries" such as telephones, glasses, and hearing aids.

Some people thrive in old age and others fail, depending upon their own personality—that complex of enduring psychologic features developed during a
lifetime of living. Given equal personal, social, and body losses in old age, one
person will adapt and another collapse.

Some people never develop a sense of the cycle of life, never expect to suffer
reverses, and are unable to adapt. To understand the kinds of changes to be expected, and to face oneself with the reality and inevitability of change, including
death, is important. If one can do this, there can be an acceptance of the precious
and limited quantity of life and the ways in which it changes. Some older persons
begin to pass on what they have learned by tutoring and sponsoring younger people; others plan, in some way, to leave a legacy. These are healthy trends.

Emotional Problems

A fiction exists that all the problems of old age are related to organic difficulties.
Not only do older people suffer the same emotional pains as younger ones, but
some serious functional disorders—specifically depressions and paranoid
states—are more prevalent. Hypochondriasis also occurs, as do psychosomatic
illnesses.

All the conditions that foster depression are present in the late years:
physical illness, losses and attendant grief states, loss of money, loss of status,
too much free time to brood, and a sense of helplessness and worthlessness. For
those who have suffered such troubles early in life, the problems may be doubled.
Depression may appear as bodily complaints or simply as confusion, which is an
important diagnostic point.

Some physicians feel impatient with patients whose disease is not readily apparent. Such patients are derisively called "crocks," or are referred to as having

the "porcelain" disease. There are always reasons for hypochondriasis, and it should never be treated as an "imaginary" illness. Rather, the emotional basis should be sought. Hypochondriasis may be a way of assuming a role, of forcing responsibility onto others, or of identifying with a person who is now deceased. It may be the emergence of a subclinical illness. In hypochondriasis too much medical concern or nursing can confirm the unfounded fears of the patient, and can be as dangerous as inadequate care. Other tangled emotional/physical illnesses, including psychophysiological (psychosomatic disorders) and conversion reactions, are also common. Unlike conversion reactions (for example, a paralyzed hand that prohibits aggressive behavior), which result in *la belle indifference* (the beautiful indifference) and which have a symbolic representation, the psychosomatic symptoms have a physiologic rather than a symbolic origin, and threaten somatic consequences. Psychotherapy is often helpful.

Psychopathology advances with age, decade by decade. Under age 15, there are 2.3 new cases of serious psychiatric disorders—either functional or organic—per 100,000, but over age 65, there are 236.1 cases per 100,000. New problems, then, are added to those that older people have accumulated during their lifetime. It is estimated that some 3 million older people, or about 15 percent, will need mental health services. A million are now in institutional settings, some 2 million more who are living in communities have serious chronic physical and mental disorders. Seven million more are at risk resulting from extreme poverty. While many elderly patients have been moved from state hospitals to community facilities, rarely are they moving closer to psychiatric care. Community mental health centers have failed to serve the elderly, as have private psychiatrists, who report only 2 to 5 percent of their time spent with persons over age 60.

ORGANIC BRAIN DISORDERS

The organic brain disorders are mental conditions caused by, or associated with, impairment of brain tissue function. The signs are: (1) disturbance and impairment of memory, (2) impairment of intellectual function or comprehension, (3) impairment of orientation, (4) impairment of judgment, and (5) shallow or labile affect. These signs may or may not be seen all at the same time. They may not all appear to the same degree; they may be barely perceptible or they may be profound. Organic brain syndromes may be either acute (*reversible*) or chronic (*irreversible*). These organic syndromes may occur at the same time as psychotic, neurotic, or behavioral disorders.

Some people are able to keep their basic personality and behavior patterns intact while suffering organic syndromes. They find ways to aid their memories and to assist themselves in getting around.

> Mrs. J, a hearty, good-natured woman of 83, compensated for her waning memory in a variety of ways. She made lists of things to remember; she tied letters to be mailed to the doorknob so that she would see them when she went out; she attached her wallet

and keys onto her belt or slip strap. She asked friends to call and remind her of appointments, and she made deliberate efforts to read and talk about the daily newspapers "to keep my brain active."

For others, any diminution of abilities is very disruptive. Not only the degree of organic disorder, but the individual's basic personality, inherited traits, and life situation affect the kind and severity of symptoms. Full treatment is often the only true test of reversibility. At times, simple measures may improve functioning. Orientation, for instance, may be improved by giving direct instructions, or by practical methods such as marking places and objects with lights, signs, and colors.

Memory changes are a common and noticeable sign of chronic brain syndrome. Although it was once thought that recent memory becomes destroyed in some manner by a deteriorative process in the brain, it now appears that brain damage interferes with registration of incoming stimuli and affects retention and recall. There is also the influence of emotions to consider, and the older person may need to forget, to deny, or to distort that which is too painful to face, or too overwhelming to admit. Depression at any age interferes with learning and memory. Organic brain disorders are caused not only by brain pathology, but also by a number of factors that operate through individual intensity or collectively with a threshold effect—the chief factor of which may be life stresses on the particular personality. They are always multidimensional and multicausal. Table 17-1 shows early signs of organic brain syndrome.

Reversible Brain Syndrome (RBS—"Acute")

Once referred to as "acute" brain syndrome, which carried the connotation of rapid onset and dramatic symptoms, it is now called reversible brain syndrome, which is more accurate descriptively. Unfortunately, it often goes undiagnosed, and if this occurs, the older person will often be thought to have an irreversible condition and will be sent to a custodial setting.

A sign of reversible brain syndrome is a fluctuating level of awareness, which may vary from mild confusion to stupor or active delirium. Often visual, rather than auditory, hallucinations are present. Typically, the person is disoriented, mistakes one person for another, and may experience impairment of other intellectual functions. Remote, as well as recent, memory is lost. Behaviorally, the person may be restless, have a dazed expression, or be aggressive. The disorientation or hallucinations may be very frightening. Sometimes anxiety or a lack of cooperation may occur. Reversible brain disorders follow, which may be associated with febrile, debilitating, or exhausting illnesses. A behavioral change in older people may signal appendicitis, although there may be no pain at McBurney's point, no fever, and no leukocytosis. The reversible brain syndrome should not be confused with transient behavioral disturbances that can accompany organic brain disease. Both may be reversible, but the latter have a chronic underlying cause not found in reversible brain syndrome.

A detailed history must be taken, and often information must be gathered

Table 17-1   Prodromal Characteristics of Organic Brain Syndrome*

Early characteristics	Potential signs and symptoms†
Cognitive	
"Intellectual" decline	Perseveration
Reduced tempo of stream of thought	Increasingly impaired comprehension
Impoverishment of ideas	
Concreteness: impaired abstraction	Increasing memory loss
	(recent and remote)
Decline of recent memory	Confabulation
Registration, retention, recall,	
organization‡	
Difficulty in maintaining attention	Perseveration, irrelevance
and set	
Behavioral and affective	
Reduced attentiveness	Progressive withdrawal and self-isolation
Reduced responsiveness	Apathy
Decreased interpersonal interaction	Pseudodepression vs. depression
Less direct, immediate affective	
expression	
Liability to "disintegration" during stress	"Inappropriate" affect
Later characteristics	
Emotional lability	Emotional incontinence
Impaired orientation	Confusion
Impaired judgment	

*Modified from S. Perlin and R. N. Butler, *In Human Aging: A Biological and Behavioral Study*, Washington, D.C.: Pub. (HSM) 71-9051, 1971.

†A one-to-one relationship between presenting characteristic and potential symptom is not implied. Other symptoms may include irritability, apathy, suspiciousness, slovenliness, etc.

‡Impaired organization refers to the inability to remember (and utilize) items in a time-related sequence.

from other people, as the patient may be unable to supply the information personally. The onset of the illness is important, and exposure to any toxic substances should be noted carefully. At times, even an over-the-counter antihistamine can cause the problem. One may see reversible disorders in association with drugs, tranquilizers, bromides, barbiturates, thiocyanates, noxious environmental substances, or even hormones.

Preexisting illness should be noted. Older persons who have reduced kidney function or arteriosclerosis, or who are undernourished, may show marked negative response to drugs. The cortisone series may cause an organic brain disorder of either the reversible or irreversible type. The steroids may affect mood, with depressive or manic presentations. Tranquilizers that are given to allay anxiety before surgery may be continued for too long, and may result in brain syndrome (iatrogenic).

Diuretics (such as the thiazides) may lead to dehydration and mental confusion. L-dopa (antiparkinsonian) and idomethacin (antiarthritic) may cause psychotic behavior. Phenothiazines are implicated in tardive dyskinesia, and in older persons, especially women, even small doses can cause this serious neurological disorder.

Some drugs bring paradoxical responses. Barbiturates, for example, may bring agitation instead of calm. Older people may also be upset by the side effects of the drugs because they may fear that the slowing of responses they are experiencing is the result of failing health.

Head trauma also accounts for reversible brain disorders. Accidents and falls plague the elderly as a result of weakness, poor coordination, or drinking. Persons over the age of 65 account for 73 percent of all fatal falls and for 30 percent of all pedestrian fatalities. Falls may bring subdural hematomas, concussion, coma, delirium, or finally, Korsakoff's syndrome. Brain tumors or surgery can also impair brain functioning.

Cerebral vascular accidents are common, and little strokes are probably quite frequent. The temporary lack of blood to the brain (ischemic attack) results in hypoxia, which is followed by aphasia and paralysis. The person becomes unconscious and, upon regaining consciousness, may pass through an acute state of confusion before a restoration of mental normality. Strokes may bring reversible syndromes, but if they are repeated or massive, irreversible brain disorders may result.

So we see that reversible brain syndromes can result from many causes: chronic respiratory disease, congestive heart failures, malnutrition, anemia, avitaminosis, pellagra, metabolic disorders, diabetic acidosis, liver failure, dehydration, uremia, emphysema, myxedema, brain tumor, general surgery, blindfolding during eye surgery (sensory deprivation), or even fatigue. Bereavement or drastic environmental changes (as when a person moves from home to a hospital) can cause confusion. Other conditions, such as hypercalcemia resulting from metastatic carcinoma of lung or breast, primary hyperparathyroidism, multiple myeloma, or Paget's disease, can cause a reversible brain syndrome. Nonketotic hyperosmolarity syndrome, in which hyperglycemia and confusion occur without any ketosis, is not uncommon as a cause of reversible brain syndrome.

Alcoholism is more common in this older group than is generally realized. Since alcohol is a central nervous system depressant that impairs intellectual and emotional functioning, and since intoxication at any age results in a reversible brain syndrome, the risk of excessive drinking is clear. While a drink in the evening or wine with a meal may be helpful to one patient as a familiar pattern or mild way to relax, such suggestions should not be extended to anyone with a pattern of alcoholism. Likewise, there is the danger of the patient's taking license from the physician and gradually increasing the intake.

Irreversible Brain Syndrome (Chronic Brain Syndrome)

Although there is a myth that all old people have damaged brains—so-called senility—this is not so. All too often any problem experienced by an older person is taken as a sign that the person is being overtaken by the invisible enemy, brain damage. This too-quick assumption has meant that emotional and physical problems, and even reversible brain syndromes, have been ignored and the person consigned to neglect before adequate treatment has even been tried. Even where definable brain damage exists and is permanent, there is a great deal that both the individual and the doctor can do to prolong independent functioning. Research has shown that a low correlation exists between the extent of an individual's decline and the degree of neuropathologic change. One person shows many symptoms and disabilities with even minimal damage, and another continues to manage despite severe brain deterioration. Anatomical changes are only a part of the picture, and here, as in so many disorders of later life, culture, personality, and environmental stress play a part. To complicate matters further, reversible brain syndromes may occur along with irreversible brain syndromes. Sometimes a patient who has been getting along fairly well in a nursing home suddenly becomes confused. One should suspect reversible brain syndrome, and full diagnostic and therapeutic work should begin at once. With the lifting of the reversible syndrome, often the patient will improve again.

In older people, there are two predominant types of irreversible brain syndrome: senile psychosis (senile dementia and senile brain disease) and psychosis associated with cerebral arteriosclerosis. The two disorders occur simultaneously in about 20 percent of the cases.

Senile psychosis refers to the chronic psychotic disorder that occurs predominantly in individuals after age 80. Associated with changes in the brain, usually the dissolution of brain cells, this disorder occurs more frequently in women than in men. Although men tend to have shorter life spans, they tend to be healthier when they do survive. Brain cells atrophy and degenerate independently of vascular changes and most strikingly in the cerebral cortex. Senile plaques and neurofibrillary tangles are found in both senile psychosis and Alzheimer's disease. Nerve cells are destroyed in a widespread manner without breaking down the structure of nervous tissue as a whole. About 20 percent of the patients also show some changes that are caused by vascular disease with moderate arteriosclerosis, but these changes are usually of minor significance.

Clinically, the person may pass from normal old age to senile psychosis with no abrupt changes. Early features of senile psychosis are errors of judgment, decline in personal care and habits, impairment of capacity for abstract thought, lack of interest, and apathy. Loosening of inhibitions may be an early sign, and emotional reactions such as depression, anxiety, and irritability are seen frequently. Depression is often of a superficial nature. Then, as time passes, the classic signs of organic impairment become apparent. Hallucinations can occur, and the person may appear restless and unable to sleep. Paranoid tendencies may appear or become worsened.

The cause of senile brain disease is unknown, although some suspect a slow-acting virus; others implicate genetics, or view it as an autoimmune disease. Some argue that senile brain syndrome is an increase in normal involutional change, and others believe it is a different process altogether.[7,8] Senile brain disease follows a steady and progressive course and eventually is fatal. Some live 10 years or more, but the average survival time is 5 years.

Psychosis associated with cerebral arteriosclerosis is a chronic disorder with an uneven and erratic downward progression. There may be "lucid" intervals—this is important in medicolegal issues, as when the validity of wills or other business transactions is being determined. It is associated with the damage done to the cerebral blood vessels by arteriosclerosis. The blood flow to the brain is interfered with, and sufficient oxygen and nutrients do not reach the brain. The age of onset is between 50 and 70 years, with the average age at about 66 years. Men outnumber women, three to one. The brain shows areas of softening, with complete deterioration of cerebral tissue over a circumscribed, limited area. The damaged area may be either anemic or hemorrhagic.

Early symptoms are dizziness, headaches, decreased physical and mental vigor, and vague physical complaints. Onset can be gradual or sudden, though in the majority of cases onset is acute, and takes the form of a sudden attack of confusion. Patients whose symptoms have a slower onset can look much like those with senile brain disease. Intellectual loss tends to be gradual, and impairment of memory tends to be spotty rather than complete. The course is up and down. The person may hallucinate and become delirious, thereby indicating the insufficiency of cerebral circulation.

The etiology of arteriosclerosis is still being debated. Some think that lipid dysfunction, heredity, diet, smoking, environmental pollution, lack of exercise, hypertension, and other elements contribute to it.

The course of the illness varies from person to person and even from time to time in the same person. A person may die quickly from a cerebrovascular accident, or may suffer a long-lasting clouded organic state. Most patients, however, live only 3 or 4 years.

Cardiac or vascular disease may cause some degree of intellectual impairment or a psychosis. The person may be more impaired physically than is usually seen with senile psychosis, and many are bedridden. The patient may need physical therapy and attention to special physical needs as well as psychotherapy. Death, when it occurs, is usually from cerebrovascular accidents, arteriosclerotic heart disease, or pneumonia.

As a general rule, in interviewing patients who are thought to have brain injury, be careful not to ask too many questions at any one time, and try to limit stress. Brain-damaged patients who are tired or overwhelmed become irritable and anxious. While such a reaction, which is called the *Goldstein catastrophic reaction*, is a diagnostic clue, it may also make it difficult to proceed, and may obscure a more precise diagnosis. The Goldstein reaction, which is caused by internal and external stress (which the patient is unable to mediate neurologically), was first noted in brain-injured soldiers during World War I.

Two puzzling and tragic conditions are Alzheimer's disease and Pick's disease. They occur in late middle age, and their causes have not been identified. Many scientists regard Alzheimer's to be an early form of senile brain disease. Few patients live longer than 5 years after the onset of Alzheimer's, which may be a familial disease.

FUNCTIONAL DISORDERS

Functional disorders appear to be emotionally based and have no apparent physical cause. The most severe functional disorders are the psychoses, and the most puzzling is schizophrenia. The latter is marked by disturbances of thinking, mood, and behavior. Hallucinations, delusions, poor reality testing, and poor interpersonal relationships are common. It is rare to see the initial onset of schizophrenia occur in an older person; however, many schizophrenics live long lives and only come to medical attention in their later years. Some have been hospitalized for 50, 60, or more years, and are virtually incapacitated. Often without their consent, they are moved to nursing homes or foster care, where they still do not receive appropriate medical care, and their condition worsens.

Neuroses are common, and may appear for the first time in old age. Although thinking and judgment may be impaired, there is no gross distortion of reality nor profound personality disorganization. Conversion reactions, obsessive and compulsive disorders, hypochondriasis, and phobic reactions fall into this group as well as disturbances in mood such as depressive and manic patterns. Paranoid states and psychophysiological reactions are common.

Psychophysiologic disorders are also provoked by anxiety; however, here the physical expression is not symbolic, but is characterized by the effects of the emotions on secretion, mobility, and vascularity in various tissue and organ systems. The signs are: (1) involvement of the autonomic nervous system, not of the somatic voluntary musculature or the sensory perceptive systems; (2) no reduction in anxiety, as there is in conversion reaction; and (3) the threat of somatic damage as a result of structural changes. In older people, common psychophysiologic reactions include skin reactions (such as pruritus ani and vulvae), psychogenic rheumatism, hyperventilation syndromes, nocturia, and cardiac neuroses (with fear of sudden death). Cultural influences as well as anxiety can cause preoccupations with bowel habits and diet. Constipation is a common complaint, and nocturia can be very disturbing.

In some cases, old age is kind, lessening the symptoms of a lifetime. For obsessive and compulsive problems, there may be some decrease in symptoms or, at least, less disruption suffered from them. The older person who was a "fussbudget" all through life may now be able to stretch minor tasks to fill a lonely day. For others, the first appearance of such symptoms may be mistakenly attributed to aging, rather than to anxiety.

Depression and Suicide

Depressions are widespread and serious in old age. Signs of depression include feelings of helplessness, sadness, lack of vitality, frequent feelings of guilt, loneliness, boredom, constipation, sexual disinterest, and impotence. With severe depressions, such symptoms as insomnia, early morning fatigue, and marked loss of appetite may be seen, and somatic symptoms are common. There are depressions that are related to a reduction in life's satisfaction, often forming what is known as a *retirement syndrome.*

There are other possible depressions, such as involutional difficulties, although many women pass through menopause without such suffering. Illnesses, particularly viruses and Parkinson's disease, are often followed by depression. Pain of any sort may breed depression, and yet families and doctors often hesitate unnecessarily to treat emotional problems while a person is physically ill. Some drugs (for example, tranquilizers and some hypotensive medication) can cause depression.

Manic-depressive reactions, either bipolar (with swings from depression to elation) or unipolar are sometimes seen.

Suicide is the end point of depression, and the elderly (although constituting only about 10 percent of the population) account for roughly 25 percent of the suicides reported each year.[9] The highest rates occur with white males in their eighties. Suicide in old age is particularly related to physical disease, isolation, and bereavement. It may be the last act under the control of a person who feels otherwise powerless. Any threat of suicide or any suspicion of such intent must be taken seriously. Treatment should begin immediately and should include frank discussion, outreach efforts, extra psychotherapeutic time, a reorganization of daily schedule, and involvement of the family.

Paranoid States

Paranoid states are not uncommon, and may be associated with grandiose or persecutory delusions. While they may be transient, they may also last a lifetime. Such adverse conditions as deafness, blindness, infections, and poverty tend to encourage such disorders. Sometimes symptoms are discrete and circumscribed. Any effort to relieve general anxiety and to improve adverse conditions may help. One woman in her late seventies thought she was being poisoned and weakened by fumes sent through her radiators at night. Investigation showed her to be frightened of being alone at night. Measures to improve her comfort and to reassure her, such as having a neighbor check to see whether she was all right, helped to stabilize her condition and to relieve her fears without ever attacking her paranoid ideas directly.

The paranoid person may get along in the community by being isolated, and most often is harmless. However, some are dangerous, and paranoid rages and murderousness or homicidal attacks do occur. Most of what appears to be paranoid behavior is a reaction to extraordinary and unbearable stress—physical, emotional, and environmental.

Sexual Issues

A distorted image of the older years has come about due to the mistaken assumption that the elderly experience a dramatic decrease in sexual desire and performance. While there is a decrease, it is usually very gradual. Individuals in their seventies and eighties can have the most gratifying and intimate sexual relations. Another distortion involves sexual deviation among the elderly. While some few young children are molested by the elderly, others are approached benignly out of loneliness. Some older men have been accused of exhibitionism when, in reality, they were merely confused and had stopped to urinate.

EVALUATION AND TREATMENT

Physicians have a lot to offer the elderly, and will be involved increasingly in their treatment. In some cases, they will have to devote additional time to seeing an older patient; in other cases, they may not. Some older patients hesitate to call a doctor for fear of being a bother. A pattern of comprehensive annual examinations should be established, particularly if the patient is deteriorating. Every avenue for improvement must be explored. The physician must be aware of personal reactions to aging, chronic disease, depression, and death, as well as the relationship of feelings about such issues to the physicians' own attitudes relative to their parents. Attitudes that inhibit the physician's treatment of the elderly can be revised. Experience will help to avoid an overemphasis on brain damage and age as limiting factors. Learning that many conditions are reversible is the best way to combat a sense of futility in working with the older patient. Older patients are fearful of losing others; sometimes they are more afraid of losing the doctor than of dying.

Evaluation

Adequate treatment can begin only after adequate evaluation. Historical data, medical, psychiatric, and social examinations should document long-standing problems as well as new ones, and find their source if possible. Goals must be set, whether for full recovery, maintenance, or support until death.

Distinctions between organic and functional disorders are particularly important. In functional disorders, mood, behavior, and thought are more likely to carry meaning and express motivation. Organic behavior is more biologic (for example, stimulus-bound) and fragmented. Table 17-2 gives key diagnostic concepts.

It is important to recognize reversible conditions so that immediate treatment can begin. Table 17-3 lists important reversible conditions.

Diagnosis must be an ongoing process. A multicausal diagnosis, with attention to both primary disease and overlays and with supportive, active treatment and concern for emotional consequences, is most helpful. For instance, treatment of a reversible brain syndrome suffered by a patient with an already-established irreversible brain syndrome can still yield substantial relief and improvement.

Table 17-2   Key Diagnostic Concepts in Brain Syndromes of the Aged

1	Insight and depression may be present in early phase of cerebral arteriosclerosis.
2	Depression may mask itself as organic confusion.
3	Reversible (acute) brain syndromes are often misdiagnosed as chronic brain syndrome.
4	Acute and chronic brain syndromes may coexist.
5	Depression and brain syndromes may coexist.
6	Retinal arteriosclerosis is *not* diagnostic of cerebral arteriosclerosis.
7	Suicide is frequent in older men.
8	Paradoxical excitatory drug reactions to barbiturate sedatives may occur.
9	Tranquilizer-induced ("iatrogenic") brain syndromes occur.
10	Tranquilizer-induced depressions are not uncommon.

Table 17-3   Important Reversible Conditions to Recognize

Certain conditions, which are recoverable and treatable, are commonly overlooked. *Look for:*
  Reversible (acute) brain syndromes
  Reversible (acute) brain syndromes superimposed on chronic brain syndrome
  Depressive reactions simulating organic brain disorders
  Paranoid states without organic brain disease
    Generalized
    Circumscribed
    Chronic paranoid state with superimposed, reversible crises
  Subdural hematomas

A comprehensive basic evaluation of the elderly person should include all the normal components of a thorough physical and psychological assessment as well as a standard mental status examination.[10] Physical examination should include rectal, pelvic, genital, and neurological examination, electroencephalogram, skull films, electrocardiograms, chest x-rays, and routine comprehensive laboratory work including such tests as a CBC, sedimentation rate, stool for occult blood, thyroid function, electrolytes, BUN, blood sugar, and serology. Some say a computerized axial tomograph should be ordered for any patient over 60. This new technique has the advantage of being both informative and noninvasive.

Hearing, vision and dental tests should be completed, and a full sociocultural assessment should be carried out. Home studies may be helpful. Evaluation and treatment of the elderly person demand skilled consultative and collaborative work with other specialties and social agencies. A physician should be familiar with all the community services available to the elderly, whether recreational, legal, or occupational, and with programs such as Meals-On-Wheels.

Common Adaptive Techniques—Defenses

Throughout life, the ability of an individual to understand his or her situation and change behavior adaptively is a major tool for living. In the absence of brain damage, this continues. Denial is often used by the older person to help ease the pain of some truths. It is helpful unless it interferes with necessary acts such as seeking treatment. Projection is common and is seen in the case of the paranoid person who projects personal feelings outward onto someone else. Counterphobia is seen with people who go to great lengths to show that they are youthful and well, even in the face of evidence to the contrary.

Families

While there are forces in our society that lead to fragmentation of the family, families have been unfairly indicted for neglect of the elderly. Families often go to extraordinary lengths to care for older relatives and, by and large, the older person without a family is at a serious disadvantage. More than half of the residents of nursing homes have no close relatives. This era is the first to have widespread experience not only with grandparents, but also with great grandparents. Nevertheless, many individuals prefer to live on their own, even though they would welcome family support and community services. Families often develop patterns for regular visits and special occasions to ensure keeping in touch. Young children who grow up in families who support and respect older relatives may develop a greater appreciation of the importance of families and of the life-span itself. Also, older relatives can be helpful to younger ones in times of crisis.

Older people without families or friends do less well. They suffer more illness and earlier deaths, to say nothing of loneliness.

When treatment plans are developed, families should, with the older person's permission, be consulted and included whenever practical. If possible, the physician should help the family understand the effects of normal aging as well as those associated with disease or trauma. Fully informed and educated families can be allies in successful treatment.

Treatment

The older person may need a dentist, nurse, occupational therapist, physical therapist, podiatrist, medical and/or psychiatric social worker, nutritionist, homemaker, shopper, and others, as well as a physician. Community resources should be used on behalf of the older person and, if necessary, such resources should be organized to provide necessary services. Seeing the needs and developing the prescription are sometimes two different things, since most communities lack a facilitator to coordinate all the services needed.

Some of the possible alternatives are limited, to say the least. Nursing homes are particularly a problem. More than a million older people live in them, and many who have psychiatric problems face an almost total lack of psychiatric services there. The best facilities have a campus approach, with a spectrum of services that allows for independent living (with supplementary services, such as meals, for as long as possible, and then gradually more complete services as needed).

Although the mental hospital offers psychiatric care, there is often no real commitment to restoring maximum functioning. Results from private mental hospitals and psychiatric units of general hospitals are better. In general, older people should be maintained on active adult treatment wards, unless it is established that custodial care is needed. Then a new, humane definition of that care should be sought. Physical space is important to the older person, since well-marked, well-lit areas; safe bathrooms; wide doors for wheelchairs; and the right to keep personal belongings can help to preserve both personality and freedom as long as possible.

Visitors are extremely important, and attention and assistance should be given to see that the patient's possessions at home are cared for. Personal possessions, especially pictures, should be brought into the patient's hospital room.

Telephones are important; patients should be allowed to make and receive calls. Doctors should remember that any calls they make to an older person could have great therapeutic significance.

Psychotherapy

All forms of psychotherapy, from Freudian to Jungian to Rogerian, can help. The elderly have often been denied such help at a time when resolving old conflicts is of great importance. Listening is important; false reassurance should be avoided. What is needed is an integrated utilization of all contemporary personality theories and practices, including a utilization of the life-cycle perspective of human life. The physician must not be destructive to the processes of illusion and denial that may be needed by the patient. The possibilities of restitution and resolution must be maintained. One must work compassionately and carefully to get behind the defenses, rather than attacking them directly. Reconciliation with siblings—and others—is possible even after 20 years of alienation. Confessions of guilt may be heard, and while the therapist does not "grant mercy" in a religious sense, he or she can listen and bear witness to the realities of life. Facing genuine guilt and other realities, such as physical illness, is difficult, and yet working with such major issues is what makes psychotherapy with the elderly an intellectually and emotionally rewarding and powerful experience.

Group therapy is very helpful, and should be part of any institutional program. Life-crisis groups with members of all ages offer a special type of learning and support between generations. Family therapy, social groups, and daytime recreational groups are valuable.

Pharmacotherapy

Pharmacotherapeutic agents can be valuable, especially in treating depressions of the elderly. However, they carry more risk with elderly than with younger persons. When utilized, unit doses should be low and then increased gradually. Tranquilizers should be used in low doses and for brief periods only and should be carefully supervised. For a full discussion of pharmacotherapy in the elderly see the section on geropsychopharmacology in Chapter 25.

Electroshock Therapy (EST)

If antidepressants and psychotherapy do not result in a lifting of depression, electroshock therapy may be indicated. While there is increased danger relative to fractures and cardiovascular stress, new techniques and safeguards have decreased this danger. Preshock sedation and muscle relaxants should be used and the number of treatments kept minimal. Exogenous reactive depressions should usually not be treated by EST, and a thorough evaluation, including consideration of organic brain damage, and extreme caution are essential. For fuller details of electroshock therapy see Chapter 26.

Treatment of Specific Conditions

Reversible Brain Syndromes   Active and adequate treatment is vital. Maintenance of adequate fluid and caloric intake should be maintained. Oxygen inhalation may be needed. Tranquilization—used briefly—can be valuable. Preferred hypnotics are nonbarbiturates, such as chloral hydrate. Bulk laxatives are preferred, if needed. With active treatment, almost 50 percent of the patients can survive and return home.

Care can prevent some reversible brain syndromes; preoperative planning can ensure the presence of familiar objects and people after surgery to enhance the patient's orientation. The incidence of so-called black patch, or cataract deliria, has been reduced by such means.

Irreversible Brain Syndromes   A prosthetic environment, one that is medically and socially supportive, is important. Allowing the patient to do as much as possible personally, but not allowing neglect, is essential. Life should be simplified, but it should be complete. Familiar patterns should be maintained as long as possible, whether the person is at home or institutionalized.

Helping the Dying Patient

Recent years have brought into focus the needs of dying patients and the ways in which the physician may help make dying an accepted and peaceful event. Cassell (Chapter 30) offers the physician a perspective and many practical suggestions for accomplishing this goal. With elderly patients, the issue of death and dying is of great importance. The knowledge that the physician will be there and will help may make this inevitable event less feared. The physician can also help to educate and prepare the family for the death of elderly relatives in ways that increase the support the family can offer the patient whose death is imminent. The physician's own attitudes about aging, death, and dying and the physician's own reaction to personal losses are critical factors in determining the nature of the support to be offered to elderly patients.

Legal Issues

As with any patient, all medical and psychiatric procedures must be explained, and consent must be received. When examining a patient for competency, this should be made clear, and the patient should be told of the right to have a lawyer present. With regard to hospitalization, voluntary admissions are always preferred although, occasionally, involuntary commitment may be the only recourse. Again, with institutionalization, freedom should be protected as long as possible, and patients should be provided with the least restrictive care possible. People do not lose their rights when they are old nor when they are ill, and all individuals should retain the right to be informed and to make important decisions about their lives as long as possible.

CONCLUSION

We are treating the elderly, and we are also treating our future selves. The fundamental issues to be dealt with are lifelong, and it is imperative to allow every person to live as fully as possible up to the moment of death.

It is not necessary to be old to understand the older person, but it is necessary to have experienced enough change, growth, and crisis to be able to empathize with the difficult tasks of growing older. An examination of society's attitudes and one's own attitudes is valuable, and will benefit not only one's patients but oneself. A grasp of the concept of a total life with its rhythms and crises, blessings and problems, and a willingness to face painful truths are necessary in working with the older person. In the United States, there has undoubtedly been an overemphasis on youth. The challenge is to take up the work and extend it throughout the entirety of life. It is both a selfish and selfless task, as it benefits others and ourselves as well.

REFERENCES

1 Brody, E. M. et al.: "Excess Disabilities of Mentally Impaired Aged: Impact of Individualized Treatment," *Gerontologist,* **11**:124–133, 1971.
2 Goldfarb, A. I.: "The Psychotherapy of Elderly Patients," in H. T. Blumenthal (ed.), *Medical and Clinical Aspects of Aging,* New York: Columbia Univ. Press, pp. 106–114, 1962.
3 Safirstein, S. L.: "Psychotherapy for Geriatric Patients," *NYS J. Med.,* **72**:2743–2748, 1972.
4 Burnet, F. M.: *Immunological Surveillance,* New York: Pergamon Press, pp. 224–257, 1970.
5 Dastur, Darab K. et al.: "Effects of Aging on Cerebral Circulation and Metabolism in Man," in J. E. Birren et al. (eds.), *Human Aging: A Biological and Behavioral Study,* Washington, D. C.: U.S. Government Printing Office, 1963.
6 Butler, R. N.: *Why Survive? Being Old in America,* New York: Harper and Row, 1975.
7 ———: "Clinical Psychiatry in Late Life," in Isadore Rossman (ed.), *Clinical Geriatrics,* Philadelphia: J. B. Lippincott, 1971.
8 Dorken, H.: "Normal Senescent Decline and Senile Dementia: Their Differentiation by Psychological Tests," *Med. Serv. J.,* **14**:18–23, 1956.
9 Resnik, H. L., and J. M. Cantor: "Suicide and Aging," *J. Am. Geriatrics Soc.,* **18**:152–158, 1970.
10 Butler, R. N., and Myrna I. Lewis: *Aging and Mental Health, Positive Psychosocial Approaches,* St. Louis: C. V. Mosby, 1977.

BIBLIOGRAPHY

Birren, J. E. et al.: *Human Aging: A Biological and Behavioral Study,* Washington, D. C.: U.S. Government Printing Office, 1963.
Brody, E. M. et al.: "Excess Disabilities of Mentally Impaired Aged: Impact of Individualized Treatment," *Gerontologist,* **11**:124–133, 1971.
Busse, E. E.: *Therapeutic Implications of Basic Research with the Aged,* Strecker Monograph Series no. IV, The Institute of Pennsylvania Hospital, 1967. Published courtesy of Roche Laboratories, Nutley, N.J.
Butler, R. N.: "The Life Review: An Interpretation of Reminiscence in the Aged," *Psychiat.,* **26**:65, 1963.
———: "Clinical Psychiatry in Late Life," in Isadore Rossman (ed.), *Clinical Geriatrics,* Philadelphia: J. B. Lippincott, 1971.
———: "Toward a Psychiatry of the Life Cycle," in *Aging in Modern Society, Psychiatric Research Report 23,* American Psychiatric Association, 1968.

————: *Why Survive? Being Old in America,* New York: Harper and Row, 1975.

————, and Myrna I. Lewis: *Sex After Sixty: A Guide for Men and Women for Their Later Years,* New York: Harper and Row, 1976.

Dastur, Darab K. et al.: "Effects of Aging on Cerebral Circulation and Metabolism in Man," in J. E. Birren et al. (eds.), *Human Aging: A Biological and Behavioral Study,* Washington, D.C.: U.S. Government Printing Office, 1963.

Dorken, H.: "Normal Senescent Decline and Senile Dementia: Their Differentiation by Psychological Tests," *Med. Serv. J.,* **14**:18–23, 1956.

Goldfarb, A. I.: "Patient-Doctor Relationship in Treatment of Aged Persons," *Geriatrics,* **12**:18, 1964.

————: *The Psychotherapy of Elderly Patients,* in H. T. Blumenthal (ed.), *Medical and Clinical Aspects of Aging,* New York: Columbia Univ. Press, pp. 106–114, 1962.

———— et al.: "Hyperbaric Oxygen Treatment of Organic Mental Syndrome in Aged Persons, *J. Gerontol.,* **27**:212–217, 1972.

Perlin, S., and R. N. Butler: "Physiological-Psychological-Psychiatric Interrelationships," in J. E. Birren et al. (eds.), *Human Aging: A Biological and Behavioral Study,* Washington, D.C.: U.S. Government Printing Office, 1963.

Resnik, H. L., and J. M. Cantor: "Suicide and Aging," *J. Am. Geriatrics Soc.,* **18**:152–158, 1970.

Safirstein, S. L.: "Psychotherapy for Geriatric Patients," *NYS J. Med.,* **72**:2743–2748, 1972.

Usdin, G., and C. K. Hofling (eds.): *Aging: The Process and the People,* New York: Brunner/Mazel, 1978.

Chapter 18

Normal Sleep and Sleep Disorders

William C. Dement, M.D.

EDITORS' INTRODUCTION

What is it like to fail to fall to sleep for several hours, night after night? What is it like to feel sleepy much of the time? To have your mate complain of your loud snoring? To experience nightmares?

What is it like to recognize that the sedative prescribed by your physician is no longer effective? To ask for "something stronger" and be told that you do not need it? To be referred to a sleep laboratory, and to meet a number of new professionals there?

How does the physician who was trained before the explosion in knowledge about sleep feel when confronted by the insomniac whose symptoms do not respond to mild sedation and brief psychotherapy? How serious does the physician consider sleep disturbances to be?

Sleep disturbances are reported by one-third of the population. Research of the past several decades has brought much understanding and order to this complex field. Narcolepsy and upper-airway sleep apnea are recognized now as seriously debilitating and potentially fatal illnesses. The differential diagnosis of the insomnias has been influenced drastically by expanding research data. The indications for and against the use of hypnotics in the different insomnias have been clarified by findings from sleep laboratories.

As research has increased our understanding of the sleep disorders, it has also made it clear that treatment must be based on accurate diagnosis, that the "routine" prescription is not congruent with the complexity of the field and that, indeed, it may have dangerous consequences.

In this chapter, a distinguished scientist and pioneer in the field of sleep research provides answers to many of the questions confronting all physicians. Normal sleep is described, and sleep disorders are considered against the background of that knowledge. There are many pragmatic suggestions for the practicing physician, and an understanding of both normal sleep and sleep disorders provides the physician with increased opportunities for a truly scientific approach to these disabling and distressing syndromes.

Sleep is an exciting new frontier of scientific and clinical research, a complex and fascinating field in which knowledge is changing and expanding rapidly. Sleep disorders medicine is the newest clinical discipline in American medicine. This chapter discusses the basics of normal sleep mechanisms as they are presently understood, and the diagnostic indicators of the sleep/wake disorders that are encountered in general medical practice.

The study and treatment of sleep disorders in medicine is based on the premise that sleep is a profoundly important area of human functioning and pathology. Recent research and clinical experience indicate that we may be dealing with *two* patients: the patient in the waking state and the patient in the sleep state.

What is known about physiology during the waking state may not be true of physiology during sleep. For example, Phillipson determined that regulation of respiration is entirely different in sleep, and that the classic Hering-Breuer reflex does not exist in sleep.[1] Heller and Glotzbach found that there is no temperature regulation during Rapid-Eye-Movement (REM) sleep—the organism is poikilothermic.[2] In the last decade, clinical research has made a number of advances: narcolepsy has been identified as a disorder of REM sleep; life-threatening sleep apnea syndromes have been described; the relationship of Sudden Infant Death Syndrome (SIDS) to sleep apnea has been documented; nocturnal myoclonus and drug dependency have been shown to be neurological and iatrogenic causes of insomnia; and life-threatening cardiac arrhythmias that occur in sleep have been discovered.

Research in biological rhythms, which is the study of the circadian and ultradian rhythms inherent in living organisms, underscores the need to understand the temporal dimension of health and pathology better. In addition to the disabling and/or deadly sleep-wake disorders, a number of other illnesses, including glaucoma, hypertension, asthma, epilepsy, endocrine pathologies, duodenal ulcers, parasitic disease, and migraine headaches, clearly reflect a significant

24-hour periodicity. The rhythmic function may also affect conventional treatment. Radiation for tumors will kill more cancerous cells in the a.m. than in the p.m.[3] An LD50 dose of amphetamine may kill 90 percent of test rats at one time, and 12 hours later it may kill only 10 percent.[3] Recent statistics reveal that more deaths occur during traditional sleep hours.[3] To many people, sleep may be the enemy, rather than the "gentle restorer."

PREVALENCE OF SLEEP DISORDERS

Hauri states that "between 12 to 15 percent of all people living in industrialized countries have serious sleep problems."[4] In a survey of health characteristics by Karacan et al., substantially more than half of 1,645 randomly selected individuals, aged 16 and over, complained about sleeping too little or too much. Based upon these data, the investigators estimated that at least 30 million people in the United States have sleep complaints.[5] In another study of 1,064,000 people who were specially selected for prospective analysis of health conditions and death rates, approximately 25 percent complained of insomnia. In addition, the death rate was lowest in individuals who habitually slept 6 hours nightly, and was dramatically elevated for those individuals who habitually slept 4 hours or less and 10 hours or more.[6] In a national survey of "selected symptoms of mental distress," sleep disturbances were reported among 32.4 percent of the adult population, and were second only to anxiety among mental symptoms.[7] A similar figure was reported by Kales et al., who participated in the 1963 Los Angeles Metropolitan Survey.[8]

Narcolepsy was once presumed to be an esoteric disorder. An extensive prevalence study carried out in the Los Angeles and San Francisco Bay areas indicated that its incidence may be dramatically high. If the findings are extrapolated to the entire nation, there may be at least 150,000 individuals with this disease in the United States, over twice as many as the number of patients with multiple sclerosis (70,000).[9]

THE DEVELOPMENT OF SLEEP DISORDERS MEDICINE

The most obvious difficulty in dealing with sleep disorders is that they are hidden by night. Today's student of medicine assimilates an encyclopedic body of empirical knowledge that is based on medical observations of millions of patients throughout the centuries. In contrast, one of the major features of normal sleep, REMs, escaped observation for thousands of years.

The existence of periodically occurring periods of REMs during sleep was first documented by Aserinsky and Kleitman in 1953.[10] This was followed by the observation that the periods of REMs were related to dreaming, and that these periods recurred on the average of every 92 minutes.[11] Jouvet found that REM sleep was also characterized by intense cortical activity and complete electromyographic suppression, or absence of muscle tonus in voluntary muscle groups. These studies destroyed the centuries-old myth that sleep was a period of uniform, passive quiescence.[12] Sleep was found to consist of discrete states, one of which, REM sleep, involved brain-wave activity that was more intense than such activity in waking.

Narcolepsy as a specific sleep disorder was described by Gelineau in 1880.[13] However, as late as the 1950s there was serious controversy about whether the various manifestations of the syndrome represented epileptic equivalents, sequelae of viral encephalitis, or were of psychogenic origin. Until the discovery of REM sleep onset in patients with narcolepsy by Rechtschaffen et al. in 1963[14] and Takahashi and Jimbo in 1964,[15] the narcoleptic symptomatology was not interpreted correctly in terms of a disturbance of the normal REM sleep processes. Further study of canine narcolepsy, through a spontaneous animal model discovered in 1973, confirmed that narcolepsy is a disease of REM sleep.[16]

The restless legs syndrome was described by Ekbom in 1944,[17] and was related to nocturnal myoclonus in the 1950s. Research on the sleep apnea symptoms is less than a decade old, and a previously unknown insomnia-sleep apnea was discovered by Guilleminault in 1972.[18]

Researchers are still trying to find a satisfactory reason for the function of sleep. No theory has fully answered the question of why we sleep, apart from a desire to prevent sleepiness.

Sleep researchers are faced with the awesome task of making the necessary empirical observations and clinical-pathological correlations that took centuries to complete in other clinical disciplines.

The development of polysomnography after World War II provided a technique for measuring, describing, and evaluating sleep objectively.

LABORATORY MEASUREMENT OF SLEEP AND NORMAL SLEEP PARAMETERS

Sleep is measured by monitoring simultaneously the electrical activity of three systems: the brain, the eyes, and the muscles. The wave forms are then interpreted by sleep technicians according to standardized definitions. The changes in form and frequency of brain waves give the experienced technician a complete picture of the night's sleep.

The record of brain activity in humans is based on the voltage fluctuations from a point on the scalp—the EEG, or electroencephalogram. The difference in electrical potential between the cornea and the retina is transmitted through electrodes attached to the face, and makes up a record of eye movements, or the EOG (electrooculogram). The electrical potentials generated in the muscle fibers are recorded by electrodes that are attached to the chin and are known as the electromyogram (EMG).

In routine outpatient evaluations, the patient arrives at the laboratory about an hour before the usual bedtime, and prepares for bed with the same bedtime ritual used at home. The sleep center provides private, specially equipped bedrooms, lavatory, and other facilities. A polysomnography technician checks equipment to ensure that adjustments that may disturb the patient's habitual sleep pattern will not be necessary during the night. Before "lights out," the patient's face and scalp are cleansed thoroughly with acetone or alcohol at the points of electrode placement. Scalp electrodes are attached by means of gauze pads that have been soaked in collodion and quick-dried with compressed air. Surgical tape is used to attach the electrodes to the face. The wires are then bundled and anchored to the scalp in a "pony tail," which the patient carries to bed. There the technician plugs each of the wires into a numbered panel on the polygraph. Special techniques may be used to measure cardiac functions, respiration, penile tumescence, or other variables, depending upon the nature of the complaint and the presumptive diagnosis.

Normal Sleep Parameters

To understand the nature of the sleep pathologies, one must first understand normal sleep structure.

The first basic fact about normal sleep is that there are *two entirely different kinds of sleep:* NREM (Non-REM) and REM sleep. Any prolonged sleep period consists of a regular alteration between these states, which are as different from one another as both are from wakefulness. REM sleep is characterized by a generalized motor inhibition, during which the organism is effectively paralyzed. Electrodes placed over muscles show a suppression of electromyographic activity, and reflexes are also suppressed. Major exceptions include breathing and the extraocular functions that give this state its name. The tremendous activity of the brain during REM sleep is in marked contrast to the body's flaccid paralysis. The brain is awake during REM sleep, for all intents and purposes, and is furiously active. It has been hypothesized that REM sleep is not sleep at all, but a third state of consciousness. Eye movements during REM sleep are in no way different from those seen during wakefulness, when a human being is actively scanning the environment. A remarkable feature of REM sleep in males is penile tumescence; nearly all REM periods in males are accompanied by erections, even in the aged and in infants. Finally, arousal of volunteer subjects during REM sleep almost invariably elicits detailed dream recall.

NREM sleep, by contrast, is a state of cerebral deactivation, a period of diminished mentation. Peripheral motor functions are not inhibited, reflexes can be elicited, and a low-grade tonic muscle activity continues, in contrast to the EMG suppression of REM sleep.

REM sleep has been summarized as a state resulting from an awake brain, which is preoccupied by the vivid hallucinations of the dream world and is inside a paralyzed body.

Normal sleep involves a cyclical shifting back and forth between NREM and REM states. In a normal individual, NREM sleep always comes first. Typically, the first NREM period lasts for about 60 minutes, and is followed by about 10 minutes of REM sleep, which makes a "sleep cycle" of one NREM period and one REM period, totaling about 70 minutes. The next cycle is usually about 110 minutes, the third about 120 minutes, and subsequent cycles are close to 90 minutes, which is the approximate mean. Five sleep cycles represent an average night's sleep, about three-fourths of which is spent in NREM sleep.

The normal human adult enters NREM Stage 1 sleep from wakefulness. (Infants may go directly into REM sleep, but sleep onset is followed by NREM when the organism matures.) The normal sleeper passes through succeeding NREM Stages 2, 3, and 4, and returns to Stage 2 again before entering the first REM period. An adult spends more time in NREM Stage 2 than in any other stage of sleep—about 40 to 50 percent of total sleep time.[19] As normal adults age, the tendency is toward lighter sleep. Age seems to be the single most powerful determinant of sleep patterns.[20]

Routine polysomnographic examination continuously measures the EMG, or muscle activity; EEG, or brain-wave activity; EOG, or eye-movement activity; the multiple respiratory functions of effort, air flow, and oxygen saturation of the blood; EKG, or heart rate and regularity; and abnormal body movements, particularly in the legs. These measurements provide the objective parameters of sleep. They allow the technician to record the precise moment of sleep onset, and thereby measure the objective sleep latency of the individual, or how long it takes to fall asleep; the objective total sleep time; and when REM sleep occurs. Polysomnography makes an objective description of the patient's sleep possible and provides direct observation of sleep-related malfunctions hidden during the waking state.

DISORDERS OF SLEEP: THE HYPERSOMNIAS

Hypersomnia is the term used widely throughout the literature to mean Excessive Daytime Sleepiness (EDS), or pathological sleepiness. The two major causes of EDS are narcolepsy and sleep apnea.[21]

The seriousness of excessive daytime sleepiness as a medical and social problem has not been fully recognized. In our work-oriented culture, sleepiness is considered to be a vice to be overcome by willpower. The individual who succumbs to sleepiness repeatedly is considered by many to be lazy. Contrary to these deeply held biases, the person who is suffering from an undiagnosed case of pathological sleepiness has a real and serious medical disorder.

Pathological sleepiness means excessive daily sleepiness without prior sleep loss at night—sleepiness that is not caused by sleep deprivation. In one series of EDS patients, excessive amounts of sleep are actually rare; the complaint is of "excessive sleepiness," or an excessive susceptibility to sleep. Ninety-five percent of the cases involving excessive daily sleepiness in a series had an identifiable pathological cause, but not a single patient had the commonly ascribed causes of hypoglycemia or hypothyroidism. Fifty to seventy percent of the patients were diagnosed as suffering from narcolepsy or from sleep apnea syndrome. Tragically, the average patient had consulted at least three physicians over a period of 10 to 15 years, and either remained undiagnosed or was misdiagnosed as "depressed," "mentally disturbed," "hypothyroid," or "hypoglycemic."[21]

Steps in Diagnosis of EDS

The first step in distinguishing pathological sleepiness is to take a good history of
the patient's sleepiness and sleep patterns: when the patient falls asleep, the duration of sleep, and when he or she feels overwhelmingly sleepy. Chronic sleep loss
should be ruled out before the physician makes a presumptive diagnosis of hypersomnia. If the patient reports a problem with daytime sleepiness, fatigue, and
lack of alertness despite what seems to be a normal amount of sleep, pathological
sleepiness should be suspected. Three simple questions will help to diagnose patients who complain of excessive daytime sleepiness:

1   Do you ever have attacks of muscular weakness or paralysis that seem to
be caused by strong emotions, such as anger or laughter? (The sleepy patient who
answers "yes" is suffering from the narcolepsy syndrome.)
2   Do you snore? (If yes, suspect sleep apnea, especially if the patient is a
male.)
3   What medications have you used chronically during the past few months
or years? (Chronic use of stimulants, hypnotics, and other drugs can result in a
complaint of EDS—usually about 5 to 10 percent of patients.)

Narcolepsy

Narcolepsy is a syndrome characterized by four symptoms: excessive daytime
sleepiness, or extreme susceptibility to sleep-inducing situations; cataplexy; sleep
paralysis, sometimes accompanied by nocturnal sleep disturbance; and hypnagogic hallucinations. The key symptom for the definitive diagnosis of narcolepsy is cataplexy. (A common error in diagnosis is to assume that excessive
sleepiness alone is narcolepsy.)

Cataplexy is loss of muscle control and muscle tone (a type of flaccid
paralysis), and is usually precipitated by strong emotion or excitement. It is a
reversible attack of quadriplegia that is most commonly caused by laughter,
stress, or anger. When muscle function is measured during a cataplectic attack,
electromyographic activity decreases sharply, and tendon reflexes disappear. Patients may have infrequent or partial attacks that involve only one muscle group
(such as sagging of the facial muscles), but some have hundreds of attacks a day
and are completely disabled.[22]

The onset of narcolepsy usually occurs about the time of puberty, although
children or mature adults over 30 may develop the disorder. The typical case
history reveals a problem with sleepiness that becomes apparent at about 8 to 12
years of age. Individuals with a narcoleptic relative have a 60 percent higher
chance of developing the disorder, and children of a narcoleptic parent have
about a 1 in 20 chance.[23] Recent research with canine narcolepsy strongly suggests
a genetic component—perhaps a recessive gene.[23,24]

Patients with narcolepsy can be described as having an excessive *susceptibility* to sleepiness and sleep-inducing situations. Commonly, sleepiness will begin to
appear at times when most people may get sleepy—in dull lectures or overheated

rooms, after a heavy meal, or during a long car ride. The patient may present as being fatigued and without energy, rather than as "sleepy," especially since sleepiness is not socially acceptable. One patient described the constant fatigue as a "continual sense of physical depletion," and stated that she would be glad to suffer both cataplexy and sleep attacks in exchange for normal periods of feeling energetic.

Sleepiness becomes "sleep attacks" when the impulse to sleep becomes overwhelming, despite the inappropriateness of the situation. The patient does not go from normal alertness into sleep suddenly, but is fighting sleep constantly until finally the patient is overcome. Patients have fallen asleep while making love, driving, eating dinner, or in the middle of a sentence. The patient, who is frequently unaware of the lapses or the extent of the sleepiness, may continue the conversation with exactly the same phrase that was being used when sleep occurred.[25]

A diagnostic gauge for narcolepsy, then, is the frequency of sleep and sleepiness in sleep-inducing situations, and the occurrence of sleep or sleepiness in inappropriate situations. The patient may describe the symptoms, however, as "fatigue" and "lack of energy"; incidents of falling asleep may have to be elicited through careful questioning. Interviewing parents, teachers, or spouses can be very helpful, since they may be aware of naps and sleepiness of which the patient is not. In the case of a child with narcolepsy, this is especially important.

Some diagnostic questions are:

1 Has the patient ever been called "lazy" or "sleepy," or given a nickname referring to laziness or sleepiness—such as "Lazy Susan," or "Sleepy"? Has there been a dramatic change in grades or performance, especially in the case of a child or adolescent?

2 Does the patient have difficulty getting out of bed in the morning? Does the patient "lose" time—go to bed and sleep through 1 or 2 days, especially after exertion?

3 Does the patient seem to be forgetful or not fully aware? Does the patient fall asleep in lectures; in a car, whether driving or as a passenger; in church; in movies; on dates; after meals; at a certain time of day?

4 Is the patient in the habit of taking naps during the day in order to continue functioning? (Female patients have reported sleeping on the toilet in restrooms in order to get through the work day. This conveys how occult and shameful sleepiness is in our wide-awake society.)

5 Does the patient have a craving for sweets, and use sweets, cigarettes, and coffee in an effort to stay awake?

In the case of patients who do not have severe cataplexy, the symptom may have to be elicited by the physician. One patient thought that weakness in the knees while laughing was normal. Patients also learn to avoid emotional or exciting situations, not to express emotions, and to tense themselves in order to avoid cataplexy. In a mild or partial attack, the jaw or neck muscles may sag momentarily, or the patient may feel weakness in the knees. Cataplexy is usually precipitated by strong emotion, but patients may experience cataplexy without such a precipitant.

During cataplexy, the patient seems to be in a third state of consciousness, where he or she is aware of external events, but is often hallucinating or experiencing "out of body" sensations while being paralyzed. Polygraphically, the attacks look like intrusions of REM sleep into waking life. Research continues to explore how closely cataplexy resembles REM sleep in humans. Polygraphic studies of dogs with narcolepsy show that EEG, EOG, and EMG during cataplexy are identical to those in REM sleep.[24]

Cataplexy is often confused with epilepsy, hysteria, or "conversion neurosis." Psychiatric literature describes cataplexy as a psychological escape from emotional stress and repressed desires.[26,27] Since cataplexy occurs spontaneously in canine narcolepsy, and is usually precipitated by excitement, play, or the anticipation of food, the evidence indicates that the symptom is neurological rather than emotional.[24]

Complete cataplexy can be dangerous in some situations, and is always frightening and embarrassing to the patient, as in the following case:

> A patient had cataplexy in a San Francisco bank. He was forced to lie helpless and speechless while employees forced a spoon down his throat, because they had confused the cataplectic collapse with epileptic convulsions. When the patient regained control (with a lacerated throat) and explained to the police and ambulance attendants that he had narcolepsy, he was arrested for possession of narcotics.

Attempts at avoidance can have a severely inhibiting effect on the patient's life. The patient may withdraw from social interaction, expressions of emotion, sexual activity, athletics, and any other situation in which cataplexy may occur. For example:

> A patient who had been a successful stockbroker was forced to inhibit his selling techniques severely because the excitement of anticipated success would elicit cataplexy in front of customers—he had to choose between success at selling and avoiding cataplexy, and eventually lost his job.

Associated, but not diagnostic, symptoms are automatic behavior, hypnagogic hallucinations, disturbed nocturnal sleep, and sleep paralysis.[28] During automatic behavior, the patient performs mechanically, without sufficient alertness to respond to new situations:

> A patient put all her best china dishes into the clothes drier instead of the dishwasher, and came to her senses to the sound of her china crashing into pieces.

> Patients frequently pass their highway exit, and arrive at an unintended destination without knowing how they got there.

> A patient who was a computer programmer spent several hours programming nonsense, while seeming to go through the normal motions of his work.

Hypnagogic hallucinations and sleep paralysis are usually associated. Sleep paralysis is the inability to move while falling asleep; hypnagogic hallucinations are extremely frightening and vivid "dreams" experienced while the patient is awake or falling asleep:

> The patient is convinced that someone is trying to get into the house, or will have a vivid sensation of threat or danger, but is unable to investigate because of the sleep paralysis.

The following history illustrates the gradual onset of the disorder and some of the clues at diagnosis:

> The patient started falling asleep at the dinner table at age 12. Teachers and school friends joked about her "laziness," but the patient did not feel herself to be unusually sleepy or lazy. In fact, she was falling asleep in class without being aware of her naps. The sleepiness increased during adolescence, but was considered to result from life changes. Gradually, she gave up activities and interests, including training for pre-Olympic sports, because she "just didn't have the energy." Employers at a part-time job told her to cut down on her social life so that she wouldn't fall asleep at work. Performance in classes deteriorated, despite an above-average IQ. The patient began falling asleep on dates, especially on long car rides. Cataplexy was limited to weakness in the knees and partial collapse of the facial muscles when laughing, which she thought was normal. She married young and left college. Her sleepiness and lack of energy were interpreted by spouse and children to be lack of concern, and the marriage ended in divorce. She was diagnosed in her late thirties after relatives sent her a magazine article on narcolepsy, and she was referred to a sleep disorders center.

A definitive diagnosis of narcolepsy can be obtained at an accredited sleep disorders center.[29] Two definitive tests are performed: sleep latency testing, and polysomnographic recording of the patient's sleep onset periods. In sleep latency testing, the patient is asked to take a nap every 2 hours in a sleep laboratory setting. The normal person who is not suffering from sleep loss may take 20 minutes to fall asleep, or will not sleep at all. The patient with narcolepsy falls asleep each time, typically in 30 to 90 seconds. Patients also go directly into REM sleep, without the normal introductory progression through the NREM stages.[30]

Narcolepsy is treated by the general family physician or internist as any other lifelong, progressive, disabling disease. Many patients are disabled completely or partially by age 40; the goal of the attending physician is to prevent this disability for as long as possible, and to help the patient achieve and maintain the maximum level of possible alertness. None of the available treatments is entirely satisfactory, so long-term management requires careful recordkeeping and continued interaction between patient and physician.

Treatment consists of life-style changes and chemotherapy that is supplemented by counseling. Life-style changes include a regular bedtime, avoiding sleep loss whenever possible, and scheduling regular naps. There is evidence that five or ten evenly scheduled naps every day can help offset sleep attacks, and decrease dependence on medication. Dangers should be identified and discussed. For example, the patient with severe cataplexy should refrain from swimming alone; auto accidents can be avoided if the patient is aware of the danger and schedules naps and medication so he or she can drive at periods of alertness.

Cataplexy should be explained to the patient and family. Family members need to learn when the patient may be in danger, pain, or may otherwise require assistance, and when the attack should be accepted as routine and the patient allowed to recover spontaneously. Cataplexy is especially frightening for the children of parents with narcolepsy, when the physician has not taken time to explain the condition.

Chemotherapy is indicated in most cases. The two major symptoms, excessive sleepiness and cataplexy, are discrete and must be treated separately. Establishing the optimal dosage for either symptom requires careful recordkeeping and interaction with the patient. Sleepiness is counteracted by alerting medications. The compounds most widely used are methylphenidate, dextroamphetamine, and pemoline. Methylphenidate is the drug of choice with which to begin treatment. The patient can begin with 1 to 2 weeks' dosage, as low as 2.5 mg daily or 2.5 mg b.i.d. The patient can use a simple sleepiness scale to evaluate the continued effectiveness of the medication by rating the level of alertness periodically during the day:

1 Fully alert
2 Slightly sleepy
3 Very sleepy
4 Asleep

If cataplexy is not a serious problem for the patient, it should not be treated. Specific compounds for the treatment of cataplexy, sleep paralysis, and hypnagogic hallucinations are the tricyclic antidepressants, which are used because they suppress REM sleep, and the monoamine oxidase inhibitors. Anticataplectic effects are almost immediate—orally within an hour, and intravenously within minutes. Side effects of the medications should be explained carefully to patient and spouse. Anticataplectic medications tend to aggravate sleepiness, and often interfere with the male's ability to have penile erections. Taking the medication at bedtime eliminates the worst effects of the sleepiness. Many male patients regularly discontinue medication for a day or two at a time, to allow erectile potential to return while the anticataplectic action is still in effect. These problems illustrate the tremendous need for more research to find better treatments for narcolepsy. Currently, protriptyline is the drug of choice for treatment of cataplexy, beginning with a dose of 5 mg twice a day and 15 mg at bedtime. Monoamine oxidase inhibitors should be used only as a last resort, because of side effects.

The most common problem in chemotherapeutic treatment of narcolepsy is the gradual development of tolerance. Though drug holidays and substituting medications can delay the development of tolerance, it is almost inevitable that the patient will reach a point when withdrawal is advisable. Methylphenidate is rarely prescribed in a dosage above 60 mg daily to counteract sleepiness, and more than 200 mg daily, in divided doses of imipramine, is rare to counteract cataplexy. The patient should be cautioned that sleepiness will increase dramatically during withdrawal from the alerting medication. Withdrawal of anticataplectic medication is more complex. A rebound effect will greatly exacerbate the symptoms. Precautions to protect the patient from physical injury should be taken if the medication is withdrawn outside a hospital setting. If the patient's cataplexy has been severe, withdrawal should take place in a hospital setting, with complete bed rest, bed rails, and hand feeding. Medication can be reinstituted within 1 to 2 weeks, at much lower levels.[31]

To cope with the considerable emotional stress that the disorder's symptoms cause, counseling for the patient and family is very important. Both patient and physician should also be aware of the activities of the American Narcolepsy Association, which include sponsoring self-help groups for patients, promoting research and a better understanding of the disorder, and publishing valuable literature and information on narcolepsy.[32] The physician's intervention may also be necessary in order to explain the disorder to the patient's employer or school authorities.

The Sleep Apnea Syndromes

The *sleep apnea syndromes* are a sleep-induced respiratory impairment. Whether or not they produce the complaint of hypersomnia or insomnia, these syndromes are serious and potentially life-threatening .

Apnea is defined as any pause in air flow that lasts longer than 10 seconds. Upper-airway sleep apnea is the most important syndrome clinically, and one that presents the most danger to the patient. Studies, and particularly those by Lugaresi et al.,[33] led to the definition of three types of apneas, or respiratory pauses. The first sleep apnea syndrome is known as *diaphragmatic or central apnea.* In patients with this syndrome, the diaphragm stops moving during sleep, presumably because there is a temporary lapse in the proper nerve impulses from the brain stem. In *obstructive* or *upper-airway sleep apnea,* the most prevalent and life-threatening of the apneas syndromes, the upper airway becomes obstructed and the air cannot move in or out. The diaphragm actually moves more forcefully than normal, and the intrathoracic pressure may double as the body attempts to overcome the breathing block. A central mechanism that affects the constrictor muscles of the pharynx has been postulated for upper-airway sleep apnea. The third type of episode is *mixed,* where the diaphragm stops moving, and then must overcome the obstruction in the airway when it begins to move again (for example, the central apnea is spontaneously relieved as the obstructive apnea begins).

Sleep apnea has been recognized for less than a decade. Much of our current understanding has come about only in the past 5 to 6 years, and is heavily indebted to data derived from studies of normal respiration and circulation during sleep. These studies have been conducted over the last 15 years in the United States, Sweden, England, and Italy.

The term *Pickwickian* was coined in 1956 by Burwell et al. to describe a patient who was markedly obese, and presented with chronic hypoventilation and daytime somnolence.[34] In 1965, Gastaut et al. reported that Pickwickian patients showed repetitive apneas during sleep.[35] In 1967 Schwartz and Escande demonstrated the tendency for the muscles around the nasopharynx, hypopharynx, and pharynx to hyperrelax in Pickwickian patients during sleep, thereby causing blockage of the airway.[36] Lugaresi et al., as well as other investigators, described the identical sleep-related respiratory impairment in nonobese patients.[37] Guilleminault concluded from a controlled study of obese and nonobese upper-airway sleep apnea patients that obesity was not part of the syndrome.[38]

Snoring is a commonplace, sleep-induced partial airway obstruction in normal subjects—the heavier and louder the snoring, the closer the person comes to a sleep-induced upper-airway obstruction. Upper-airway sleep apnea has been popularly known as "the snoring disease." The typical upper-airway sleep apnea patient has 300 to 400 repetitive apneas during a single night,[38] and it is possible to have as many as 600 to 700 a night. These apneas may last from 30 seconds to almost 3 minutes. Upper-airway sleep apneas are also accompanied by abnormal, flailing body movements; vocalization, such as moaning or groaning; sleepwalking; and of course, extremely loud snoring. This kind of apnea can often be diagnosed by having the spouse or bed partner describe the patient's behavior during sleep.

There are three types of Upper-Airway Sleep Apnea (UASA), based on their relationship to REM and NREM sleep. Type A UASA is the most common and life-threatening; with this sort, the cycles of apnea are continuous throughout the night, regardless of REM or NREM sleep. This type has the worst prognosis, because the episodes are continuous and the patient's body never has a chance to normalize. These patients are hypoxemic all night, with PAO_2 dropping to as low as 25 mm mercury and fluctuating to a high of 50 or 75 mm, but never returning to normal. In Type B UASA, the apneas occur in NREM sleep, but respiration is normal in REM. The patient has a chance to normalize the respiratory physiology approximately every 90 minutes during REM periods. In Type C UASA, the apneas are most frequent during REM and during transitions between sleep stages, such as sleep onset, or transition from NREM to REM. Respiration is normal in NREM stages 3 and 4. The patient has multiple opportunities to normalize respiration during the night.[39]

The first consequence of the physiological changes that occur during UASA is disabling daytime sleepiness. Although the patient may seem fully awake in the physician's office, the hundreds of arousals, the night-long hypoxemia, and the disturbed nature of the sleep lead to a relentless, continuous daytime sleepiness, with the same profoundly disabling effects as in the case of patients with narcolepsy.[38]

The second consequence, which is also seen in diaphragmatic or central apnea and mixed apnea, involves changes in blood pressure. There is a precipitous rise in blood pressure during the apneas, which finally persists in the waking state as unexplained hypertension. The third major consequence, which is not detectable in the waking state, is cardiac irregularity during sleep. The apneic episodes are accompanied all night long by bradycardia during the apneas, and tachycardia during the hyperapneas. Heart block is also seen in UASA; the most serious arrhythmia is ventricular tachycardia, which can occur several times in a single night in some patients. Any serious arrhythmias, when not reversed or self-limiting, can lead to sudden death during sleep.[40]

If the patient who complains of excessive daytime sleepiness also has hypertension and is a male, there is a 50 percent chance that he has UASA. Although UASA can also occur in women and children, with especially disabling effects on intelligence and growth in the case of children, over 95 percent of one series were men.[21] The spouse or bed partner should be questioned about other symptoms—history of extremely loud snoring, repetitive sleep disturbance, sleepwalking, and abnormal movements. If there is a history of heavy snoring punctuated by pauses, it is extremely likely that the patient has UASA. The services of a sleep disorders center and polysomnographic examination are absolutely indicated at this point, to confirm the diagnosis and evaluate the condition quantitatively. A thorough ENT examination should be performed to rule out any potential physical obstruction. Hypertrophic tonsils and adenoids in a child, macroglossia, or a deviated nasal septum in adults can also cause obstruction of the airway.[21]

Polysomnographic examination will provide a definitive diagnosis and will also indicate the seriousness and urgency of the condition. Respiratory effort is measured by recording the patient's endoesophageal pressure, which is roughly equivalent to intrathoracic pressure. Airflow is measured by a CO_2 probe positioned in the posterior nasal pharynx; blood gases are measured by an ear oximeter that measures O_2 saturation. It is important to remember that the patient's respiration will be completely normal during waking hours.

Type A UASA patients in whom the apneas occur both during NREM and REM sleep are at high risk. No chemotherapeutic treatment is yet available. Weight loss, if the patient is obese, will not affect the apneas significantly or reduce the danger to the patient. The first approach of choice is surgical correction of any upper-airway defect that has been uncovered by careful and thorough examination. One example of such surgery is the removal of hypertrophic tonsils and adenoids. In children with UASA, this may produce sufficient relief to make further surgical treatment unnecessary. In most adults, however, the 100 percent effective treatment of choice is a permanent tracheostomy.

A tube is inserted into the trachea, and is opened by the patient upon going to sleep at night, thus completely bypassing the upper-airway problem and enabling the patient to have normal respiration all night long. In the morning, the patient closes the valve. The tube itself has an opening in the upper portion, so the patient can breathe and talk normally in the waking state with the valve closed. This treatment is followed by a dramatic reversal of daytime sleepiness, and usually of the hypertension, and resolution of cardiac arrhythmias during sleep, thereby reducing the risk of sudden death during sleep.[41]

The patient may need counseling and support to adjust to the permanent tracheostomy, as the following history shows. The benefits to the patient, however, are considerable.

> The patient, a 15-year-old girl, was hospitalized for periodic reevaluation of recurrent migraine headaches, daytime sleepiness, and enuresis. She was considered to have intelligence in "the borderline retardation range" and was receiving psychotherapy and many medications, including imipramine, destroamphetamine, and methylphenidate, without relief of symptoms. At the time of the evaluation, the patient had been in individual and family psychotherapy for some years, and was taking 75 mg of methylphenidate and 300 mg of diphenylhydantoin. Sleep evaluation revealed an upper-airway sleep apnea syndrome. Tracheostomy was performed. Sleepiness, enuresis, and headaches disappeared completely. All medication was stopped. The patient had to deal with an initial emotional depression because of peer and school personnel attitudes toward the tracheostomy, but changing schools and receiving moral support from her mother enabled her to adjust. This adolescent girl, who had been severely disabled previously, is now taking ballet and horseback riding lessons, and is dating and attending school normally. Her IQ tests have only improved slightly, however. It is not known whether this indicates a permanent learning impairment.

Ease in adjusting socially to the tracheostomy is often proportional to the severity of symptoms before the operation. One patient stated that the morning after the tracheostomy was the first morning of his life in which he had awakened feeling well-rested and refreshed.

UASA should never be overlooked by the physician, as the following case history illustrates:

> A lawyer consulted a sleep clinic because of disabling daytime sleepiness. His sleepiness had persisted for a long time, but at first only troubled him in the evening. When he began to fall asleep in the courtroom and his job was seriously jeopardized, he sought professional assistance. The patient was diagnosed as suffering from upper-airway sleep apnea syndrome, with hypertension and serious cardiac arrhythmias during sleep. Surgical treatment was recommended with urgency. The patient was warned that weight loss would probably not be helpful, but he chose this course to avoid surgery. He was found dead one morning by his family, and his death was classified by the coroner as a heart attack. The assumption of the attending physician at the sleep clinic is that the patient died during sleep of an asystole, or heart block.

In one series of UASA patients, the incidence of sudden death during sleep over a 2- to 3-year follow-up period was 25 percent among patients who refused surgical intervention. Other patients developed congestive heart failure as a result of the high blood pressure. Many sleep clinicians regard UASA as a terminal disease when it is not treated.[42]

THE INSOMNIAS

Insomnia is one of the most frequent complaints in medical practice. It is a complaint with a multiplicity of causes, rather than a syndrome in itself. To deal effectively with this complaint, the physician must regard each patient as a unique and individual clinical problem, determine which of many possibilities is the cause of the complaint, and devise the best possible treatment. Unfortunately, the average physician spends about 3 minutes on this complaint, and usually writes a prescription for sleeping medication. A superficial approach may result in diagnostic or treatment errors. Prescribing sleeping pills without careful consideration may create a problem where none really existed—a true iatrogenic disorder.

Differentiating the conditions involving insomnia should always begin with the possibility of *drug dependency*. Many Americans habitually use hypnotics or tranquilizers. With chronic use, these medicines nearly all impair sleep, because the user almost invariably develops tolerance and dependency.

Drug-Dependency Insomnia

Initially, a patient's sleep time increases , but within a week or two total sleep will decline, and may even drop below the premedication baseline. A higher dosage is needed, and results in a repetition of the vicious cycle. Within a few months, a patient may be taking thousands of milligrams of barbiturates every night. Sleep clinics have treated patients who were ingesting 7,000 mg of barbiturates and 1,000 mg of amphetamines daily. If the patient tries to withdraw abruptly at this point, he or she will not be able to sleep, or sleep will be disturbed with large amounts of intense REM sleep. Kales et al. have demonstrated that convulsions and nightmares may occur after precipitous withdrawal from barbiturates.[43]

In addition to the barbiturates, other compounds that produce drug-dependency insomnia include glutethimide, methyprylon, ethclorvynol, methaqualone, and certain sleep-inducing antihistamines. Insomnia is also a major consequence of chronic alcohol ingestion.

Treatment of drug-dependency insomnia can be surprisingly complex. The patient usually believes strongly in the necessity for the drug; the schedule of administration often involves multiple drugs and is very inconsistent; and the program demands interaction between physician and patient and the use of behavior-change contracts.

The solution is gradual withdrawal. The first step is to educate the patient. The patient should be counseled about the effects of the drug and about the fact that normal sleep parameters will return when withdrawal is complete. The second step is stabilization of the drug dosage. The physician should assume complete control of the patient's medication. Prescriptions should be issued to the patient on no more than a weekly basis, and the dose should be taken at a specific time. The third step is actual withdrawal. If more than one drug is being used, all should be withdrawn, one at a time, and the dose reduced by one unit each week. If a patient were taking one gm of sodium pentobarbital, for the first week he or she would take 900 mg, and 800 mg the second week. At each step, the patient will experience a slight decrease in total sleep time, followed by an improvement in normal sleep parameters. If the withdrawal can be accompanied by polygraphic monitoring, the patient can be recorded and confronted with objective data of better sleep with fewer drugs. Symptoms gradually improve over a

4- to 6-week period after complete withdrawal. For about 20 percent of the patients in one series, withdrawal from sleeping medication solved the sleep problem. In 50 percent of the case series, drug-dependency insomnia was at least part of the problem.[44]

Two neurological causes of insomnia, nocturnal myoclonus and central sleep apneas, should be eliminated before others are investigated, particularly before treatment with hypnotics is instituted.[44] The first is a bizarre syndrome, which was found in 17 percent of insomniac patients in one series.

Nocturnal Myoclonus

This disorder may occur alone or in association with the "restless legs syndrome." The "restless legs syndrome," which was first described by Ekbom in 1944,[17] consists of a crawling sensation in the legs, which the patient can relieve only by moving the legs or walking. At night, "restless legs" patients must get out of bed and walk around before falling asleep again. In nocturnal myoclonus, the patient's anterior tibialis muscles periodically contract during sleep, causing pronounced leg jerks. The myoclonus is highly rhythmic, and occurs simultaneously in both legs. The leg jerks periodically awaken the patient, who is usually unaware of the movements but complains instead of insomnia. It is useful to interview the spouse or bed partner about the symptom. If the services of a sleep clinic are available, polysomnographic recording will clearly show the myoclonus.

There is no satisfactory treatment for nocturnal myoclonus, but definitive diagnosis will save the patient from needless anxiety and inappropriate treatment. Symptomatic relief has been obtained with diazepam, 5 to 20 mg before bedtime. Carbamazepine has been used successfully for "restless legs," but medication must be followed very carefully because of occasional bone marrow depression. One tablet of oxycodone before bedtime can also be useful, but it is important to avoid tolerance and the development of addiction.[44]

It is not understood what causes this syndrome. No evidence has been found that it is epileptic in orgin, and none of the cases in one series was associated with depression or other secondary causes of insomnia.[45]

Central or Diaphragmatic Sleep Apnea

Central or diaphragmatic sleep apnea was described briefly in the section on hypersomnia, and produces a complaint of sleeplessness. Central sleep apnea as a cause of insomnia was first described in 1972 by Guilleminault et al.[18] In central sleep apnea, the diaphragm periodically stops moving after the patient has fallen asleep. The patient awakens continually during the night in order to breathe. The presence of snoring and its observation by the spouse or bed partner are helpful indicators of this disorder. Symptomatic treatment should be avoided with heavy snorers. *Since most currently available hypnotics are respiratory depressants, ingestion by a patient with central sleep apnea may be fatal.*

No satisfactory chemotherapeutic treatment has been found. The complaint and incidence of apneas have been reduced with chlorimipramine, but effectiveness is lost with chronic administration.[18]

Circadian Rhythm Disturbances

Studies by Kleitman, Aschoff, Webb, Agnew, and others emphasize the prominent 24-hour periodicity of the sleep/wake cycle, and that performance and body temperature also maintain a 24-hour periodicity, regardless of sleep.[46,47,48] Disturbances of these 24-hour rhythms may cause complaints of insomnia. In *jet lag,* the individual has difficulty adjusting the internal body clock to a new external time zone. The body will readjust within a few days, but airline personnel and others who frequently cross time zones often complain of insomnia. In *phase lag syndrome,* the patient cannot fall asleep until early in the morning, and then cannot awaken at a time considered normal by society. In *phase lead syndrome,* the patient falls asleep too early and awakens too early. There is some evidence that insomnia complaints in the elderly are actually phase lead disturbances. Frequent travel across time zones, working on irregular shifts, or an erratic schedule can cause circadian rhythm disturbances.

Treatment consists of attempting to synchronize the patient's internal body rhythms with external time by gradually shifting the patient's bedtime and wake time to normal hours, or to hours considered normal by society.

Pseudoinsomnia

A substantial number of patients who complain bitterly of insomnia have completely normal sleep recordings. In a recent study of 122 chronic complainers, total sleep time was seriously underestimated, and sleep latency was overestimated.[49] The diagnosis of pseudoinsomnia is applied to patients who sleep 6 hours or more, and in whom no cause can be established for the complaint, including insomnia secondary to illness or chronic pain. Patients in this subgroup respond positively to the knowledge that their sleep is normal. Chemotherapeutic treatment is likely to compound the problem, but counseling, reassurance, and suggestions about sleep hygiene will usually be effective:[19]

> The patient, a 61-year-old single college professor, had suffered chronically from insomnia since college. At the age of 58, he felt unable to continue teaching, because of the insomnia, and retired officially. During evaluation at a sleep clinic, the patient stated in a sleep diary he kept for 2 weeks that his average daily sleep time was 3 hours and 59 minutes. His average sleep time on four consecutive nights of sleep recording in a sleep laboratory, however, was 8 hours and 9 minutes. The patient was also recorded on two additional nights after a hypnotic; sleep time averaged 7 hours and 58 minutes. After counseling and reassurance that his sleep was normal, the patient reported much less anxiety and depression about his complaint.

Insomnia Secondary to Psychiatric Disturbances

Kales and others have found that over 80 percent of 200 insomniac patients had one or more major scales in the pathologic range on Minnesota Multiphasic

Personality Inventory (MMPI) tests.[50] Estimates vary from 30 to 85 percent, but emotional and psychiatric disturbances are the underlying cause of the complaint of insomnia in a significant number of patients. Hauri comments that the patient who presents with a complaint of insomnia, when other emotional difficulties are present, has made a statement about self. The patient may be a "repressor" who prefers to describe him- or herself as an insomniac rather than as an individual who is suffering from emotional difficulties.[4] The physician should keep in mind that "normal insomniacs" exist—individuals who sleep 4 hours or less a night, and who do not complain.[51,52] Sleep deprivation alone does not cause psychopathology, though poor sleep and psychopathology potentiate each other. Periodic sleep deprivation has been used as a treatment for depression with some success, and Vogel et al. have found that selective deprivation of REM sleep may be an effective treatment for depression.[53] Hauri recommends that the clinician search carefully for signs of depression in intractable cases of insomnia. If depression is suspected, an antidepressant regimen is preferable to treatment with hypnotics.[4]

Other Causes

Almost any medical problem, including chronic pain, can cause the complaint of insomnia. Behavioral conditioning, an uncomfortable sleep environment, poor sleep hygiene, and weight loss may also produce this complaint. Hauri's "Checklist for the Work-Up of an Insomniac" is recommended for use by the clinician in dealing with insomnia.[4]

Treatment Alternatives

Where a diagnosable cause can be found, the underlying condition should be treated. Patients should be made aware of the "Ten Rules to Better Sleep Hygiene," and should be encouraged to use them.[4] Various kinds of behavioral therapy, including meditation, biofeedback, stimulus control, and relaxation therapy are available. Changing the conventional sleep environment may be helpful if the patient associates it with anxiety and sleeplessness. Obviously, much more research is needed to understand the manifestations of insomnia and to discover effective treatments.

This leaves the question of when hypnotics should be used, and how to determine their efficacy. If short-term symptomatic relief seems urgently desirable, a hypnotic could be prescribed with the following precautions:

1   Only hypnotics proven to be effective in laboratory tests should be used. Use should be consistent with demonstrated effectiveness: flurazepam currently is the most widely used, and apparently the most effective, hypnotic drug, and can be prescribed for 28 consecutive nights. Secobarbital, in contrast, should be given for no more than 2 to 3 days. (The use of barbiturates has decreased markedly, and they may soon become a drug of the past for the treatment of insomnia.)

2   The hypnotics should be withdrawn when the short-term cause of stress has terminated, no more than 2 to 4 weeks after the initial prescription.

3 If daytime anxiety is also a complaint, a tranquilizer may be more appropriate than a hypnotic.

4 Hypnotics should never be prescribed to heavy snorers without prior polysomnography—snoring is frequently a sign of sleep apnea syndrome, and administration of hypnotics can be fatal.

5 The dose should never be escalated. If the hypnotic is ineffective in the therapeutic dose range, the patient does not have true insomnia.

6 Drug accumulation should be avoided to prevent daytime sedation. Doses should be kept at the minimum level, and it may be appropriate to schedule "drug holidays."

7 Counseling and reassurance, when insomnia is uncomplicated by drug dependency, psychosis, or an organic cause, is often the most effective treatment. Relaxation and behavioral therapies can also be used in place of hypnotics.

8 Every patient for whom hypnotics are prescribed should clearly understand the way sleeping medications affect their sleep, and the danger of drug addiction.

The general trend is for use of the benzodiazepines, although they are not the final or ideal drug for symptomatic relief. With these drugs, fatal overdoses are less common, withdrawal is easier, and long-range effectiveness of up to 1 month has been established.[4,54]

The Parasomnias

Parasomnias or *dyssomnias* have been defined as activities, such as walking or urinating, which are normal when performed during wakefulness, but are abnormal during sleep.[20] This general category includes the childhood sleep disorders—sleepwalking, sleeptalking, bruxism (tooth-grinding), night terrors or *pavor nocturnus,* head-banging, and enuresis. (Sleep clinics also occasionally see adults who suffer from somnambulism, severe nightmares, and sleep epilepsy.)

Somnambulism, night terrors, and enuresis cause a great deal of concern in families. None of them really requires treatment, though counseling is often useful. The childhood sleep disorders have been studied extensively by Broughton, Fisher, and others.[55,56] All these disorders have characteristics in common, and are now seen as "disorders of arousal" that occur during NREM sleep and may be caused by neurological immaturity, which the child will outgrow.[57] Children usually stop sleepwalking within a few years; meanwhile, general security measures can be taken to prevent the sleepwalking child from harm. Drugs that suppress Stage 4 sleep, such as flurazepam or diazepam, can be used if necessary. Although the emotional impact of night terrors seems to be intense, the syndrome is associated with NREM State 4 sleep rather than with dreaming sleep. The child does not remember the incident in the morning, and dream recall is not associated with the syndrome. The frequency of episodes can be reduced by administering diazepam at bedtime, but the treatment is for the family rather than for the patient.[56] Enuresis may be a consequence of limited bladder capacity during the deep sleep typical of children. If no organic defect can be found, reassurance may be the best treatment. Techniques of bladder training may also be instituted. If bed-wetting is a severe inconvenience, 75 to 125 mg of imipramine twice daily may bring relief.[4] In the case of tooth-grinding, rubber guards may be worn over the teeth at night. Biofeedback has also been used with some success in controlling this symptom.[4] Violent rhythmic movements during sleep, such as head-banging, will probably also be outgrown. Neurological examination is indicated if the symptom continues into adulthood, however.[4]

CONCLUSION

Sleep disturbances are a cause of distress for many patients, and in cases of narcolepsy and sleep apnea, are severely debilitating and life-threatening. The physician need not be a specialist to become familiar with the diagnostic indicators of sleep disorders. Although the field is new, appropriate treatments for many sleep disturbances are now available. In contrast, inappropriate treatment or diagnosis may cause lifelong disability, drug addiction, or death.

Accredited sleep disorders centers are now available for evaluation of sleep disturbances, and can be an important tool in definitive diagnosis of sleep problems or in determining the efficacy and urgency of treatment. These centers are referral and research centers, however. The best care for the patient with sleep problems is provided by the concerned, well-informed physician who is knowledgeable and who uses the specialized services of sleep disorders centers.

REFERENCES

1 Phillipson, E. A. et al.: "Ventilatory and Waking Responses to CO_2 in Sleeping Dogs," *American Review of Respiratory Diseases,* **115**: 1977.
2 Heller, H. C., and S. F. Glotzbach: "Thermoregulation during Sleep and Hibernation," *Int. Rev. Phys. II,* **15**: 1977.
3 Luce, G. G.: "Biological Rhythms in Psychiatry and Medicine," *U.S. Public Service Publ. #2088,* NIMH, 1970.
4 Hauri, Peter: "The Sleep Disorders," in *Current Concepts,* Kalamazoo: Upjohn MS-5595, 1977.
5 Karacan, I. et al.: "Prevalence of Sleep Disturbance in the General Population," *Sleep Res.,* **2**:158, 1973.
6 Hammond, E.: "Some Preliminary Findings on Physical Complaints from a Prospective Study of 1,064,004 Men and Women," *Am. J. Public Health,* **54**:11–22, 1964.
7 "Selected Symptoms of Psychological Distress," *Public Health Service Publ. #1000, Series 27,* Washington, D. C.: Superintendent of Documents, 1970.
8 Kales, A. et al.: "Incidence of Insomnia in the Los Angeles Metropolitan Area," *Sleep Res.,* **3**:139, 1974.
9 Dement, W. C. et al.: "The Prevalence of Narcolepsy, II," *Sleep Res.,* **2**:147, 1973.
10 Aserinsky, E., and N. Kleitman: "Regularly Occurring Periods of Eye Motility and Concomitant Phenomena during Sleep," *Science,* **118**:273–274, 1953.
11 Dement, W. C., and N. Kleitman: "Cyclic Variations in EEG during Sleep and Their Relation to Eye Movements, Body Motility and Dreaming," *Electroencephalogr. Clin. Neurophysiol.,* **9**:673–690, 1957.

12 Jouvet, M.: "Paradoxical Sleep: A Study of Its Nature and Mechanisms," in W. A. Himwick and J. P. Schade (eds.), *Sleep Mechanisms: Progress in Brain Research,* vol. 20, Amsterdam: Elsevier Publishing Co., 1965.

13 Gelineau, J.: "De la Narcolepsie," *Gazette d'Hopitaux (Paris),* **53**:626–628; **54**:635–637, 1880.

14 Rechtschaffen, A. et al.: "Nocturnal Sleep of Narcoleptics," *Electroencephalogr. Clin. Neurophysiol.,* **15**:5909–609, 1963.

15 Takahashi, Y., and M. Jimbo: "Polygraphic Study of Narcoleptic Syndrome with Special Reference to Hypnagogic Hallucinations and Cataplexy," *Fol. Psychiat. Neurol. Jap.,* **7** (Suppl):343, 1963.

16 Mitler, M. et al.: "Narcolepsy-Cataplexy in a Female Dog," *Exp. Neurol.,* **45**:332–340, 1974.

17 Ekbom, K.: "Asthenia Crurum Paraesthetica (Irritable Legs)," *Acta Med. Scad.,* **118**:197–201, 1944.

18 Guilleminault, C. et al.: "Insomnia with Sleep Apnea: A New Syndrome," *Science,* **181**:856–858, 1973.

19 Dement, W. C.: *Some Must Watch While Some Must Sleep* (The Portable University Series), San Francisco: W. H. Freeman, 1977.

20 Williams, R. L. et al.: *Electroencephalography (EEG) of Human Sleep: Clinical Applications,* New York: Wiley, 1974.

21 Guilleminault, C., and W. Dement: "235 Cases of Excessive Daytime Sleepiness," *J. Neurol. Sciences,* **31**:13–27, 1977.

22 Guilleminault, C. et al.: "A Study on Cataplexy," *Arch. Neurol.,* **31**:255, 1974.

23 Kessler, S.: "Genetic Factors in Narcolepsy," in C. Guilleminault et al. (eds.), *Narcolepsy,* New York: Spectrum, 1976.

24 Mitler, M., and W. Dement: "Canine Narcolepsy," in J. F. Cummings (ed.), *Spontaneous Animal Models of Human Disease,* New York: Academic Press, in press.

25 Dement, W.: "Daytime Sleepiness and Sleep Attacks," in C. Guilleminault et al. (eds.), *Narcolepsy,* New York: Spectrum, 1976.

26 Zarcone, V., and H. Fuchs: "Psychiatric Disorders and Narcolepsy," in C. Guilleminault et al. (eds.), *Narcolepsy,* New York: Spectrum, 1976.

27 Bourgignon, A.: "Narcolepsy and Psychoanalysis," in C. Guilleminault et al. (eds.), *Narcolepsy,* New York: Spectrum, 1976.

28 Guilleminault, C. et al.: "Altered States of Consciousness in Disorders of Daytime Sleepiness," *J. Neurol. Sci.,* **26**:377–393, 1975.

29 For the latest information on accredited sleep disorders centers, write to: Association of Sleep Disorders Centers (ASDC), TD 114, Stanford University Medical Center, Stanford, CA 94305.

30 Dement, W. et al.: "Daytime Sleep Recordings in Narcoleptics and Hypersomniacs," *Sleep Res.,* **1**, 1972.

31 Dement, W., and W. Baird: *Narcolepsy: Care and Treatment—A Guide for the Primary Care Physician Whose Patient is Afflicted With Narcolepsy,* Stanford: Stanford Univ. School of Medicine, 1977.

32 For Information on the American Narcolepsy Association, write to: P. O. Box 5846, Stanford, Calif., 94305.

33 Sadoul, P. and E. Lugaresi (eds.): "Hypersomnia with Periodic Breathing," *Bull. Physiol-Pathol. Respir.,* **8**:976–1288, 1972.

34 Burwell, S. et al.: "Extreme Obesity Associated with Alveolar Hypoventilation—A Pickwickian Syndrome," *Am. J. Med.,* **21**:811–818, November, 1956.

35 Gastaut, H. et al.: "Etude Polygraphique des Manifestations Episodiques (Hypniques et Respiratoires) Diurnes et Nocturnes du Syndrome de Pickwick," *Rev. Neurol.,* **112**:573–579, 1965.

36 Schwartz, B., and J. Escande: "Etude Cinematographique de la Respiration Hypnique Pickwickienne," *Rev. Neurol.,* **116**:667–678, 1967.

37 Lugaresi, E. et al.: "La 'Maledizione di Ondine' il Disturbo del Respiro del Sonno Nell' Ipoventilazione Alveolare Primariea," *Sist. Nerv.,* **20**:27–37, 1968.

38 Guilleminault, C. et al.: "The Sleep Apnea Syndrome," *Ann. Rev. Med.,* **27**:465–484, 1976.

39 Guilleminault, C. et al.: "Autonomic Dysfunction and Central Nervous System Involvement in Upper Airway Sleep Apnea Syndrome," *J. Neurol. Neurosurg. Psychiatr.,* in press.

40 Tilkian, A. et al.: "Sleep-Induced Apnea Syndrome: Prevalence of Cardiac Arrythmias and Their Reversal after Tracheostomy," *Am. J. Med.,* **63**: September, 1977.

41 Simmons, F. B. et al.: "Surgical Management of Airway Obstructions during Sleep," *Laryngoscope,* **27**(3):326–338, March 1977.

42 Dement, W. C.: *The Sleep Apnea Syndromes* (IMPACT Workbook, Sleep Disorders Series), Stanford: Stanford Univ. School of Medicine, 1978.

43 Kales, A. et al.: "Chronic Hypnotic Drug Use. Ineffectiveness, Drug Withdrawal Insomnia and Dependence," *JAMA,* **227**:513–517, 1974.

44 Dement, W. C. et al.: "The Pathologies of Sleep: A Case Series Approach," in Donald B. Tower (ed.), *The Nervous System, vol. 2, The Clinical Neurosciences,* New York: Raven Press, 1975.

45 Guilleminault, C. et al.: "Sleep-Related Periodic Myoclonus in Patients Complaining of Insomnia," *Trans. Ann. Neurol. Ass.,* **100**:19–22, 1975.

46 Kleitman, N.: *Sleep and Wakefulness,* Chicago: Univ. of Chicago Press, 1963.

47 Aschoff, J.: "Desynchronization and Resynchronization of Human Circadian Rhythms," *Aerosp. Med.,* **40**:844–849, 1969.

48 Webb, W. and H. Agnew: "Sleep and Waking in a Time-Free Environment," *Aerosp. Med.,* **45**:617–622, 1974.

49 Carskadon, M. et al.: "Self-Reports Versus Sleep Laboratory Findings in 122 Drug-Free Subjects with Complaints of Chronic Insomnia," *Am. J. Psychiatry,* **133**:13, 1382–1387, December 1976.

50 Kales, A. et al.: "Personality Patterns in Insomnia," *Arch. of Gen. Psych.,* **33**:1128–1134, September 1976.

51 Jones, H. S., and I. Oswald: "Two Cases of Healthy Insomnia," *Electroenceph. & Clin. Neurophysiol.,* **24**:378–380, 1968.

52 Meddis, R. et al.: "An Extreme Case of Healthy Insomnia," *Electroenceph. & Clin. Neurophysiol.,* **35**:213–214, 1963.

53 Vogel, G. et al.: "REM Pressure and Improvement of Endogenous Depression," in M. Chase et al. (eds.), *Sleep Research,* vol. 5, Los Angeles: Brain Information Service/Brain Research Institute, University of California, 1976.

54 Dement, W. et al.: "Sleep Laboratory and Clinical Studies with Flurazepam, in *The Benzodiazepines,* New York: Raven Press, 1973.

55 Broughton, R.: "Sleep Disorders: Disorders of Arousal?," *Science,* **159**:1070–1078, 1968.

56 Fisher, C. et al.: "A Psychophysiological Study of Nightmares and Night Terrors: The Suppression of Stage 4 Night Terrors with Diazepam," *Arch. Gen. Psychiatry,* **28**:252–259, 1973.

57 Pedley, T. and C. Guilleminault: "Episodic Nocturnal Wandering Responsive to Anticonvulsant Drug Therapy," *Ann. Neurol.,* **2**:30–35, 1977.

BIBLIOGRAPHY

General

Dement, William C.: *Some Must Watch While Some Must Sleep.* (The Portable University Series), San Francisco: W. H. Freeman, 1977.

Hartmann, Ernest L.: *The Functions of Sleep,* New Haven: Yale University Press, 1973.

Hauri, Peter: "The Sleep Disorders," in *Current Concepts,* Kalamazoo: Upjohn MS-5595, 1977.

Usdin, Gene L. (ed.): *Sleep Research and Clinical Practice,* New York: Brunner/Mazel, 1973.

Weitzman, Elliot D. (ed.): *Advances in Sleep Research,* vol. 2, New York: Halsted Press, 1976.

Williams, Robert L. et al.: *Electroencephalography (EEG) of Human Sleep: Clinical Applications,* New York: Wiley, 1974.

Insomnia

Coates, Thomas, and William Thoresen: *How to Sleep Better: A Non-Drug Approach to Overcoming Insomnia,* Englewood Cliffs, N.J.: Prentice- Hall, 1977.

Luce, Gay, and J. Segal: *Insomnia: The Guide for Troubled Sleepers,* New York: Doubleday, 1969.

Chapter 19

Emergency Situations

Shervert H. Frazier, M. D.

EDITORS' INTRODUCTION

What is it like to be in a busy hospital emergency room, to be bewildered, confused, frightened, and to have the doctor question you about who you are, where you are, how you are? What is it like to feel vague or unreal, and be in a hospital room wanting somebody to explain things, and not have any hospital personnel come in? What is it like to feel violent, to feel that you must attack someone? How does it feel to believe that you are in danger of being persecuted and attacked? What is it like to have unexplained anxiety, an apprehensive feeling about the unknown or the possibility of physical or mental illness? How does it feel to be frightened for no apparent reason and to have the doctor tell you that unconscious sexual feelings are the cause? What is it like to be immobile and unable to talk, and yet to have a doctor who is both trying to talk to you and encouraging you to talk yourself?

Regardless of the individual patient's idiosyncratic experience, a second group of factors may complicate the emergency. These factors involve the setting in which the emergency services are rendered. Here we refer not just to the physical setting, but in particular to the attitudes of the professional staff. How kind, considerate, supportive, and caring are they? How clear is the structure of the emergency service? Is clarity purchased at the cost of rigid rules that dehumanize patients and staff alike? Is there a sense of clear and flexible structure, or is there an element of chaos that adds to the patient's confusion and fear?

What is it like to be a physician or other professional who is working in an emergency room, feeling overwhelmed by the sheer volume of patients, and to have to make quick decisions and offer appropriate care to a demanding young man with acute panic, who comes to the emergency room at the same time as patients with bleeding ulcers, severe trauma, coronary occlusions, or ingestion of toxic substances? Fortunately, physicians often have experiences that are useful in understanding the psychiatric patient's emergency dilemma. Their training as medical students and later as physicians provides them with a wide range of professional experiences.

Or at a personal level, anyone who has sought emergency care for physical illness in a strange city can imagine how a person with a psychiatric emergency must feel. To such a person the strange mental state makes any place seem strange. To be considered different from the patient with chest pain or a broken leg in a general hospital emergency room creates a foreign world for many persons in emotional crises.

In this chapter, a prominent psychiatric clinician and administrator presents the reader with an overview of psychiatric emergencies. Familiarity with its contents will provide physicians with the knowledge base from which to evaluate and treat these patients. Hopefully, the experiential orientation of this book, together with the broad perspective of this particular chapter, will increase the reader's sense of competence in dealing with psychiatric emergencies appropriately.

INTRODUCTION

Why do there now appear to be so many more psychiatric emergencies than in the past? One answer is population growth; another is increasing concern about illness and the accessibility of health services. Still a third is the possibility that our accelerated pace of living produces problems, many of which are seen by the patient as being of an emergency nature. A fourth reason is that emergency medical services have developed extensively during the last two decades, and as a consequence many persons in our technological society are relying upon 24-hour per day emergency rooms for immediate treatment in times of need or crisis.

The term *psychiatric emergency* is a misnomer, because it implies only one kind of emergency. In fact, there are two types of psychiatric emergencies: (1) the *intrapsychic emergency,* which is caused by an individual's inability to function, and (2) the *social emergency,* which is brought about by the malfunctioning of a group.[1]

Systematized emergency psychiatric care is a recent development; 69 percent of emergency psychiatric services in this country were established after 1950.[2] Although these services are increasing rapidly, the psychiatric emergency probably has the lowest priority in the training of psychiatric residents, and often is the most avoided area of psychiatric practice. In many instances, the hospital's emergency psychiatry staff is poorly trained, or the duty falls either to first-year residents or to nonmedical personnel. Furthermore, psychiatrists' reluctance to become involved with emergencies may be attributable in part to training that has been oriented toward long-term therapy and not toward the sudden and immediate treatment needed in a crisis. Finally, the emergency psychiatric patient often exhibits raw emotions—threats of assault, homicide, suicide, or domestic upheaval—to such an extent that even professionals have difficulty grappling with the intensity of these emotional experiences hour-by-hour each day. Although most psychiatrists do handle the emergencies that arise in their own practices, only a few have a constant case load of frank emergencies.

DEFINITION OF A PSYCHIATRIC EMERGENCY

There is only general agreement about the definition of a psychiatric emergency. Linn states that a psychiatric emergency exists when there is a disturbance of thoughts, feelings, or actions for which immediate treatment is deemed necessary.[3] Miller defines the emergency patient as any individual who "develops a sudden or rapid disorganization in his capacity to control his behavior or to carry out his usual personal, vocational, and social activities."[4]

From the point of view of crisis theory, Parad and Resnik state that the inability to deal with stress by means of habitual coping patterns creates a crisis state in which the person attempts to find new ways to cope with or to solve problems.[5] When confronted with a new or an overwhelmingly distressing problem, a person usually responds with a temporary state of emotional disruption. Exploring new methods for coping may lead to problem solving. If, however, the person is unable to find new methods for dealing with the problem, the inability to master it may lead not only to increased inner turmoil, but also, in time, to diagnosable mental illness. Typically, the crisis-prone individual lacks or is unable to utilize the personal, familial, and social supports that most people depend upon to cope with stress while functioning in everyday roles.

A survey of criteria used by psychiatric hospitals and community mental health centers to define emergencies showed that an emergency is:

1   Any urgent condition, functional or organic, for which immediate treatment would increase or contribute to the patient's likelihood of recovery, or provide urgently needed protection
2   The appearance of symptoms of uncontrollable distress or behavior, analogous to acute exacerbations of physical illness that constitute emergencies
3   Any problem that a referring source feels incapable of handling[4]

Conceptually, the psychiatric emergency can be viewed from several distinct frames of reference. The first is the *psychodynamic*. The person may be emotionally deprived and have unbearable feelings of helplessness and futility. The patient may be impulsive, lack control of aggressive urges, and also be confused, anxious, and frightened. Often the situation is compounded by the use of drugs or alcohol. Another frame of reference is the *organic;* cerebral dysfunction may be contributing to poor impulse control. The person may have had a seizure or may be suffering from psychomotor epilepsy, head trauma, metabolic disturbances, or other physical illnesses that are complicating factors.

A third frame of reference includes the *personal, interpersonal, developmental,* or *situational* factors. In the emergency room the doctor is compelled to think: "Is the person's distress only individual—perhaps the result of an exacerbation of mental illness?" or, "Is the person's anguish and disturbed behavior produced by interactions with others?" or, "Is the person affecting others deleteriously?" or "Has a situation beyond the individual's control, a natural disaster or an act of fate, produced emotional distress?"

PRECIPITATING EVENTS

The use of this latter frame of reference enables us to classify events that precipitate emergencies. For example, at the *personal* level, failure to take prescribed medications, the use of alcohol, or fantasied threats lead to disequilibrium or to conflict that can result in symptoms and behaviors requiring emergency treatment. *Interpersonally,* many events can precipitate emergencies; the most common are family conflicts (including marital discord, impending divorce, desertion, or concern about children). *Developmental* problems, such as the difficulties of adolescence or of old age, also can be precipitants. Or a *situational* problem, such as job loss through no personal fault, the death of a loved one or a colleague, or a natural disaster such as a tornado or flood, can precipitate emotional reactions necessitating emergency care.

Tolerance of stressors is highly variable. The emergency patient may appear to be unusually sensitive even to minor stressors, but in reality many of these people have experienced a number of stressful events concurrently or in rapid sequence; and even the emotionally stable individual has a breaking point, a point beyond which additional stressors create anxiety and limit coping ability. Furthermore, reactions to stressors depend not only upon the individual's emotional and physical capabilities but also upon coping resources, both human and material, that can mediate the effects of stressors.

EVALUATING THE EMERGENCY PATIENT

Basic principles for the evaluation of the emergency patient include:

1 Gathering data about what happened, when, and who was involved. For example, has the person under treatment for mental illness been neglecting to take medications or been having an adverse reaction to them?

2 Determining whether the person is suffering from a physical illness. A sudden change in personality or behavior should lead one to suspect that organic

factors are responsible for the emergency, especially when the family setting and the social environment have been warm and supportive, and when the patient has no history of mental illness. Also, rapid and periodic fluctuations in behavior and mental status may signal organic illness. Obviously, a history of recent central nervous system (CNS) disease or trauma, drug use or abuse, and the medical history are critically necessary factors in the evaluation. Therefore, as soon as the doctor has obtained basic information about the nature of the emergency, at least a superficial physical examination should be conducted at once. And in many cases, steps should be taken to carry out a more complete physical examination and to obtain laboratory tests.

    3 Carrying out a Mental Status Examination. This is needed to differentiate between mental and physical illness and is absolutely necessary to determine whether the patient is in early delirium. Slight trauma, transient disorientation, or disturbance of memory are common signs of early delirium that are produced by drugs or disease; in contrast, the acute schizophrenic or manic patient usually remains oriented even though he or she is somewhat confused. Visual hallucinations suggest organic brain disease, whereas auditory hallucinations are much more likely to be present when the patient is schizophrenic.

    4 Conducting a detailed neurologic examination of the cranial nerves and the motor system. The physician should look for tremor, asterixis, and signs of autonomic hyperactivity. If at all possible the visual fields should be examined.

    5 Collecting information from family, friends, or others about possible precipitating events, and rechecking the patient's psychiatric and medical history if at all possible.

    6 Assessing the quality and quantity of the person's interpersonal relationships and the presence or absence of social support systems.

    7 Working quickly with the patient to assure him or her concretely that the emergency situation can be handled.

PRESENTING BEHAVIOR

The psychiatric emergency can present with any form of behavior, ranging from stupor or quiet anguish to assaultive acts. Such behavior can be classified into three broad categories: (1) that which threatens life, (2) that which threatens existing life patterns, and (3) that which indicates impaired ability to negotiate life's tasks.

Life-Threatening Behaviors

The most common behaviors that fall into this first category are suicidal plans, gestures, or attempts, and violence or assaultiveness. The most critical factors in the evaluation of the seriousness of such behaviors are: (1) the past history, (2) the patient's explicit intent to die or to do harm to others, and (3) the patient's perceptual and reality-testing capacities.

Behaviors Threatening Existing Life Patterns

Behaviors that upset the pattern of life are produced by schizophrenia, affective disorders, anxiety, and various physical or psychosomatic conditions.[2] In the emergency situation, a physician should focus on the specific symptoms to be treated. For example, if the patient has a primary depressive disorder, the clinician should work initially with the symptoms of depression; immediate symptomatic relief is the therapeutic objective. In the emergency room, the doctor should always be aware that behavior that disturbs existing life patterns can quickly become life-threatening behavior when, for example, the patient searches, often frantically, for some type of symptomatic relief from what seems to be intolerable stress.

Behaviors Impairing Function

The behaviors that make it difficult to function are most often caused by such organic brain dysfunctions as toxic drug reactions, drug use or abuse, other types of central nervous system (CNS) dysfunction, or metabolic disorders. However, depressive stupor, hypomania, catatonia, and other schizophrenic symptoms and behaviors can impair a person's ability to function.

Although diagnosis is important, the doctor who is treating the emergency is compelled to focus on the manifest symptomatology. Muller et al. gathered data on 5,000 psychiatric emergencies in hospitals, and found that physicians confront a broad variety of syndromes when they are dealing with psychiatric emergencies.[6] The diagnostic categories are less important, however, than the behaviors that are displayed by emergency patients: that is, extreme agitation, attempted suicide or homicide, alcoholism, emotional withdrawal, or isolation. Thus the patient's behavior is the key to evaluation, and ultimately to successful management.

GENERAL PRINCIPLES OF MANAGEMENT

The evaluation of a psychiatric emergency obviously is complex; moreover, it is only the first step in management. How the doctor evaluates the psychiatric emergency and deals with the patient and others at this time can influence further treatment and the prognosis. When the evaluation is conducted skillfully, the groundwork is laid for successful management.

When the physician is called upon to work with a psychiatric emergency, the following general principles usually serve as valuable guidelines for patient care.

1 As one approaches, observe the patient and those with him or her. Often the verbalization and the body language as well as the more obvious actions of all involved can alert the doctor to diagnostic and treatment possibilities.

2 Separate the patient from those who have brought him or her to the emergency room. When it is at all possible, place the patient in a quiet setting, listen carefully, and allow the person to ventilate.

3 Evaluate the patient by gathering a brief history, by observing the person's general physical condition, and by conducting a physical examination.

4 Reassure the patient, simply but firmly, that help is at hand and that even though the problem may be a difficult one, there are few problems that are truly unsolvable.

5   Ascertain whether one can rely upon familial or other support systems, or whether the person needs to be removed, at least temporarily, from interactions with others.

6   Call for assistance and consultation from one's medical and surgical colleagues, from other personnel on duty in the emergency room, or on occasion, even from the security officer.

In caring for a psychiatric emergency, the doctor must take prompt action. Another fundamental requirement is that a disturbed, excited, panicky, or unruly patient must be accepted as is, rather than being scolded, resented, or punished. Remember that the patient should be informed about what is happening. Importantly, the emergency patient should never be left alone; the physician or some other qualified person should stay with the patient at all times. Finally, as a general rule, it is usually better to do too much rather than too little. Most patients who are acutely disturbed have regressed and are unable to utilize many of their normal capacities.

COMMON PSYCHIATRIC EMERGENCIES

Suicide Plan or Attempt

Assessing the emergency patient's suicide risk is a crucial, difficult task for the doctor. For full details see Chapter 20. Indicators of high risk for suicide are the history of a previous attempt, a definite plan, poor impulse control, the use of drugs and/or alcohol, recent familial disturbance, and the absence of social support systems. Most patients who are planning suicide are depressed, although schizophrenic patients are also suicide risks, and even the "hysterical" patient who intends to make only a suicidal gesture may succeed. Therefore, when the risk of suicide is present, the doctor generally should hospitalize the patient. Usually the depressed patient's lowered mood, sadness, history of difficulty in eating or sleeping (any change in normal patterns), and feelings of despair indicate that depression is the fundamental condition. On occasion, however, one encounters the grim, smiling, depressed patient who is usually taciturn and cooperative, but regardless of appearance is a high-suicide risk. When these depressed patients are being hospitalized, the physician in the emergency room should alert all the personnel to the possibility of suicide during the course of admission to the inpatient unit; suicide precautions should be instituted promptly.

Risk of Homicide

Most homicidal patients have been violent or have expressed their intention to be violent. All threats of violence and homicide should be taken seriously. Usually, violent patients are brought to the emergency room by police or by others in authority. The doctor in the emergency room should find out immediately whether the patient is armed or has access to weapons. If the patient is armed, the doctor should ask him or her to surrender the weapon; usually a concealed weapon will be given to a doctor who evinces an attitude of understanding and support, but upon occasion the patient will adamantly refuse to do so. When that occurs, the doctor who is handling the emergency should obtain help from the security officers and others, and should use overwhelming force to obtain the weapon.

Although many homicidal patients are paranoid schizophrenics who are carrying weapons to protect themselves against the fantasied attacks of others, the physician should always recall that an organic disorder may produce violent behavior. The physician should consider the possibility that the patient has psychomotor epilepsy or the minimal brain dysfunction syndrome. According to Lion, limbic system dysfunction provides a possible organic basis for violent behavior.[7] Experimental and clinical data have shown that the limbic system is involved in the expression of aggression; neoplasms of the limbic system have been known to produce aggressive behavior. Epileptic foci within the limbic system or at the surface of the temporal lobe can produce seizures and violent behavior. However, the diagnosis of limbic system dysfunction is difficult to make and requires extensive clinical and laboratory studies.

Most physicians fear violent patients, and rightly so. These patients usually exhibit an intense emotional state that may evoke a defensive reaction or negative attitude on the part of the physician. Although most patients with mental illness are not violent, their strong internal emotions are communicated to others, who react defensively. Either a belligerent or a too-defensive attitude toward the potentially violent patient may provoke violence in one seeking desperately to prevent such loss of control. Therefore, a professional attitude that is characterized by calm objectivity is required.

In a recent study, Madden et al. reported that there had been a number of cases of assault against psychiatrists.[8] Most of these occurred while the psychiatrist was in residency training, and most of the patients were undergoing treatment at the time. All physicians must be prepared for possible assault by a violent patient. Such assaults include: (1) the sudden, unexpected assault that could occur at any time, (2) the crescendo assault that builds up over time, (3) the undirected maniacal assault, or (4) the directed assault. Most importantly, the physician should have time to talk to the patient, and when possible, a team of qualified coworkers (of both sexes) should relieve each other; they provide assurance of safety for both the patient and the staff. Having a female nurse or physician in the room can have a softening, mollifying effect on a belligerent patient. In this study of reported assaults, the precipitating factors were: (1) failure to meet a patient's request, (2) forcing a patient to take medication, (3) setting too many or not enough limits on the patient, and (4) insistence that the patient confront upsetting or painful martterial too quickly.[8] Whitman and his colleagues surveyed psychotherapists in psychiatry, psychology, and social work. They found that 9.2 percent of all patients seen by 101 therapists in 1 year presented a threat to others, 1.9 percent posed a physical threat to the therapist, and 0.63 percent actually assaulted the therapist. They stressed the need for interchange of ideas between therapists, which could be promptly applied in these crisis situations.[9]

All homicidal and violent patients should be hospitalized. The physician must reassure the patient that no one is trying to get rid of him or her. Generally, most violent patients accept hospitalization after they have been given a little bit of time to "think it over"; they are afraid of their own impulses and want controls to be established. When hospitalization is presented in a nonpunitive manner and the staff approaches the patient honestly and compassionately, anxieties, fears, and threats usually diminish. Finally, it is important that the doctor should explain to the patient that the responsibility for hospitalization rests with the physician and not with the family. Many patients believe that their families or other persons want to "put them away." Taking responsibility for the hospitalization prevents further fracture of potentially meaningful, familial, or other interpersonal relationships.

On some occasions, the patient's inner turmoil is so great that medications are indicated. The medications of choice are an injection of a phenothiazine or of haloperidol. Every effort should be made not to restrain the violent patient. In particular, when the violent patient is psychotic, restraints usually intensify the terror. Following the administration of medication it is necessary to monitor the vital signs.

All too frequently, the doctor in the emergency room sees the *victim* of an assault. Usually this patient is suffering from emotional stress that is equal to the physical harm that has been inflicted upon him or her. Patients who have been mugged, assaulted, or raped are often in a tense, shocklike state. They may keep mumbling, "Why did it happen to me?" Sometimes they think that they have been at fault, that they have either invited the attack or that they have placed themselves in vulnerable positions. Thus, in addition to emotional shock, which is characterized by detachment and suppressed fear, often the patient is burdened by guilt. Although state laws vary, all such victims are required to have clinical examinations, and the assaults must be reported. But taking care of the victim physically is only one part of the emergency room physician's task; he or she also should be alert to the emotional distress that the patient is undergoing. Placing the victim in a secure, friendly environment, asking sympathetically what has happened, and reassuring the patient that the danger has past usually has a calming effect. The emergency room physician should make sure that the victim obtains comfort, solace, and protection from others, as well as referral to various specialty centers, clinics, or practitioners. It is best to tell the victim that an emotional reaction to assault and violation is normal, and that psychiatric and mental health assistance can diminish the intensity and duration of the reaction.

Anxiety

Overwhelming anxiety frequently impels patients to seek emergency care. The anxiety may be manifest, and characterized by overt nervousness, tremulousness, fear, autonomic hyperactivity, and even a panicky state. Generally, anxious patients begin to calm down when the doctor in the emergency room starts to work with them—to ask about precipitating factors and symptomatology and to supply reassurance. Usually, conducting the physical examination is beneficial; it assures the patient that he or she is in the hands of a professional. Thus, a professional approach, ventilation, and often the administration of an antianxiety agent will produce prompt relief of the anxious patient's most extreme symptomatology. But these therapeutic measures suffice only for the management of the emergency; it is imperative therefore to refer patients who experience extreme anxiety for intensive psychiatric evaluation and therapy.

Some of these patients are suffering from the *hyperventilation syndrome.* After a few minutes of overbreathing, respiratory alkalosis sets in as a result of excess carbon dioxide output. The patient complains of altered consciousness, and specifically of giddiness, faintness, trembling, and blurred vision. These symptoms add to the patient's apprehension and increase the rapid breathing, which after a while is accompanied by tingling sensations in the lips, fingers, and toes. Treatment of the hyperventilation attack consists of reassuring explanations that instruct the patient to relax and to breathe (actually rebreathe) into a paper bag. Although the hyperventilation attack subsides quickly and the patient expresses gratitude for prompt relief of symptoms, the physician should explain that emotional factors produce such attacks, that the attacks are likely to recur unless adequate treatment is obtained, and that the prognosis is good but that psychiatric therapy is necessary.

Many patients with severe *phobias* present in emergency rooms with anxiety symptoms. Usually these patients are aware that they have become overwhelmed by fear, but do not know why the fear has become so distressing. Agoraphobia is receiving national attention; most of the agoraphobic patients are women who suffer from intense anxiety symptoms when they are shopping or in strange places. The emergency treatment of a patient with a phobia is similar to that of the anxious patient, but it is important that the patient be referred for psychiatric therapy to prevent the condition from becoming chronic.

Homosexual panic is a sudden, acute onset of severe anxiety that is precipitated by an unconscious fear or conflict about one's homosexual impulses. A person who is experiencing such panic may be concerned about destructiveness, blinding anger, confusion, or "going crazy." When the panic has been precipitated by a situation of intimacy with people who threaten sexual equilibrium, the patient should be removed immediately from the situation, whether it be a prison, military barracks, or a college dormitory. When it is not possible to place the patient in a supportive, nonthreatening environment, hospitalization may be required.

Hypomanic and Manic Episodes

These episodes occur in persons who are suffering from bipolar affective conditions. The symptomatology of the manic disorder contrasts with that of depression. Manic patients are elated, bursting with joy, "on top of the world," irritable, and flighty; but their judgment is poor, their timing is inappropriate, and often they engage in excessive spending or other activities. Such patients are easily identifiable, because they are aggressive, overactive, energetic, impulsive, and uninhibited. However, when they are frustrated, irritability appears and quickly turns to hostility or often to suspicion. They are extremely talkative, and generally evince increased psychomotor activity and a rapid stream of thought. Manic patients are true emergencies; they may hurt themselves, or the manic episode may be followed by a serious, precipitous bout of depression and suicide attempts. Hospitalization with treatment for the mania and then lithium is indicated.

Psychoses

The affective disorders and schizophrenia are the two most common types of psychoses that present as emergencies. As mentioned previously, many depressed patients are high suicide risks. When the patient is in a *depressive stupor,* in addition to having a life-threatening illness, that patient's ability to negotiate the everyday tasks of living is impaired. The inner urge toward self-punishment can result in the depressed patient's becoming the victim of an accident. Unless the depressed patient can be cared for supportively and unambivalently by the family or other social support system, hospitalization is indicated.

Schizophrenic patients who appear as emergencies usually manifest one of three common syndromes: (1) agitation, confusion, and bewilderment; (2) paranoid schizophrenic thinking; or (3) catatonic stupor or excitement. The confused, upset schizophrenic patient usually is classified as suffering from *undifferentiated schizophrenia.* Such a patient often appears to be highly anxious and generally bewildered, has a flattened affect, and exhibits a loosening of associations or other disturbance of thought processes that makes the conversation difficult to follow. These patients require hospitalization. Although they may have been on drug therapy and will "compensate" after they are given sufficient antipsychotic medication, they may become the victims of assault, harm themselves, or become involved in dangerous situations. As soon as the diagnosis is made, the patient should be reassured firmly and concretely that he or she can be helped and that immediate hospitalization is necessary.

Patients with *paranoid ideation* imagine that "enemies" are out to get them. Most of them have a history of suspiciousness and of difficulties with interpersonal relationships. Their thoughts are dominated by illogical and often changeable persecutory delusions. They usually tell about various plots and conspiracies, or express delusions of grandeur in which they believe themselves to be famous or well-known personalities. Many have auditory hallucinations; their judgment is poor, and their behavior can become dangerous. The extremely disturbed paranoid patient, for example, may strike out against imagined foes, and in so doing may harm or even kill innocent bystanders. Hospitalization is necessary.

Patients with *catatonic schizophrenia* may appear either semistuporous and negativistic or extremely excited. Catatonic excitement is difficult to manage as a psychiatric emergency.[3] The patient may shout excitedly and incoherently, pace back and forth rapidly, or attack others impulsively. Catatonic patients are frenzied and are extremely dangerous to themselves and others, because they attack suddenly. Many catatonic patients alternate between periods of stupor and excitement; therefore, although the patient may be stuporous at one moment, the physician should be aware that excitement may supervene "in a split second." Hospitalization is necessary.

Amnesia

Particularly in large city hospitals, the police or other public officials bring amnesic patients to the emergency room. Such patients appear to be "dazed" and bewildered, and complain of a loss of memory for a period of time lasting from several hours to several months. Sometimes they have forgotten all personal identification. Generally these patients are suffering from hysterical dissociative reactions or fugue states. Often they are fleeing from a stressful emotional situation. In almost all instances, they should be reassured that they will recover quickly and that hospitalization is necessary. Usually it is unwise for the emergency room physician to attempt to "break through" the patient's amnesic defenses.

Hysterical Psychosis

This type of mental illness is related to the fugue state. It is a psychotic reaction of acute and sudden onset and is related to an upsetting event or circumstance such as witnessing violence or a sexual threat. Clinically, patients with this illness may suffer from delusions, hallucinations, and symptoms of unreality, and may exhibit unusual behavior. When such patients are given supportive social and psychiatric treatment, they recover quickly. The emergency physician's role is to maintain a calm professional stance with them, arrange for hospitalization, and reassure relatives and friends. After the patient has been admitted to the hospital, special studies may be needed to rule out organic brain disease.

Delirium

Delirium is always evidence of biochemical or structural brain disease. In the early stages, the delirious patient is apprehensive, nervous, and agitated; and in the stage of frank delirium, the patient is disoriented, confused, often hallucinating (visual hallucinations), and has a rapid pulse. Delirium is produced by multiple etiologic factors; emotional and other stressors may be precipitants, but generally the patient is suffering from an infectious disease (lungs or kidneys), has been injured, has a metabolic disorder or a circulatory disturbance, and/or has been drinking. In young delirious persons, drugs are often the real culprits, although again the physician should always suspect multiple etiologic factors. Since the delirious patient will require an intensive physical examination and diagnostic evaluation, and since delirium is a true medical emergency, the physician should hospitalize the patient promptly. The attending staff should be aware that these patients can be suffering from delusions, illusions, and hallucinations, and that frequently they may harm themselves accidentally. For example, they may mistake a window for a door and attempt to leave the strange, disorienting atmosphere of the hospital. The staff on the ward should be notified by telephone that a delirious patient is being admitted.

Alcohol and Drugs

A large number of emergency patients are suffering from various alcohol- or drug-induced conditions. These range from simple drunkenness to alcoholic hallucinosis, or may include the toxic affects of medications such as digitalis, insulin, antidepressants, antianxiety agents, or street drugs. When these patients are conscious, the physician should rely primarily on the general principles of emergency treatment. The first step is to gather essential information about the amount and type of alcohol or drugs ingested and the circumstances surrounding their use. Then, one should ascertain whether the patient has had a mental or physical illness. Evaluation of the patient's physical and mental status should be accomplished promptly and noted, so that subsequent evaluations will indicate changes in the level of consciousness. If the patient has a history of ingestion of drugs or if medications or drugs have been taken with an intent to commit suicide, it is necessary to empty the patient's stomach. Such patients should be kept in the emergency room until one is sure that they are stable physiologically; their vital signs should be monitored closely. If the patient is semiconscious or unconscious, the emergency room physician should take immediate steps to provide life-support systems; these include an airway, an intravenous catheter, and careful monitoring. The number and variety of street drugs that are taken singly or in combinations are so great that it is best not to attempt to use an antidote unless there is clear-cut evidence that the patient has taken an opiate derivative. Generally, the utilization of life-support systems will pull the patient through the acute episode. Many, however, will require psychiatric therapy after recovery. The doctor who is taking care of psychiatric emergencies is referred to Shader's *Manual of Psychiatric Therapeutics,* which describes the management of such conditions in detail.[10]

Bereavement

Acute grief is a distinct syndrome that has both psychologic and somatic symptomatology; it appears shortly after bereavement, 2 to 3 months later, or sometimes on the anniversary of the death. Lindemann's report on a series of 101 psychiatric interviews with grief-stricken patients is the definitive work on this topic.[11] He describes the grief syndrome and its various stages. The syndrome includes sensations of somatic distress that occur in waves of choking, tightness in the throat, sighing, an empty feeling in the pit of the stomach, weakness, and distress that is described as tension or pain. The symptomatic wave usually lasts from 20 to 30 minutes and often is precipitated by mention of the deceased, an offer of sympathy, or a visit from a friend or relative. Typical complaints about lack of strength by the bereaved person are: "It's impossible to climb stairs" or "Everything is so heavy" or "The slightest effort exhausts me." These patients often mention that they have no appetite or that food does not taste good, and frequently they say that they have no feelings or are emotionally detached from others. A preoccupation with guilt can be apparent. Sometimes patients feel that the death of the loved one could have been prevented, and they may accuse themselves of negligence or may exaggerate minor omissions in care. The grief-stricken person's relationships with others are characterized not only by some degree of emotional detachment, but also by irritability, anger, and loss of warmth.

A bereaved person often is restless, talks incessantly and repetitively about the deceased, appears to be somewhat disorganized, and seems to be carrying out everyday activities only with extreme difficulty. The person is surprised to find out how many of the normal daily activities revolved around the deceased, and becomes dependent upon anyone who offers sympathy or will encourage activity.

Morbid grief reactions are distortions of normal grief. Their intensity and duration depend upon how well the bereaved adjusts to life without the deceased and forms new relationships. Of course, the presence of a strong social support system usually benefits the patient. A major obstacle, however, is the bereaved patient's refusal to discuss the grief experience or to express emotions. Such patients maintain that they want to avoid the distress of going through the process.

Emergency work with the grief-stricken person can be particularly beneficial. Parkes found in a carefully controlled study that the morbidity and mortality rates for bereaved persons during the year after their loss were significantly higher than rates for those in the age-controlled group.[12] Furthermore, proper therapeutic reactions may prevent prolonged and serious alterations in the patient's social adjustments.

The physician should encourage the patient to accept the pain of bereavement, review the relationship with the deceased, cry, grieve openly, and ventilate anguish. Delayed reactions can occur at any time, and may be mistaken for the onset of mental and/or physical illness. Generally, careful questioning will reveal that the delayed grief reaction has been triggered at a particular time by a meaningful event or anniversary that reawakens the bereaved person's memories of and emotions about the deceased. The emergency room physician should rely primarily upon psychotherapeutic measures when working with these patients, and should refrain from giving them antianxiety or other psychotropic medications. If medication is required, adequate nighttime sedation is generally beneficial.

Hypochondriasis

The doctor in the emergency room should be alert to the possibility that some patients who are seeking or demanding immediate medical assistance are suffering from hypochondriasis. Hypochondriacal neurosis is characterized by a preoccupation with bodily sensations and a fear of diseases of various organs. These preoccupations and fears persist despite repeated reassurances from physicians. Often, hypochondriasis is related to depression. Clues to the diagnosis of hypochondriasis can be obtained during the interview with the patient. For example: (1) Does the patient give a vague history of the illness? (2) Does the patient complain specifically of abdominal pain or pains in the head, neck, or chest? (3) Are the complaints of pains and aches great? and (4) Is the sense of pain predominately subjective and overinclusive? Since the treatment of hypochondriasis is difficult and the results are variable, it is wise for the emergency room physician to attend only to the patient's most pressing complaints. He or she should make sure that the patient is not suffering from a life-threatening medical illness, and then should refer the patient to the family physician. In general, the emergency room physician should be wary about prescribing medications for these patients.

Anorexia Nervosa

Anorexia nervosa usually occurs in adolescent females from upper- or middle-class families. These patients have an obsessional preoccupation with the desire to be thin, and adamantly refuse to eat. The compulsion to avoid food may occasionally result in death from starvation. The patient with anorexia nervosa may be brought to the emergency room by frightened parents who are concerned about a deteriorating physical condition; or, upon occasion, the patient may become so negativistic that the parents feel completely helpless. Sometimes the patient is critically emaciated and dehydrated.

Hospitalization is mandatory in severe cases of this life-threatening disorder. In the hospital, a regimen can be established to reward the patient in direct proportion to weight gain. Treatment is complex, but the immediate goal is the ingestion of food to prevent death; sometimes this requires intravenous or tube feeding.

Reactions to Natural Disasters

The emergency room physician should be aware that the initial reaction to natural disasters (tornadoes, floods, hurricanes, and fires) is stunned dismay. The full impact is not realized immediately, but after a day or two, some of the persons appear to be wandering about aimlessly, as if in a catatonic state. Full realization of the extent of the disaster evokes several symptom patterns: (1) panic, (2) retardation, (3) overreactivity, or (4) somatic reactions.

Panic can be particularly maladaptive. Not only does it sometimes result in harm to the person, but it also can be contagious. One panic-stricken individual can panic many others.

Some patients suffer retardation. They respond to the initial shock with dismay, followed by listlessness and apathy. For days they appear to be markedly slowed down, and their helplessness burdens the community.

Overreactions are manifest by rapid speech and inappropriate joking, as well as by frenetic movement. Such persons have a limited attention span and are unable to contribute to the general welfare of others. Sometimes they show signs of grandiosity that are accompanied by denial of reality. Many of them are frustrated easily, and their manic-like reactions may give way to feelings of demoralization.

Disaster victims may exhibit somatic manifestations such as trembling, vomiting, and sweating. These autonomic reactions may subside and be replaced by symptoms of conversion hysteria, which are characterized by loss of sensation or motor activity. Such symptoms are reactions to intolerable anxiety, and in a sense they represent a maladaptive psychological defensive maneuver.

After the first impact of the disaster has subsided, many people become inordinately suggestible, and tend to react anxiously or even with panic to the destruction surrounding them and to the losses they have sustained. Generally the level of emotional maturity throughout the community diminishes, so that many seem to be regressed.

The role of the clinician in administering psychiatric first aid should be parental. Hostile, punitive attitudes are futile. Firm but gentle leadership is required. Assigning tasks to those who show self-control is often therapeutic, since it eases terror and restores confidence. Sedation of a terror-stricken person in times of disaster should be avoided, because evacuation of a sedated person can be dangerous. If sedation is absolutely necessary, it should be noted on the person's identification tag so that others will be aware of the person's limited ability to follow instructions.

After a disaster strikes a community, the doctor and the medical staff often have a primary responsibility for the psychological aspects of disaster control. They should establish an advisory committee that is made up of community professionals. The role of each specialist should be defined, and plans should be developed for evacuation of the helpless or uncontrollably disturbed. Also, the community should be informed about provisions for emergency care. To prevent the emergency services from being overloaded, mental health clinics should maintain longer hours, and public officials and professionals should mount educational programs designed to alert the people to the emotional reactions to disaster.

PSYCHIATRIC EMERGENCIES IN CHILDREN

Psychiatric emergency situations that involve children are often difficult to manage because of the relative shortage of child psychiatrists and the child's panic or inability to respond because of immaturity. An emergency exists when the adults involved are unable to cope with the child's behavior and can no longer provide the necessary control and support.

The Battered Child

There may be no physical evidence of deliberate injury to a child, but when a physician suspects abuse the child should be hospitalized immediately. Top priority should be given to separating the child from the potentially dangerous environment. The parents should be interviewed to determine the cause of the abuse. Child abusers often have been abused when they were children. The children who are most likely to be mistreated are stepchildren, and those who are precocious, hyperactive, or adopted. All state governments require child abuse to be reported. Parents of the abused child need psychiatric help; many communities have self-help groups for this purpose. If the family is not cooperative or cannot be rehabilitated, arrangements for a foster home for the child are necessary.

Accidental Poisoning

Self-poisoning attempts in children can be accidental, experimental, suicidal, or can involve complicated pathological mother-child interactions.[3] Swallowing poison may often be an act of defiance on the part of the child. Ascertaining the poison that has been ingested is, of course, of primary importance. If steps for remedial action are not available in the emergency room, information can be obtained by calling a poison control center. After the child is comfortable, consultation with a child psychiatrist may be a good precautionary step.

Bereavement

Many of the children who are seen in emergency psychiatric consultation have lost a parent, sibling, or other person close to them. The symptoms that may develop are suicidal behavior, acute phobias, hysterical conversion, hypochondriasis, fear of death and dying, regression in toilet training, fire setting, cruelty to animals, and occasional psychotic reactions. Drug or alcohol abuse and sexual promiscuity may be seen in teenagers.

If the family is disturbed, the child will be also. The bereaved adult may not be able to pay sufficient attention to the child during this difficult time; consequently, the youngster may feel that love has been withdrawn. He or she goes through various stages of bereavement; the resulting behavior should be explained to the parent. The child needs to be given the opportunity to mourn the loss, but should not be permitted to become overwhelmed by it. If one parent has died, the surviving parent must spend as much time as possible with the child to alleviate fears of abandonment and feelings of vulnerability to death.

School Phobia

A child may suddenly refuse to go to school without giving any reason for such behavior and, when pressured, may become panicky unless permitted to stay at home. This is a serious emergency, since the longer the child is allowed to stay out of school, the more afraid he or she will be to return. The more severe the social and educational impairments become, the harder the child is to treat. Lassers et al. suggest a plan for managing a child with school phobia.[13] After a thorough physical examination, a psychiatric examination is performed to determine the precipitating events that produced the phobia. A therapeutic ally should be found to assist the family on a daily basis, if necessary. A firm back-to-school plan should be drawn up, with the alternative being hospitalization with classroom facilities. The child should be allowed to return to school gradually, if that is the only solution. In some cases, complete resumption is advised. A mild tranquilizer can be given to the child to help through the transitional period. Continuing support should be maintained, and follow-up visits should be recommended even after school has been resumed.

Sexual Assault

Two emergency categories of sexual assault are the act of exhibitionism and indecent exposure by an adult and acute physical contact and rape.[3] The child who has been raped or sexually molested has suffered serious emotional trauma, particularly if the person committing the crime is someone the child has trusted. This is more likely to be the case than not, since most rapes and indecent exposures are committed by family members or friends.

The physical needs of the child who has been raped must be attended to immediately and must include repair of injured tissue, prevention of venereal disease, and, if the child is an adolescent girl, prevention of pregnancy.

The physician should be sensitive to the child's emotional state, and should make a concerted effort to abate the child's panic. It is best to avoid hospitalization and instead to refer the child to a family-centered treatment program on an outpatient or home-treatment basis.

CONCLUSION

This chapter has been devoted to a discussion of the common psychiatric emergencies, and has been directed specifically toward the treatment of the emergency. Emergency treatment in itself is a necessary but usually incomplete method for handling emotionally disturbed and troubled persons. The skill with which the doctor deals with the psychiatric emergency is not only beneficial to the patient, but also can pave the way for successful therapy in the hospital, outpatient clinic, or practitioner's office. Therefore, in addition to basic knowledge about the care of psychiatric emergencies, the doctor who is working with them needs to know about the psychiatric and mental health facilities in the community, so that patients can be referred efficiently and effectively.

Emergency psychiatric situations will be faced many times by all physicians, whether or not they are psychiatrists. These situations will vary in urgency and severity, and often will require ingenuity and initiative on the part of the physician. Any emergency situation brings with it increased anxiety for the physician, but the satisfactory handling of such a situation can be rewarding for the physician and crucial for the patient.

REFERENCES

1 Frazier, S. H.: "Comprehensive Management of Psychiatric Emergencies," *Psychosomatics,* **9**: January–February 1968.

2 Tucker, G. J.: *The Psychiatric Emergency,* Weekly Psychiatry Update Division Series 28, Princeton, N.J.: Biomedia, 1977.

3 Linn, L.: "Other Psychiatric Emergencies," in A. M. Freedman, H. I. Kaplan, and B. J. Sadock (eds.), *Comprehensive Textbook of Psychiatry,* Baltimore, Md.: Williams and Wilkins, 1967, pp. 1785–1797.

4 Joint Information Service of the American Psychiatric Association and the National Institute for Mental Health: *The Psychiatric Emergency,* Washington, D. C., 1966, p. 4.

5 Parad, H. and H. L. P. Resnik: "The Practice of Crisis Intervention in Emergency Care," in H. L. P. Resnik and H. L. Ruben (eds.), *Emergency Psychiatric Care: The Management of Mental Health Crises,* Bethesda, Md.: National Institute of Mental Health, 1975, pp. 25–34.

6 Muller, J. J. et al.: "Acute Psychiatric Services in the General Hospital: Statistical Survey," *Am. J. Psychiat.,* 124:46–57, 1967.

7 Lion, J. R.: *Evaluation and Management of the Violent Patient,* Springfield, Ill.: Charles C Thomas, 1972.

8 Madden, D. et al.: "Assaults on Psychiatrists by Patients," *Am. J. Psychiat.,* 133:422–425, April 1976.

9 Whitman, R. J.: "Assault on the Therapist," *Am. J. Psychiatry,* 133:4, 426–429, April 1976.

10 Shader, R. I. (ed.): *Manual of Psychiatric Therapeutics,* Boston, Mass.: Little, Brown, 1975.

11 Lindemann, E.: "Symptomatology and Management of Acute Grief," *Am. J. Psychiat.,* 101:141–148, 1944.

12 Parkes, C. M.: "The Psychosomatic Effects of Bereavement," in O. W. Hill (ed.), *Modern Trends in Psychosomatic Medicine,* vol. 2, New York: Appleton-Century-Crofts, 1970, pp. 71–80.

13 Lassers, E. et al.: "Steps in the Return to School of Children with School Problems," *Am. J. Psychiat.,* 130:265–268, 1973.

BIBLIOGRAPHY

Ackerman, S. H., and E. J. Sachar: "The Lactate Theory of Anxiety: A Review and Re-evaluation," *J. Psychosom. Med.,* 36:69–81, 1974.

Anderson, W., and J. Kuehnle: "Strategies for the Treatment of Acute Psychosis," *JAMA,* 229:1184–1189, September 30, 1974.

Bakwin, H., and R. Bakwin: *Clinical Management of Behavior Disorders in Children,* 3d ed., Philadelphia: Saunders, 1966.

Beck, A.: *Depression,* Philadelphia: Univ. of Pennsylvania Press, 1967.

Brown, G. W. et al.: *Influence of Family Life on the Course of Schizophrenic Disorders,* London: Oxford Univ. Press, 1966.

Bruch, H.: *Eating Disorders,* New York: Basic Books, 1973.

Campbell, J. D.: *Manic-Depressive Disease,* Philadelphia: Lippincott, 1953.

Dimsdale, J. E.: "The Coping Behavior of Nazi Concentration Camp Survivors," *Am. J. Psychiat.,* 131:792–797, July 1974.

Engel, G. L. et al.: "Hyperventilation: Analysis of Clinical Symptomatology," *Ann. Int. Med.,* 27:683, 1947.

Frazier, S. H.: "Comprehensive Management of Psychiatric Emergencies," *Psychosomatics,* 9: January–February 1968.

Gelenberg, A. J.: "The Catatonic Syndrome," *Lancet,* 1:1339–1341, 1976.

Grinker, R., and J. Spiegel: *Men Under Stress,* New York: Blakiston, 1945.

Hagen, D. Q. et al.: "Aggression in Psychiatric Patients," *Comp. Psychiat.,* 13:481–487, 1972.

Holmes, T. S., and T. H. Holmes: "Short-Term Intrusions into the Life Style Routine," *J. Psychosom. Res.,* 14:121–132, 1970.

Jenkins, R. L.: "The Varieties of Children's Behavioral Problems and Family Dynamics," *Am. J. Psychiat.,* 124:1440, 1968.

Jung, C. G.: *The Psychology of Dementia Praecox,* New York: Nervous and Mental Diseases Publishing, 1917.

Kaplan, H. I., and B. J. Sadock: "The Status of the Paranoid Today: His Diagnosis, Prognosis, and Treatment," *Psychiat. Quart.,* **45**:528, 1971.

Kenyon, F.: "Hypochondriasis," *Internat. J. Psychiat.,* **2**:308–334, 1966.

Knudson, A. G., and J. M. Natterson: "Participation of Parents in the Hospital Care of Fatally Ill Children," *Pediatrics,* **26**:482–490, 1960.

Kolb, L. D.: *Modern Clinical Psychiatry,* Philadelphia: Saunders, 1973.

Langfelat, G.: *The Schizophreniform States,* London: Oxford Univ. Press, 1939.

Lazarus, R.: *Psychological Stress and the Coping Process,* New York: McGraw-Hill, 1966.

Lion, J. R. et al.: "The Self-Referred Violent Patient," *JAMA* **205**:91–93, 1968.

Lipsitt, D. R.: "Medical and Psychological Characteristics of 'Crocks,' " *Psychiat. Med.,* **1**:15–25, 1970.

Pilowsky, I.: "Dimensions of Hypochondriasis," *Brit. J. Psychiat.,* **113**:89–93, 1967.

Pincus, J., and G. J. Tucker: *Behavior Neurology,* New York: Oxford Univ. Press, 1973.

Roche Report: "Aftercare: Chicago Clinic Copes with the 'Difficult Patient,' " *Frontiers of Psychiatry,* **7**:13, 1977.

Slater, E., and M. Roth: *Clinical Psychiatry,* Baltimore, Md.: Williams and Wilkins, 1969.

Spinetta, J. J.: "The Dying Child's Awareness of Death: A Review," *Psych. Bull.,* **81**: 256–260, 1974.

Swanson, D. W. et al.: *The Paranoid,* Boston: Little, Brown, 1970.

Winokur, G. et al.: *Manic-Depressive Illness,* St. Louis, Mo.: Mosby, 1969.

Chapter 20

The Physician and
the Suicidal Patient

Gene Usdin, M.D.
Jerry M. Lewis, M.D.

EDITORS' INTRODUCTION

What is it like to wish you were dead? To feel that life is hopeless? What is
it like to feel that there is no way out of a painful problem? To feel helpless
week after week? What is it like to want to die and open your medicine
cabinet and wonder if any of its contents are lethal? To pick up your pistol
and know that it is loaded?

What is it like to find yourself meticulously planning to commit suicide
and to imagine what those "significant others" will think and feel? What is
it like to let "slip out" how bad you feel and what you are planning to do and
to get no response from your mate, child, parent, or friend? To try to talk
about it during your annual physical examination and find that your doctor
does not seem to notice?

What is it like for a physician to hear a patient make an indirect and
fleeting reference to suicide, but to be uncertain whether or not to question
the patient aggressively? After all, it was a tiny and oblique reference, and
your patient has always been a competent, productive person. Will he or
she be offended if you pursue the remark?

How does a physician feel when a patient commits suicide? Does he or
she experience it as a loss? Is there a lingering doubt—"Did I miss a clue?

Could I have prevented it?" Has the physician ever felt suicidal? Has he or she lost a loved one to suicide?

Suicide is an emotionally charged issue for most physicians. Many react to patients' suicides as a failure of medical care, with the possible exception of fatally ill patients. Depressed patients are the greatest risks, and yet their depression can be masked by physical symptoms, alcoholism, drug dependency, or other symptoms. Often, the recognition of a masked depression occurs only after a suicide or an unsuccessful suicide attempt. Too often the presence of depression or a subtle cry for help goes unnoticed.

Physicians should be aware of their reactions to suicidal potential in patients. Many physicians take the suicidal ideation or the suicide attempts of their patients as personal rebukes. Physicians' reactions frequently interfere with their capacity to appraise objectively the suicide risks involved.

This chapter is intended to help the clinician understand the etiologic factors behind suicide and suicide attempts. It should enable the physician to better evaluate the potential for suicide and to deal more comfortably with the suicidal patient. It is indeed a difficult task to care for anguished and desperate individuals and to provide both empathy and appropriate detachment. Some physicians have the unique qualities required; others should strive to recognize and minimize their limitations in this emotionally charged area, so that they can offer their patients greater support with these life or death problems.

INTRODUCTION

In 1976, 25,200 suicides were *reported* in the United States.[1] This translates into a rate of 11.7 per 100,000 population. Suicide statistics have not changed significantly in the past couple of years. In recognition of the fact that many suicides are unreported, a more realistic figure for the actual number of suicides in the United States would seem to be about 50,000 annually, with a rate of 23 per 100,000 population. While suicide has moral, religious, legal, and sociocultural components and involvements, the primary responsibility for the prevention of suicide and for the treatment of suicide attempts clearly falls into the domain of the medical profession. It becomes an important responsibility of any clinician to be aware of the prevalence of suicide, the importance of the physician's involvement, and preventive measures that can and cannot be taken. Too often the physician has not recognized suicide potential, has minimized its intensity, and has responded ineffectually. Many suicidal patients give warnings, almost as a cry for help, to persons in their immediate environment. When the physician does not heed these warnings, and fails to search further for their significance, it may lead to tragedy. Repeated studies have confirmed that many persons who commit suicide have seen a physician within a reasonably short period before the suicide or suicide attempt.

Quite often potentially suicidal patients consult their physicians with physical complaints and do not verbalize their suicidal ideation. The greatest danger of suicide is with the patient who has a depressive reaction, and the depression may be either masked or not verbalized directly. The physician should be alert to the potential of depression when, in doing the review of systems, he or she learns that the patient has anorexia, weight loss, decreased libido, and insomnia—the so-called vegetative signs and symptoms of a depression. The clinician should become even more concerned when the patient expresses feelings of hopelessness, helplessness, or worthlessness. When to this are added numerous physical complaints with no apparent organic basis or when the patient is alcoholic, the physician should recognize that a serious suicidal risk is present.

How does the physician proceed further in questioning? What other studies are indicated? Should consultation be involved? What warning should be expressed to the patient and family? What safeguards should be initiated?

Some physicians will avoid involvement for a complex set of personal reasons. These may vary from physician to physician as well as from patient to patient. The important fact is that the sensitive physician may play an important role in suicide prevention as well as in helping the patient and family after an attempted or successful suicide. It narrows down to the central thrust of this text, which is that physicians need heightened awareness and willingness to become involved with their patients, particularly during suicidal crises.

The further intent of this chapter is to aid the physician in recognizing patients with increased suicide potential; to help them appreciate the importance of questioning patients about suicide (and to suggest an appropriate means of doing so); to understand the basic psychodynamics involved in suicide (including which persons are especially vulnerable to serious attempts); and to recognize which patients may be treated as outpatients, which require protective hospitalization, which may require consultation and further studies, which may be considered less serious, and what psychotherapeutic, psychopharmacological, and other treatment modalities may be utilized.

EPIDEMIOLOGY

Statistics regarding suicide are notoriously unreliable. To a certain extent they are contrived; their variation from country to country or locale to locale may reflect overt to covert underreporting. The reporting of a death as suicide varies by country, religion, socioeconomic group, and the particular society involved. Table 20-1 shows suicide rates for selected countries for 1973 and 1974. Such reporting often reflects the frame of reference and theoretical predisposition of the interpreter. One thing certain is that suicides are never overreported. The statistics often are misused to prove or disprove certain points. The availablility of insurance plays no small role in Western society because many life insurance policies specifically exclude suicide as a basis for payment. The Roman Catholic Church will not provide a requiem Mass for someone who is known to have committed suicide. There continues to be a social stigma attached to suicide, and this

Table 20-1   Suicide Rates, Selected Countries: 1973 and 1974 (Crude rate per 100,000 population).

Country	1973			1974		
	Total	Male	Female	Total	Male	Female
United States	12.0	17.7	6.5	12.1	18.1	6.5
Austria	22.1	31.6	13.6	24.1[1]	35.5[1]	13.9[1]
Australia	11.6	15.7	7.5	11.7	16.0	7.4
Belgium	14.9	20.7	9.3	15.6	21.4	10.1
Canada	12.6	18.0	7.1	12.9	18.7	7.1
Denmark	23.8	29.2	18.5	24.1[1]	29.9[1]	18.4[1]
Finland	23.5	37.6	10.3	25.1	40.6	10.5
France	15.5	22.6	8.7	15.6	22.7	8.8
Germany, Fed. Rep. of	20.8	27.4	14.7	21.0	27.9	14.7
Greece	3.0	4.0	1.9	3.4	4.6	2.4
Ireland	3.4	5.0	1.9	3.8	5.9	1.7
Israel	6.4	6.9	5.8	5.5	7.0	4.0
Italy	5.7	8.1	3.4	5.4	7.3	3.5
Japan	17.3	20.1	14.7	18.0[1]	21.4[1]	14.6[1]
Mexico	.7	1.1	.3	2.1	3.4	.8
Netherlands	8.7	9.9	7.4	8.9[1]	10.8[1]	7.0[1]
Norway	8.6	13.1	4.3	10.4	16.3	4.5
Philippines	1.4	1.6	1.1	1.2	1.3	1.0
Poland	11.7	19.6	4.3	11.3[1]	19.3[1]	3.7[1]
Portugal	8.6	13.5	4.2	8.5[1]	13.4[1]	4.2[1]
Puerto Rico	9.1	15.0	3.5	7.7	12.5	3.0
Spain	4.2	6.2	2.3	4.0	5.8	2.2
Sweden	20.8	29.5	12.1	19.4[1]	27.7[1]	11.2[1]
Switzerland	18.8	27.4	10.6	22.5[1]	32.5[1]	12.9[1]
United Kingdom:						
England and Wales	7.8	9.4	6.2	7.9	9.5	6.4
Northern Ireland	4.5	4.2	4.9	4.0	5.1	2.9
Scotland	8.4	10.1	6.8	8.2[1]	9.0[1]	7.4[1]

[1]For 1975.

Source: United Nations World Health Organization, *World Health Statistics,* annual.

is felt frequently by the survivors. Family members and close friends often feel they have failed, and that they are responsible for the suicidal act. Although these widely held social attitudes have diverse implications, a particularly important implication is the way in which they interfere with accurate reporting of suicidal deaths. Table 20-2 gives data on suicide rates in the United States broken down by sex, race, and age. Table 20-3 ranks the states by suicide rate.

While many attempted suicides have no truly serious death intent, many persons obviously go to great lengths to conceal their suicide attempts. Considering

Table 20-2. U.S. Suicide Rates, by Sex, Race, and Age Groups: 1965 to 1975

(Rates per 100,000 population. Beginning 1970, excludes deaths of nonresidents of the United States)

Age	Male White 1965	1970	1974	1975	Male Black and other 1965	1970	1974	1975	Female White 1965	1970	1974	1975	Female Black and other 1965	1970	1974	1975
All ages	17.4	18.0	19.2	20.1	7.7	8.5	10.2	10.6	6.6	7.1	7.1	7.4	2.5	2.9	3.0	3.3
5–14 years	.5	.5	.8	.8	.2	.2	.4	.1	.1	.1	.2	.2	.1	.2	.2	.2
15–24 years	9.6	13.9	17.8	19.6	8.5	11.3	12.9	14.4	3.0	4.2	4.8	4.9	3.1	4.1	3.9	3.9
25–34 years	17.7	19.9	23.3	24.4	14.2	19.8	22.9	24.6	7.6	9.0	8.7	8.9	6.0	5.8	6.3	6.5
35–44 years	23.4	23.3	23.8	24.5	15.0	12.6	15.6	16.0	12.0	13.0	12.1	12.6	4.2	4.3	4.5	4.9
45–54 years	30.8	29.5	28.3	29.7	13.5	14.1	11.9	12.8	13.6	13.5	14.1	13.8	4.1	4.5	4.0	4.5
55–64 years	39.7	35.0	32.1	32.1	14.2	10.5	12.5	11.5	12.3	12.3	11.0	11.7	2.8	2.2	3.4	4.1
65 years and over	43.3	41.1	38.9	39.4	15.0	10.8	15.3	11.8	9.1	8.5	7.7	8.5	3.2	3.6	2.3	3.0

Source: U.S. National Center for Health Statistics, *Vital Statistics of the United States*, annual.

Table 20-3   Ranking of States by Suicide Death Rate,* 1976

Rank	State	Suicide death rate
1	Nevada	26.7
2	Alaska	19.4
3	New Mexico	18.3
4	Wyoming	17.7
5	California	17.5
6	Florida	17.4
7	Colorado	17.3
8	Arizona	17.1
9	Montana	17.1
10	Idaho	16.4
11	Virginia	15.9
12	Vermont	15.5
13	Oregon	15.0
14	Washington	14.8
15	Georgia	13.5
16	Tennessee	13.2
17	District of Columbia	13.0
18	Michigan	13.0
19	Missouri	13.0
20	New Hampshire	13.0
21	Utah	13.0
22	Wisconsin	13.0
23	Oklahoma	12.7
24	Maine	12.6
25	Ohio	12.6
26	Kentucky	12.6
27	North Carolina	12.4
28	Delaware	12.2
29	Rhode Island	12.0
30	Texas	11.9
31	Arkansas	11.7
32	Maryland	11.5
33	Pennsylvania	11.5
34	Louisiana	11.3
35	Kansas	11.2
36	South Dakota	11.1
37	Iowa	11.0
38	North Dakota	10.9
39	Indiana	10.7
40	Alabama	10.4
41	West Virginia	10.0
42	Connecticut	10.0
43	Hawaii	10.0
44	Minnesota	9.9
45	Nebraska	9.7
46	South Carolina	9.7
47	Illinois	9.4
48	New York	9.3
49	Mississippi	9.2
50	Massachusetts	9.0
51	New Jersey	7.5

*Death rates are per 100,000 population
Source: Table 1-14, *Vital Statistics of the United States, Volume II, Mortality, Part A,*
published annually.

the aforementioned factors, the figure of 50,000 suicides annually in the United States appears quite realistic. Many of the over 100,000 deaths per year that are attributed to accidents may, in reality, be suicides.

This point leads to the complex interface between suicide and accidents. Many suicides are reported as accidents in an effort to reduce the stigma or to collect life insurance that may have provisions against reimbursement for suicidal death. In other situations, there is reason to suspect that what appears to be an accident was, in reality, suicide. The case of the car speeding into the concrete bridge support is the classical example. There are many situations in which it is difficult to know whether death was accidental or suicidal. This concern with pinpointing the individual's intentions is often reflected in a psychologic autopsy, in which an attempt is made to reconstruct the circumstances, conflicts, and feelings that preceded an individual's death. Awareness of this gradation of intention seems to emphasize the degree of personal involvement, either conscious or unconscious, that each person has in his or her own death.

Statistics about suicide produce striking figures. The World Health Organization (WHO) reported that in 1973 1,000 persons committed suicide, and at least 10 times that number attempted suicide daily. They noted further that suicide rates are rising, especially among youths. Hungary consistently has the highest reported suicide rate, most recently at 36.9 per 100,000 population. However, the city of West Berlin, which reports individually, has an even higher rate.[2] A year earlier, Winnik maintained that a half million people die by their own hands annually.[3] West Germany, Hungary, Japan, Denmark, Sweden, Finland, and Switzerland report rates of over 25 per 100,000 population, and Italy, Spain, and the Netherlands report rates of under 10 per 100,000 population.[4] Whatever the difference in reporting, it is apparent that there is no simple relationship between the nature of the large social system and that social system's suicide rate.

SOCIAL ASPECTS OF SUICIDE

Suicide has been viewed differently at various stages of history. Before the Christian era in classical Rome, life was held to be rather cheap, and suicide was not viewed negatively; but with the advent of the Christian era the social attitude came to be negative, and suicide has been viewed as either a sin or a crime. However, in many countries or societies today, suicide may be considered honorable under certain circumstances (hara-kiri, seppuku, suttee, etc.).

The scientific study of suicide received initial emphasis at the beginning of this century with the work of Durkheim and Freud.[5,6] Their emphases were different: the former studied the sociological aspects and the latter the psychology of the individual patient. Durkheim viewed suicide as the result of society's strength or weakness of control over the individual. Freud considered suicide as intrapsychic, within the mind. These two major approaches have continued, the resulting data are complementary, and both approaches are important in understanding the phenomenon of suicide. The complementary nature of the two aspects is important to keep in mind, because there has been a long philosophical argument about whether the blame or responsibility for suicide rests primarily with society or with the individual.

Gender, age, and ethnicity are important variables. In this century, more men than women commit suicide, the ratio being about 3:1. Women, however, make more suicide attempts, and again the ratio is about 3:1 (three women to one man). Suicide attempts among the general population are frequent. A reasonable estimate is that there are eight to ten attempts that fail for each "successful" suicide.

Age is another important variable. Although few children commit suicide, some do, and the rate goes up in adolescence, while continuing to escalate into adult life.[1] When considered from the perspective of rank, however, suicide is one of the leading causes of death in young people. It is, for example, second only to accidents for white males between the ages of 15 and 19.

The suicide rate for whites is higher than for blacks, although the rate for the latter is said to be climbing closer to that for the former.[7]

There are many intriguing social correlates and differences among suicide patterns, and those factors that have been presented are but a modest sample. It is important to keep in mind that these broad social variables interact with each other in complex ways, and no simple, linear causality can be assumed. They may be considered the important, broad brush strokes on the canvas of suicide. In order to understand suicide as completely as possible, we must narrow the focus and try to understand what goes on in the mind of the person who commits suicide.

PSYCHOLOGICAL ASPECTS OF SUICIDE

The study of the psychologic characteristics of suicide, particularly as influenced by psychoanalytic investigations, has resulted in the accumulation of rich and diverse clinical data. Those who wish for a simple psychologic explanation, however, have been disappointed. It becomes quickly apparent that there are many roads to suicide. Many different emotions, intrapsychic conflicts, and interpersonal problems may lead to a suicidal crisis. The early psychoanalytic position, for example, focused on the role of hostility. Suicide was considered to represent a homicide against an introjected person toward whom the suicidal individual had both a strong emotional connection and intense hostility. Committing suicide was seen primarily as a way of murdering an ambivalently loved object. In later years, Karl Menninger expanded this early concept of the role of hostility in suicide to include the wish to kill, the wish to be killed, and the wish to die.[8]

Although hostility can play a significant role in many suicides, other feelings can play the dominant role. The feeling of utter hopelessness is powerfully conducive to suicide. Many individuals cannot tolerate days, weeks, or months of feeling profoundly hopeless, and come to feel that death is preferable by far. Shame, a consuming dependency, intense helplessness, guilt, and sadness may all be involved, and in some persons these may be the major feelings leading to suicide. The physician must be aware that patients who communicate these feelings need to be involved in an exploration of their potential for suicide.

Certain individuals with a variety of psychodynamic conflicts reach a point of intense conflict in an emotionally important, often strongly ambivalent, interpersonal relationship, and develop an intense feeling state. The feeling state can be dominated by one strong feeling or by a combination, but frequently intense hopelessness, helplessness, and/or hostility is present. Under these circumstances, some individuals come to think of suicide as a solution. With a feeling of ambivalence about dying, some may turn the dilemma over to fate, others may commit suicide, and many will turn to a physician for help. Again, the request for help may be disguised, and the physician must respond in ways that facilitate exploration.

Shneidman has described three important general characteristics of the suicidal patient.[7]

1 The acute suicidal crisis, or period of great lethality, is typically of short duration. It is measured in minutes, hours, or days, and is a peak of self-destructiveness.

2 Suicidal patients are often intensely ambivalent about their death. They both want and do not want to die. This factor accounts for the frequent chance-taking suicidal behavior, such as playing Russian roulette. The ambivalence about dying is resolved, for the moment, by chance.

3 Most suicidal tensions are between two people who know each other well: husband and wife, parent and child, or lover and lover. The suicide can be understood, in part, as an act of grave interpersonal significance. It is something that occurs between people, and it is often an act that is motivated by a wish to hurt, punish, or escape from a significant other.

There are additional psychologic clues. If, for example, the physician recognizes the presence of a major mental illness in a patient who fits some or all of the characteristics noted above, there is an increased likelihood of suicide. Guze and Robins reviewed 17 studies and found that affective disorders were associated with suicide rates that were approximately 30 times the rate in the general population.[9] Tsuang contrasted the suicide rates in schizophrenic, manic, and depressed patients.[10] Although major depressive conditions carry a marked additional suicidal potential, this study demonstrated that there was increased risk for all the psychiatric groups (except for female schizophrenic patients). The group with the greatest risk was male patients with depressive syndromes. A recent, significant, major study reported that 15 percent of depressed people committed suicide.[11] The implication for the clinician is clear; the presence of major psychiatric disturbances, especially depressive syndromes, should raise the index of suspicion regarding the possibility of suicide.

Another pertinent factor involves the patients' social support systems, their relatives and meaningful friends. Those individuals who are connected to others and can, therefore, receive and give support, share interests, and combat loneliness are less apt to commit suicide than those with little or no social support. The elderly white male without a family who lives alone and is in poor physical health is considered a high risk, particularly because of the lack of any social support system. The implication of this finding for the physician is the need to inquire specifically about a patient's involvement with others. Those who have little or no involvement with others have an increased suicide potential.

Another factor involves the concept of *partial death* or slow suicide. There is a growing awareness that certain chronic processes or life-styles can be understood to reflect self-destructive or suicidal themes. Alcoholism, drug addiction, and risk-taking behavior in general are often considered to be examples of slow suicide. Menninger writes of *chronic* suicide (for example, alcoholism), *focal* suicide (for example, multiple surgery) and *organic* suicide (for example, the self-punishing tendencies of some patients with organic diseases in neglecting to follow recommended therapeutic regimes for the management of their illness).[8] Some of these patients can be understood as expressing suicidal equivalents. Modlin has brought together a set of clues concerning suicide potential. These clues may be garnered from standard data that the office or hospital clerk has secured from patients: age, race, sex, marital status, living arrangements, condition of employment, and state of physical health.[12] From a review of these data, he concludes that the patient in suicide jeopardy is most nearly typified as an aging, white male who is divorced, living alone frugally, unemployed, and in poor health. The suicide rate increases along a married-, single-, widowed-, divorced-continuum. The divorced may contemplate themselves with feelings of failure and residual self-recrimination. The psychosocial supports of a person who is living alone are often lacking. Unemployment brings with it not only diminished self-respect, but also a lack of the wherewithal to enjoy the pleasures of life, as well as a decreased opportunity to procure the necessities of life. Poor health is discouraging, especially if the person perceives it as chronic, hopeless, and painful. The implication for the physician is the need to consider an underlying suicidal motivation when evaluating patients with such syndromes.

EVALUATION OF THE SUICIDE ATTEMPT

Most physicians see patients who have made suicide attempts. Each patient should be evaluated carefully, and the physician who sees the patient initially bears the responsibility for commencing the evaluation. Treating the patient's physical condition (that is, suturing a wrist, pumping out a stomach), and then not evaluating the attempt and the subsequent risk carefully is hazardous. All too frequently, suicide patients are dismissed as "only wanting some attention." The fact that some suicide attempts have nothing to do with the wish to be dead and may clearly reflect the patient's attempt to manipulate others should not blind the physician to the need to evaluate carefully the specific patient who has made an attempt.

A number of factors must be considered in the evaluation of such a patient.

The central factor is the necessity to evaluate the patient's continuing potential for self-destruction. Litman and Farberow have presented a format for the assessment of self-destructive potential.[13] Factors such as the time of onset for the self-destructive behavior, history of recent personality change, a history of repetitive self-destructive behavior over a long period of time, the method of self-injury, the recent loss of a loved one, recent serious medical illnesses, evidence of depression (that is, anorexia, weight loss, insomnia), and the nature of important relationships are but some of the areas to be explored.

Particularly important is the lethality of the suicide attempt. The more serious the attempt, the greater the patient's need for intervention and protection. It is important, however, not to dismiss attempts of lower lethality as conclusive evidence that a patient's suicide attempt was not serious. Tabachnick and Farberow constructed an objective scale of lethality by asking psychiatrists and other professionals to rank the lethality of common suicide attempts.[14] There was much agreement, and the list (from most to least lethal) was: (1) firearms and explosives, (2) jumping from high places, (3) cutting and piercing vital organs, (4) hanging, (5) drowning (if unable to swim), (6) poisoning (solids and liquids), (7) cutting and piercing of nonvital organs, (8) drowning (if able to swim), (9) poisoning (gases), and (10) analgesics and soporific substances. In addition, these authors advise consideration of two other factors. The first is the "point of no return," by which they mean the speed with which the suicide attempt can produce death. The second involves the feasibility of intervention. This factor attempts to clarify whether or not the method of the suicide attempt allowed for the possibility of rescue.

Although females attempt suicide more frequently than males, and the prototype of the patient who attempts suicide without desire for death is a young white female of hysterical temperament who cuts her wrists or takes a small overdose of a sedative after breaking up with her boyfriend, the physician should guard against stereotyping all such females who have attempted suicide. Some are genuine in their suicidal intent, and others may succeed "accidentally."

MANAGEMENT OF THE SUICIDAL PATIENT

The physician who makes the active effort to explore with his or her patients their feelings and life experiences will save the lives of some patients. The specific interviewing technique (collaborative exploration) that accomplishes this goal has already been described (see Chapter 1). This approach encourages the patient to explore with the physician what is on his or her mind, and consequently it may probe beyond the initial and often unfocused complaints ("I'm just tired," "Life is not worthwhile," "Have a lot on my mind," or "Been awfully worried lately"). After a period of exploration, the physician must decide whether or not to conduct a brief, directive inquiry regarding the patient's suicidal potential. This inquiry should be conducted with all patients who are depressed; who show symptoms or signs of a major psychiatric disturbance; who experience intense hopelessness, hostility, helplessness, shame, or guilt; or who have a past history of suicide attempts. The physician should not be hesitant about this directive inquiry. It is an important part of the evaluation of the patient, and contrary to folklore, it will not suggest suicide to the nonsuicidal patient. If the patient has been considering suicide, he or she usually will be relieved by the physician's inquiry. Even the inquiry, when expressed appropriately, may convey an attitude of acceptance of the patient as a worthwhile individual.

One approach is to acknowledge how difficult life has been recently for the patient, and then start the directive inquiry with a question about death wishes. "As bad as it's been lately, have you found yourself wishing you were dead?" Either a positive response ("Yes, I have") or a significantly qualified response ("Well, not really") mandates continuing with the inquiry.

The next inquiry moves to the level of suicidal ideation. "Have you thought of doing it yourself?" may lead to either an affirmative or a suggestive response. If so, it then becomes obligatory for the physician to explore the frequency, intensity, and duration of the suicidal thoughts.

It is also useful to ask questions about whether the patient has been able to share the suicidal thinking with a family member or friend. It is important to ask about the patient's view of his or her control over the suicidal urges. "Do you feel in control of these thoughts, or do you wonder if you'll be able to control your behavior completely?"

Once this has been accomplished, the physician shifts the inquiry to the specificity of method of suicide. "Have you considered how you would do it?" If the patient has a method in mind, and if the method is of high lethality, it is important to ask the patient whether he or she has actually made an attempt.

The answers to these questions must be interpreted in light of the physician's knowledge and understanding of the patient. In this way the physician can best evaluate the suicide potential.

The physician must also evaluate the strength of the physician-patient relationship. He or she must ask (silently), "How well do I know this patient?" "Is the patient willing to relate honestly to me?" "Does the patient trust and have confidence in me?" "Does the patient's current emotional status indicate that he or she can work collaboratively with me in managing this crisis?" "What support or stress is there for the patient in the family or circle of close friends?" The physician must process all the information about the patient and the crisis in order to formulate a treatment plan. The soundness of the physician's evaluation and treatment, including the manner in which the physician relates to the patient, may mean the difference between life and death for the patient.

In formulating a plan of action, it is good for the physician to bear in mind the myths about suicide in order to minimize their impact on the required clinical judgment. Shneidman has presented eight myths about suicide.[7]

1 *Fable:* Persons who talk about suicide do not commit suicide. *Fact:* Of any ten persons who will themselves commit suicide, eight have given definite warnings of their intentions.

2 *Fable:* Suicide happens without warning. *Fact:* Studies reveal that the suicidal person gives many clues and warnings regarding suicidal intentions.

3 *Fable:* Suicidal people are fully intent on dying. *Fact:* Most suicidal people are undecided about living or dying, and they gamble with death, thus leaving it to others to save them. Almost no one commits suicide without letting others know how he or she is feeling.

4 *Fable:* Once a person is suicidal, that person is suicidal forever. *Fact:* People who wish to kill themselves are suicidal only for a limited time.

5 *Fable:* Improvement following a suicidal crisis means that the suicidal risk is over. *Fact:* Most suicides occur within approximately 3 months after the beginning of "improvement," when the subject has the energy to put morbid thoughts and feelings into effect.

6 *Fable:* Suicide strikes much more often among the rich—or, conversely, it occurs almost exclusively among the poor. *Fact:* Suicide is neither the disease of the rich nor the curse of the poor. Suicide is represented proportionately among all levels of society.

7 *Fable:* Suicide is inherited or "runs in the family." *Fact:* It is an individual pattern.

8 *Fable:* All suicidal persons are mentally ill, and suicide is always the act of a psychotic person. *Fact:* Studies of hundreds of genuine suicide notes indicate that although the suicidal person is extremely unhappy, he or she is not necessarily mentally ill.

To these may be added the following myths:

1 *Fable:* Belief in religion is a safeguard against suicide. *Fact:* Clergy of all persuasions who are in the throes of mental illness or even of situational crises have committed suicide. Roman Catholicism, which clearly considers suicide a mortal sin, has a higher suicide rate than Reform Judaism, which has an essentially soft attitude toward suicide.

2 *Fable:* Children do not commit suicide. *Fact:* Children do commit suicide, and the rate has been increasing.

3 *Fable:* You should not question the patient about suicide because it might put the idea in his or her mind. *Fact:* Suicide ideation is not fortuitous. It stems from deep, internal psychological processes or a major crisis.

With these myths dispelled from the mind, the physician must formulate a treatment plan. The major factors to be considered include the assessment of the intensity of the patient's suicidal wish, the presence or absence of a major psychiatric syndrome that impairs judgment, the nature of the patient's supportive social network, the quality of the physician-patient alliance, and the availability of a spectrum of treatment resources. Most patients will fall into three treatment categories.

1 Patients requiring protective hospitalization. These patients have intense suicidal wishes, concrete and highly lethal plans, impaired judgment, few (if any) supportive others, and no effective treatment alliance with a competent professional. They must be hospitalized for their own protection, for further evaluation, and for the implementation of a treatment plan. If necessary, the physician should institute whatever legal steps are necessary to protect the patient. Excessive drinking increases the suicide potential for persons with such drives.

2 Patients who can be treated as outpatients. These patients have less intense suicidal wishes, no concrete or highly lethal suicidal plans, reasonably intact personalities, a supportive social network, and an effective alliance, or the beginning of such, with a competent professional. Some physicians choose to enter into "contracts" with such patients. The patient agrees to certain procedures, such as calling the doctor if the suicidal wish becomes overwhelming. The physician, needless to say, makes it clear to the patient that the contract is important to the physician, and the clear expectation is that the patient will fulfill the contractual obligation.

3 Patients who do not fall clearly into either group 1 or 2. These patients are the source of greatest concern and a difficult responsibility for the physician. The physician is uncertain which course to take. Often the physician is responding to an intuitive sense that the patient is hiding some aspect of his or her history. For the nonpsychiatrist, a psychiatric consultation may be helpful. If that cannot be arranged as an emergency procedure, it is best to hospitalize the patient in order to evaluate the patient's condition more completely. Often it is found that such patients have serious underlying psychiatric disturbances that were not apparent initially. On other occasions, the patient is gradually able to share personal material that did not come out during the initial evaluation.

In the evaluation and formulation of a treatment plan for the suicidal patient, it is important to interview spouse, family members, and friends who may accompany the patient. This measure can result in valuable information for formulating a treatment plan, and can provide the physician with the opportunity to evaluate the potential of the significant others to offer the patient the necessary emotional support.

The physician should also be aware of the availability of specific support systems, such as Suicide Prevention Centers. These agencies are staffed by both professionals and trained nonprofessionals, and can offer valuable help to patients.

Suicidal patients who pose a strong risk and/or present evidence of an underlying serious psychiatric disturbance require a psychiatric evaluation.

The management of the suicidal patient includes the treatment of any underlying psychiatric disturbance. Antidepressives should be prescribed for severely depressed patients and neuroleptics for significantly agitated patients. Occasionally the physician is reluctant to prescribe medication for fear of its use in a suicide attempt. Although the physician may prescribe small amounts or assign the responsibility for the medication to a spouse or friend, this degree of uncertainty or distrust on the part of the physician should bring to mind the possible need for hospitalization.

Suicidal patients can be helped through crises that threaten their lives. Physicians are often involved with such patients. Whether the patient's condition suggests a collaborative approach or mandates a directive and protective "taking-over," the physician can often make a crucial difference.

SPECIAL ISSUES

Two special issues in particular require emphasis. The first has to do with the rate of physician suicides. Rose and Rosow reviewed the published studies of physician suicides in the United States.[15] They conclude that contrary to the popular notion, the data do not support the notion of higher rates than those of the general population. Most studies, however, suffer from serious methodologic flaws. Rose and Rosow present data collected in California that indicate that physicians and health care workers as a group are twice as suicide-prone as the general population. Age and divorce are significantly correlated with physician suicide, and drugs are the most common method. These authors also point out that contrary to popular opinion, there are no reliable data in the literature to suggest that one medical speciality is more prone to suicide than others.

Physicians are often resistant to assuming the role of patient, and consequently may not present themselves as formal patients. Clues about depression or a suicidal crisis may be communicated at staff meetings or in social circumstances. The performance, appearance, and manner of suicidal physicians may make it obvious that there have been significant personality changes and/or that such physicians are deeply depressed. They may have become more reclusive, or they may have begun drinking excessively. Often a spouse may call and share concern about the physician's suicidal potential. Physicians should be sensitive and responsive to these clues. The reluctance to get involved or to seem intrusive must be overcome if physicians are to offer their colleagues the help that they may not be able to ask for directly.

A second special issue involves the physician's role with the surviving family of the completed suicide. Much can and should be done. Most survivors struggle with a variety of strong feelings. Shock, disbelief, sadness, shame, and anger are common, but ultimately most family members experience intense guilt. There is a painful period of dealing with the many ways in which the survivors could have treated the deceased relative differently. Each family member tends to personalize the suicide. Although the physician may feel that there is some truth in these guilt-laden ruminations, his or her job is to assist the family members to deal with their feelings as effectively as possible. Once a patient has committed suicide, the physician must shift attention to the family.

Helping the surviving family members deal with the suicide may be difficult if the physician is struggling with intense feelings about suicide. Most physicians experience the suicide of a patient at some point in their career. Certain specialities are more exposed than others: psychiatry, oncology, and gerontology are examples. The impact of this experience varies from physician to physician. If there had been a good doctor-patient alliance over time, and if the physician had been actively involved in treating the patient during the suicidal crisis, there is apt to be an intense reaction. Holden, for example, studied the reaction of psychotherapists to the suicides of patients who had been involved with them in psychotherapy.[16] He points out that their reactions to patient suicides were highly personal, including shock, pain, anger, and the tendency to blame others, much as any other individual would do when faced with such a loss. The physician's grief was often slow to abate, and there was often considerable guilt and temporary impairment in the sense of competence.

Although these were physicians who had been involved in long-term and intensive psychotherapeutic relationships with their patients, and therefore the finding cannot be extrapolated broadly to other doctor-patient relationships, their reactions help us to understand the reluctance of many physicians to be involved with suicidal patients. Physicians, like all others, do not want to be hurt. Most view suicide as a personal defeat of their therapeutic efforts. Patients in suicidal crises have the potential to hurt. If they commit suicide, the act may injure many. It is, therefore, somewhat understandable for the physician to be self-protective and to overlook subtle clues of a suicidal crisis. In doing so, the physician refrains from becoming involved in the chain of events. This may protect the physician from pain if the patient commits suicide, but it removes the physician from a position of potential helpfulness. In the final analysis, there is a risk-gain element in dealing with suicidal patients, much as there is in dealing with patients suffering from other potentially fatal diseases. This, of course, is the challenge of practicing medicine.

REFERENCES

1. U.S. Department of Health, Education, and Welfare, *Vital Statistics Report Annual Summary for the U.S.,* Hyattsville, Md.: National Center for Health Statistics, 1976.
2. Aalberg, Veikko: Paper presented at the Ninth International Congress on Suicide Prevention and Crisis Intervention, Helsinki, 1976. Reported in *Psychiat. News* of the American Psychiatric Association, October 1977.
3. Winnik, H. Z.: Paper presented at Eighth International Congress on Suicidal Prevention and Crisis Intervention, Jerusalem, 1975. Reported in *Ment. Health Soc.,* 3:175–177, 1976.
4. World Health Organization, *World Health Statistics Report,* 29:7, Geneva, Switzerland, 1976.
5. Durkheim, E.: *Suicide,* Glencoe, Ill.: Free Press, 1951.
6. Strachey, J. (ed.): "Mourning and Melancholia," in *The Complete Works of Sigmund Freud,* vol. 18, London: Hogarth Press, 1955.
7. Shneidman, E. S.: "An Overview of Suicide," *Psychiat. Ann.,* 6:11, November 1976.
8. Menninger, K.: *Man Against Himself,* New York: Harcourt, Brace, 1938.
9. Guze, S., and E. Robbins: "Suicide and Primary Affective Disorders," *Brit. J. Psychiat.,* 117:437–438, 1970.
10. Tsuang, M. D.: "Suicide in Schizophrenics, Manics, Depressives, and Surgical Controls," *Arch. Gen. Psychiat.,* 35(2):153–155, Febuary 1978.
11. Pokorny, A.: "Suicide in Depression," in W. E. Fann et al. (eds.) *Phenomenology and Treatment of Depression,* Chapter 12, New York: Spectrum, 1977.
12. Modlin, H. C.: "Cues and Clues to Suicide," *The Five Minute Hour,* Summit, N.J.: Geigy Pharmaceuticals, September 1975.
13. Litman, Robert E., and Norman L. Farberow: "Emergency Evaluation of Self-Destructive Potentiality," in Norman L. Farberow and Edwin S. Shneidman (eds.), *The Cry for Help,* New York: McGraw-Hill, 1961, pp. 48–59.

14 Tabachnick, Norman D., and Norman L. Farberow: "Assessment of Self-Destructive Potentiality," in Norman L. Farberow and Edwin S. Shneidman (eds.), *The Cry for Help,* New York: McGraw-Hill, 1961, pp. 60–77.
15 Rose, K. Daniel, and Irving Rosow: "Physicians Who Kill Themselves," *Arch. Gen. Psychiat.,* **29**:800–805, December 1973.
16 Holden, L. Dwight: "Therapist Response to Patient Suicide: Professional and Personal," *J. Cont. Ed. Psychiat.,* pp. 23–32, May 1978.

Chapter 21

Diseases and Illnesses Specific to Women

Carol C. Nadelson, M.D.
Malkah T. Notman, M.D.

EDITORS' INTRODUCTION

What is it like to be a 33-year-old divorcee who is sitting across the physician's desk and hears that a radical mastectomy is necessary? What thoughts go through the patient's mind as a surgeon uncomfortably ruffles those papers on the desk and takes a phone call from another patient? Will she die? What about postoperative loneliness? Who will take care of the children? Where will the money come from? What will be the reaction of the 38-year-old executive she is just getting to know?

To whom can she talk about these questions? Can it be the physician, who may be in a unique position to help her explore the answers to her questions? The way the physician handles a patient in this crisis may well influence her capacity to cope. The physician has a unique opportunity to be of service. This help may abort a major depression or other psychiatric illness. The brief psychotherapy by the physician at the time of crisis may have results equivalent to the satisfactory results achieved by psychiatrists only after long periods of treatment with some psychiatric illnesses.

The majority of physicians, however, are male, and women are increasingly dissatisfied with medical care that does not treat them as competent collaborators in the treatment process. The rhetoric of the feminists has impacted the way in which the American woman regards the manner of her physician's treatment. Her perception of her role and her autonomy has changed. This change in her attitude toward herself has increased the perception of her needs and rights as a patient. The time-honored paternalistic stance of many physicians is increasingly found lacking.

For today's physician, this new awareness by women of their own physiological and psychological imperatives demands increased understanding of physical life experiences that are unique to women—such as menarche, conception, and menopause—and the psychological functioning of women during key life phases. The physician must be aware of the knowledge and changes in reproduction and sexual patterns that have been ushered in within the past 20 years. But most of all, physicians must come to terms with deep-rooted personal attitudes toward women in order to assimilate and adapt to the needs of women patients, without recourse to stereotyped reactions.

It is not as simple as deciding to treat men and women patients alike, although an understanding of the life phases of the male patient would also foster a more sympathetic, understanding attitude toward their unique needs as men. However, if the traditional relationship between physicians and women patients is moving away from the parent-child model, it is possible to anticipate the development of a more mature collaborative partnership between doctors and patients of both sexes.

It is hoped that this chapter by Nadelson and Notman, two leading female psychiatrists, will help both male and female physicians become more introspective about their role in treating women patients—the good they can accomplish and the bad they can avoid.

INTRODUCTION

It is significant that texts on psychiatry have not included special sections that consider differences in function between men and women. These are important, not as a means of dichotomizing or further separating the two genders, but as a means of recognizing certain uniquenesses about the male and female body, with the resultant potential for physical diseases and illnesses that are specific to these differences, and as a means of recognizing their impact. While an individual's sense of identity is closely tied to the appearance, function, and intactness of his or her body, the implications of anatomic and physiological differences can be psychologically significant. For most women, breasts are identified with attractiveness, sexuality, nurturing, and femininity. Diseases of the breast are not rare, and surgery on the breast is frequent.

The reproductive organs are also part of the feminine self-image. They may be specific sites for significant pathology, and hysterectomy is usually felt as a specific phase of aging, as well as the loss of an organ that is closely identified with inherent values of motherhood and femininity.

So pathology of organs that are unique to a female is bound to bring with it significant emotional repercussions, and possibly precipitate psychiatric illnesses.

To the extent that the caring physician pays attention to the implications of this, there may be dramatic differences in how the woman patient responds. Certain crises in our lives may have long-term, serious implications. Some of the potential for untoward complications may be greatly diminished by the physician's taking a little time to contemplate, to offer the patient a listening ear, and then to provide a little personal input.

Current understanding of the psychological aspects of those physiological functions relating specifically to women has evolved from early work that considered the relationship between psychological experience and somatic manifestations.

In 1931, Horney and Frank published separate papers on premenstrual tension.[1,2] Eight years later, Benedek and Rubenstein[3] first published their work correlating ovarian activity and psychodynamic processes. Lindemann's report of pre- and postoperative evaluations following hysterectomies, which emphasized the specific meaning of the loss of the uterus, was an impetus for investigation of women's responses to the range of physiological and pathological conditions involving reproductive organs.[4] This work was expanded by Renneker and Cutler, who reported on the postmastectomy mourning process, and stressed the meaning of the loss of the breast to women.[5] A vast literature has developed in this area, but very little has been written about the less dramatic and more universal experiences of women, including menarche, conception, and menopause. Recently, attention to abortion and rape has stimulated new interest and controversy.

Since the obstetrician-gynecologist or family physician functions as the primary physician for the majority of women during their reproductive years, he or she cares for women during a number of critical life phases. Thus, it is necessary for the physician to have an understanding of the psychological functioning of women during these phases.

Mathis comments: "Sex, reproduction, and the reproductive system are almost synonymous with emotional reactions in our culture. The emotional charge invested in the genitalia makes that area peculiarly vulnerable to symptoms arising from any conflictual aspect of living. The woman who seeks medical attention for her reproductive system deserves a physician who understands the total significance of femininity as well as he knows the anatomy and physiology of the female. The physician who assumes this responsibility automatically becomes involved in emotional processes unequaled in any other branch of medicine, psychiatry not excepted."[6]

Physicians are vulnerable to emotional responses to sexuality and reproduction, and may avoid investigating these concerns with patients. They often refer emotionally related problems to the office nurse or hospital social worker. In medical school, students have generally not been taught about human sexuality within the context of human interaction, nor have they had training in dealing with their responses to emotionally charged areas. Much of the information that is communicated is divided and separated into its "appropriate" discipline, and is not integrated in such a way that it relates to the real problems faced by practicing physicians.[7]

In addition to the resistance to taking up the issues created by emotional responses in physicians, there is evidence from recent critical discussions that much of the data on which prevailing attitudes towards reproductive functioning are based, and which have been cited in the past, are questionable.[8,9,10,11] For instance, the concept that a depression inevitably follows an abortion has been shown to be incorrect.[12]

CHANGES IN REPRODUCTIVE AND SEXUAL PATTERNS

The social changes of recent years have affected women and their families significantly. Birthrates have declined, families are smaller, more women choose not to marry, to marry late, and to remain childless, and an increasing number of nulliparous women in their early twenties are seeking sterilization.[13,14]

The pregnant woman has less social support available to her now than she did 15 or 20 years ago, when prevailing social norms favored larger families and there were fewer nondomestic options for women. In fact, the shift in values has swung to the opposite pole; women having a third or fourth child describe outright hostility from peers, and occasionally encounter doubts from obstetricians as well. Many women are postponing pregnancies until their education and training are completed, or until their careers are established. The "older" pregnant woman often has difficulty gaining support from medical people.

Many of the problems that have emerged for patients are complex and have major social, legal, and ethical implications. For instance, family planning, abortion, and sterilization have an impact far beyond their meaning to the individual.

The fact that sexual mores have changed is self-evident. Sexual relations outside marriage are more widespread. Homosexual relationships are more open, and may be an expression of political ideology or of an alternate pattern of intimacy.[15] The physician has had to become accustomed to new realities, including the possibility of venereal disease in a wide cross-section of patients, requests for contraceptives and sexual counseling for unmarried couples, and gynecological care of patients identifying themselves as bisexual or homosexual.

In addition, the physician is asked to assess and even treat such complex interactional problems as sexual dysfunction, or problems requiring an understanding of a wide range of psychological principles, from psychological reactions to "normal" phenomena (such as pregnancy), to response to a complex mutilative surgical procedure.

THE CHANGING DOCTOR-PATIENT RELATIONSHIP

Certain aspects of the doctor-patient relationship emphasize the potential problem between physicians and patients. The expectation that the doctor, who has usually been male, is informed, helping, authoritative, and protective fits especially well with the conventional view of women as naive, compliant, and dependent "girls." This parent-child model has received some attention in medical

literature, and has been the subject of feminist writing. The potential depreciation is inherent in the model.

Communication fails when the doctor-patient relationship is not a true partnership. Indeed, in many instances decisions about a patient's care have been,
and still are, based on a paternalistic view that assumes the doctor's understanding of the patient's best interests, without sufficient participation of the patient.
For instance, decisions about female sterilization and abortion have until recently
been made largely on the basis of physicians' attitudes. They also required the
consent of the husband, which reflected traditional views of wives and children as
property. Generally, male sterilization had not required the consent of the wife.

In recent years, there has been a movement toward involving women more
actively in their own care. An interest in home delivery among some women has
reflected not only discontent with the institutional atmosphere of a hospital, but
also the wish to include husbands, other family members, and friends in the
childbirth process. The movement toward self-examinations and self-knowledge
is a response to the wish to rely less on trained medical personnel and more on
oneself and one's peers.

A traditionally trained physician is apt to become defensive and frustrated in
response to these departures from what has been considered good medical care.
Self-help movements threaten established medical roles, and seem to dispense
with valuable professional experience. The physician who is able to understand
and respond positively to the reactions of women who feel anxious, poorly
understood, or excluded and put off by the stereotypes and attitudes that have
predominated in the field will be able to offer better care.

In addition, the full impact of gynecological procedures on a woman's self-
image and sexuality must be attended to, and in some areas, notably in the
management of normal pregnancy, contraceptive counseling, and sexual dysfunction, the illness model may be inappropriate. A collaborative educational model
may be more effective.

PROBLEMS FOR THE PSYCHIATRIC CONSULTANT

The kinds of problems generally presented for psychiatric consultation include
questions about the management of a variety of social-psychological as well as
psychiatric problems. The problems of psychiatric patients range from addiction
and psychoses to difficulties resulting from disorganized families and different
cultural backgrounds. Patients who have received fragmented care in the past
(for example, patients with histories of incest and other sexual abuse) also present
problems that often require consultation.

An example of the range of consultations in one hospital (Beth Israel
Hospital, Boston, Massachusetts) during 1 year is shown in Table 21-1. These
data concur with the reports of others who discuss the high level of "psychological distress" in medical patients.

We will turn now to some specific areas where emotional issues are of particular importance.

Table 21-1 Consultations and Their Frequencies

	Consultation	Frequency (%)
1	How to manage patients presenting with psychiatric symptoms such as bizarre ideation, depression, and intense anxiety, as well as patients with a psychiatric history	36
2	How to understand the emotional reactions to an obstetrical or gynecological experience, such as the birth of a defective child or the diagnosis of malignancy	25
3	How to evaluate the potential response to specific procedures such as an abortion where the patient is ambivalent, or a tubal ligation in a young woman	20
4	The assessment of "psychosomatic" problems, somatic presentation, or forms of psychiatric disorders, such as pelvic pain or abdominal pain, that are unexplained by organic disease	11
5	The assessment of patients with nonspecific emotional issues	8

PREGNANCY

The complex interaction of physical and psychological factors in pregnancy may make demands upon physicians that their training has often not addressed, and that may conflict with their individual values and attitudes. A paradigm for understanding the evolving role of the psychiatrist in gynecologic care is the problem of the pregnant teenager, whose management requires a complex integration of expertise in a number of fields. The gynecologist is asked to help her make a decision about her pregnancy, and to treat her in a sympathetic, unbiased manner, often without the necessary understanding of the problem or objectivity required in the situation. If the teenager decides to abort the pregnancy, the physician is asked to perform a procedure that may not have been legal or considered ethical during his or her training, and about which he or she may have conflicted feelings. Physicians delivering babies of teenagers find themselves frustrated by the teenagers' seeming inability to use contraceptives effectively. Such physicians often feel uncomfortable dealing with young women who may have a very different concept of pregnancy and motherhood from the one physicians have grown accustomed to understanding.

Until recently, the major questions that were considered in understanding a pregnancy included the patient's acceptance or rejection of her "feminine" role in pregnancy, and the likelihood of postpartum depression or psychosis. The questions that have become increasingly important are more complex concerns about the impact and motivation for contraception, pregnancy, motherhood, and abortion.

The idea of pregnancy as a disease is an old concept that has been perpetuated by some of the restrictive practices and some of the advice that has been given. Recent moves toward more active participation of both parents, and even toward home delivery in uncomplicated situations, have led a trend toward an alternative view that considers pregnancy to be a normal function, with special characteristics that make it similar to other important nodal points in the life cycle, such as puberty and menopause.[16,17] These experiences confront the individual with new issues and challenges requiring adaptation. They also precipitate the reemergence of earlier unsettled conflicts, and offer the possibility of further growth and maturation through mastery of these earlier conflicts. Bibring et al. point out that pregnancy involves both physical and psychological changes that are immutable.[18] Thus pregnancy, like puberty and menopause, is a milestone.

For most pregnant women, "routine care," including physical attention, factual information, and support, is sufficient. However, for many women the physician may be the only person in a position to observe and respond to failing psychological defenses that may result in decompensation. Bibring and Valenstein studied a group of "normal pregnant women" and found that a "surprising" number of young women were diagnosed initially as borderline personalities, or were considered to be seriously disturbed because of their emotional lability.[19] They noted, however, that therapeutic results could be obtained with greater ease than would have been expected from the severity of the presenting disturbances, and that the adjustment to pregnancy and parenthood was not necessarily so difficult as had been anticipated. They concluded that pregnancy could be considered a developmental crisis, and that upheaval and even regression, which eventually served the process of maturation, could be expected.

When the diagnosis of pregnancy is made, even when the pregnancy is desired and the overall feelings are positive, fear and ambivalence are experienced frequently, as would be expected with any new and major life change. The beginning is simple, but the implications are lifelong, and the changes are permanent and progressive. Areas that had previously seemed conflict-free may no longer be experienced in the same way. Anxiety and questions may arise about one's future role and responsibility in marriage or career. Pregnant women often describe feeling alienated from a physician who does not acknowledge the possibility of negative feelings, or permit expression of ambivalence. They feel criticized and guilty.

Also basic to pregnancy are the emergence of feelings concerning the woman's early experience of having been mothered, and her current relationship to her mother as she changes roles from daughter to mother. Past difficulties may cause feelings of guilt, anger, ambivalence, and remorse.

A pregnancy has multiple meanings for both partners together, as well as for each of them individually. They must conceptualize themselves as parents, which revives feelings toward their own parents. In addition, the father may feel threatened if he sees the child as a potential competitor for the attention and affection of the mother. The child's sex or position in the family may also have particular meaning for parents.

Sexual problems may be manifested for the first time during pregnancy. These often relate to feelings about pregnancy and about change in status, or they occur because of the physical changes of pregnancy and the postpartum periods. Bearing a child also represents a hastening toward full adulthood for adolescents.

Motivation for Pregnancy

The motivations for pregnancy are complex and multiple, and are not limited to feelings about a specific relationship. They may be different from those relating to actual wishes to start a family and care for children, and may represent an attempt to resolve questions about the reality or endurance of a particular relationship; they may also serve to affirm sexual identity, especially in adolescents and younger women.[20,21] However, while the occurrence of a pregnancy provides the physical evidence of femininity or adulthood, the psychological aspects of adulthood and femininity are not necessarily resolved, and thus become part of the task of the period of pregnancy. Concerns about the ability to love or be loved may be motivating factors. Women at times express the feeling that a child would guarantee them love. Even an adult woman may want a child because she wants a mother and needs to master an early life experience of deprivation.[21] The pregnancy may provide in fantasy a means of having a child and at the same time being a child who is taken care of. It may also be an unconscious attempt to seek a resolution of early Oedipal conflicts.

Pregnancy in the Adolescent

Although people generally are having fewer pregnancies, the number of teenage parents is increasing rapidly. Each year more than one million 15- to 19-year-old women, and 30,000 under the age of 15, become pregnant; one-third of these pregnancies are intentional.[22,23] The implications of this increase are extremely important. In addition to the problems created by the superimposition of two developmental phases, that is, adolescence and adulthood, the long-term consequences for the teenage mother and her child must be considered.

Both physical and psychosocial consequences are considerable. Teenage mothers have a higher risk of toxemia, premature birth, perinatal loss, pre- and postnatal infection, and complications of labor and delivery. These appear to be related to poor prenatal care, which is often correlated with socioeconomic factors. Dropping out of school and repeated failures in jobs and other life situations, as well as a high pregnancy recidivism rate, occur.

Early in adolescence, teenagers handle sexual fantasies and feelings by direct expression in action, by symptom formation, or by repression, withdrawal, or denial. At times the adaptive and defensive measures employed are extreme, and severe regression may occur. Inconsistency, unpredictability, and ambivalence are part of the evolutionary process toward maturation. In the course of the development of a self-concept, the young adolescent girl does not necessarily integrate a perception of herself as a physiological woman who is capable of procreation in the same way that an adult woman is. The possible consequences of sexual activity may not be perceived. Pregnancy, for example, may be a vague, unintegrated, and unreal possibility; a baby may seem to be a doll to play with, it may express a regressive wish, it may be the representation of a childlike self-image, or it may be a plea for caring. Schaffer and Pine consider pregnancy in adolescents as an expression and solution of the conflict between the wish to be mothered and the urge to mother.[24] It may be a response to a loss, or an attempt to facilitate separation from parents and/or to resolve problems in relation to them.[25]

Bernard described the interplay of social and familial forces, and pointed to the significance of disorganization and deprivation in the families of many young pregnant adolescents.[25] At present, however, pregnancy occurs in a wide range of families and social groups. Deutsch pointed out that no specific dynamic constellation is present for all pregnant adolescents.[20] She emphasized unconscious motivation, and mentioned flight from incestuous fantasies by means of intimacy with the first man encountered. Also important are passivity, identification with the pregnancy of a mother or sister, revenge toward the family, and depression.

Young noted that the pregnant adolescent's failure to apply her sexual knowledge to herself was evidenced by nonuse of contraception and lack of anticipation of pregnancy.[26] The adolescent may be unwilling or unable to give up comforting and supporting fantasies, and may thus be unmotivated to avoid pregnancy. She may be terrified to face her own emptiness.

Once pregnant, the problems of loss may be intensified further because the putative father (also frequently an adolescent) may abandon her, or she may provoke rejection to alleviate her guilt and mollify her parents. The resultant feelings of despair and unworthiness result in further lowering of self-esteem.

For the pregnant adolescent, the conflict resonates between the positive aspects of conception and pregnancy and the frustration and sadness of making a choice either to terminate the pregnancy, to continue it and by so doing change the course of her life, or to confront a permanent separation by giving up the child. There is no conflict-free alternative.

This conflict is of particular developmental significance since it may represent the first time a decision with lifelong implications must be faced. Even passive acceptance represents a decision to continue the pregnancy. The resolution of a decision about an unwanted pregnancy is often complicated by a regressive response because there is a lack of firmly established, effective means for dealing with the problem, a lack that includes the limited decision-making capacity in the adolescent. This lack may be reinforced by family strife.[27]

Since denial is a major ego defense mechanism of the young adolescent, it is not surprising that acknowledgment of the reality of a pregnancy is often delayed. In addition, inexperience, fear, and anxiety play a major role in preventing the teenager from seeking help. Many adolescents are uncertain about where to turn. Others are fearful and guilty about confronting their parents, or they are overly influenced by peer pressures.

A teenager who has become pregnant and has not worked through maturational issues is more at risk to repeat a pregnancy. Data have been accumulated on the recidivism rate for unwanted pregnancy, and its relationship to nonuse of contraceptives. Some authors report a 20 to 40 percent repeat within 3 years after a pregnancy.[23] In a study of teenage pregnancy Sarrel reported that, of 63 primigravidas who delivered an out-of-wedlock baby, 36 delivered another baby 1 year later.[28] In a follow-up of 100 teenage (13- to 17-year old) unwed mothers over a 5-year period, he found that there was a total of 349 pregnancies and 9 abortions; only 5 girls did not become pregnant again.

Abortion Versus Continuation

Recent research on the psychiatric risks of abortion generally reveals that the contraindications to abortion are not specific. Some psychiatric sequelae of abortion exist, but they are not major or permanent; they are related to personality dynamics, stress tolerance, and degree of ambivalence.[29] It is important to note that there appear to be fewer problems related to guilt when abortion is legal and available than when illegal abortion is the only recourse.[30]

Those who choose to carry a pregnancy to term do so for a variety of reasons, including the desire to have a baby, the inability to bear the abortion loss, or the inability to make a decision for abortion on religious or ethical grounds. There may be fear of ostracism by a peer group or family; or there may be a feeling of guilt for sexual behavior, and the continuation of pregnancy is seen as a deserved punishment.

In an attempt to separate from her parents and differentiate herself, the adolescent may polarize her behavior and even her ideas. She may choose a solution primarily because she feels her family wants the opposite. The parents, on the other hand, may be angry and seek to punish their daughter. Since the adolescent most likely will continue to live with her family, it is difficult to help her to make a decision without their participation. The adolescent who is making a decision whether to have an abortion or to continue a pregnancy needs help to understand her motivations, explore her ambivalence, and consider the alternative solutions as objectively as possible. This may not be easy if she is frightened, suspicious, or angry. Discussion about future prevention of pregnancy can sometimes be facilitated because of the experience with an unwanted pregnancy.[29]

The legalization of abortion has permitted more open consideration of choice, and has made it possible for counseling to be an active part of the decision-making process. Since the adolescent's capacity for delay and tolerance of anxiety may be severely tested by an unwanted pregnancy, she may want to avoid counseling, and reach a rapid decision to reduce the tension she experiences. This pressure toward action, although realistic, can also serve to deny the implications of the pregnancy.

In the counseling situation, there are two primary goals: (1) short-term intervention, including decision-making about the pregnancy; and (2) the beginning of integration of the experience, which necessarily includes some understanding of motivation and the precipitating social and family circumstances. Although pregnancy may be considered a crisis in a teenager, it is not in itself either an indication of psychopathology or a reason for long-term psychotherapy.

MENSTRUAL FLUCTUATIONS AND PREMENSTRUAL SYNDROME

New information on the female reproductive cycle has brought into question some established ideas about the menstrual cycle. Recent critical examinations of existing data, as well as new studies, have indicated that connections between the endocrine and other physiological changes and behavioral and emotional symptomatology are not as well established as had previously been thought.[31]

The existence and basis of behavioral and mood fluctuations with phases of the menstrual cycle has been debated for years. Although many women experience no changes premenstrually, it is apparent clinically that for others the days before each period are characterized by irritability, lability, or depression. For those who experience it, the symptoms disappear with the onset of the menstrual period.

Premenstrual tension has been considered responsible for a wide variety of social behavior and psychological phenomena. Crimes, suicide attempts, the misbehavior of schoolgirls, and psychiatric admissions in emergency rooms and walk-in clinics have been related to the premenstrual period. Studies of suicidal attempts have indicated that a majority occurred in the bleeding phase of the cycle, and were minimal in the postbleeding and preovulatory phase of the reproductive cycle.[32,33] Self-reports of functioning during the menstrual cycle indicate that a small percentage of women feel their judgment or mental faculties are impaired to some extent, particularly in the premenstrual phase of the cycle.[31]

Sommer and Parlee, in reviewing studies of cognitive and perceptual-motor behavior in relation to menstruation, point out the methodological problems in much of the research.[31,8] The problem of determining the hormonal status of the subjects, the selection bias toward women with regular cycles, the use of self-reports, and the compounding of objective with subjective data complicate evaluation of results. Many studies have not been replicated. A majority of studies using objective performance measures have failed to demonstrate significant cyclic fluctuation in performance.

Sommer concludes: "It appears that those instances in which a cyclic effect occurs are those in which responses are mediated by social and psychological factors. Subjects express feelings in interaction with their social environment in ways consonant with their expectations about themselves and about the demands and expectations of the social milieu in which they move. Where social or psychological expectations of menstrual debilitation are altered, the effect disappears."[31] Thus, when a woman expects that her behavior and responses will be affected by her menstrual cycle, and lives in a setting where these expectations are shared, it is likely that her perception of her functioning will reflect this. Nevertheless, the large body of data suggesting some behavioral effects of menstrual phases needs further exploration. Recently there has been some data suggestive of the possibility that there are electroencephalographic responses to varying hormones.[34] These data deserve further research.

Clinical observations of menstrual variations may reflect responses of the individual to her own and to social expectations, to identification with important women in her life, or to somatic expressions of a wide variety of feelings about herself, her femininity, and her body. Family patterns in menstrual responses indicate a strong tendency for girls to repeat the patterns of their mothers in their premenstrual reactions, the presence of dysmenorrhea, and the extent of morbidity around the menstrual period.[35]

It is important that the physician avoid an "either/or" approach to evaluation and treatment of these symptoms, and maintain awareness of the individual and social context that may lead to certain patterns of response. The expectation that a woman is likely to have "premenstrual tension" may also lead to relying on this explanation for emotional symptoms that may be unrelated, thus closing off further exploration or understanding.

Menopause

Recently, increasing attention has been paid to the middle years of adult development, including the menopausal period. Here too, endocrinological and social-psychological data indicate that many misconceptions have existed about the nature and extent of the symptomatology directly ascribable to the menopause.[36,37] Perlmutter states, "There are multiple disorders that have been ascribed to the changing hormonal balance and are equated with menopause. In reality, not all the changes that are noted are due to hormonal imbalances . . . ."[38]

Research in this area suffers from such methodological problems as relying on case histories, clinical impressions, or analyses of data from selected samples of women who are under the care of gynecologists or psychiatrists. Those studies that are more reliable show that "psychosomatic and psychological complaints were not reported more frequently by so called 'menopausal' than by younger women."[39]

Vasomotor instability, which is "manifested as hot flashes, flushes, episodes of perspiration or attacks" has been one of the consistent symptoms accompanying menopause. This is present in up to 75 percent of women reporting some type of symptomatology.[38,40] McKinley and Jefferys, in a review of symptoms of women aged 45 to 54, found that hot flashes and night sweats were "clearly associated with the onset of a natural menopause and that they occur in a majority of women."[39] The other symptoms that were investigated, "namely headaches, dizzy spells, palpitations, sleeplessness, depression, and weight increase, showed no direct relationship to the menopause, but tended to occur together."

The etiology of the hot flashes is unclear. Although there is general agreement that estrogen therapy will alleviate the symptomatology in most women, other disease processes in which estrogen levels are low (for example, stress amenorrhea and anorexia nervosa) are not characterized by hot flashes.[38] Thus, the etiology of the symptoms appears to be more complex than simple estrogen deficit. Psychological factors such as anger, anxiety, and excitement are considered important in precipitating "flashes" in susceptible women, as are activities giving rise to excess heat production or retention, such as a warm environment, muscular work, and eating hot food.[40] However, the symptoms may arise without any clear psychological or heat-stimulating mechanism.

Other problems accompanying menopause are atrophic changes in skin, subcutaneous tissue, and mucosa, which are part of the aging process. Since vaginal lubrication may be slower to develop in the menopausal woman, sexual symptoms may result.

The age of menopause varies from the late thirties to the middle or even late fifties. This variation supports the tendency to assign a variety of symptoms occurring in these years to a woman's menopausal status. In a study of menopausal age, McKinley, Jefferys, and Thompson found that "The median age at menopause in industrial societies now occurs at about 50 years of age, and there is no firm evidence that this age has increased at least in the last century, nor any indication of any close relationships between the age at menopause and the age at menarche or socioeconomic status."[41]

Many other mid-life symptoms have been attributed to menopause, and many menopausal symptoms have been attributed to estrogen deficiency or hormonal changes. The range of symptomatology that is considered part of the menopausal syndrome includes insomnia, irritability, depression, diminished sexual interest, headaches, dizzy spells, and palpitations.[39] Neugarten and her coworkers studied 100 women aged 43 to 53 by using menstrual histories as an index of menopausal or climacteric status. They found "climacteric status to be unrelated to a wide array of personality measures." They also found "very few significant relationships between the severity of somatic and psychosomatic symptoms and these variables."[42,43] Kraines found that women who previously had low self-esteem and life satisfaction were likely to have difficulties with menopause.[44] Menopause is then possibly one of the important experiences for women, but one which is best understood in the context of their entire lives.

Thus, women's reactions to such turning points in their lives as menarche and pregnancy are consistent with their reactions to menopause. While this is not surprising, a surprising finding, which is supported by cross-cultural data, is that women with "high motherliness" scores on scales, who have invested heavily in their childbearing and rearing, are more likely to experience depression during menopause.[36] Women who have not had children do not have the most difficulty with menopause, perhaps because many of them have had to come to terms with their childlessness earlier than the biological menopause.

Social class is an important variable. Middle- and upper-class women appear to find the cessation of childbearing more liberating, because more alternatives are open to them. Neugarten and her coworkers report that middle- and upper-class women tended to minimize their reactions compared to lower-class women.[45] From their data, younger women anticipating menopause were more concerned than women who were actually menopausal. Postmenopausal women generally took a more positive view, "with higher proportions agreeing that the menopause creates no major discontinuity in life and agreeing that except for the underlying biological changes, women have a relative degree of control over their symptoms and need not inevitably have difficulties." Another study confirms that middle-class women are less anxious about the menopause than working-class women, but generally "menopausal status is not associated with measurable anxiety."[46] There is also a postmenopausal rise in energy and activity, possibly deriving from the diminished time and energy needed in caring for children.[47]

A developmental impetus may occur for women whose lives offer them opportunities for growth. When their major role and source of self-esteem has been perceived as centering around reproductive life, the ending of childbearing creates a real loss. The concomitant changes of aging and the devaluation of the aged and aging, especially in women, leads to lowered self-esteem and to potential depression. However, although mid-life depression in women is an important clinical entity, it appears that the group most at risk for depression are married women, and specifically those with young children living at home.[37,47]

Family experiences of this period are important. The mid-life transition for men, who are often the husbands of menopausal women, brings new stresses. This period for men is often accompanied by sexual problems, which sometimes lead to affairs, marital disruption, and the abandonment of the women. Adolescent children may be sexually and aggressively provocative, challenging, or disappointing. Children leaving home for school or marriage change the family balance. This has been described generally as loss. However, some women view it as extension or expansion of parenting to include the wider interests of their children.[48] Although change and transition do cause stress and require new adaptations, which are sometimes accompanied by symptoms, Bernard, in her studies on marriage, indicated that marital satisfactions increase as children leave the home.[49] The "empty nest syndrome" does not appear to be universal.

SURGICAL PROCEDURES

Several surgical procedures have particular significance for women, since they often involve reproductive or sexual organs and hence affect the woman's concept of her feminine identity. Hysterectomy and mastectomy have major impact on body and self-image. In addition, they are often superimposed on a serious malfunction or malignancy. Other procedures such as sterilization or amniocentesis may be elected for positive prevention, but at the same time can be experienced as assaults. To understand reactions to surgery, a history of the individual's response to other stressful situations may be helpful for assessing coping capacity.

An individual who has suffered any traumatic experience may tend to repeat aspects of the experience to gain mastery. This includes talking about it, reconstructing the circumstances, and exploring alternate responses. However, in an attempt to reduce discomfort, create an atmosphere of optimism, or encourage the patient to feel well, physicians may promote for the patient an environment that minimizes the significance of what is happening.

Hysterectomy

It was estimated that in 1973, 690,000 hysterectomies were performed in the United States.[50] This represents a higher rate than for any other major operation, and the numbers are rising. The fact that it is performed more than twice as frequently in the United States as in England and Wales suggests the lack of substantial agreement about indications.

For women, the experience is psychologically significant for many reasons. Although a hysterectomy can leave minor or no scars, the experience of mutilation, and the sense of damage to femininity, can be profound. Conscious and unconscious influences must be differentiated. Thus, a woman who consciously fears further pregnancies may experience conscious relief following a hysterectomy. However, the unconscious desire for more babies might result in a postoperative depression.[6] While this may be an unavoidable response, depressive reactions can be prevented or minimized by preoperative preparation and postoperative support where the physician appreciates the significance of sterilization as a possible loss to the particular woman.

Attitudes toward hysterectomies vary, and the surgeon making a decision to perform a hysterectomy may not consider the alternatives, and take into account the impact on the individual or her family. In many sociocultural groups, men feel that a woman is "damaged" and less desirable if she has had a hysterectomy, and she may be rejected because of it. Myths about the effect of hysterectomy on sexual responses may also affect her and her relationships with men. The loss of the uterus may signal the beginning of the aging process, as does natural menopause, since the ovaries may also be removed.

Posthysterectomy depression is a generally recognized clinical entity. In a number of studies, a higher incidence of depression following this procedure as compared with other surgical procedures is reported.[51,52,53] Although sampling and methodological problems complicate these studies, they do demonstrate overall vulnerability of women to posthysterectomy depression. The most vulnerable women are those without organic pathology in the uterus, those who are under age 40, and those whose marital supports have been disrupted. Women with previous emotional disturbance also seem more likely to become depressed. Some of the considerations that are important in understanding menopause are also applicable in this situation. If there is a malignancy, however, then clearly there is an additional stress.

The loss of an organ with important unconscious symbolic significance, especially if the preparation has been insufficient, can produce psychological symptoms, particularly if there is anxiety about the underlying diagnosis. Since the importance of reproductive intactness for a woman's self-esteem is affected by sociocultural values and feelings regarding her role, the reaction to hysterectomy may be less severe if her reproductive life is considered as only one component of her femininity and self-esteem.

Sterilization

Another area where changes in patient populations and their problems have brought new issues into focus is the increase in sterilization requests. When a woman is young and nulliparous, a psychiatrist is often asked to consult in order to evaluate both her competence to make the decision and her awareness of its implications, as well as to assess her motivation and potential reaction.

Although there are few studies on this subject, those that do exist indicate that the decision is generally a carefully considered one. Lindenmayer, in a small study of nulliparous women in their early twenties who were seeking voluntary tubal ligation, indicated that the women had all taken time to make the decision, and had based the wish for childlessness on negative feelings toward children, on their assessment of their incapacity to be mothers, and on a strong desire for independence.[13] Lindenmayer felt it was not possible to explain the decision solely in intrapsychic terms. He noted the importance of assessing the decision-making process in these circumstances, and determined that there should be no outside pressure, no major conflict, and the agreement of both partners if the woman is married or involved in a stable relationship.

Kaltreider and Margolis, in a study of women under 30 who requested sterilization, found that these women had a strong motivation for sterilization and a history of family disruption, fear of motherhood, and dislike of children.[14] In a follow-up of these women up to 10½ months after tubal ligation, they reported "no regrets, a sense of increased control in their own lives, and more sexual pleasure." The authors suggest that for this group, "the choice to be barren was multidetermined, persistent over time, and ego-syntonic."

The physician, however, must be aware of the developmental potential of the patient, and of the possibility that life events will bring about a change in the balance of her priorities. Thus, an irreversible procedure may prove to be self-destructive. The studies cited indicate that at least for some women the motivation for childlessness may be deeply rooted and consistent with other directions in which they see their fulfillment. If the patient is fully aware of the implications of the decision, respect for the patient's autonomy and decision making is paramount.

Mastectomy

Breast surgery involves many of the same anxieties about body image, femininity, intactness, and mutilation as does hysterectomy. Recently, the efficacy of radical mastectomy for malignancy has been questioned.[54] Modified radical surgery, simple mastectomy, and even "lumpectomy" have been performed with good results. For some women, the knowledge that a disfiguring operation is not inevitable has made it easier to seek medical attention for breast masses.

Breasts are important symbolically and realistically to both men and women. For many women, they represent an important component of femininity and self-esteem because they combine nutrient maternal potential with sexual attractiveness.

A mastectomy raises a number of issues since it is both a confrontation with a life-threatening illness and the loss of an important body part. For the physician, the predominant aspect usually is first the life-threatening illness, then the morbidity associated with both the malignancy and the cure, and finally the patient's physical and emotional response to the whole experience. Many physicians feel that they protect the patient by not communicating their concern about prognosis fully to her. There may be a discrepancy between what the physician knows and what he or she tells the patient and family, and therefore what the patient must deal with. There may also be a discrepancy between what the doctor thinks he or she is doing, namely helping the patient, and how the patient perceives this, namely not only as a helpful procedure for her survival and cure but also as an attack.

The acuteness of the situation has a considerable effect on the kind of trauma that a mastectomy represents. A sudden change from a state of apparent good health to one in which a major loss has occurred creates great potential for disorganization. There are psychological advantages in allowing the patient an adequate time for psychological preparation between diagnosis and surgery.

A major component of the reaction to mastectomy is a reaction to loss and the restitutive efforts made. Although this is true of other surgery, the visibility of the breast makes it particularly important. The reaction to the loss of a breast may also revive earlier losses, or it may reflect the patient's concern about dying. The loss of sexual attractiveness is a concern of many women, not only those who are young. A menopausal woman who is worried about the effects of aging on her physical attractiveness may be particularly vulnerable to the effects of a mastectomy.

Concerns about disfigurement from the loss of a breast may be considerable, even though the absence of the breast may be hidden under clothing and by prosthesis. Reconstructive surgery in suitable patients following mastectomy may create a positive emotional reaction.[55] It also conveys the physician's belief in her recovery since he or she thinks it worthwhile to invest in reconstruction. For suitable patients, it does represent a significant contribution toward restitution and recovery.

As with hysterectomy, family factors are extremely important in the reaction to mastectomy. The stability of a marriage, reassurance of sexual attractiveness, the capacity of family members to tolerate the truth, and the anxiety of uncertainty about the future are pivotal in the amount of support the patient has in regaining her emotional balance.[56] In the rehabilitation of the postmastectomy patient, the family or other supportive people are highly important in determining her acceptance of the loss of the breast and in the reintegration of her self-image as a person with a changed body who still feels no less worthy of love.[57]

AMNIOCENTESIS

Recent advances in genetics have increased our capacity to make prenatal diagnosis, and hence to be more involved in reproductive decisions. A number of disorders can be detected *in utero*, with minimal risk to mother or fetus. While the use of this procedure is relatively restricted at this time, the possibility of future advances, as well as the use of abortion, has raised serious ethical, social, religious, and economic questions. While a thorough discussion of these issues is beyond the scope of this chapter, it is important to emphasize the complexity of the issues to be considered. These include the possibility of monitoring all pregnancies for chromosomal abnormalities, criteria for abortion after amniocentesis, and decisions about who should be responsible for making the decisions. Some authors have speculated that the choice of genetic qualities and traits will result in the choice of children of a certain sex, or that "gene shopping" will occur to produce children with more desirable traits.[58]

Transabdominal amniocentesis is done between 16 and 20 weeks of gestation, and carries a risk of 0.5 percent. This includes all complications, for example, spontaneous abortion, vaginal bleeding, and fetal injury.[59] In 95 percent of the cases, the procedure yields favorable genetic results.[60] Thus, it represents a significant psychological reassurance to people at risk.

Although most families who have a positive genetic diagnosis choose abortion, some elect to continue the pregnancy. In one study, of 115 mothers who were concerned about x-linked genetic traits and were undergoing amniocentesis to determine fetal sex, 54 were carrying a male fetus. Of these, 40 women chose to be aborted, while 14 decided to continue the pregnancy.[60] The decision not to abort was based on several factors including: (1) the fact that 50 percent of these male fetuses would be unaffected, (2) religious reasons, (3) inadequate genetic counseling, and (4) the prospective parents felt that the disability was not severe enough for them to choose abortion as a solution. Families making the choice to continue a pregnancy under these circumstances usually require a great deal of support during the pregnancy.

This field is new enough to have few guidelines. Davis points out that termination of pregnancy may be questioned when a treatable disorder is discovered, for example, phenylketonuria, or when there are unknown and unproved risks but strong popular opinion, for example, with the XYY fetus.[61] Physicians are increasingly concerned that they will be obliged to provide amniocentesis to any patient who requests the procedure.

RAPE

Rape has recently received serious attention from medical professionals. In the past, physicians felt that they had little to offer, or shared the popular view that the victim was acting out conscious or unconscious sexual fantasies, and therefore was not "really" a victim. Thus, the victim of rape was not offered the empathy and understanding that are usually extended to people in crisis. The increased incidence of rape and changing ideas about it have confronted health professionals with the necessity to become more involved. The link between the physical and psychological aspects of medicine is particularly emphasized in the approach to the rape victim. Rape is both a medical and a psychiatric emergency.[62]

Rape is a violent crime that is expressed sexually. The absence of consent is crucial to the definition of rape. Since the possibility of serious harm or death exists, the victim's prime concern is to protect herself from injury.

Rape is a stressful situation in which a traumatic external event disrupts the balance between ego adaptation and the environment. Since it is an interaction between an extreme environmental stimulus and the adaptive capacity of the victim, it is similar to other traumatic situations, such as those experienced by victims of community disasters, war, or certain surgical procedures.

Victims range widely in their initial responses to rape. Some appear to be calm, without overt evidence of fear and anxiety; others react with confusion, agitation, and terror. Following the experience, as behavioral control and memory are regained, the woman may experience a profound sense of failure and inadequacy if she perceives criticism of her response pattern or mistrust of her story. Retrospectively the victim often blames herself for her lack of perception of the potential for danger at the time of the rape.

Affective Responses

Burgess and Holmstrom describe a rape crisis syndrome, which consists of an acute disorganizational phase with behavioral, somatic, and psychological manifestations, and a long-term reorganizational phase with variable components depending upon the ego strengths, social networks, and specific experiences of the woman who confronts this situation.[63] They also emphasize the guilt and self-blame seen in rape victims.

Societal support for the idea that the victim may have, in some way, participated in the rape encourages repression of anger and fosters guilt and shame that are concomitant with feelings of helplessness and vulnerability. The victim often feels that she should have been either more active or more passive in order to have prevented the attack. The societal tendency to emphasize the sexuality rather than the violence also supports guilty feelings.

Problems in resolving the rape crisis may result in the development of a traumatic neurosis, with symptoms including repetitive nightmares, phobias, sleep and eating disturbances, inability to concentrate or function effectively, regression, and depression.

Life State Considerations

The single woman between the ages of 17 and 24 is the most frequently reported rape victim. In this age group, rape victims frequently have prior knowledge of the rapist, who may be a relative or a neighbor. If this is the case, the victim may reproach herself, particularly feeling that she should have been able to prevent the rape. Her sense of helplessness may reinforce fears of relationships with men. This is especially true for the young woman whose first sexual experience may have been a rape. Parents, friends, and relatives can invite regression with suggestions that she stay at home or leave school. This reaction often derives from their guilt about not having been protective enough, and although it may be an expression of concern, it may not be helpful to the victim in mastering the trauma and restoring independence.

The gynecological examination may pose particular problems for the rape victim. Since she may have suffered physical trauma, been exposed to venereal disease, or become pregnant, an examination is necessary. The examination may, however, be perceived as another rape, especially by an inexperienced or severely traumatized woman who is examined by a nonempathic physician.

The divorced or separated woman has additional concerns, because her apparent sexual availability makes her more vulnerable. She may also experience rape as a confirmation of her feelings of inadequacy and her inability to be independent. If she has children, she may worry about her ability to protect and care for them. She must also deal with the problem of how to handle herself in the community in which she lives, if the rape is reported. Many women feel ostracized and accused of complicity.

For the "middle-aged" woman, the issues of control of her life and reaffirmation of her sexual identity are important. She may be in a period of reassessment of her role and future goals, particularly as her relationships to her family change. Husbands, who are in their own mid-life crises, may not be responsive and supportive.

Long-Term Responses

The experience of rape confronts many women with their ambivalent feelings about men, feelings which may have evolved from past developmental experiences and expectations. The sense of betrayal by the rapist, as well as by the husband, father, or lover who had been seen as a potential protector, has a profound effect. Almost all victims describe the experience of trusting men less for varying periods of time following the experience.

It is difficult to predict the long-term reactions or needs of the rape victim, since the experience and the working through of the trauma are so individually determined. Some of the issues that emerge at a later date are:

1 Mistrust of men, with avoidance of or hesitation about contact
2 Sexual disturbances
3 Phobic reactions
4 Anxiety and depression, which are often precipitated by seemingly unrelated events that in some small details bring back the original trauma

Counseling

Adequate counseling requires an understanding of the victim's life adjustment as well as her ego functions, including relationships, stress tolerance, and adaptive resources. The current life situation of the victim and the kinds of supports available to her are also important.

Initially, the rape victim needs reassurance about the way in which she handled the encounter and about her efforts to cope with her feelings about the experience. She may be defensive or may displace her anger onto those who are attempting to help, such as friends, doctors, or the police. They may react directly to her behavior, and often reject her without understanding the underlying issues. The more subdued victim may need to be encouraged to communicate her feelings as best she can, rather than to receive approval for her ability to be "cool" and a "good patient." Rape victims may need the opportunity for counseling in the future if they reject it initially.

Since the psychological issues may be the most critical variables in the ultimate recovery of the victim, they must be given high priority. The anxiety and anger of those who provide the initial care for the rape victim often cause them to focus more on medical and legal issues, and they may fail to perceive the magnitude of the emotional stress. This is particularly true if the woman has a response in which she attempts to restore self-esteem by being in control.

CONCLUSION

The physician has an abundance of new data to assimilate, and has to adapt to changing information and attitudes. Because of the nature of the issues of reproduction and sexual functioning, physicians who treat women have a wide range of responsibility and great emotional and physical demands. The physician should be willing to take the time, and must be comfortable with an active role in providing emotional support and understanding to women and their families. Time must be taken to listen to the patient in order to avoid responding with stereotyped reactions. These challenges must be met if women are to receive the quality of care they deserve.

REFERENCES

1   Horney, K.: "Premenstrual Tension," in H. Kelman (ed.), *Feminine Psychology,* New York: Norton, 1967.
2   Frank, R.: "Hormonal Causes of Premenstrual Tension," *Arch. Neurol. Psychiatry,* **26**:1053–1057, 1931.
3   Benedek, T., and B. Rubenstein: "Correlations between Ovarian Activity and Psychodynamic Processes, (1939)," in T. Benedek (ed.), *Studies in Psychosomatic Medicine: Psychosexual Functions in Women,* New York: Roland, 1952.
4   Lindemann, E.: "Hysteria as a Problem in a General Hospital," *Med. Clin. N. Amer.,* May 1938.
5   Renneker, R., and M. Cutler: "Psychological Problems of Adjustment to Cancer of the Breast, *JAMA,* **148**:833, 1952.
6   Mathis, J.: "Psychiatry and the Obstetrician-Gynecologist," *Med. Clin. N. Amer.,* **51**:6, 1375–1380, 1967.
7   Lief, H. I.: "Sex Education of Medical Students and Doctors," in C. E. Vincent (ed.), *Human Sexuality in Medical Education and Practice,* Springfield: Charles C Thomas, 1974, pp.19–33.
8   Parlee, M. D.: "Psychological Aspects of Menstruation, Childbirth, and Menopause: An Overview with Suggestions for Further Research," paper prepared for the conference *New Directions for Research on Women,* Madison, Wisc., 1975.
9   Lennane, K. J., and R. J. Lennane: "Alleged Psychogenic Disorders in Women—A Possible Manifestation of Sexual Prejudice," *NEJM,* **288**:6, 288–292, 1973.
10   Glasser, M., and R. Pasnau: "The Unwanted Pregnancy in Adolescence," *J. Fam. Pract.,* **2**:2, 91–94, 1975.
11   Pasnau, R. O.: "Psychiatry and Obstetrics-Gynecology: Report of a Five Year Experience in Psychiatric Liaison," in R. O. Pasnau, *Consultation-Liaison Psychiatry,* New York: Grune and Stratton, 1975.
12   Payne, E. et al.: "Outcome Following Therapeutic Abortion: 100 Cases," *Arch. Gen. Psy.,* **33**:6, 725–733, June 1976.
13   Lindenmayer, J. P.: quoted in "Roche Report," *Frontiers of Psychiatry,* June 15, 1976.
14   Kaltreider, N. B., and A. Margolis: "Childless by Choice: A Clinical Study," *Am. J. Psych.,* **134**:2, 179–182, February 1977.
15   Defries, Z.: "Pseudo-Homosexuality in Feminist Students," *Am. J. Psych.,* **133**:4, 400–404, April 1976.

16 Seiden, A.: "The Sense of Mastery in the Childbirth Experience," in C. Nadelson and M. Notman (eds.): *The Woman Patient: Medical and Psychological Interfaces,* New York: Plenum Press, 1978.

17 Bibring, G.: "Some Considerations of the Psychological Processes in Pregnancy," *Psychoanal. Study of the Child,* **14**:113, 1959.

18 Bibring, G. et al.: "A Study of the Earliest Mother-Child Relationship," *Psychoanal. Study of the Child,* **16**:9, 1961.

19 Bibring, G., and A. Valenstein: "Psychological Aspects of Pregnancy," *Clin. Obs. Gyn.,* **19**:2, 357–371, 1976.

20 Deutsch, H.: "The Psychology of Women," *Motherhood,* vol. 2, New York: Grune and Stratton, 1945.

21 Benedek, T.: "Sexual Functions in Women," in S. Arieti (ed.), *American Handbook of Psychiatry,* vol. 1, New York: Basic Books, 1959, Chap. 37.

22 Planned Parenthood League of Masssachusetts, *Report #34,* February 1977.

23 Mecklenberg, F.: "Pregnancy: An Adolescent Crisis," *Minn. Med.,* **56**:2, 101–104, 1973.

24 Schaffer, C., and F. Pine: "Pregnancy, Abortion, and the Developmental Tasks of Adolescence," *J. Child Psych.,* **14**:511–536, 1975.

25 Bernard, V.: "Psychodynamics of Unmarried Motherhood in Early Adolescence," *Nervous Child,* **4**:25, 1944.

26 Young, L.: *Out of Wedlock,* New York: McGraw-Hill, 1954.

27 Notman, M., and J. Zilbach: "Family Factors in the Non-Use of Contraception in Adolescence," presented at the 5th International Congress on Psychosomatics in Obstetrics-Gynecology, Tel Aviv, Israel, 1974.

28 Sarrel, P.: "The University Hospital and the Teenage Unwed Mother," *Am. J. Public Health,* **57**:8, 1308, 1967.

29 Nadelson, C.: "Abortion Counselling: Focus on Adolescent Pregnancy," *Pediatrics,* **54**:6, 765–769, 1974.

30 Budwell, M., and L. Tinnin: "Abortion Referral in a Large College Health Service," *JAMWA,* **27**:8, 1972.

31 Sommer, B.: "Menstruation and Behavior: A Review," *Psychosom. Med.,* **35**:515–533, 1973.

32 Mandel, A., and M. Mandell: "Suicide and the Menstrual Cycle," *JAMA,* **200**:792–793, 1967.

33 MacKinnon, H. et al.: "Lethal Hazards of the Initial Phase of the Menstrual Cycle," *Brit. Med. J.,* **1**:1015–1017, 1959.

34 Vogel, W. et al.: "EEG Responses in Regularly Menstruating Women and in Amenorrheic Women Treated with Ovarian Hormones," *Science,* **1972**:388–391, 1971.

35 Perlmutter, J.: Personal Communications.

36 Bart, P., and M. Grossman: "Menopause," in C. Nadelson and M. Notman (eds.), *The Woman Patient: Medical and Psychological Interfaces,* New York: Plenum Press, 1978. Also published in *Women and Health,* **1**:3, 3–10, 1976.

37 Barnett, R., and G. Baruch: "Women in the Middle Years: Conceptions and Misconceptions," from *Symposium: Toward an Understanding of Adult Development in Women,* Eastern Psychological Assoc. Meetings, April 1976.

38 Perlmutter, J.: "Menopause," in C. Nadelson and M. Notman (eds.), *The Woman Patient: Medical and Psychological Interfaces,* New York: Plenum Press, 1978.

39 McKinley, S. M., and M. Jefferys: "The Menopausal Syndrome," *Brit. J. of Preventive and Social Med.,* **28**:2, 108–115, 1974.

40 Reynolds, S.: "Physiological and Psychogenic Factors in the Menopausal Flush Syn-

drome,'' in W. Kroger (ed.), *Psychosomatic Obstetrics, Gynecology, and Endocrinology,* Springfield: Charles C Thomas, 1962.

41 McKinley, S. M. et al.: "An Investigation of the Age at Menopause,'' *J. Biosoc. Science,* **4**:161–173, 1972.

42 Neugarten, B.: "Adult Personality: Toward a Psychology of the Life Cycle,'' in W. Sze (ed.), *Human Life Cycle,* New York: Aronson, 1975.

43 Neugarten, B., and N. Datan: "The Middle Years,'' in S. Arieti (ed.), *American Handbook of Psychiatry,* 2d ed., vol. 1, New York: Basic Books, 1974.

44 Kraines, R. J.: *The Menopause and Evaluations of the Self: A Study of Middle-Aged Women,* unpublished doctoral dissertation, University of Chicago, 1963. Quoted in reference 36.

45 Neugarten, B. et al.: "Women's Attitudes Toward Menopause,'' in B. Neugarten (ed.), *Middle Age and Aging,* Chicago: The Univ. of Chicago Press, 1968.

46 Levit, L.: *Anxiety and the Menopause: A Study of Normal Women,* unpublished doctoral dissertation, University of Chicago, 1963. Quoted in reference 36.

47 Benedek, T.: "The Functions of the Sexual Apparatus and Their Disturbances,'' in F. Alerduder (ed.), *Psychosomatic Medicine,* New York: Norton, 1950.

48 Zilbach, J.: "Some Family Developmental Considerations of Midlife,'' paper presented at American Psychiatric Association panel, *New Look at the Midlife Years,* 1975.

49 Bernard, J.: *The Future of Marriage,* New York: World Publishing, 1972.

50 Braun, P., and E. Druchneder (eds.): "Public Health Rounds at the Harvard School of Public Health,'' *NEJM,* **295**:264–268, July 29, 1976.

51 Barber, M. G.: "Psychiatric Illness After Hysterectomy,'' *Brit. Med. J.,* **2**:91–95, 1968.

52 Richards, D. H.: "Depression after Hysterectomy,'' *Lancet,* **2**:430–433, 1973.

53 Polivz, J.: "Psychological Reactions to Hysterectomy: A Critical Review,'' *Am. J. Obstetrics-Gynecology,* **118**:417–426, 1974.

54 Tishler, S.: "Disease of the Breast,'' in C. Nadelson and M. Notman (eds.), *The Woman Patient: Medical and Psychological Interfaces,* New York: Plenum Press, 1978.

55 Goldwyn, R.: "Esthetic Surgery in Women,'' in C. Nadelson and M. Notman (eds.), *The Woman Patient: Medical and Psychological Interfaces,* New York: Plenum Press, 1978.

56 Asken, M. J.: "Psychoemotional Aspects of Mastectomy: A Review of Recent Literature,'' *Am. J. Psychiatry,* **132**:56–59, 1975.

57 Gifford, S.: "Emotional Attitudes Toward Cosmetic Breast Surgery: Loss and Restitution of the 'Ideal Self,''' in R. M. Goldwyn (ed.), *Plastic and Reconstructive Surgery of the Breast,* Boston: Little, Brown, 1976, pp. 103–122.

58 Etzioni, A.: *Genetic Fix,* New York: Harper and Row, 1973.

59 Davis, J.: "Symposium on Amniocentesis,'' *Am. J. Pediatric,* October 20, 1975.

60 Milunsky, A.: *The Prenatal Diagnosis of Hereditary Disorders,* Springfield: Charles C Thomas, 1973.

61 Davis, J.: "Genetic Counselling,'' in C. Nadelson and M. Notman (eds.), *The Woman Patient: Medical and Psychological Interfaces,* New York: Plenum Press, 1978.

62 Notman, M., and C. Nadelson: "The Rape Victim: Psychodynamic Considerations,'' *Am. J. Psychiatry,* **133**:4, April 1976.

63 Burgess, A. W., and L. L. Holmstrom: "Rape Trauma Syndrome,'' *Am. J. Psych.,* **131**:9, 981–986, 1974.

Chapter 22

Disturbances of
Intellectual Functioning

George Tarjan, M.D.
Steven R. Forness, Ed.D.

EDITORS' INTRODUCTION

What is it like for parents to be told by a physician that their cute, plump, attractive child is probably mentally retarded, and that they, the parents, will have to adapt to limited goals of intellectual performance and personal adjustment for their cherished 1½-year-old daughter? What is it like to contain a fear about your child within and not discuss it with your spouse? How does it feel to be a 9-year-old and to recognize that you are in a special school for "slow learners"? Or what is it like for a child to be in a regular school, struggling to keep up with other students and behaving badly to relieve tension or achieve attention? It is not easy for the parents or for the child—for that matter, it is not easy for any of the nuclear family. It involves a great deal of readjustment on the parents' part, a special tolerance for difficulty, and constructive effort to have the child achieve what is possible and to strive for the impossible. It involves faith.

More recently, an old but relatively newly discovered phenomenon, learning disabilities, has become of special interest to caregivers, as well as to those who are afflicted themselves or are close to people afflicted with these conditions. The awareness of the prevalence of learning disabilities has emerged, and rather dramatic strides have been taken toward the recognition, treatment, and adjustment of these disabilities. Once disabilities are discovered, it becomes important to achieve maximum benefits from the newer treatments which are coming forth dramatically.

How painful it can be for the physician to have to help a family accept that they have to adjust to limited goals and accomplishments for their child! What degree of empathy can the physician have for both the parents and the child? Can the physician avoid recognizing the effects on the entire family system, and what can be done to make the effects less harmful? Can the physician help the family recognize the satisfaction in dealing with a child who may be limited intellectually? The physician may reflect on his or her own children, or on close relatives or friends who have had to deal with the problem. It is hoped that the reader of this chapter by Tarjan and Forness, acknowledged leaders in the field, may think a little more deeply, and feel more secure about these difficult situations. Physicians (especially pediatricians) and teachers should be sensitive to the possibility of learning disabilities, and should refer children with possible disabilities for evaluation and possible treatment.

Dealing with either mental retardation or learning disabilities requires tact, good judgment, and a reasonable amount of knowledge about the conditions involved. The earlier the correct diagnosis is established, the sooner treatment can be initiated and the greater the possibility of maximum treatment benefits. This chapter is intended to supply background to enable the physician to meet this responsibility better.

The physician is often the first person to whom a family turns when a child fails to develop normally or has problems in school. It is not at all uncommon for parents to suspect learning difficulties long before the school becomes aware of their child's problem, and to seek out their family physician for answers. The physician who is unfamiliar with disorders of learning often compounds the problem, since early recognition is crucial. The longer such difficulties remain undiagnosed, the more difficult treatment or remediation becomes. The child's emotional response to prolonged failure may complicate both school progress and family adjustment, and more serious interventions may be required. Clinical expertise in this area enables a physician both to provide early detection and to coordinate treatment efforts with other professionals.

Approximately 12 percent of all children fail to learn through normal means of instruction in school. Excluding primary physical, sensory, or emotional impairments, two disorders of intellectual functioning remain, mental retardation and learning disabilities. Each is a highly prevalent and complex syndrome. Discussion of both in a single chapter reflects recent trends toward placing retarded and learning-disabled children together in the same classrooms because of increasing recognition of their similar educational needs.[1] Recent federal legislation on developmental disabilities also treats mental retardation and learning disabilities under the same rubric, as overlap often occurs with diagnostic procedures, parental reactions, associated behavioral problems, and treatment.[2]

While mental retardation usually presents as a global functional impairment, a learning disability often manifests itself as a disorder in a single area of functioning. Etiologic agents common to both suggest that differences may also reside in the degree of impairment. This chapter contains separate discussions for each syndrome, which opens with a statement of definition, followed by sections on epidemiology, classification and etiology, and procedures for diagnosis and treatment. The chapter concludes with comments on the role of the nonpsychiatrist, and what psychiatry has to offer.

MENTAL RETARDATION

Mental retardation is a syndrome and not a single disease entity. Commonly used clinical definitions stress the following features: (1) significant impairment in intellectual performance, (2) concurrent deficits in general adaptation, and (3) onset before mental maturity (that is, before age 18).[3,4] Intellectual impairment is generally determined by an individual's performance on a psychometric test. Mental retardation is not diagnosed unless the intelligence quotient (IQ) is at least two standard deviations below the mean, that is, approximately below 70. Considerable controversy centers around the use of intelligence tests with ethnic minority children because of the inordinately high number of such children who fall within the retarded range. Unfortunately, success in school is still measured against the performance of middle-class children who have a good command of the English language. In fact, the tests were primarily standardized against the performance of such children.

For an individual to be diagnosed as mentally retarded, general adaptation must also be deficient. Adaptation refers to the ability to perform daily tasks with acceptable success. Such tasks are age- and environment-specific. Although attempts have been made to develop measures of general adaptation, assessment in this area remains a clinical skill that is highly dependent upon diagnostic acuity and experience. During the school years, general adaptation and intelligence tend to be closely related. Prior to and after this period, many people with relatively low IQs manage to adapt adequately to their environments. Even when examined, they cannot be diagnosed as mentally retarded. Likewise, many individuals show poor general adaptation in spite of relatively high intelligence. The diagnosis of mental retardation therefore depends upon *concurrent* deficits in both intelligence and adaptation.

The third criterion pertains to the time of onset. Since it is a developmental disorder, mental retardation should not be diagnosed when impairments occur during adult years. Examples are those whose deficits originate from adult types of schizophrenia, are sequelae of central nervous system injury sustained after age 18, or are the result of an aging process. On the other hand, when impairments in measured intelligence and general adaptation are observed concurrently in early childhood (as is usually the case in autism), the diagnosis of mental retardation is appropriate.

Epidemiology

Approximately 3 percent of the United States population scores below 70 on customary IQ tests, simply as a function of test "standardization." This represents over 6 million individuals. Of greater importance epidemiologically is that only one-third of the 6 million, or 1 percent of the population, would be found mentally retarded.[5] Clinical examination would reveal adequate general adaptation in the remainder. Mildly retarded people, with IQs between 50 and 70, usually are not identified until after entrance into school when their intellectual differences are most obvious. As these individuals leave school, their differences become less evident to society, and many disappear from the identified population. On the other hand, it is correct to say that approximately 3 percent of the newborn are apt to be diagnosed as mentally retarded at some time during their life. The more severely retarded, with concomitant somatic symptoms, are usually diagnosed during the preschool years, and continue to remain identified. The rate of diagnostic ascertainment rises sharply for the mildly retarded during the early school years, and then tapers off. Caution against excessive pessimism is thus appropriate for the latter group.

These prevalence and incidence rates are uneven within sex and socioeconomic class. In the mentally retarded population, males predominate at a ratio of approximately 65 to 35. Although significant, this difference is still somewhat less than one finds among child psychiatric patients. The most common biological explanation concerns the X chromosome "advantage" of the female. Not all the disparity, however, can be explained by this phenomenon. It is likely that higher social-role expectations for males and lesser tolerance toward deviant behavior in this sex have contributed to a greater extent than somatic variations.

Mental retardation is also highly social-class dependent. It has been estimated that children who are born and reared in urban ghettos or impoverished rural environments are 15 times more likely to be diagnosed as mentally retarded than their age mates from suburbia.[6] Prevalence rates among middle- or upper-income neighborhoods are substantially lower, and are often considerably less than 1 percent. Public agencies have in fact been shown to identify poor or ethnic-minority children living in deteriorated housing as mentally retarded, far more frequently than they identify white children living in middle-class neighborhoods.[7]

Vulnerability to superimposed handicaps is especially high in the mentally retarded population. The prevalence of secondary handicaps is, in general, inversely related to measured levels of intelligence. The lower the IQ, the greater the probability is that the patient will have impairments in speech, vision, hearing, neuromuscular function, or seizure disorders. This vulnerability extends to emotional and behavioral disorders as well.

Classification and Etiology

Mental retardation may be classified according to either severity of intellectual impairment or etiology.[8] The terms moron, idiot, and imbecile have been abandoned for classification. They are pejorative and stigmatizing, and have become part of a derogatory common parlance. Attempts to classify by level of adaptation have yet to meet with clinical acceptance. Classification by intelligence is based on standard deviations from the mean IQ of 100. Beginning with two standard deviations below the mean, the retarded are classified as mild, moderate, severe, and profound, with the size of the group decreasing as severity increases. Brief descriptions of these levels are provided in Table 22-1. In practical terms, only some 5 percent of the retarded population are so severely impaired that they cannot distinguish between safety and danger, and thus require constant care for survival. Approximately 20 percent can make such distinctions, but fail daily tasks that require symbolic communication (reading, writing, and arithmetic). In public school terms, this latter group is classified as "trainable." Some 75 percent can acquire basic symbolic communication, but fail when abstract thinking or complex judgments are required. In school terms, this last group is described as "educable," since ordinarily they can attain academic levels commensurate with those of elementary school children.

Etiologic classification of mental retardation is a complex issue. Despite rapidly expanding knowledge in this area, one can establish a definitive etiologic biomedical factor for only about 20 to 25 percent of mentally retarded individuals. Among the majority, who fall in the mildly retarded range, no demonstrable somatic pathology is evident. Two additional cautions should be noted. First, even when a clear-cut syndrome is identified, the exact relationship between somatic pathology and manifest behavioral deficits remains undetermined. Second, behavioral symptoms generally reflect the complicated interplay among biologic, cognitive, social, and psychiatric factors.

Biomedical classification commonly groups mental retardation into 10 etiologic clusters.[3] The first includes infections and intoxications. Examples of prenatal infections are cytomegalic inclusion disease, rubella, syphilis, and toxoplasmosis. Postnatal infections include the viral encephalitides and the bacterial meningitides. The last group contains children who paradoxically, as a result of progress in antibiotic therapy, survive the infection, but often at the cost of significant neurologic sequelae. Major examples of intoxication are toxemia of pregnancy, maternal phenylketonuria, hyperbilirubinemia, and lead poisoning. The devastating effects of chronic maternal alcoholism have also gained recent attention.[9]

The second group includes trauma or physical agents, such as injury to the pregnant mother, perinatal mechanical injury, and hypoxia during or after birth. Cyanosis at birth is not necessarily the result of obstetrical complications, but may arise as a function of a poorly developed brain that fails to take over the respiratory function after birth.

The third cluster contains cases resulting from disorders of metabolism or nutrition, including inborn errors of metabolism, mineral and endocrine disorders, and severe forms of malnutrition. In the first group are the neuronal lipid storage diseases (for example, Tay Sachs disease), the carbohydrate disorders (for example, galactosemia), the amino acid disorders (for example,

Table 22-1   Levels of Mental Retardation

Level	IQ Range*	Expected adaptive behavior	Expected educational attainment	Adult outcome
Profound	Below 25	May eventually be able to feed self and to interact with others in simple play activities, but speech and toileting remain at a primitive level.	Capable of some preschool activities.	Will require continued custodial care.
Severe	25–39	May eventually be able to feed, toilet, and dress self adequately; carry on rudimentary conversation; and run errands or do simple household chores.	Capable of some skills at kindergarten level such as recognizing words and basic number concepts.	Will need to live in closely supervised environment.
Moderate	40–54	May eventually be able to feed, dress, and groom self adequately; carry on simple conversations and interact cooperatively with others; and be responsible for simple routines of daily living.	Capable of 1st or 2nd grade learning such as reading simple sentences and basic addition and subtraction.	Able to live independently but needs periodic supervision, can work in sheltered situations.
Mild	55–69	May eventually be responsible for all feeding and personal grooming activities, communicates effectively in everyday conversation, enjoys friendships and group social activities, travels with ease in hometown.	Capable of 2nd to 7th grade learning such as reading stories, communicating in writing, and handling simple financial transactions.	Able to live independently, may marry or have children, and hold unskilled or semiskilled jobs, but will need occasional assistance in all these areas.

*Note that these levels are determined using the Wechsler Intelligence Scales and that IQ values for other individual intelligence scales may be slightly different.

503

phenylketonuria), and the nucleotide disorders (for example, Lesch-Nyhan disease). Mineral disorders include two types of abnormalities in copper metabolism and one involving calcium metabolism. Endocrine disorders include two forms of cretinism: one due to enzymatic defects in the production of thyroid hormone, and the other caused by the absence or underdevelopment of the thyroid gland. Severe malnutrition (for example, kwashiorkor and marasmus) can impair cognitive functions, particularly when it occurs during critical periods of brain growth. Effects of milder degrees of malnutrition are less clear.

Mental retardation is also associated with gross brain disease, such as the neurocutaneous dysplasias (for example, von Recklinghausen's disease, Sturge-Weber's disease, and tuberous sclerosis), nonfatal brain tumors, degenerative disorders of the cerebral white matter (for example, the leukodystrophies), other degenerative diseases of the central nervous system, and hemorrhage or thrombosis involving the cerebral vascular system.

A fifth group is malformations that involve the central nervous system and that are of unknown prenatal influence. Many occur sporadically, though some can be transmitted genetically. The most common include craniofacial anomalies (for example, the Cornelia de Lange's and Crouzon's syndromes), the various dysraphic states, hydrocephalus, and microcephaly.

Chromosomal abnormalities include the most common somatic entity in mental retardation, that is, Down's syndrome (formerly termed mongolism).[10] Incidence is approximately 1 in 600 births, and increases with maternal age. Common symptoms include brachycephaly, oblique palpebral fissures, epicanthal folds, small low-set ears, furrowed tongue, simian lines, fifth-finger clinodactyly, abnormal dermatoglyphics, and hypotonia. Congenital abnormalities of the heart and the gastrointestinal tract are also frequent. Mental development is most often in the moderately retarded range on psychometric tests. The overwhelming majority of Down's syndrome cases involve trisomy of chromosome 21. The remaining few are accounted for by translocation of excess material to another chromosome. Trisomies and deletions of other chromosomes result in different somatic syndromes. Sex chromosome abnormalities (for example, Turner's, Klinefelter's, XYY and XXX syndromes) are less often associated with mental retardation than those involving other chromosomes.

Gestational disorders include prematurity, low birth weight, postmaturity, and placental dysfunction syndrome. Of significance is the fact that gestational disorders occur at least twice as frequently among mothers of low socioeconomic status.

The eighth category represents an interface between early childhood psychoses and mental retardation. Considerable controversy exists over issues of diagnosis and classification. When mental retardation and some form of childhood psychosis are noted concurrently, the diagnosis is customarily "mental retardation following psychiatric disorder," specifying the type of psychosis (for example, early infantile autism or childhood schizophrenia).

Mental retardation is also associated with adverse environmental influences in early childhood, in cases where there is no demonstrable organic pathology.

The most frequent is that which results from "psychosocial disadvantage," which is discussed later. However, prolonged isolation, severe environmental restrictions, and gross maternal deprivation may also produce retardation, even without the presence of psychosocial disadvantage.

The final category is called "other conditions," and involves cases where causation cannot be assigned to any of the specific agents enumerated so far. Included in this category are children in whom retardation appears to exist because of sensory handicaps (for example, blindness or deafness), or because of the occurrence of several biologic or social forces, without any single variable being primarily responsible.

From a practical standpoint, one can also consider the mentally retarded as consisting of two dichotomous groups.[11] The first involves so-called *clinical mental retardation.* In this group, diagnosis is established at birth, or shortly thereafter, and remains unaltered. Children from all socioeconomic levels are affected. Somatic pathology is evident, with mortality rates well above average. Degree of retardation generally ranges from moderate to profound.

The second group involves mental retardation resulting from psychosocial disadvantage, or *sociocultural retardation,* and comprises some 75 percent of all cases. Retardation is generally mild, often is not diagnosed until entrance into school, and is rather specific to the school milieu. The term "six-hour retarded child" has been coined as a consequence.[12] Since current biomedical technology cannot pinpoint specific somatic etiologies, three factors are suggested. The first involves current controversies around polygenic inheritance. However, a second set of factors, involving noninheritable environmental somatic forces, appears more important. At risk are children born to mothers whose general nutrition and health care has been poor. Such mothers also tend toward multiple pregnancies over brief periods, and often have premature deliveries. Obstetric and pediatric care is substandard. Cumulative effects of such organic insults can often produce impaired intellectual functioning without concomitant somatic signs. The third factor relates to early parenting experiences. Involved are children from broken homes or with physically or emotionally unavailable mothers. Parents often inhibit exploratory behavior or serve as poor language models. The resultant mixture of deprived or ill-timed sensory inputs, suppressed exploratory and language experiences, and unstable nurturing all serve to explain the presence of mental retardation.[13]

Diagnosis and Treatment

Diagnosis of mental retardation involves two phases: determining that the individual is retarded, and establishing an etiologic diagnosis, if possible. A detailed developmental history is of key importance. Focus should be on landmarks of motor, cognitive, self-help, social, and adaptive skills. Though physical examination may not be very revealing, except in the well-defined clinical syndromes, it should be conducted with care and with a focus on the nervous system. Laboratory studies can range from routine procedures, such as urinalysis, to more complex tests, such as amino acid chromotography or cytogenetic studies.

Caution should prevail in ordering any test, since a tendency toward overutilization of laboratory examinations often exists, and invasive studies of the brain should be used with particular parsimony.[14] On the other hand, rapidly developing diagnostic techniques in genetics, including amniocentesis and concomitant genetic counseling, are often underutilized. Today these techniques are readily available in major medical centers. Psychometric and other psychologic tests, developmental scales, education readiness and achievement tests, and assessments of vision, hearing, speech, and language are all of vital importance in establishing the level of retardation and planning case management.

Diagnosis should lead to a treatment plan. The first phase often requires counseling, and at times psychotherapy, for the parents. A retarded child places major psychological stresses upon parents who value intellectual achievements. In response, parents commonly mobilize such defense mechanisms as denial, projection, magical expectation, reaction formation, and sublimation. Parents may also manifest guilt, depression, rejection, overprotection, and alienation, and may often engage in costly and exhausting therapeutic or diagnostic "shopping."[15]

Careful diagnosis may uncover associated conditions that are amenable to therapeutic interventions. Acute disorders should be treated in accordance with standard practices, and should be modified to fit the retarded child. Comprehensive management plans should also provide for treatment of certain chronic conditions, such as congenital malformations, sensory deficits, neuromuscular handicaps, speech impairments, seizure disorders, and emotional disturbances.

Behavior modification is currently a particularly popular mode of treatment.[16] Based on systematic application of reinforcement theory to clinical problems, the technique is used both in acquisition of self-help, social, or academic skills, and in elimination of maladaptive behaviors. It is used with individual patients as well as in management of groups or classrooms. A recent development is the involvement of parents or siblings as auxiliary therapists.[17] Substantial benefits are often noted, but two cautions are in order: first, generalizability of skills acquired through behavior modification is as yet unproven, and second, use of aversive procedures should be restricted to particularly difficult situations, and used only after other treatment approaches have failed.

Special education has become a central focus in long-term care of the mentally retarded child.[18] Severely retarded children have traditionally been placed in separate schools, and mildly retarded children in special classes located in regular schools. Today the field of education for the retarded student is in flux. Recent federal legislation has mandated education for all levels of retarded children, ages 3 to 21, and has provided that individual plans for each child's schooling be developed jointly by parents and teachers.[19] Unfortunately, some school systems remain inadequately prepared to provide meaningful education for severely or profoundly retarded children. Recent emphasis has been on efforts that provide "early stimulation," both within and outside the schools, to infants and young children, even those with severe impairments. There is also a trend toward "mainstreaming" mildly retarded school-age children into regular classrooms, whenever possible, though benefits of this approach remain as yet unvalidated. Although mildly retarded children have been shown to do better academically in regular classes, their general social adjustment may suffer.[20]

Most retarded children can and do remain at home on a continuous basis; however, for a variety of reasons, some may have to be placed in alternative settings. Separation from the family is particularly stressful for the child, as well as for the parents. Intensive counseling, similar to that employed during the diagnostic phase, is often necessary during these and other developmental changes in the child's life. Other periods of stress revolve around developmental delays, attainment of school age, onset of puberty, transition from school to adult life, and relocation of the family. Growing public awareness of mental retardation continues to lead to understanding and acceptance of these problems. The physician plays an important role in prevention and continuing care.

LEARNING DISABILITIES

In contrast to mental retardation, the subject of learning disabilities is of fairly recent origin, less well understood, vaguely defined, and still controversial. A wide variety of other terms, such as minimal brain dysfunction, dyslexia, hyperactivity, and perceptual handicaps, has been applied to these disorders. A consensus definition, which was recently included in federal legislation on schooling, stresses the following features: (1) dysfunction in one or more of the basic psychologic processes involved in understanding or using written or spoken language; (2) discrepancy between intellectual ability and attainment in reading, writing, spelling, calculating, listening, or speaking; and (3) absence of sensory or motor handicaps, mental retardation, psychosocial disadvantage, or primary emotional disturbance.[21] The first part of the definition reflects origins of the syndrome in early work on brain injury (for example, Strauss's syndrome).[22] In practical terms, lack of pathognomonic criteria renders specific diagnosis of presumed neurologic dysfunction quite difficult.[23] Patients with similar neurologic symptoms may or may not present with learning difficulties, and learning-disabled children are frequently found with negative medical histories and absence of neurologic signs. Current technology does not allow precise description of basic psycholinguistic or perceptual processes, though clinical experience suggests that combined neurologic and psychometric findings may supply evidence of dysfunction in some cases.[24]

To be diagnosed as learning disabled, a child must exhibit a severe discrepancy between actual and expected performance in a single area, such as reading, though disorders in associated areas are not uncommon. Differentiating a learning-disabled child from a retarded child depends upon the fact that children with learning disabilities are generally competent in most other areas. They have at least average or near average intellectual functioning (IQ above 70), but do not perform as expected in one or more of the basic school skills. For example, an otherwise normal 8-year-old may be suspected of having a learning disability if the child has not mastered basic reading by the third grade. The physician should be cautious in making a diagnosis with young children, however, since the concept of maturational lag suggests that different abilities may normally develop at different rates within the same child. Identification before age 6 or 7 is particularly hazardous. Determination is generally made by the child's poor school progress and low performance on individual tests of academic achievement. When performance on intelligence tests is near normal, and achievement testing is well below expected grade level in one or more areas, a learning disability is likely.

The third criterion relates to differential diagnosis. Deficits in visual or auditory acuity, or other correctable physical conditions, must be ruled out. More difficult are distinctions between learning disabilities and mild mental retardation or psychosocial disadvantage. Most problematic is the question of primary emotional disorder. Psychiatrists sometimes fail to consider that a behavior problem may be secondary to brain dysfunction, or to the frustrating effects of learning failure. Motivational problems or inappropriate choice of previous teaching methods, while more difficult to rule out, should likewise be considered.[25]

Epidemiology

Estimates of learning disability in the United States range from 1 percent to over 15 percent, a fact that reflects both inconsistencies in definition and the heterogeneity of the learning-disabled population. While prevalence rates of children's underachievement in reading are among the higher figures, more conservative estimates of the number of children requiring special remedial education range from 1 to 3 percent.[26] Most incidence and prevalence estimates are derived from meager empirical data, and little is available on the numbers of children presenting with disorders in arithmetic, spelling, or other disability areas. Of practical significance, federal legislation attempted to limit numbers of learning-disabled children who can be served by public schools to 2 percent, a measure apparently designed to ensure careful diagnostic evaluation.[27] Because the disorder relates primarily to educational growth and development, children are rarely diagnosed before school age, and incidence drops sharply after early adolescence.

In the learning-disabled population, males predominate at a ratio of approximately six to one, which reflects both genetic and social-role factors. It is not uncommon for learning-disabled girls to present with a slightly different clinical picture that features more severe levels of disability and fewer associated behavioral problems. Unlike mental retardation, excessive numbers of learning-disabled children have come from middle- and upper-class families. Children of impoverished families are more likely to be diagnosed as mentally retarded. Clinical experience, however, suggests that poorer parents tend to be less aware of learning disabilities, and less apt to press for its attention as a clinical entity. As diagnosis becomes more precise, a more equitable distribution should be found across social class and ethnic groups.[28]

Other handicapping conditions in learning-disabled children are emotional behavior disorders that are frequently found as secondary reactions. Hyperactivity, perceptual problems, motor awkwardness, and seizure disorders constitute associated handicaps. Mildly retarded children may occasionally be given a secondary diagnosis of learning disabilities when specific deficits are found relative to mental-age expectations.[29]

Classification and Etiology

While there is no widely accepted classification system for learning disabilities, most approaches classify them either by specific type of disability or by underlying disorder.[30] The consensus definition lists several types of disability, which can be grouped under three major headings: reading disability, verbal communication disorders, and visual-motor problems. Reading failure is the major referring complaint for children who are later diagnosed as learning disabled. Difficulties may occur in letter and word recognition, word attack skills, comprehension, or retention. A diagnosis of reading disability is usually reserved for children with adequate intelligence, who fail to read after normal exposure to teaching techniques that are successful with most children. The term dyslexia implies a severe reading disability with presumed neurologic etiology. Verbal communication disorders include disturbances in expressing or comprehending spoken language (expressive or receptive developmental aphasia) or more specific problems in auditory discrimination or memory (auditory agnosia). Visual-motor problems refer to difficulties in spelling or handwriting (dysgraphia), calculation (dyscalculia), or other functions involving visual monitoring or perception integrated with motor coordination. Etiology of each type of disability is presumed to derive from at least one of the following areas: neurologic, psychodynamic, or functional.

Strauss's syndrome represents a neurologic disorder underlying learning disabilities. Diagnostic criteria include an absence of family members with mental retardation, a history of neurologic impairment, soft neurologic signs, perceptual problems, difficulty in organizing thoughts or materials, and perseveration (a tendency to pursue a single activity excessively). Also associated are hyperactivity and so-called catastrophic reaction, in which the child is hyperresponsive to minor frustrations or to changes in environment. A diagnosis of Strauss's syndrome may be given to children displaying the behavioral manifestations without neurologic signs or a history of impairment. In such cases the diagnosis falls under the category of suspected neurologic impairment.

Other suspected neurologic disorders are minimal brain dysfunction[31] and the hyperactive child syndrome.[32] Though both are essentially variants of Strauss's syndrome, the former is defined more broadly, and the latter focuses on specific behavioral manifestations. It is important to note that diagnosis of minimal brain dysfunction often rests on a cluster of symptoms, among which are learning and perceptual problems, coordination deficits, hyperactivity, impulsivity, emotional lability, distractibility, equivocal neurologic signs, and EEG abnormalities. A given child may present with deficits in relatively few of these areas and still receive the diagnosis, particularly if basic perceptual and inhibition deficits are found.

The hyperactive child syndrome is manifested by four cardinal symptoms:

hyperactivity, impulsivity, distractibility, and excitability. The term denotes a behavioral syndrome with no etiologic implications. Hyperactivity as a symptom does not necessarily imply a greater amount of motor activity, but rather a different type, which is often described as restless, tense, or fidgety. Distinction must be made between such behaviors and transient situational reactions to boredom, lack of readiness for group situations, or natural curiosity. In some cases, aggressive or antisocial behavior may be present as a secondary reaction. Learning disabilities occur with approximately 50 to 75 percent of hyperactive children. Such disabilities are thought to occur when symptom behavior disrupts acquisition of new information or interferes with decision-making processes, which results in more impulsive, less reflective decisions.[33] Follow-up studies of hyperactive children suggest that hyperactivity eventually diminishes but that other symptoms persist into adolescence, with significant psychiatric and social pathology in adulthood a frequent possibility.[34]

Because they describe overlapping groups, the terms Strauss's syndrome, minimal brain dysfunction, and hyperactive syndrome are often used synonymously, or are referred to jointly as attentional disorders.[35] Although the etiology of these learning disorders is commonly said to be neurologic, multiple factors will be discovered when detailed scrutiny is undertaken.[36]

Genetic transmission is strongly implicated in minimal brain dysfunction,[37] in hyperactivity,[38] and in reading disabilities,[39] though exact mechanisms are as yet undetermined. As in mental retardation, maternal infections, prematurity, obstetrical complications, perinatal hypoxia, postnatal encephalitides, head trauma, malnutrition, and environmental deprivation are all high-risk events. Anatomic sequelae are most often presumed to focus on the regions of the angular gyrus or the reticular system.[40] Structural abnormalities of the brain are less commonly detected.[41] Low physiologic arousal of the central nervous system has been found in hyperactive children,[42] with evidence suggesting that the catecholamines, dopamine and norepinephrine, are crucial neurotransmitters in the etiology of the disorder.[43] Certain stimulant medications, such as amphetamines and methylphenidate, enhance catecholamine activity, and thereby produce the so-called paradoxical effect of reducing hyperactivity. Maturational lag, in which specific neurologic functions develop at slower rates, also predisposes a child to learning disabilities. Further etiologic classification of underlying neurologic disorders largely depends upon future research.

Psychologic factors, both primary and secondary, may contribute to learning problems. While inadequate resolution of intrapsychic conflict may be etiologic in learning disturbances, no specific type of internal or external conflict seems to characterize the child with a learning disability.[44] Although young children normally have fears when approaching the learning situation, those with a history of disturbed family relations may develop neurotic responses. Refusal to learn is seen as a defense against anxieties that are more fearful than school failure itself. For boys in particular, identification with the masculine role and conflicts with aggressive impulses are at issue. Through faulty resolution of basic conflicts, a child may be unable to achieve in areas seen as the parents' "turf," though this may also be related to general family tendencies to suppress or deny aggressive instincts. Also implicated are disturbed family communication patterns that involve nonmention or minimal mention of shame-ridden family secrets. Inability of the developing child to integrate such events can lead to anxieties that are centered around "knowing" or "active looking," and thus to neurotic inhibition of the learning process. Finally, children may fail to learn because unmet dependency needs become fulfilled by assuming a helpless role, which is often abetted by parents' own unresolved conflicts about the growing child.

The possible contribution of parental psychopathology to children's learning anxieties and inhibitions needs to be underscored, but care should be taken to exclude other possibilities before pursuing psychogenic factors. Particularly demanding are distinctions between learning neuroses and secondary emotional reactions to the educational process. It is also possible that parents who themselves have been poor readers provide poor models for children who are learning to read. Parents with a history of poor progress in school may not support their children's efforts as readily as other parents who enjoy books, read aloud to their children, and take an active interest in their children's reading.

Another group of children who are at risk for learning disabilities are those whose temperament or style is dissonant from significant features of their environment. Recent work by Thomas and Chess on the constitutional temperament of schoolchildren is instructive in this regard.[45] Just as children's development can be jeopardized when their temperaments differ from that of their parents, so can their academic progress when temperamental traits conflict with a teacher's classroom standards. The "difficult" child who distracts easily and reacts strongly to new situations may experience more problems in a permissive, unstructured classroom than one with a predictable routine. The "easy" or the "slow-to-warm-up" child may find it difficult to learn in classrooms that stress group conformity or quick adaptability. Other factors relate to subtle interactions between learning style and instructional methods. A child with auditory-discrimination deficits may be disadvantaged in reading programs that stress phonics. Certain instructional materials may cause difficulty for a child with visual-perceptual problems. Though current knowledge does not allow prediction of which approaches benefit which children, lack of fit between child and classroom variables may create difficulty where none need exist.[46] Children from impoverished environments that provide inadequate opportunity for perceptual or cognitive development are greatly at risk, since classroom demands may be discontinuous with previous learning in specific areas.

Diagnosis and Treatment

The diagnosis of learning disabilities involves two phases: establishing that a learning disability indeed exists, and determining an etiologic diagnosis whenever possible. As in mental retardation, a detailed parental interview is essential. Focus should be on developmental and family medical history, with particular care given to genetic, obstetric, and psychologic precursors. Though preschool development may be revealing, there are often subtle difficulties in language, perception, and coordination. School history should be thorough, and should be related to concurrent psychologic events in the family. Especially revealing are school records and phone or personal interviews with school personnel. Symptom inventory should include social, behavioral, and neurologic aspects. The child interview affords an opportunity to evaluate self-perceptions, preoccupations, and approaches to reading or other school-related tasks. Disparities are not uncommon, however, between behavior described by parents or teachers and children's demeanor in interview sessions.

Though physical examinations are usually normal in learning-disabled children, neurologic workup may reveal minor types of abnormalities.[47] Laboratory and EEG studies are recommended only when examination reveals definite physical or neurologic disorder.[48] Psychometric studies are vital, both in establishing discrepancies between measured intelligence and academic achievement, and in assessing related language and perceptual processes. The Peabody Individual Achievement Test is especially helpful in the assessment of a variety of academic skills.[49] Correctable defects in speech, hearing, and vision should be ruled out early in the diagnostic workup.

Diagnostic studies have clinical significance since, in most cases, treatment primarily involves appropriate school placement or other educational interventions.[50] Children with neurologic disorders may require drug management of seizure disorders or hyperactive behavior. The latter remains a complex area both in pediatrics[51] and in psychiatry.[52] Amphetamines and methylphenidate may reduce hyperactivity and impulsivity in some hyperactive children, though increases in classroom learning are less predictable. Principal side effects are weight loss and sleep disturbances; nausea, headache, pallor, and depression have also been reported. Magnesium pemoline is longer-acting, but titration may be difficult because of longer latency of onset. Tricyclic antidepressants have been effective in some cases, but have greater toxic potential. Minor tranquilizers and phenothiazines are contraindicated until stimulant medications have been tried. Proper drug treatment should be initiated only after therapeutic changes in school and home environments have failed, and such treatment should be subject to thorough monitoring. Families should be prepared for a trial-and-error process, and close attention should be paid to firsthand observation of the child's progress in school. A note should be added about current claims that attribute hyperactivity to synthetic food additives. These have yet to be substantiated, and nutritional management beyond normal attention to diet remains unwarranted.[53]

Psychotherapy as a primary treatment for learning-disabled children is rarely indicated, but it may be required for secondary emotional symptoms. Considerable effort, including psychotherapy, should be directed toward helping both the child and the parents understand the nature of the individual's learning difficulties and the function of therapeutic interventions. Behavior modification has been used increasingly with learning-disabled children, and the contribution of motivational deficits to learning disabilities should not be overlooked. Not only can academic skills be improved through use of proper incentives, but behavioral techniques have been shown to rival drug therapy in improving classroom behavior.[54] Of course drugs and behavior modification may complement each other and may therefore be indicated concurrently.

Educational approaches have recently focused on maintaining learning-disabled children in regular classrooms, with ancillary services from special resource personnel.[55] Occasionally, children may need at least partial assignment to special classes or to resource rooms when their disabilities involve complex remediation or associated behavior problems that require special management. As is the case with mental retardation, recent legislation has mandated education for learning-disabled children, with certain restrictions. Education of learning disabilities remains controversial, since research has not favored certain approaches over others.[56] Despite the benefits of early education, detection of learning disabilities before school age is fraught with methodological difficulty. Not only is the relationship of etiologic disorders to disability areas unclear, but programs addressed to specific language or perceptual deficits have had only limited success. The key to educating learning-disabled children remains individualized clinical teaching, with careful monitoring of progress.

THE ROLE OF THE NONPSYCHIATRIST

The physician has several important responsibilities in the care of children with disorders of learning. One is recognition that such problems exist, and that their solution often depends upon close and continuing cooperation with other professionals. There is no question that early screening will be a primary role for the family physician. Physicians will be called upon increasingly to share diagnostic information with school personnel, and to assist parents in securing appropriate special education. After children with disorders of learning are identified and evaluated, the school plays a primary role in subsequent treatment. As indicated previously, school programs for children with learning handicaps are undergoing considerable transformation. Early identification, increased opportunity for preschool intervention, interdisciplinary evaluation, cooperative educational planning with parents, and protection of the rights of handicapped children are recent innovations that call upon the physician to support and assist families in significant ways as they relate to the school system.

The physician acts as advocate for families, as they relate to other systems as well. Parents face continuing difficulties in raising a learning-disabled or retarded child. While the physician can provide first-line support and guidance, referral for psychiatric consultation is periodically needed, along with case management by regional centers for the developmentally disabled, financial aid, vocational counseling, residential placement, and the like. The physician can be an effective and trusted liaison between the family and other sources of assistance.

Although health maintenance is the physician's primary role, parents commonly complain that some physicians are either unwilling or unable to deal with children who are retarded, hyperactive, or present similar difficulties in behavioral management. The unique problems of such children demand a certain sensitivity as well as an ability to coordinate treatment with other professionals. The physician with clinical knowledge and expertise in learning disorders is usually less apprehensive about caring for such children. Indeed, continued medical practice with retarded or learning-disabled children tends to emphasize the similarity between such children and normal children, and proves to be particularly challenging and rewarding.

THE ROLE OF PSYCHIATRY

The past few years have witnessed the increasing involvement of psychiatry in disorders of learning, since the mainstay of both evaluation and treatment in this area is recognition of interdisciplinary contributions. With its dual tradition in both medicine and behavior, it is natural that psychiatry become an important pivot around which issues of differential diagnosis and treatment are resolved. The psychiatrist may best understand the complex interplay of the biologic and psychologic variables that determine prognosis in individual children. Since treatment frequently proceeds on many fronts, psychiatry is in a unique position to play a pivotal role. Recognition of precipitating events in families can often lead to early detection and preventive treatment well before the school years, thereby diminishing the effects of secondary symptoms. Psychiatric expertise is often needed in choosing from among several possible interventions. The field is particularly prone to faddism, and families need to be protected from prematurely embracing unproven approaches.

Over the entire course of development, necessary decisions may include those involving school, therapy, drug management, hospitalization, or access to various service systems. A collaborative multidisciplinary model should be maintained. In many cases, the psychiatrist serves both as an advocate for families and as a consultant to other professionals. The psychiatrist and other physicians must be aware of particular community resources, and must be willing to intercede if a child's progress appears jeopardized through inaction or ill-advised approaches. Open lines of communication with school or other agencies are required. Through training or through personal inclination, many psychiatrists are prepared to serve as consultants to both programs and individuals in understanding the unique needs of such children, the necessity for professional interchange, and the limitations of current knowledge.

REFERENCES

1 Forness, Steven R.: "Implications of Recent Trends in Educational Labeling," *J. Learning Disabil.,* 7:445–449, August 1974.
2 Hewett, Frank M., and Steven R. Forness: *Education of Exceptional Learners,* Boston: Allyn and Bacon, 1977.
3 Grossman, Herbert J. (ed.): *Manual on Terminology and Classification in Mental Retardation,* rev. ed., Washington, D.C.: American Association on Mental Deficiency, 1973.

4 American Psychiatric Association: *Diagnostic and Statistical Manual of Mental Disorders,* 2d ed., Washington, D.C., 1968.

5 Tarjan, George et al.: "Natural History of Mental Retardation: Some Aspects of Epidemiology," *Am. J. Ment. Defic.,* **77**:369–379, January 1973.

6 Tarjan, George: "Some Thoughts on Sociocultural Retardation," in H. Carl Haywood (ed.), *Sociocultural Aspects of Mental Retardation,* New York: Appleton-Century-Crofts, 1970, pp. 745–758.

7 Lei, Tzuen-jei et al.: "Agency-Labeled Mentally Retarded Persons in a Metropolitan Area: An Ecological Study," *Am. J. Ment. Defic.,* **79**:22–31, July 1974.

8 Valente, Mario, and George Tarjan: "Etiologic Factors in Mental Retardation," *Psychiat. Ann.,* **4**:22–37, February 1974.

9 Jones, Kenneth L. et al.: "Outcome in Offspring of Chronic Alcoholic Women," *Lancet,* **7866**:1076–1078, June 1974.

10 Crandall, Barbara F.: "Genetic Disorders and Mental Retardation," *J. Am. Acad. Child Psychiat.,* **16**:88–108, Winter 1977.

11 Tarjan, George, and Charles V. Keeran: "An Overview of Mental Retardation," *Psychiat. Ann.,* **4**:6–21, February 1974.

12 President's Committee on Mental Retardation: *The Six-Hour Retarded Child,* Washington, D.C.: U.S. Government Printing Office, 1970.

13 Tarjan, George: "Sensory Deprivation and Mental Retardation," in Leo Madow and Lawrence H. Snow (eds.): *Psychodynamic Implications of Physiological Studies on Sensory Deprivation,* Springfield, Ill.: Charles C Thomas, 1970, pp. 70–89.

14 Smith, David W., and F. Estelle Simmons: "Rational Diagnostic Evaluation of a Child with Mental Deficiency," *Am. J. Dis. Childr.,* **129**:1285–1290, November 1975.

15 Group for the Advancement of Psychiatry: *Mental Retardation: A Family Crisis—the Therapeutic Role of the Physician,* Report no. 56, New York: Group for the Advancement of Psychiatry, 1963.

16 MacMillan, Donald, and Steven R. Forness: "Applied Operant Programs in Mental Retardation," *Monographs of the American Association on Mental Deficiency,* no. 4, Washington, D.C.: American Association on Mental Deficiency, 1979.

17 Patterson, Gerald, and M. Elizabeth Gullion: *Living with Children: New Methods for Parents and Teachers,* Champaign, Ill.: Research Press, 1973.

18 Forness, Steven R.: "Education of Retarded Children: A Review for Physicians," *Am. J. Dis. Childr.,* **127**:237–242, February 1974.

19 Torres, Scottie (ed.): *A Primer on Individualized Educational Programs for Handicapped Children,* Reston, Va.: Foundation for Exceptional Children, 1977.

20 MacMillan, Donald: *Mental Retardation in School and Society,* Boston: Little, Brown, 1977.

21 U.S. Congress: *Public Law 94-142: Education for Handicapped Children Act,* Washington, D.C.: Federal Register, August 23, 1977.

22 Strauss, Alfred A., and Laura Lehtinen: *Psychopathology and Education of the Brain-Injured Child,* New York: Grune and Stratton, 1947.

23 Wender, Paul H., and Leon Eisenberg: "Minimal Brain Dysfunction in Children," in Silvano Arieti (ed.): *American Handbook of Psychiatry,* vol. 2, New York: Basic Books, 1974, pp. 130–146.

24 Kirk, Samuel A., and Winifred D. Kirk: *Psycholinguistic Learning Disabilities: Diagnosis and Remediation,* Urbana, Ill.: University Press, 1971.

25 Dunn, Lloyd M.: *Exceptional Children in the Schools,* 2d ed., New York: Holt, Rinehart and Winston, 1973.

26 Kirk, Samuel A.: *Educating Exceptional Children,* 2d ed., Boston: Houghton Mifflin, 1972.

27 U.S. Congress: *Public Law 94-142: Education of Handicapped Children (Children with Specific Learning Disabilities),* Washington, D.C.: Federal Register, November 29, 1976.

28 Burke, Arlene A.: "Placement of Black and White Children in Educable Mentally Handicapped Classes and Learning Disability Classes," *Except. Childr.,* **41**:438–440, March 1975.

29 Cruickshank, William M.: "Myths and Realities in Learning Disabilities," *J. Learning Disabil.,* **10**:51–58, January 1977.

30 Johnson, Stanley W., and Robert L. Morasky: *Learning Disabilities,* Boston: Allyn and Bacon, 1977.

31 De La Cruz, Felix F. et al. (eds.): "Minimal Brain Dysfunction," *Ann. NY Acad. Sci.,* 205:5–396, February 28, 1973.

32 Cantwell, Dennis P. (ed.): *The Hyperactive Child: Diagnosis, Management, Current Research,* New York: Spectrum, 1975.

33 Keogh, Barbara K: "Hyperactivity and Learning Disorders: Review and Speculation," *Except. Childr..,* **38**:101–109, October 1971.

34 Cantwell, Dennis P.: "Natural History and Prognosis in the Hyperactive Child Syndrome," in Dennis P. Cantwell (ed.): *The Hyperactive Child,* New York: Spectrum, 1975, pp. 51–64.

35 Schain, Richard J.: *Neurology of Childhood Learning Disorders,* Baltimore: Williams and Wilkins, 1972.

36 Black, F. William: "Neurological Dysfunction and Reading Disorders," *J. Learning Disabil.,* **6**:313–316, May 1973.

37 Omenn, Gilbert S.: "Genetic Issues in the Syndrome of Minimal Brain Dysfunction," *Seminars in Psychiatry,* **5**:5–19, February 1973.

38 Cantwell, Dennis P.: "Familial-Genetic Research with Hyperactive Children," in Dennis P. Cantwell (ed.): *The Hyperactive Child,* New York: Spectrum, 1975, pp. 93–105.

39 Klasen, Edith: *The Syndrome of Specific Dyslexia,* Baltimore: University Park Press, 1972.

40 Dykman, Roscoe A. et al.: "Specific Learning Disabilities: An Attentional Syndrome," in Helmer R. Mykelebust (ed.): *Progress in Learning Disabilities,* vol. 2, New York: Grune and Stratton, 1971, pp. 56–93.

41 Werry, John S.: "Organic Factors in Childhood Psychopathology," in Herbert C. Quay and John S. Werry (eds.): *Psychopathological Disorders of Childhood,* New York: Wiley, 1972, pp. 85–121.

42 Satterfield, James H.: "Neurophysiologic Studies of Hyperactive Children," in Dennis P. Cantwell (ed.): *The Hyperactive Child,* New York: Spectrum, 1975, pp. 67–82.

43 Moskowitz, Michael A., and Richard J. Wurtman: "Catecholamines and Neurologic Diseases," *N. E. J. Med.,* **293**:332–336, August 1975.

44 Heinicke, Christoph M.: "Learning Disturbance in Childhood," in Benjamin B. Wolman (ed.): *Manual of Child Psychopathology,* New York: McGraw-Hill, 1972, pp. 662–705.

45 Thomas, Alexander, and Stella Chess: *Temperament and Development,* New York: Brunner/Mazel, 1977.

46 Bryan, Tanis H., and James H. Bryan: *Understanding Learning Disabilities,* Port Washington, N.Y.: Alfred, 1975.

47 Werry, John S. et al.: "Studies of the Hyperactive Child: Neurological Status Compared with Neurotic and Normal Children," *Am. J. Orthopsychiat.,* **42**:441–451, April 1972.

48 Gerson, Samuel: "Pediatric Psychopharmacology—Clinical Laboratory Standards," *Psychopharmacology Bulletin,* Special Issue, Washington, D.C.: Department of Health, Education and Welfare, 1973, pp. 167–181.

49 Dunn, Lloyd M., and Frederick C. Markwardt: *Peabody Individual Achievement Test,* Circle Pines, Minn.: American Guidance Service, 1970.

50 Hamish, Nichol: "Children with Learning Disabilities Referred to Psychiatrists: A Follow-Up Study," *J. Learning Disabil.,* **7**:118–122, February 1974.

51 Baldessarini, Ross J. et al.: "Symposium: Behavior Modification by Drugs," *Pediatrics,* **49**:694–715, May 1972.

52 Bosco, James J., and Stanley S. Robin (eds.): *The Hyperactive Child and Stimulant Drugs,* Chicago: University Press, 1977.

53 Spring, Carl, and Jonathan Sandoval: "Food Additives and Hyperkinesis: Critical Evaluation of the Evidence," *J. Learning Disabil.,* **9**:560–569, November 1976.

54 Christensen, Donald E.: "Effects of Combining Methylphenidate and a Classroom Token System in Modifying Hyperactive Behavior," *Am. J. Ment. Defic.,* **80**:266–276, November 1975.

55 Forness, Steven R.: "Educational Therapy," in Dennis P. Cantwell and Peter E. Tanguay (eds.): *Clinical Child Psychiatry,* New York: Spectrum, 1979.

56 Hammil, Donald D., and Nettie R. Bartel: *Teaching Children with Learning and Behavior Problems,* Boston: Allyn and Bacon, 1975.

Part Five

Treatment

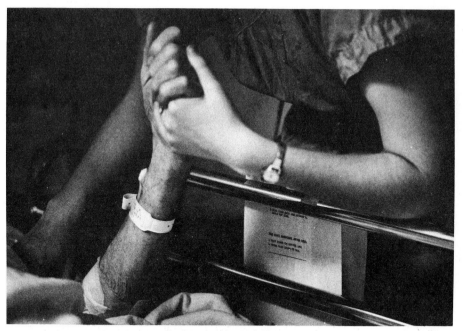

Courtesy of Sherry Suris/Photo Researchers, Inc., NYC.

Chapter 23

The Physician
as Psychotherapist

Judd Marmor, M.D.

EDITORS' INTRODUCTION

Patients often turn to their physician with life's problems. The pain in the shoulder, insomnia, "just not feeling right," or a request for a "complete physical" may be the device by which the appointment is obtained. The need to talk over a concern, worry, or fear with a trusted expert who knows how to keep confidences can be a compelling urge. The physician is placed in the position of counselor or psychotherapist, whether or not the physician desires it. The initial issue is whether the physician will recognize the unavoidable psychotherapeutic aspect of his or her role as physician. If the recognition is avoided, if the physician denies that psychotherapy is a part of all doctoring, the range of helpfulness that can be provided for patients is seriously constricted—and the patient, in finally confiding a personal worry or problem, is rejected and may be unwilling ever again to take the risk of confiding deep, intimate, personal problems.

Too often, medical school and postgraduate training does not prepare the physician adequately for the recognition and successful accomplishment of the psychotherapeutic function. The physician may have to rely only on intuitive skills, without having had the opportunity to learn to use the self as a therapeutic instrument. To do so involves not only the capacity for objective analysis of the patient's dilemma, but also the ability from time to time to place oneself in the patient's position. The physician's life experiences provide a base for the empathic part of the psychotherapeutic role. Physicians, after all, have grown up in families, struggled with adolescent worries and concerns, fought to gain entrance to medical school, experienced the stress of the input overload of the first year, most often have married and have had to work to make that relationship an effective one, frequently have become parents and experienced the joys, sorrows, and fears of that role. In short, physicians have lived and are living, and in the process have come to know something of what life is about. Although this knowledge may be restricted somewhat by social class and ethnic factors, much of it is useful in the process of being helpful to patients.

In this chapter, Marmor, one of this country's foremost clinicians, presents the reader with a clear structure with which the physician's psychotherapeutic function can be augmented. He presents phases of the psychotherapeutic relationship, the process of therapy, and concepts of what goes on within the physician as well as within the patient in a manner that will be helpful to both nonpsychiatric and psychiatric physicians.

Only those physicians who never see a live patient can fail to find reason to question their current methods of treatment. For the remainder, this chapter offers both a theoretical overview of psychotherapy and practical suggestions to increase the physician's psychotherapeutic competence.

INTRODUCTION

Fifty to seventy-five percent of all people who consult physicians for physical complaints have complicating or contributing mental or emotional problems that may be precursors of more serious psychiatric disorders. Thus, the primary practitioner of medicine is in a unique position to offer a front-line defense against mental illness.

Indeed, the family practitioner enjoys certain advantages over the psychiatrist in dealing with a patient's emotional problems. The family physician is apt to have had a continuity of relationship with the patient and his or her family over prior years that the psychiatrist usually does not have, and is therefore more likely to have an intimate knowledge of the patient's family and life situation, and of significant others in the patient's life. In addition, the medical practitioner's more direct knowledge of the patient's physical and physiological history constitutes an important edge not only in distinguishing between somatic and functional complaints on the part of the patient, but also in knowing what kind of medication the patient tends to respond to, favorably or unfavorably. Finally, the very fact that the physician is *not* a psychiatrist is a positive factor in the minds of many patients, who still tend to feel that needing the help of a psychiatrist means that they are crazy or, at the very least, that there is something seriously wrong with them mentally. Thus, patients are more apt to be initially defensive and emotionally tense in an interview with a psychiatrist than they are with their family practitioner. Consequently, the fact that the primary physician is not a psychiatrist but a familiar helping figure allows patients to present their problems to him or her, at least at the outset, with a more open attitude and with a greater initial trust and expectation of being helped. To put it in psychiatric parlance, this enables the primary physician to establish a therapeutic alliance with the patient more rapidly.

THE INITIAL INTERVIEW AS THE BEGINNING OF THERAPY

In Chapter 1, Lewis and Usdin described the techniques of the initial interview. In the context of the present chapter, it can be added that the initial interview is also a psychotherapeutic transaction, even though neither the physician nor the patient may consciously regard it as such. The very fact that the patient is able to discuss a personal problem in an ambience of hope and positive expectancy is the beginning of a therapeutic experience. Moreover, the interest and warmth that hopefully are conveyed by the physician as he or she listens to the patient constitute additional psychotherapeutic elements.

DIAGNOSIS AS A BASIS FOR THERAPEUTIC PLANNING

Still another point needs to be made, however. The initial interviews and the diagnostic evaluation that emerges furnish the basic groundwork for subsequent psychotherapeutic planning. Whether or not the patient can be helped directly by the primary physician or should be referred to a psychiatrist, whether and what medication is indicated, whether the therapeutic task will be to try to educate the patient to cope more effectively with life problems, or whether it will be to attempt to modify certain stresses in the patient's life, are decisions that depend on an appropriate diagnostic evaluation.

As Lewis and Usdin have indicated, the most important thing that a physician can do in the initial interviews is to give the patient an opportunity to present personal problems as fully and spontaneously as possible, within the limitations of the physician's time. This should enable the physician to arrive at a decision concerning the nature of the presenting stresses in the patient's life, and the way in which the patient is coping with these stresses. The ratio between the magnitude of life stresses (see Chapter 9) on the one hand, and the effectiveness of the patient's coping ability ("ego strength") on the other, offers a rough gauge of prognosis to therapeutic response. In general, the greater the magnitude of life stresses and the greater the patient's ego strength, the more we can expect a favorable response, either with short-term psychotherapeutic interventions or with modifications of the life stresses. On the other hand, when we deal with individuals whose histories show inadequate coping mechanisms throughout most of their lives, and who break down in the face of relatively minimal life stresses, we face a much more difficult therapeutic challenge.

In the course of accumulating this information, the physician is not just searching for a diagnostic label that can be attached to the patient's condition;

more importantly, the physician is probing for, and attempting to reach, an understanding of the circumstances that lie behind the patient's complaints.

EVALUATING LIFE STRESSES

The magnitude of a patient's life stresses is generally fairly recognizable. Many rating scales have been developed to relate stresses to the emergence of physical or emotional illness. One much-used scale is that of Holmes and Rahe, who have shown that such events as the loss of a love object, loss of a job, the taking on of a new job, moving to a new location, financial difficulties, divorce, separation, or other life changes all involve significant emotional stress.[1] Their rating scale attempts to rank-order the impact of these life events (see Table 23-1). Of course, not infrequently a patient may be experiencing more than one of these stresses simultaneously. Not only the number of such events, but also their duration in time and their qualitative importance in the patient's mind contributes to the degree of the stress that the patient feels. (See Chapter 9 for a more complete description.)

EVALUATING PERSONALITY STRENGTH

Coping abilities, on the other hand, can be evaluated by the way in which patients have dealt with the usual sequential events in their lives. Many of these may be known to the primary physician by reason of previous contacts with the patient. They include such matters as developmental vicissitudes of early childhood (feeding problems, thumb sucking, enuresis, etc.), adaptation to school, educational level, employment history (frequency of job change, length of time that jobs were held, progress and promotion in chosen work), sexual history (attitudes about masturbation, menstruation, first sexual experiences, presence or absence of sexual dysfunctions, nature of sexual fantasies, etc.), interpersonal relationships (with peers, employers, same and opposite sex, marital partner, children, etc.), and the way in which the individual has coped with responsibilities.

RECOGNIZING MASKED DEPRESSION

In addition, in the diagnostic evaluation of the patient, there are certain other specific things that the physician should look for that have an important bearing on the kind of treatment to be offered. One of these is the presence or absence of vegetative symptoms, such as insomnia, anorexia, weight loss, loss of sexual desire, fatigue, listlessness, dry mouth, gastrointestinal complaints, and diurnal mood variation (especially feeling worse in the morning but better as the day goes along). The reason for asking about these in particular is that often such symptoms mask a depressive state. The presence of such symptoms should alert the physician to ask about underlying mood, and particularly about feelings of hopelessness or helplessness. Should evidence of depression be found, questions regarding suicidal thoughts would then be in order (see Chapter 20).

Another important diagnostic differentiation that physicians should make

Table 23-1   Social Readjustment Rating Scale

Rank	Life event	Mean value
1	Death of spouse	100
2	Divorce	73
3	Marital separation	65
4	Jail term	63
5	Death of close family member	63
6	Personal injury or illness	53
7	Marriage	50
8	Fired at work	47
9	Marital reconciliation	45
10	Retirement	45
11	Change in health of family member	44
12	Pregnancy	40
13	Sex difficulties	39
14	Gain of new family member	39
15	Business readjustment	39
16	Change in financial state	38
17	Death of close friend	37
18	Change to different line of work	36
19	Change in number of arguments with spouse	35
20	Mortgage over $10,000	31
21	Foreclosure of mortgage or loan	30
22	Change in responsibilities at work	29
23	Son or daughter leaving home	29
24	Trouble with in-laws	29
25	Outstanding personal achievement	28
26	Wife begin or stop work	26
27	Begin or end school	26
28	Change in living conditions	25
29	Revision of personal habits	24
30	Trouble with boss	23
31	Change in work hours or conditions	20
32	Change in residence	20
33	Change in schools	20
34	Change in recreation	19
35	Change in church activities	19
36	Change in social activities	18
37	Mortgage or loan less than $10,000	17
38	Change in sleeping habits	16
39	Change in number of family get-togethers	15
40	Change in eating habits	15
41	Vacation	13
42	Christmas	12
43	Minor violations of the law	11

From Thomas H. Holmes and Richard H. Rahe, "The Social Readjustment Scale," *J. Psychosom. Res.*, **11**:216, 1967.

early in their work with patients is whether they are dealing with a neurosis, a personality disorder, or a psychosis (see Chapters 9, 10, and 11). Such a diagnostic differentiation will, of course, be of considerable importance in enabling physicians to decide whether the patient's problem is one that they can treat themselves, or whether the patient should be referred to a psychiatrist for more specialized therapy.

WHAT MAKES PSYCHOTHERAPY WORK?

Let us now assume that the physician has decided that the patient's problem is one that can be approached psychotherapeutically. At this point, it might be useful for the physician to have some idea about what makes psychotherapy work. The psychotherapeutic process generally involves 10 basic factors.[2] These are: (1) a good patient-physician relationship, (2) ventilation or "catharsis," (3) cognitive insight, (4) operant conditioning through implicit or explicit approval-disapproval cues, (5) operant conditioning through a corrective emotional relationship, (6) identification, (7) suggestion, (8) persuasion, (9) rehearsal or practice of new coping techniques, and (10) consistent emotional support.

1 Patient-Therapist Relationship

The basic matrix of all successful psychotherapies is a relationship of trust and rapport between the therapist and the patient. If the patient perceives the physician as a genuine, trustworthy, warm, interested, empathic, and knowledgeable person, faith in the latter's ability to help, and positive expectancy of receiving help, will be greatly increased. If, on the other hand, the patient experiences the physician as impatient, disinterested, cold, insensitive, or lacking in judgment, the working basis of a good psychotherapeutic relationship will not be forthcoming. It is of major importance, therefore, that the physician should give the patient unqualified interest and attention. It is not so much the length but the quality of the time that a physician spends with the patient that makes a major difference in what the patient will obtain from psychotherapy.

2 Ventilation or "Catharsis"

A second factor in all psychotherapies is the opportunity to "ventilate" one's problem to a person who, by virtue of professional status and training, is endowed with the attributes of a helping person and who will maintain the patient's confidence. Most patients come to a physician with the hope and expectancy of receiving relief; unburdening themselves of their anxieties, fears, and symptomatic complaints is the first step in the psychotherapeutic transaction. Most patients experience a discharge of tension from this unburdening process, which is why Freud likened it to catharsis.

3 Cognitive Insight

In the course of listening to the patient's story and obtaining a history, the physician can form a diagnostic impression not only of what the patient is suffering from, but also of the reasons for the patient's complaints. The physician then tries not only to help the patient understand these reasons and etiological factors, but also confronts the patient with any perceptual or emotional distortions that become apparent as they go along. These efforts at explanation and confrontation constitute what is called the giving of cognitive "insight" to the patient. By virtue of such insight the patient is enabled, in a way not previously possible, to understand the reasons for the symptoms and/or difficulties, and thus is in a position to cope with them more constructively.

4   Operant Conditioning: Reward-Punishment

Often, however, mere understanding does not in itself enable the patient to change coping patterns that have been long established through habitual use, and the patient may keep repeating the old maladaptive patterns. In the course of the therapeutic relationship, however, the physician implicitly or explicitly reflects approval or disapproval of how the patient is behaving. Because the physician is a respected authority figure whom the patient consciously or unconsciously wishes to please, the latter tends to respond by attempting to give up the disapproved patterns of behavior and adopting those that are approved. This is a kind of operant-conditioning process in which the "reward" of the physician's approval and the "punishment" of his disapproval operate as conditioning responses that, over time, gradually influence the patient toward more adaptive coping techniques. These conditioning responses may be explicit, in the form of specific statements of approval or disapproval, or they may be implicit, and reflected only in the expression on the physician's face or the tone of the physician's voice.

5   Operant Conditioning: Corrective Emotional Experiences

Still another type of operant conditioning that takes place in psychotherapy is that which Alexander called "corrective emotional experience."[3] By this is meant that the patient often experiences a healthier and more rational set of reactions and responses in the relationship with the physician than in relationships with significant authority figures from the past. Thus a patient who may have felt rejected or demeaned by his or her own parents, but is accepted and respected by the physician-therapist (a type of parental surrogate), or one who in the past has been intimidated by the anger encountered from parents whenever a mistake was made, but who now meets with a more tolerant and understanding response from the physician under similar circumstances, is experiencing a corrective response that helps to shape behavior toward healthier and more effective patterns.

6   Identification: The Physician as a Model

Another factor in the psychotherapeutic process is that over time the respected physician-therapist, wittingly or unwittingly, becomes an implicit model after whom patients unconsciously tend to pattern themselves. Thus, to the extent that physicians behave maturely, react adaptively, and function with understanding, they set an example for more adult and adaptive behavior with which patients can identify.

7 Suggestion

Suggestion is an indirect way of trying to influence a person's patterns of thought or behavior. Some degree of suggestion is implicit in every psychotherapeutic transaction, simply by virtue of the things in which the therapist shows interest or disinterest, and by virtue of the things treated as normal and those that are reacted to as being neurotic, as well as in the specific interpretations or explanations that the therapist offers. In these diverse ways the therapist, often unwittingly, conveys a personal value system and views about how the patient should or should not be behaving. Thus, suggestion is an inevitable part of every psychotherapeutic process. In nondirective psychotherapies, it tends to be implicit; in directive therapies, it is more explicit. Patients who have the greatest need to please the therapist will, of course, be most suggestible.

8 Persuasion

In contrast to suggestion, persuasion involves a more conscious and deliberate effort to urge the patient toward certain patterns of behavior or thought in preference to certain others. Techniques that tend to be directive obviously employ persuasion more frequently than those that are essentially nondirective in character.

9 Rehearsal or Practice

In all psychotherapies, as patients begin to learn new adaptive techniques, the application of these new techniques does not come readily. There is a tendency to fall back automatically on old coping habits and, indeed, there is even some resistance to trying the new techniques of adaptation. This might be likened to the way in which a person who has been playing golf poorly keeps falling back on an old "maladaptive" swing, in spite of the fact that the pro has demonstrated what is wrong with the swing. Nevertheless, the old swing feels more comfortable and the new one, the correct one, still feels awkward to the golfer. Thus it often requires a good deal of repetition, practice, or rehearsal on the part of the student to master the new techniques. Similarly, in psychotherapy, only as the new ways of behaving are tested repeatedly does the patient eventually begin to feel more comfortable with them and realize that the fears on which the old behavior was based are no longer valid. For example, a patient who has been harboring the assumption that assertive behavior will lead to rejection, when in fact a healthier pattern of assertiveness will result in greater respect, will learn this only through repeatedly attempting to be more assertive and finding out that it "works." This is part of what psychiatrists sometimes call the "working through" process.

10 Emotional Support

Finally, for all of this to take place effectively, a climate of consistent emotional support on the part of the physician is essential. The patient is encouraged to move forward in the new coping techniques, not only by means of trust in the physician, but equally importantly, by the evidences of the physician's trust and confidence in the patient's capacity for change. This consistent emotional support on the part of the physician validates the patient's worth as a person, and since the lack of self-worth is often a major element in the self-image of emotionally disturbed individuals, the ability to enhance a patient's self-esteem is often a crucial factor in successful psychotherapy.

THE PROCESS OF PSYCHOTHERAPY

The psychotherapeutic process may be conveniently divided into three stages: a beginning phase, a middle phase, and a termination phase. Each of these phases presents its own unique problems, and each makes special demands on the technical skill and understanding of the physician-therapist.

The Beginning Phase of Therapy

The opening phase of therapy generally involves four basic elements. The first of these is sometimes referred to in psychiatric parlance as the *contract* between the therapist and the patient. This should not be understood in any legal sense, but rather it refers to an understanding established at the very outset about what the therapeutic work entails and what each of the participants in the therapeutic work may expect of one another. Basic to all effective psychotherapy is the understanding that the patient will endeavor to be completely frank and honest in the presentation of thoughts or problems, and that in return the therapist will protect any information received with the utmost confidentiality. A schedule of appointments is set up, and every effort should be made on both sides to adhere to that schedule as closely as is humanly possible. The physician who is planning to do adjunctive psychotherapy should set a certain amount of time aside for that purpose. Although the vicissitudes of a physician's schedule are quite different from those of the average psychiatrist, the physician-therapist should nevertheless be aware of the fact that keeping patients waiting for long periods of time for their appointments can create serious obstacles to psychotherapeutic progress.

The length of interviews should be clearly specified wherever possible, particularly since the physician's time is apt to be quite limited. If the physician is setting time aside specifically for this purpose, it may be advisable to have an understanding with the patient that last-minute cancellations will be charged for, unless they have been caused by circumstances clearly beyond the patient's control. The reason for this is that psychiatrists have learned through long experience that if they do not do so, patients may use such cancellations capriciously in the service of unconscious resistance to therapy.

Closely related to this first element in the beginning phase of therapy is the necessity for achieving what psychiatrists have come to call a *therapeutic alliance* with the patient. This involves engaging the healthy part of the patient's ego in a cooperative working relationship with the therapist for the purpose of accomplishing the therapeutic goal. For a therapeutic alliance to become operative, a climate of mutual trust and confidence needs to be established. The genuine interest, the empathic concern, and the warmth conveyed by the therapist are major elements in establishing the atmosphere of rapport in which a therapeutic alliance can flourish. In this context, the quality of time spent with the patient is considerably more important than the quantity. Whatever the time set aside for a session, it is imperative that the physician's undivided attention be given to the patient during that period. Nothing is more destructive to an atmosphere of rapport than a physician who is impatient or who is constantly stealing glances at the clock.

The third element in the opening phase of therapy involves the development of a *therapeutic focus*. This refers to the physician's effort to formulate the aims of therapy in terms of a particular area or specific problem that needs to be worked through. The working through of this problem becomes the limited aim of therapy from the beginning, and the therapist tries to help the patient to focus attention on that area. The determination of this focus is achieved by careful history taking in the initial interview. In the process of gathering information, the physician endeavors to evaluate the various sources of stress in the patient's life and to focus on those areas that seem to be most critical in producing the patient's distress or maladjustment. These focused areas are sometimes referred to as the *core problem* that the patient presents.

Finally, on the basis of the evaluation of the core problem and the factors involved in it, the physician-therapist tries to establish a *therapeutic plan*. This will involve such questions as whether the patient's problem can be resolved most easily by such supportive measures as reassurance, drugs, and making certain changes in the environment, or whether a more basic reeducational process will be necessary to improve the patient's coping abilities.

These objectives of the initial phase of therapy can sometimes be achieved in a first interview, but more often than not several interviews may be necessary for this purpose. The therapy then shifts to the middle phase.

The Middle Phase of Therapy

In the middle phase of therapy, the physician-therapist concentrates on helping the patient to face the focal problem and to understand it in all of its ramifications. One of the most effective ways of doing this is to enable the patient to see the connection between the *historical determinants* of the focal problem, the way it is manifesting itself in the *current life* of the patient, and the way in which it manifests itself in *relationship to the therapist*. This tripartite effort at clarification has been called "the triangle of insight" by Karl Menninger.[4] It is during this middle phase also that the physician is apt to encounter resistance on the part of the patient, in that the patient often is unconsciously reluctant to face or accept the implications of the insights that are being given. The reason for this is that the old adaptive patterns, neurotic and maladaptive though they may be, were originally shaped by life experiences for which they had a certain validity, but they have now become habitual, like the poor golf swing, and the patient finds it either fearful or uncomfortable to change them. The patient therefore "defends" against these insights in a number of ways. Some patients give intellectual lip service to what they are being told, but clearly have no emotional reaction to it; thus, the insight fails to have the change-inducing impact that is hoped for. Others manage to "forget" or repress the clarifications they have received, and come back the next time as though they had never heard them. Others manifest their resistance by coming consistently late to appointments or "forgetting" them. In each instance it is part of the physician-therapist's task to point out patiently and nonjudgmentally what is happening and why, so that the patient can finally arrive at a greater awareness of the nature of the underlying emotional conflicts and their implications for the presenting problem.

A fundamental phenomenon that the physician will encounter during this middle phase of therapy revolves around the transference distortions that the patient may present in the work with the therapist. By *transference distortions,* psychiatrists mean that patients inevitably react to important authority figures in ways that are based upon their perception of the significant authority figures of their childhood. Thus, if a patient felt unloved by parents in the past, he or she is apt to assume automatically that the therapist also will be unloving. Patients whose parents were very critical and judgmental often assume automatically that the therapist, too, is critical and judgmental, even when that is not so. One of the most common and troublesome forms of transference distortion involves the exaggerated dependency upon, and idealization of, the therapist, much as a child reacts to an important parent figure. This emotional dependency can become a profound resistance when the patient is confronted with the necessity for developing more mature and independent patterns of adaptation. The patient may stubbornly resist thinking or functioning autonomously, and may want the therapist to make all the important decisions. It is easy for a therapist to be seduced into doing this by the patient's obvious gratitude and idealization, and yet, if it is the purpose of therapy to enable the patient to function maturely and autonomously, such an approach on the part of the physician becomes antitherapeutic. This is why psychotherapists only rarely tell people what to do. Rather, after the underlying psychodynamic factors have been clarified, they try to help patients to identify and weigh the various options that are available, and encourage them to make independent decisions. This is an important approach to take, not only because no physician is omniscient, but also because the decisions that are sometimes sought are of a major nature for which only patients themselves can take responsibility. Thus the question of whether or not to break up a marriage, quit a job, or move from one location to another can often have such major ramifications that it would be unwise for a therapist to accept or take on the responsibility for making such decisions.

Another manifestation of transference that occurs not infrequently, particularly between a patient and physician of opposite sexes, is an erotic idealization of the physician by the patient, which may result in seductive advances toward the physician. It is very tempting for the physician to be taken in by such an eroticized idealization, and to succumb to it. Such a response is not only counter to the Hippocratic oath, but is also inevitably destructive to the psychotherapeutic process. Such erotic transference reactions are more often than not a subtle kind of resistance on the part of the patient. It is a way of saying, "Don't try to change me. That is too difficult for me. Just love me and then everything will be all right.'' Sometimes such seductive behavior is also an unconscious way of trying to demean the physician and reduce the physician's authority, which is experienced as threatening by the patient. It is extremely important, therefore, that the physician recognize reactions of this kind as transference manifestations and not as reality-based reactions. Such recognition will make it possible to deal with these reactions constructively, in the interests of the psychotherapeutic process.

The Termination Phase of Therapy

The termination phase of psychotherapy is extremely important. If it is handled badly, it can often undo much of the good work that has gone before. In approaching this phase, the physician should understand that the process of separating from someone who has become important to us is a major psychological event in all human existence. It is, indeed, one of the major tasks of the maturational process. Learning to walk by oneself as a child, then to play alone in a room, then to go off to school without mother, then finally to leave home and make an independent life for oneself are all different phases of development that involve the process of separation and individuation. The ways in which people handle the loss of a loved one or the move to a strange city are other examples of this capacity to handle separation. In the course of psychotherapy, with the close trust and intimacy that is involved, it is not surprising that patients will often find it very difficult to give up the relationship with the therapist. Recognizing this fact, when the physician feels that the patient has made sufficient progress to go on alone, the issue of termination should be broached well in advance, and the patient should be given an opportunity to work through his or her feelings with regard to the termination process. Not infrequently, when a patient is faced with the prospect of terminating what has become an important supportive relationship, there may be a transitory recurrence of earlier symptoms or other indications of a temporary setback. The physician should recognize these as a reaction to the separation process, and interpret them so. If this is done empathically and supportively, the patient's symptoms tend to disappear quickly, the patient's anxieties can be discussed openly, and a smooth transition to termination can be finally achieved.

THE QUESTION OF TIME

The physician may well be prompted to respond, ''This is all very well, but how am I, a busy physician, going to be able to devote the kind of time to a patient that such psychotherapy requires? With a waiting room full of people, I am in no position to give each patient 45 or 50 minutes of my time as a psychiatrist does.''

This is, indeed, a legitimate concern, but it is important to realize that a great deal of psychotherapy can be accomplished with much lesser amounts of time. As has already been indicated, it is not so much the quantity of time as it is the quality of the time spent with a patient that is decisive in achieving psychotherapeutic goals. The warmth, empathy, and genuineness that a physician reflects in dealing with a patient can make even a short amount of time helpful psychotherapeutically. Furthermore, a certain amount of interview time has already been spent merely in the normal procedure of obtaining a medical history. The physician who is willing to spend an extra 15 minutes with a troubled patient will be gratified to find how helpful that additional amount of time can be.

THE QUESTION OF FREQUENCY

As for frequency, unless a patient is unusually troubled, a scheduled visit of once or twice a week will suffice for the large majority of patients. Studies have shown that 97 percent of patients who are seen by psychiatrists (excluding psychoanalysts) are seen twice a week or less;[5] on the average, a patient is seen about 26 times a year.[6] For the particularly disturbed patient, a twice-a-week frequency is more than twice as good as a once-a-week visit because it permits greater continuity of effort, and there is less tendency for the patient to "put a lid" on the psychotherapeutic work between visits.

FOCUSING ON THE CORE PROBLEM

As experience is gained, the physician will become able to zero in on the patient's core problems more rapidly. Making these the central focus of therapeutic efforts and working with them only, the physician may find it possible to help the patient psychotherapeutically in a relatively short period of time. This will be particularly true in those instances in which the physician is able to delineate a specific stress factor in the patient's life situation that is responsible for the patient's emotional distress. Enabling patients to understand the source of their emotional symptoms and helping them to deal more effectively with the stressful life situation will often prove quite gratifying in terms of therapeutic response.

Thus, the young housewife who is suffering from headaches and some elevation in blood pressure may be reacting to an upsetting interpersonal relationship with a dominating and interfering mother-in-law; the middle-aged minor executive with ulcer symptoms may be reacting to an increased workload and the pressure of increased responsibilities; the lawyer with extrasystoles may be responding to friction with law partners; the middle-aged housewife with a wide variety of somatic pains and complaints may be reacting to a growing estrangement from her husband, etc.

SHOULD ONE BE DIRECTIVE OR NONDIRECTIVE IN THERAPY?

The question of whether the physician should be directive or nondirective in his or her relationship with the patient hinges to some degree on what the therapeutic objectives are. Where the problem is essentially one of recognizing a stress situation such as those described above, and of enabling the patient to deal with it more effectively, a warm, explanatory, and gently directive approach may give the patient the kind of support and strength that is needed for coping with the life situation and for resolving more effectively the emotional disequilibrium that is responsible for the symptoms.

On the other hand, when the difficulty seems to be more in terms of the patient's inability to cope with ordinary problems of living, then a direct approach on the part of the physician may well backfire. The reason for this is that such a directive approach is very apt to be repeating the kind of dominating or controlling relationship that has made such patients unassertive, ineffective, or rebellious in their personality development. Under such circumstances, the physician would do better to be supportively nondirective and, by virtue of such a nondirective relationship, to convey faith in the patient's capacity to eventually become a more autonomous and effectively functioning human being. Such a "corrective emotional relationship" shows a greater respect for the patient's worth and human dignity, and is therefore more apt to encourage a favorable therapeutic response.

THE AUXILIARY USE OF OFFICE PERSONNEL

At times the physician can augment therapeutic efforts by making use of auxiliary personnel from the office staff. This is particularly useful when it is important to mobilize a support system for a patient whose own support system is either crumbling or inadequate. Thus a sympathetic secretary, office nurse, or social worker can often be of great assistance to the physician in making the time-consuming phone calls that are occasionally necessary in order to mobilize help from community resources on behalf of a patient. It is worth noting in this context that an empathic and understanding office assistant makes a substantial contribution to the total psychotherapeutic ambience of the physician's office. Conversely, an abrasive, unsympathetic, or impatient office assistant may have the contrary effect.

THE USE OF DRUGS

The issue of whether or not drugs are indicated, and under what circumstances, is discussed in Chapter 25. The point to be made here is that the use of drugs for the purpose of ameliorating distressful symptoms more rapidly should not be considered a substitute or an alternative to going ahead with a psychotherapeutic effort to help the patient understand the source of personal difficulties and reach better ways of resolving them. To prescribe psychopharmacological agents for the control of symptoms, without attempting to understand and deal with the source of these symptoms, is akin to prescribing medication for pain without treating its underlying causes. For example, Greenblatt and Shader have correctly emphasized that the use of hypnotics without attempting to diagnose the cause of the patient's insomnia constitutes an irrational use of drugs.[6] Accurate diagnosis is particularly important with insomnia because its sources may be either physical or psychological. Thus, hypnotics or sedatives are contraindicated in patients whose insomnia is caused by respiratory insufficiency or hypoxia, while insomnia resulting from somatic pain should be treated by analgesics rather than by hypnotics. Insomnia resulting from depression will often respond more favorably to the use of antidepressant medication than to hypnotics, while insomnia resulting from anxiety may respond more effectively to the use of minor tranquilizers than to the use of hypnotics. Thus, in every instance it is essential to try to determine the cause of the insomnia before proceeding to prescribe a hypnotic (see Chapters 18 and 25).

WHEN TO REFER THE PATIENT TO A PSYCHIATRIST

Finally, under what circumstances should the physician consider referring the patient to a psychiatrist, assuming of course that a psychiatrist is available for referral? Five major circumstances come to mind:

1 One basis for such referral would be a circumstance in which a patient is developing an *acute psychotic reaction.* Such patients are best treated in a psychiatric inpatient situation, in which the entire milieu is set up for such treatment. On the other hand, chronically psychotic individuals, particularly those who are in a state of remission or who are maintaining some kind of homeostatic balance, however precarious, with their environment, can often be managed by the family physician. Such patients require, in addition to their maintenance medication (see Chapter 25), some ongoing emotional support and efforts to see that their outside support system is reasonably adequate. It is with regard to exploring and furthering the latter that a physician's auxiliary office team can often be very helpful.

2 A second reason for referral would be the circumstance of a patient who presents an acute danger of *suicide* (see Chapter 20). Such patients should be referred to a psychiatrist, and in most instances are best treated in a psychiatric inpatient setting.

3 Patients with *severe personality disorders* or *long-standing, severe psychoneurotic patterns,* whose symptoms are not related to specific traumatic stress in the current life situation but instead go back a long way, are usually candidates for long-term psychotherapeutic intervention, and the choice of technique and methodology are best left, in most instances, to a psychiatrist.

4 *Psychosomatic disorders or other emotional difficulties that are failing to respond* to the physician's own psychotherapeutic efforts should, after a reasonable amount of time and effort, either be referred to a psychiatrist for treatment or, at the very least, a consultation should be sought with a psychiatrist to explore the reasons for the lack of progress.

5 One very important factor that can often emerge as an obstacle to a physician's efforts to treat a patient personally is the phenomenon of *countertransference.* This involves an arousal in the physician, in the course of psychotherapeutic work with the patient, of feelings that are irrational or inappropriate, and that are usually based on events in the physician's own past life or on subjective needs unrelated to the patient's welfare. Such feelings might be an emotional overinvolvement with a patient, a temptation to become implicated with the patient erotically, or an inexplicable irritation or resentment toward the patient. This tendency to countertransference exists in all people, and indeed is one of the major reasons why psychiatric treatment is advocated as part of the training of all psychiatrists. It is hardly to be expected or recommended, however, that all physicians should undergo psychiatric treatment in order to minimize such potential in themselves. Nevertheless, the physician should be constantly on the alert for such countertransference manifestations. If the manifestations are recognized, the physician may indeed be able to control them, and continue to work effectively with the patient. On the other hand, if these feelings are getting out of control and are interfering with efforts to help the patient, it would be most advisable to refer that patient to a psychiatrist for treatment.

CONCLUSION

We have learned in psychiatry that one of the most important instruments in the psychotherapeutic process is the personality of the therapist. Physicians must learn to apply their own personalities to the therapeutic styles that are most compatible for them within the kind of framework of understanding that this volume is endeavoring to provide. The process of psychotherapy does not always run smoothly. Faith and patience are no less important for the physician than they are for the appropriately named "patient." Equally important is an awareness of the limitations imposed both by the conditions of the practice and the boundaries of the physician's psychiatric knowledge. When these limitations are exceeded, the physician should have both the wisdom and the humility to refer the patient for appropriate psychiatric therapy or consultation. Nevertheless, the family physician will be gratified by how often significant help can be provided, much more often than might have been anticipated.

REFERENCES

1 Holmes, Thomas H., and Richard H. Rahe: "The Social Readjustment Scale," *J. Psychosom. Res.,* **11**:216, 1967.
2 Marmor, Judd: "The Nature of the Psychotherapeutic Process," in G. Usdin (ed.), *Psychoneurosis and Schizophrenia,* Philadelphia: J.B. Lippincott, 1966, pp. 66–75.
3 Alexander, Franz: "The Scope of Psychotherapy," in F. Alexander and T.M. French (eds.), *Psychoanalytic Therapy,* New York: Ronald Press, 1946, p. 22.
4 Menninger, K.A., and P.S. Holzman: Theory of Psychoanalytic Technique, (2d ed.), New York: Basic Books, 1973, p. 152.
5 Marmor, Judd et al.: *Psychiatrists and Their Patients,* Washington, D.C.: Joint Information Service, 1975, p. 77.
6 _____: *Psychiatrists and Their Patients,* Washington, D.C.: Joint Information Service, 1975, p. 84.
7 Greenblatt, D.J., and R.I. Shader: "The Clinical Choice of Sedative-Hypnotics, *Ann. Int. Med.,* **77**:91–100, 1972.

Chapter 24

Psychiatric Treatment

Jerry M. Lewis, M.D.
Gene Usdin, M.D.

EDITORS' INTRODUCTION

What is it like to be a psychiatric patient? To be anxious, depressed, fearful, or feel you are "going crazy," and be referred to a psychiatrist? Despite your personal physician's reassurance, how does it feel to go to a strange office and meet a new doctor who asks all sorts of questions?

What is it like to be asked to say everything that comes to your mind; to have previously unnoticed connections pointed out between thoughts and feelings, present and past, and intentions and impact? How must it be to discuss for the first time the painful memory of a parent's death, an early seduction, or an embarrassing failure?

What is it like to go to group therapy for the first time? To find a room full of strangers who seem to talk about things you never heard discussed openly before? To have other group members tell you that, although you feel sad, you come across mad? To listen and watch another person sob painfully as he recalls the death of his wife?

What is it like to be referred to a new doctor for treatment of migraine headaches? How must it be to wonder how learning about the temperature of your hand can have anything to do with the headaches? What is it like to try hard to learn a new kind of deep relaxation?

To be a psychiatric patient almost always introduces a number of new experiences. Many of them seem strange; often it appears that one is being asked to do the impossible. The psychiatrist's approach seems very different from that of all the doctors the patient has previously seen. Invariably there is anxiety about the newness, which adds to the symptoms leading to the referral.

The physician who is trained in psychiatry also handles a great deal of complicated data when first seeing a new patient. He or she is partly the detached expert—observing, listening, and searching for patterns in what the patient says. At other moments, however, the psychiatrist is "listening" to the feelings, thoughts, and memories that push into his or her own consciousness. Why does this patient make me feel sad, anxious, or hostile? Why do I find myself remembering a forgotten event as I listen to this depressed man? These questions, and many other data, are synthesized into a formulation of the patient's dilemma that allows treatment to be planned. Should this patient be seen in individual therapy? In group, marital, or family therapy? Should an antidepressive or other medication be used? Is there a suicidal risk? Should the patient be hospitalized? What strengths does the patient have? What are the strengths of the spouse, family, and friends?

In this chapter, the authors introduce the reader to the process of clinical decision making in psychiatry, and present a concise overview of many of the current treatment modalities.

Psychiatric disorders, like all other illnesses, are caused by multiple etiologic factors. Heredity, developmental trauma, family conflict and dysfunction, social stress, hormonal disturbances, alterations in brain chemistry—these and other factors, working in concert, produce clearly defined syndromes. The multiplicity of causation allows many different perspectives. In evaluating a patient, some psychiatrists will focus selectively on one of the causative factors: social stress, developmental trauma, or brain chemistry. As a consequence, the treatment prescribed will be slanted by the psychiatrist's perspective on etiology. That may lead to confusion for the nonpsychiatric physician, who wonders why psychiatrist A treats one middle-aged, depressed man with an antidepressive drug, while psychiatrist B treats a similar patient with individual psychotherapy. The issue, of course, is that both treatments are acceptable approaches, and that the situations in which there are conclusive data about the preferred or most effective treatment are yet to be determined for many psychiatric disorders.

Psychiatric treatment can be divided into two basic groups: the organic or biologic, and the psychologic or psychotherapeutic treatments. Treatments from each of these categories may be used jointly or separately. The status of treatment in psychiatry undergoes continual reassessment, as both clinical work and research provide new concepts, techniques, and therapeutic agents. Historically, however, the recent past has seen a series of significant developments.

Prior to World War II, American psychiatry, for the most part, concerned itself with patients in remote state hospitals who, at best, were treated with kindness, respect, and sedation; at worst, they were treated with dehumanized custodial care. The introduction of both convulsive treatments and insulin therapy provided a fulcrum for the movement toward an active "do something" approach that added to the important concept that severe psychiatric illness could be treated effectively.

Following World War II, there was a dramatic growth in psychoanalysis in this country. The insights into human behavior that psychoanalysis provided were so superior to all that preceded them that there was broad acceptance of the basic psychoanalytic constructs. The importance of the unconscious, the significance of childhood developmental events, the central role of conflict and anxiety, free associations, the therapeutic power of interpretation, and other constructs were incorporated into the mainstream of psychiatric thinking and into the folklore of the culture itself. Psychoanalytic leaders played a prominent role in military psychiatry during that war, and their influence upon young military physicians was considerable. In the ensuing 30 years, there have been ongoing modifications in psychoanalytic theory and technique, and the influence of this perspective continues to play a dominant role in psychiatric thinking.

Another major post-World War II development was the discovery of new psychopharmacologic agents. Starting with chlorpromazine, a number of antipsychotic compounds were developed that have influenced the treatment of many major mental disorders dramatically. Shortly thereafter, a new group of antianxiety drugs were introduced, and these proved valuable in the treatment of anxiety and some of the neurotic disturbances. This was followed by the development of antidepressive medications and, more recently, by the discovery that an older drug, lithium, has a specific role in the treatment of manic-depressive illness.

Each of these important developments gave rise to a renewed hope that a single, specific form of treatment had been found that would cure all forms of mental illness. This hope, of course, has lead to waves of enthusiasm and, often, to unwarranted pronouncements. However, the magnitude of the problem of mental illness, the tremendous amount of human suffering involved, the number of lives shattered, and the economic cost all combine to produce a climate in which there is inevitably the deep and searing wish for a simple, easy, and broadly applicable treatment. The present state of knowledge, however, does not suggest that a powerful "silver bullet" is at hand or on the horizon. Rather, there are a wide variety of therapeutic techniques available, many of them of unusual strength. The mark of the skilled psychiatrist, like that of any skilled physician, is in the fitting of specific treatments to individual patients, based on a careful understanding of the factors involved in each patient's psychiatric disturbance. This individualized approach to each patient is the foundation upon which all psychiatric treatment is based. It underscores the need for a painstaking evaluation of the patient.

THE EVALUATION OF THE PATIENT

A psychiatric evaluation is the process by which the psychiatrist arrives at a diagnosis and a formulation of the factors responsible for the patient's symptoms. It is much more, therefore, than a labeling process. The basic components of the evaluation process include the exploratory interview (see Chapter 1), the psychiatric history (see Chapter 2), the mental status examination (see Chapter 2), physical and neurological examinations, and special studies. The last may include a joint interview with the patient and spouse, an exploratory family interview, psychological tests, and special laboratory procedures.

Through the use of these procedures, the psychiatrist not only arrives at a diagnosis, but obtains data with which to answer a number of questions, including the following:

1 What has been the course of the patient's symptoms? What stressful events or developmental crises appear to play a precipitating role?

2 What is the degree of disability produced by the patient's disorder?

3 What strengths or coping mechanisms does the patient have?

4 What is the intensity of the patient's motivation? What are his or her goals for treatment? Does the patient appear capable and interested in exploring himself or herself?

5 What is the patient's social reality?

6 How supportive or stressful are the significant others in the patient's life?

7 Is there evidence for biologic factors, for example, organic brain disease or hormonal disturbances?

8 Can this patient be treated more effectively in group, marital, or family therapy?

9 Should the patient be treated psychotherapeutically? If so, what type of individual psychotherapy is best suited for this patient?

10 Will the patient benefit from a psychopharmacologic agent? If so, which one?

11 Are there clues as to the risk of suicide or aggression toward others?

12 What helpful role can the family doctor play?

This list is by no means all-inclusive, but perhaps communicates something of the highly individualized nature of the psychiatric evaluation. The answers to these and other questions give psychiatric treatment its form and structure for the individual patient.

With this brief overview of the psychiatrist's approach to the patient in mind, let us turn now to descriptions of the various treatment modalities.

THE PSYCHOTHERAPIES

There is a profusion of specific psychotherapeutic techniques. This, combined with considerable overlapping between techniques and the tendency of most psychiatrists to develop a personal amalgam involving many techniques, often leads the nonpsychiatrist to feel confused about the psychotherapies. There is, however, some order behind the apparently chaotic profusion. To appreciate this, it is necessary to understand the evolution of the four major schools of psychiatry, for each gives rise to specific psychotherapeutic techniques. Havens has clarified this progression.[1]

The oldest school, *objective-descriptive psychiatry,* involves careful observation of the patient, emphasis on symptoms and signs, and above all else, correct diagnosis. The psychiatrist, more the emotionally detached expert than anything else, uses his or her authority to encourage, exhort, and in many other ways direct the patient. The doctor is in complete control of treatment, and therapy is based on a specific diagnosis.

Some current psychotherapies are related clearly to objective-descriptive psychiatry. Much of supportive psychotherapy follows this model. Behavior therapy and hypnosis also can be understood as modern derivatives of this school of psychiatry.

Freud's development of *psychoanalysis* was next, and represented an entirely new direction. Here, the psychoanalyst was the careful monitor of the patient's associations and was detached, neutral, and concerned primarily with making conscious that which had been repressed. Interpretation of resistance, unconscious conflicts, and the intrusion of the past in the form of transference were the techniques designed to separate out and remove the neurotic process. The emphasis was on the patient's psychological mechanisms, conflicts, and relationships with others, rather than on the signs and symptoms of the psychiatric illness.

Psychoanalysis in "pure" or modified form continues to be the major model for the most frequently used forms of individual psychotherapy. It also provides a structure for a form of group psychotherapy called *analytic group therapy.*

Two additional major schools of psychiatry have evolved, both responsive in part to psychoanalysis. *Existential psychiatry,* which is European in its roots, was in part a reaction to what its leaders considered to be psychoanalytic deficiencies. Psychoanalysis, they thought, was too intellectual, too detached, too neutral, too interpretive, too concerned with sexuality, and insufficiently tuned to the central importance of the patient's affect or feelings. For the existential psychotherapist, the major technique was "being" with the patient in all that he or she felt. This major focus on empathy was supplemented by the technique of therapist self-disclosure, with license given to the therapist to share deeply his or her inner world, as long as such sharing seemed to be in the service of "being" with the patient. Psychoanalysts reacted often to this form of psychotherapy as "wild," undisciplined, and chaotic. It is probable, however, that existential psychiatry's emphasis on feelings influenced other schools, including psychoanalysis, to reevaluate the role of affect in psychiatric disturbances.

What some considered to be the freedom suggested by existential psychiatry provided the impetus to the development of a number of newer therapies. Encounter groups, Gestalt therapy, primal therapy, and some forms of psychodrama are representative.

Interpersonal psychiatry, which is the only purely American development, evolved in part as a reaction to the heavy emphasis in psychoanalysis on the role of the past in shaping the present and future. The interpersonal therapist focuses on the patient's hear-and-now relationship style, and attempts to interfere with the patient's distorted ways of responding and relating to the therapist. This here-and-now focus has influenced the development of a number of therapies. Transactional analysis, many forms of group therapy, and family therapy are examples.

It is possible, therefore, to relate most of the newer psychotherapies to one of the major schools, and to understand their emphases, basic theories, and techniques as derivatives of a major school.

There are two basic questions about psychotherapy. The first is, "Does it work?" and the second is "If so, how?" Psychotherapy research has attempted to answer these questions. The question of the effectiveness of psychotherapy has been considered by outcome research. Meltzoff and Kornreich reviewed the outcome-research literature exhaustively, and concluded that over 70 well-designed studies demonstrate that a variety of individual and group therapies are better as contrasted to control groups.[2] The first question is answered positively; outcome research demonstrates the effectiveness of psychotherapy.

The second question, however, is as yet unanswered. Process research—How is psychotherapy effective?—has not resulted in a body of data that demonstrate conclusively what processes make psychotherapy effective.

Psychoanalysis

The word *psychoanalysis* has three different meanings. It is used to describe an official organization comprised of psychoanalysts, a treatment technique, and a school or system of psychology.

The greatest impact of psychoanalysis has been as a school or system of psychology. It has provided an extensive and rich view of human beings and their functioning, and other schools of psychology do not begin to compare with it. Beginning with Freud's discoveries, a series of psychoanalysts have continued to elaborate theoretical constructs from clinical observations. There have been disagreements, and splinter groups have developed, usually by following an outstanding leader. Despite this splintering, psychoanalysis has provided psychiatry with a comprehensive model of intrapsychic life in humans. The unconscious, the impact of childhood development upon adult life, the constructs of conflict and anxiety, the elaboration of psychological defense mechanisms, the study of object relationships, the importance of dream life—all these, and many more, have sprung from psychoanalysis. Most of what has come to be known as dynamic psychiatry, or psychodynamics, is attributed directly to psychoanalysis.

As a therapeutic technique, psychoanalysis has made an indelible imprint on the development of psychotherapy. The concepts of free association, resistances, interpretation, transference and countertransference, insight, and working through are but a few treatment fundamentals that, in one form or another, have been incorporated into the major body of psychotherapeutic work.

As a treatment technique, psychoanalysis has continued to evolve. Fundamentally, the patient is encouraged to free-associate, and the psychoanalyst, who is seated behind the couch, listens attentively to the patient's associations, and notes in particular the resistances to the flow of associative material. These resistances are pointed out to the patient, and an effort is made to clear the way for the emergence of repressed feelings, early memories, and other mental material about which the patient has been unaware. The analyst's relative inactivity and neutrality encourage the patient to project feelings and conflicts having to do with important individuals from early life onto the analyst. The clarification and working through of this transferred material is an essential part of psychoanalysis.

Early in the development of psychoanalysis, it was felt that the crucial process involved in cure or resolution of the patient's neurosis was the patient's increased understanding of himself or herself, which was termed "insight." Although this aspect of treatment continues to be an important element, there is perhaps less certainty about its central role. Some psychoanalysts, for example, have stressed the importance of the patient's emotional experience with the analyst as one that clarifies and corrects conflicts arising from earlier relationships.

Psychoanalytic training is separate from, and in addition to, the physician's residency training in psychiatry. It occurs at one of the approved psychoanalytic institutes, and includes course work on theory, technique, and analyzing, with close supervision, a small number of "control cases." A central aspect of the psychoanalyst's training is his or her own analysis, which must be done by a senior psychoanalyst designated as a "training psychoanalyst."

As a treatment technique, psychoanalysis has been criticized for being lengthy (four or five sessions per week for several years or longer). Those people who are sensitive to the high prevalence of emotional disturbance in the general population have pointed out that psychoanalysis can help only a tiny fraction of such people and that this fraction will be exclusively from the more affluent segments. This view is of course correct, but underestimates the value of the extrapolation from what is learned in the intensive work of psychoanalysis to other treatment modalities.

Although the specific indications for psychoanalytic treatment are unclear, it appears that patients with lesser and moderate disturbances, such as neuroses and some personality disorders, form a group that is particularly suitable for this intensive and demanding treatment.

Individual Psychotherapy

Marmor (Chapter 23) has outlined the essentials of individual psychotherapy for the nonpsychiatric physician, and stressed the multiplicity of factors that account for its effectiveness. That material will not be repeated; rather, the varieties of psychotherapy, as practiced by psychiatrists, will be described briefly.

Supportive Psychotherapy This form of psychotherapy is characterized by less frequent sessions (once a week or, more likely, once every several weeks). The psychiatrist plays a more active role and, in addition to the techniques of more intensive psychotherapy, encourages, suggests, offers advice, disapproves, offers approval, and in many ways directs the patient. It is, of course, based on a relationship of trust and confidence, but the psychiatrist does presume that he or she "knows what is best" for the patient, and is willing to accept the responsibility for playing an important role in the management of the patient's life. There is little sustained effort to help the patient develop anything but superficial insight. The therapist-patient relationship is generally not talked about or explored. The therapist uses his or her own personality strengths, problem-solving abilities, and reality testing. It is these features of supportive psychotherapy that make it much like counseling, and the work done by other professionals.

The danger of supportive psychotherapy is that it may preclude the patient's growth and development of skills, and may produce instead a dependent, childlike relationship with the therapist. For this reason, supportive psychotherapy should not be offered to a patient without a painstaking appraisal of the severity of the patient's disorder, its chronicity, and the patient's personality strengths. For very disabled patients, however, this type of therapy may bring order into a chaotic life and prevent further decompensation or regression. There are some psychotherapists who insist that supportive psychotherapy should not be offered unless a trial of more intensive exploratory therapy has failed. At the minimum, however, supportive psychotherapy should be a carefully considered modality of treatment.

Exploratory or Intensive Psychotherapy   This type of psychotherapy can be seen in many ways to occupy a position between psychoanalysis and supportive psychotherapy. It is the most frequent therapeutic activity of many psychiatrists and some psychoanalysts. The patient is seen one to three times a week, and the goals of the treatment are to produce relief from symptoms and basic changes in the patient's pattern of relationships with others. The goals of this form of therapy, which include basic change in some dimensions of the patient's personality, distinguish it from supportive psychotherapy.

Much of what transpires in this type of psychotherapy is exploratory in the sense that the therapist uses a number of techniques to assist the patient to explore previously unrecognized feelings, conflicts, and memories. Insight is one of the major goals. Therapeutic techniques include following trains of associations, empathic responsiveness, clarification, confrontation, interpretation, and other techniques derived from psychoanalysis. The patient's resistances to exploration are clarified. However, in contrast to psychoanalysis, transference material is usually clarified and interpreted as it arises, in an effort to avoid the development of what is called a transference neurosis. *Transference* is the pervasive tendency to project feelings and conflicts from early, important people to current relationships. A *transference neurosis* is the patient's projection of all aspects of a conflicted early relationship to the analyst. Psychoanalysis encourages the development of a transference neurosis and its subsequent resolution. In intensive psychotherapy, a transference neurosis is not encouraged, although it may develop. This is an important distinction between intensive psychotherapy and psychoanalysis.

The psychotherapist is generally more active in intensive psychotherapy than in psychoanalysis, but less so than in supportive psychotherapy. He or she does not want a decisive, managerial role in the patient's life, but encourages the growth of the patient's strengths and coping abilities. Since many people want advice, answers, and direction, and are accustomed to receiving it from other physicians, the psychotherapist often frustrates the patient by being unwilling to play that role. The patient's feelings of disappointment are, however, explored, and often form the basis for explorations into earlier relationships involving disappointment.

In intensive psychotherapy the psychotherapist attempts to develop a collaborative relationship (see Chapter 1) with the patient, a relationship in which the patient may come to experience his or her own strengths and abilities. This contrasts with the nature of the therapeutic relationship in supportive psychotherapy, where the therapist may assume a much more powerful position.

An important aspect of intensive psychotherapy is the therapist's use of his or her feelings, thoughts, and life experiences. These are particularly important in the development of the ability to be empathic, to place oneself in the patient's situation. The therapist's recognition of idiosyncratic responses to the patient, which often result from memory traces of the therapist's earlier relationships (countertransference), is important. If recognized and thought through, this material can be used to understand the patient's problems better.

Intensive psychotherapy involves the therapist in repeatedly moving from "being with" the patient, as in moments of empathy, to a more detached, analyzing, "what is the meaning of this" position. These moment-to-moment alterations in the way in which the therapist experiences the patient and their relationship are a central part of learning to be a therapist.[3]

Most psychiatrists who do intensive psychotherapy evolve a personal amalgam of techniques. Although the general model may be more psychoanalytic than anything else, techniques from existential psychiatry and interpersonal psychiatry, as well as some of their derivatives (transactional analysis and Gestalt therapy) are frequently included. At the core, however, the psychotherapist must have the capacity for both intimate and disciplined relating. It is often taxing and exhausting work. The growth of the patient is often slow, and considerable patience is required. Strupp has remarked that psychotherapy's focus on the individual patient and his or her needs, feelings, and experiences is an oasis of individualism in an increasingly collectivistic society.[4]

Intensive psychotherapy has broader indications than either psychoanalysis or supportive psychotherapy. Patients with lesser disturbances, such as the neuroses, are treated effectively by means of intensive psychotherapy, but it is also important in the treatment of severe psychiatric disorders. Although its usefulness in the treatment of schizophrenia and other psychoses is questioned by some, others feel it is the cornerstone of effective treatment, and that psychopharmacologic approaches are but important adjuncts. Intensive psychotherapy is the only approach currently available for the treatment of the more severe personality disorders.

The most frequent criticism of intensive psychotherapy is that it is time-consuming, slow, and expensive. The critics point out that lower-income groups seldom receive intensive psychotherapy. The basic problem seems to be social, and to involve the distribution of this country's resources. The dream behind the community mental health movement, the provision of quality mental health care to lower-income groups, has, depending upon the perspective, achieved only limited reality or none at all. There is, unfortunately, little to suggest that many patients in community mental health centers receive highly individualized, intensive forms of psychotherapy.

Group Psychotherapy

Group psychotherapy has wide applicability and a continuously expanding number of indications. The community mental health clinics and innovative newer psychotherapies have found group therapy highly useful. In addition, experience and careful study have markedly increased our knowledge of how and when group therapy is helpful, as well as introducing new techniques. In more recent years, group therapy principles have found broad application in dealing with many chronic physical disorders (for example, dialysis, cancer, colostomy, ulcerative colitis, diabetes), juvenile delinquency, and drug abuse. They have extended into everyday problems of parenting, executive management, and personnel interworkings. Group therapy has been used in treating eating disorders, smoking, and alcoholism. It has been used in large institutions for dealing with ward management, with patients' relatives, with schizophrenics, and with patients who have other mental disorders. Actually, it is likely that a basic healing mechanism behind Alcoholics Anonymous is that of group dynamics. Business executives have used T or sensitivity groups to understand themselves better and to function more effectively. Unfortunately, group therapy has experienced more than its share of misuse, with inexperienced, unknowledgeable nonprofessionals frequently conducting it. Sometimes through personal charisma, they become successful in developing groups and in exerting considerable influence on the individual members of the groups.

Ideally, group therapy involves a trained therapist's treatment of carefully selected people who meet regularly to help one another effect personality changes. Most early group leaders worked within a psychodynamic framework, but more recently, interactional or experiential groups have become popular. This section will concern itself only with groups that include patients with physical or emotional disorders.

The therapist is the most important member of the group, with responsibility for:

1 Carefully selecting group members, that is, determining suitability of the patient for the group, as well as of the group for the patient
2 Determining the frequency and length of sessions
3 Deciding whether the group will or will not admit new patients (closed or open-ended groups)
4 Deciding whether or not the group will be time-limited insofar as the number of sessions are concerned

5 Deciding when a patient may be discharged from the group (some suggest that this should be based on a joint opinion of the therapist, the member involved, and the other group members)
6 Being the group leader

In psychodynamic groups, the therapist is relatively passive, and functions as a screen on which group members can project their thoughts and feelings. The therapist essentially controls the members as minimally as possible, and is primarily a facilitator. He or she may be looked upon as a catalyst for group interaction, with the group members themselves being the source of change and cure. Groups develop an esprit de corps and, with the mechanisms of social reinforcement and consensual validation, members can develop increased self-reliance. Patients have a unique opportunity to learn about their interpersonal impact upon others. This type of social feedback appears especially important in a cohesive group that is experienced as basically caring and supportive.

At times, the therapist helps members to focus on pertinent problems and situations, and to avoid irrelevant material. There may be a need to point out connections between the present and earlier periods of life. If the group becomes nonproductive, the therapist may have to stimulate the discussion by attempting to help the group understand the reasons for the nonproductiveness.

In many experiential groups, the therapist may have a different role, and may no longer be only a facilitator. Now he or she may be an active participant who is directing the group, provoking, interacting, overtly experiencing and, at times, setting up roles. In some groups, the therapist actively criticizes and is criticized. Various degrees of emotional reactions may be elicited through touching or feeling in some experiential groups. This should be carefully considered and is not the usual technique. In the "here-and-now" therapies, interpretation or intellectualization is minimized. The emphasis is on the present and, especially, current feelings.

Structural Organization Groups may have as few as 3 or as many as 15 members. Most therapists consider about 8 members to be optimal. Too few members may not be productive of enough interaction, and the ratio of patients to therapist is too small. With larger groups, members may not have enough opportunity to talk about personal conflicts, and may also withhold or retreat readily. However, in some situations (for example, ward management, drug regulation, and chronic illness), the groups may be much larger. There is some question whether this can be considered group therapy.

Most groups are conducted on a weekly basis, but this is not necessarily so. Especially with inpatient groups, the sessions may be more frequent. Sometimes there is a system of alternate sessions in which the group meets twice weekly, once with and once without the therapist. In a time of crisis for a group member or the group as a whole, an extra meeting may be indicated. Group sessions usually are of 1 to 2 hours in duration, with the average length being $1\frac{1}{2}$ hours. The time limit should be constant to help teach the setting of limits and to help avoid manipulation by group members. In the past 8 years, there has emerged a prolonged type of group therapy (usually termed *marathon group therapy*), in which the group may meet continuously for periods ranging up to 6 days.

Indications for Group Therapy   There are definite indications for group therapy, which at times make it more beneficial than other forms of therapy for the patient. At other times, it may be combined with individual psychotherapy or pharmacotherapy. Unfortunately, group psychotherapy is used too often for the sake of expediency. That is, unavailability of personal, individual, or other forms of therapy, or the fact that it is less expensive than other forms of therapy, frequently influences the choice of group therapy unduly.

What are some of the advantages of group psychotherapy?

1   Members of the group may receive needed interpersonal support.

2   The group can re-create a family surrogate situation for patients, so that they can receive "family" input and rework some of their earlier family conflicts as well as their present ones.

3   Members may become less intolerant of deviations from "normal" in others and in themselves.

4   Hearing others discuss suppressed material may enable a patient to bring up the same inner conflicts.

5   Receiving insight from peers (group members) may be more helpful than receiving interpretations or insights from seers (the therapist).

6   Members can learn to give and take positive and negative thoughts and feelings from others in a controlled situation.

7   In time, members may develop a sense of trust and come to rely on the group as a whole.

8   A group may help the member with reality testing, since the member's perceptions are subject to consensual validation or invalidation by other group members.

9   Transference feelings may be developed, noted, and possibly resolved. This transference may be to the therapist, to other members, or to the group as a whole.

10   Members may experience a closeness, connectedness, and intimacy never before experienced. Observing others risk such closeness without destructive impact may provide the impetus for a patient to chance such an experience. This may be a "first" for the patient.

11   There is group pressure to improve and to change, without the therapist's assuming a directive role. In this way, there may be less of an attempt to please a parental surrogate.

12   Abreaction with more intense emotions may occur because of a group setting and permission from one's peers.

13   Intellectual understanding may be augmented by emotional experiences in the group in ways that are often not possible in individual therapy.

At this time, group therapy is utilized increasingly in nonpsychiatric situations. As previously noted, it may be helpful with chronic physical disorders. Group therapy has also been helpful with the relatives of patients who are seeing physicians.

Physicians who desire to improve their capacity or to develop an ability for group therapy may find it helpful to do considerable reading in this field, and to become a member of a group. At other times, there are opportunities to be cotherapist with an experienced therapist. Many nonpsychiatric physicians have good "psychologicalmindedness," whereby the development of group therapy skills is not difficult.

There are conflicting opinions about the specific indications and contra-indications of group therapy for the various psychiatric syndromes. Many group therapists perceive it as a broadly applicable treatment technique. Others consider it most useful for patients who have pronounced interpersonal difficulties. Many consider the presence of a gross or incipient psychosis or severe, manipulative personality disorder a contraindication. Neurotic patients and those with mild or moderate personality disturbances are considered the most favorable candidates for a positive therapeutic effect.

Family, Marital, and Sexual Therapies

Innovations in family, marital, and sexual therapies are presented in Chapters 4, 26, 27, and 28. They are more recent developments, and have been more significantly incorporated into the main body of psychiatry than have most of the newer therapeutic modalities.

Family and marital therapies are based on the concept that in some clinical situations the important or central problem is in the marital relationship or in the entire family system. This type of treatment focuses more clearly on the ongoing relationship, rather than on the individual's intrapsychic problems. As a consequence, in properly selected instances, change can be effected more quickly and economically. These therapeutic modalities have great strength but, at the present time, there is little carefully controlled outcome research to demonstrate their effectiveness. Currently, however, a number of psychiatric residency programs are training psychiatrists in individual, marital, and family therapy (as well as in group therapy). This generation of psychiatrists will be able to fit the treatment to the clinical situation more effectively than earlier psychiatrists who, for the most part, were trained only in individual psychotherapy.

Sexual therapy continues to be a rapidly changing field. Starting with the work of Masters and Johnson [5,6] and, more recently, of Kaplan,[7] the current trend is to include both the experiential, educational components and the treatment of the nonsexual aspects of the couple's relationship (see Chapter 28). An increasing number of psychiatric training programs are offering residents introductory training in sexual therapy, but most reliable training still occurs in a few established sexual therapy centers.

PSYCHIATRIC HOSPITALIZATION

There has been an unfortunate tendency in some circles to equate all psychiatric hospitalization with long-term, essentially custodial care. Despite this tendency, there has been a significant growth in the number of psychiatric units in general hospitals and in the number of free-standing psychiatric hospitals.

It is useful to think in terms of three types of hospitalization for active treatment. These are short-term (up to 30 days), intermediate (30 to 90 days), and long-term (over 90 days). Short-term hospitalization occurs most often in psychiatric units of general hospitals. Its emphasis is on crisis resolution, and several types of patients are commonly treated—the individual with an acute, severe psychiatric disturbance, and the chronically ill patient who has undergone a sudden further decompensation. Also admitted are patients who present difficult diagnostic problems or management problems to general medical and surgical units. Patients who have made unsuccessful suicide attempts, or who represent suicidal or homicidal problems, are another group. Although there are differences, in many short-term units the major treatment modality is psychopharmacologic in nature. Often the psychiatrist is able to form an effective relationship with the patient, which then becomes the basis for continuing outpatient treatment.

Intermediate hospitalization occurs often, both in psychiatric units in general hospitals and in free-standing psychiatric hospitals. Here the emphasis is apt to be both on psychopharmacologic and psychotherapeutic treatment. Often treated are patients who have the same type of disturbances as those treated with short-term hospitalization. They have, however, failed to respond to the crisis-oriented brief hospitalization, and are unable to move back into the community without further treatment.

Long-term active treatment most often is accomplished in free-standing psychiatric hospitals. The patients admitted fall into several groups. One group includes treatment failures from short-term or intermediate hospitalization, who continue to be disabled significantly by their disorders. A second group are patients who have severe psychiatric disorders that are not amenable to psychopharmacologic approaches, and who are unable to adjust or survive outside a hospital. Many of these patients have severe personality disorders or chronic psychotic conditions. Treatment is pluralistic in the sense that psychopharmacologic drugs are often used, but the major emphasis is most often on intensive psychotherapy and milieu therapy. *Milieu therapy* is the structuring of the patient's entire day with potentially therapeutic experiences. The ward or unit treatment team provides support and confrontation regarding the patient's behavior, such special activities as psychodrama and group discussions are provided, and patients are encouraged to provide each other with feedback about their behavior.

The appropriate use of psychiatric hospitalization can be seen as a series of interventions. If hospitalization is required, it is well to consider the possibility of short-term care. If the patient does not respond, the next step might be intermediate care. For some, however, treatment will have to include long-term, active, inpatient care. Occasionally, the psychiatrist knows the condition of the patient well enough to move directly to intermediate or long-term hospitalization.

Another related development is the day care or partial hospitalization concept. Patients go to such facilities for part or all of each day, and spend nights at home. During the day, patients are involved in numerous therapeutic activities. Some authorities see this concept as replacing all psychiatric hospitals, but most feel that it is a complementary treatment modality with specific indications and usefulness for some, but not all, patients who otherwise would require hospitalization.

Despite the economic forces mobilized in some states to close hospitals and treat all patients in their home communities, there continues to be a need for custodial care. With a few patients, it is humane to reevaluate repetitious and failing treatments, and to provide the patient with a kind, respectful environment where there will no longer be pressure from treatment efforts. Such decisions must be considered carefully, but are applicable for a few patients with chronic, severe disorders, where all treatment has failed. Doing away with all custodial hospitals has resulted in the "dumping" of patients into communities that neither want nor care for them. Some such patients lead lives of great isolation, deprivation, and loneliness, little of which is helped by the notion that they are "in the community."

PSYCHODRAMA

Psychodrama derives from group therapy, and its founder is considered to be Moreno. It has been modified by different psychological schools. Its basic tenet is that the acting of a role within a group, with a director (therapist) who constantly instructs group members about their roles, helps correct the patient's pathological patterns and may provide a corrective emotional experience with insight that would be unobtainable through merely verbal means. Soliloquies, role playing, and role reversal are some of the techniques used. Because of the necessity for a cast, psychodrama is utilized most often in hospitals or in partial hospitalization programs.

HYPNOTHERAPY

Hypnosis involves inducing a state of hypersuggestability. Therapeutically, it is used for accelerating the relating of information and securing more compliance from the patient. At the present time, hypnotherapy seems to find its greatest usefulness in some patients with such habit disturbances as overeating or smoking. Although the hypnotized patient usually appears to be in various levels of sleep, the patient's concentration is focused acutely on listening and relating to the hypnotist. In deep hypnosis, the patient submits executive control, and regresses to a dissociated state. Peripheral awareness is markedly reduced.

Not all people are hypnotizable, and the degree of hypnotizability (the level of the trance state) varies markedly in individuals. Hypnosis should not be used casually, although it often is. More pertinently, hypnotherapy should be used only with carefully selected patients and with specific goals in mind.

Hypnosis may help through aberaction, but at times complex exploration with direct suggestions may be necessary. Often, just suggesting increased memory recall may result in the emergence of emotionally charged, previously repressed material. Hypnosis, while surprisingly easy to do, should be utilized carefully, and those wishing to use it should take courses and do considerable reading to be aware of the indications, techniques for evaluating and performing hypnosis, the precautions, and contraindications.

BIOFEEDBACK

Biofeedback is a relatively new treatment modality that is useful in a variety of disorders. The method involves recording with electronic instrumentation, which simultaneously provides the patient with an external signal reflecting an internal physiologic process. Given the opportunity to recognize and identify certain bodily states (for example, brain waves, heart rate, and skin temperature), the patient can learn to modify functions that were previously considered involuntary.

Biofeedback has enjoyed much success in teaching patients to recognize and modify the physical states associated with anxiety. The patient's learned ability to monitor physiologic reactions has also proven to be a valuable tool in managing aspects of certain physical diseases, apart from anxiety. Biofeedback has proven to be a significant addition to the armamentarium in the management of muscular, paralytic, and spastic disorders, some cardiac arrhythmias, uterine and intestinal contractions, some peripheral vascular diseases, hypertension, and especially tension and migraine headaches.

Although only slightly over 10 years in clinical usage, biofeedback shows great promise of being valuable in the diagnosis and treatment of many medical conditions. It is apt to become a routine medical treatment in the offices of many nonpsychiatrists. Like many new procedures, its full impact is yet to be realized.

BEHAVIOR THERAPY

Behavior therapy, or behavior modification, is the use of the principles of learning theory to treat a variety of behavior disorders. Its fundamental premise is that behavior is caused or maintained by environmental events, and thus can be modified by systematic manipulation of responses to the behavior. It is based upon a thorough analysis of the behavior in question, which describes it in terms that are as quantitative as possible (for example, frequency, degree, amount). The analysis of the behavior is based only on what is directly observable, and attempts to understand the behavior in terms of its dynamic meaning are not a part of the treatment process.

A central technique of behavior therapy is systematic desensitization. This technique is used when it is determined that the patient's anxiety is precipitated by specific situations or objects (for example, heights or snakes). The patient and therapist construct a list of imaginary scenes, starting with those that produce mild anxiety and extending to those associated with severe anxiety. Next the patient is taught a deep form of muscular relaxation. When this is learned, the patient is asked to imagine a mild anxiety-producing scene. The deep state of muscular relaxation is antithetical to the experience of anxiety or, at the minimum, blunts the reaction. When a mild anxiety-producing scene can be imagined without anxiety, the next and more severe imaginary scene is dealt with. The pairing of the anxiety-inducing scene and deep muscular relaxation is considered the means by which the anxiety is deconditioned. The patient is encouraged to enter between sessions the actual anxiety-producing situations that have been imagined during the treatment session, and receives strong positive reinforcement from the therapist for doing so.

This form of treatment is useful in some situations where the factors precipitating the patient's anxiety can be identified clearly. Some patients with psychophysiologic reactions, well-defined phobias, and certain sexual problems have benefited. In other patients, however, the desensitization alone is insufficient, and relief may be obtained by combining it with psychotherapy or psychopharmacologic agents.

The use of operant conditioning in the form of positive reinforcement is found in certain aspects of milieu therapy, token economies (for example, weekend passes from the hospital in reward for increased participation in group therapy), and the treatment of isolated neurotic symptoms. In each of these forms of treatment, the pathologic behavior is disregarded, and nonpathologic behavior is rewarded with staff attention, tokens with which desirable privileges can be purchased, or other positive reinforcement. Another example of positive reinforcement occurs in some forms of marital therapy, where each partner is taught to reward the other's positive or pleasing behavior rather than responding negatively to displeasing behavior.

The use of behavior therapy is growing in psychiatry and, although much work needs to be done and controlled outcome studies need to be elaborated, the techniques hold much promise for well-selected patients. The concern that such techniques would be curing symptoms without approaching underlying problems, a view held by many dynamic psychiatrists, has, to a large extent, proved groundless.

NEWER THERAPIES

In the past two decades, there has been a broad profusion of the newer therapies. Most of these have taken their roots outside the mainstream of psychiatry, and are derivatives of either existential or interpersonal schools of thought. Most stress "here-and-now" reactions. Each has its enthusiastic adherents, usually a vigorous originator, and offshoots. Two important factors regarding these newer therapies are: (1) The fact of their acceptance by a considerable number of people who are searching for personal change or answers says something about our culture's failing to provide satisfaction and meaning to many. (2) The second point is that, although some people are undoubtedly helped, there is a lack of systematic attempts to assess the effectiveness of these therapies. There is considerable potential for harm.

These therapies are often led by individuals who have little training or understanding of human behavior, and who frequently accept all clients or patients who apply. Many of these newer therapies have had but a brief period of prominence, and soon fade into oblivion. Others persist, and certainly help some, or their techniques become incorporated into a movement generally called the *human potential movement*. Several, however, have had some apparently lasting impact on the mainstream of psychiatry, often by providing techniques or logical constructs.

Transactional Analysis

Transactional analysis, which was developed in the mid-1950s, originally was used as an adjunct to group psychotherapy. It has continued to enjoy great popularity, especially among nonprofessionals. A large portion of this popularity is attributable to several popular books that have achieved a broad readership.

Transactional analysis's founder, Berne, was a classical psychoanalyst who was influenced by the avant garde group therapies, rejected the Freudian treatment model, and developed a treatment system that he believed was easy to understand, faster, and therefore less costly to the patient.[8,9] A medical background is considered unnecessary. There now are a number of transactional analysis institutes in this country, with many of their graduates (or readers of the books) applying transactional analysis in their daily living. Berne had a relatively simplified three-layer strata of ego states: the child, the adult, and the parent. The child ego state represents archaic elements that were fixed in early childhood but remain operative throughout life. This state is considered to be dynamic, conscious, readily observable, intuitive, and greatly influential in determining our behavior. It is imaginative, creative, essentially uninhibited, and pleasure-seeking.

The adult state possesses the rational thinking component and thus decreases the effectiveness of the child state. Likewise, the parent state, with its directive, ethical, moral, often prejudicial manner, often hampers what Berne considered crucial in ego functioning, the intuitive assets of the child.

The important concepts in this modality concern the terms transactions, games, strokes, strips, and contracts. Considerable attention is paid to nonverbal communication, including expression, movements, and pauses.

A transaction is a stimulus-response reaction from the ego state of one person to another. The communication may be manifest or latent. In a complementary transaction, the communication is from one state of a person to the same state in another, for example, child to child or adult to adult. In a crossed transaction, communication is between different states (see Figure 25-1).

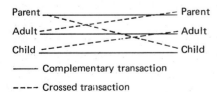

——— Complementary transaction

- - - - Crossed transaction   **Figure 25-1.**

Communication may continue indefinitely in a complementary transaction, but ceases immediately in crossed ones.

Games   Throughout life, people learn *game* patterns. Many individuals learn them early in childhood, but continue the game patterns throughout life, destructively and repetitively. Berne provided a clever group of readily recognized game vignettes in which pathological themes were played. The therapist proposes oppositional moves to alter the patient's customary game playing.

Strokes   *Strokes* are the positive and negative feelings or thoughts we receive from others. Strokes guide behavior, and the therapeutic goal is to make the patient aware of them and their effect. There can be a stroke or stimulus deficit, which can lead to increased game playing and bizarre behavior.

Scripts   Some game plans are developed by transactions in early childhood (for example, the need to achieve, to please parents) and are often passed from generation to generation. A *script* is a mini-story that someone else has written for us, which we follow but which may need to be changed.

Contracts   Transactional analysis uses *contracts,* which are directive agreements that the patient accepts from the therapist. The contract may be simple, and usually involves agreement of the patient to break up at least one part of the patient's usual script or game plan (for example, not to be lured into lengthy arguments with one's spouse about anger concerning in-laws).

In essence, transactional analysis provides a framework or system for understanding human functioning with a minimum of jargon (except for its own simple concepts). It gives many the security of believing that they have a handle on their problems.

Gestalt Therapy

Gestalt therapy evolved from the principles of Gestalt psychology in early twentieth-century Germany. Gestalt therapy is a "here-and-now," self-oriented therapy emphasizing humanistic and holistic views. Authenticity, experimentation, self-enhancement, directness, and openness, with a sharing of innermost feelings and thoughts, are emphasized. Taking care of oneself is to lead ultimately to the benefit of all. The immediate experience is stressed, and the immediate goal is the restoration of unobscured, full awareness by the patient. Emphasis is not on the why of actions, but on the how of actions. One deals with one's most pressing need (gestalt) and, as that need is resolved, the next most pressing need is to come forth, which permits an ever-expanding accretion of new life experiences (growth).

The therapist is active in combating the patient's attempts to avoid problems and to use the therapist as a dependency-enhancing support. Basically, confrontation and frustration, as well as support for autonomy and authenticity, are considered crucial in promoting personal growth.

At times, the therapist discloses his or her own immediate reactions to the patient, and this becomes very important. Dreams are used not for interpretation, but to be relived during the session—to be acted out by role playing of people as well as objects.

It is easy to recognize that Gestalt therapy can be highly charged emotionally, and can involve many open, direct interpersonal reactions as well as role playing aberactions. The patient takes full responsibility for his or her own feelings, thoughts, and actions. It is interesting to note that Alcoholics Anonymous emphasizes the same basic principle of personal responsibility; that is, the alcoholic, in taking a glass or bottle to his or her lips, is personally responsible—not the mate, job, good or bad news, or fate.

It is easy to recognize the relationship and role that Gestalt therapy has played in the development of transactional analysis and the interrelations between Gestalt and other existential psychotherapies.

ORGANIC TREATMENTS

The organic treatments occupied a major role in psychiatry prior to World War II. They were supplanted by the various psychotherapies in the years after the war, and by the development of psychopharmacology in the years since the 1950s. Currently, the psychotherapies and psychopharmacology are the two major treatment modalities.

Psychopharmacology (see Chapter 25) has provided psychiatry with a wide spectrum of effective treatment agents and, to a considerable extent, has replaced the older organic treatments. There is, however, a place for several of the organic treatments in carefully selected patients.

Electroshock

In this form of treatment, a current of electricity is passed briefly between two electrodes placed laterally on the forehead. Under usual circumstances, the patient is administered a short-acting barbiturate anesthetic and a muscle relaxant intravenously, immediately prior to the electroshock treatment. There is both a tonic and clonic phase to the patient's response and, upon regaining consciousness, the patient is usually amnesic for the treatment. Proponents of the use of unilateral electroshock (administered to the nondominant hemisphere) emphasize that fewer side effects occur and that the treatment is as effective as bilateral electroshock. Unilateral electroshock is the more prevalent form of electroshock in England but not in the United States, although its use has been steadily increasing.

A series of treatments is administered, usually given 3 or 4 days each week. The number of individual treatments in a series varies with the patient and the nature of the disorder being treated. Some patients respond to as few as 4 treatments, but many require 12 to 15.

Electroshock is useful in the treatment of severe depression, where it can be life-saving. It has also been effective in treating some patients with severe manic disturbances in which the patient may become exhausted to the point of endangering life. It has also found some use in the treatment of acute, agitated schizophrenic disorders, although here it is being replaced by other treatment modalities. Currently, however, most patients with severe depression are treated with antidepressive agents and psychotherapy. The question of the use of electroshock in such patients arises when the patient does not respond to either tricyclic and monoamine oxidase inhibitors or psychotherapy, and continues to pose a grave suicidal risk.

The effectiveness of lithium in manic-depressive disorders has distinctly diminished the indications for electroshock in severe manic disorders. Occasionally, however, a patient will not respond to or tolerate lithium, and is inaccessible to psychotherapy. Under such circumstances, electroshock should be considered.

Electroshock has been criticized by some as producing permanent brain damage. The evidence for this is conflicting at this time. Many clinicians feel that when it is administered in moderate amounts (up to 12 or 15 treatments), the associated confusion and memory loss clear rapidly. Part of the problem is that the mechanism of action is unknown, and much folklore is based on the erroneous notion that the treatment helps by producing memory impairment.

There have been some attempts in several states to outlaw electroshock as but one form of what some critics call "psychiatric assault." This is unfortunate for, although like most treatment modalities it can be misused, it has helped many patients and remains, in a few instances, a life-saving procedure.

Psychosurgery

Psychosurgery is the attempt to alleviate symptoms of certain mental disorders by the direct destruction of brain tissue. During the past several years, it has been outlawed in several states as a result of the activity of groups of laypersons concerned about its misuse. A recent federal commission addressed the issue as one part of its report, and found no evidence to substantiate that concern. During the 1940s, however, the early psychosurgery procedures were practiced on many patients without sufficient evaluation; these procedures were relatively crude, and resulted in considerable destruction of brain tissue.

Occasionally, the procedure is undertaken for the relief of intractable pain. In addition, 400 to 500 patients with mental illness are operated on each year. These patients are suffering primarily from severe treatment-resistance anxiety that disables them; the procedure is considered a "treatment of last resort." The newer techniques allow precise localization of the tissue to be destroyed, and do not result in the broader tissue destruction of the earlier procedures.

The issue appears to be whether a procedure should be allowed that is helpful to a small group of patients with disabling symptoms when they are unresponsive to other treatment, or whether the concern regarding its potential for misuse should preclude its limited use. Assuming its continued use, a second question concerns the nature of the safeguards to be established regarding its use. At the present time, the future of psychosurgery for mental illness is uncertain.

Other Organic Treatments

There is a small group of little-used procedures that, at this point in time, are mostly of historical interest. Insulin treatments were of two types: *insulin coma* for schizophrenia and *subcoma insulin* for anxiety states. The use of insulin in these conditions had no etiologic implications, but represented, in addition to electroshock, another facet of the movement to treat mental illness actively and vigorously. Some patients were benefited, but it was not established whether this resulted from the intensive nursing care associated with the treatment, a placebo effect, or some not-understood pharmacologic action.

Carbon dioxide treatments enjoyed a brief vogue as a form of convulsive treatment. Earlier, prolonged sleep was used to treat severe mental illness. These, and other forms of treatment, were never subjected to rigorous, controlled evaluation, and have passed from the scene.

CONCLUSION

In this chapter, many of the forms of psychiatric treatment have been described. Often, the individual patient is treated with a combination of treatment approaches. At the core of psychiatric treatment, however, is the belief that each patient's treatment must be based on as complete an understanding as possible of the biologic, developmental, family, and social factors that together produce a disorder in the individual patient.

REFERENCES

1 Havens, Leston L.: *Approaches to the Mind: Movement of the Psychiatric Schools from Sects toward Science,* Boston: Little, Brown, 1973.
2 Meltzoff, Julian, and Melvin Kornreich: *Research in Psychotherapy,* New York: Atherton Press, 1970.
3 Lewis, Jerry M.: *To Be a Therapist: The Teaching and Learning,* New York: Brunner/Mazel, 1978.
4 Strupp, Hans H.: *Psychotherapy: Clinical, Research, and Theoretical Issues,* New York: Jason Aronson, 1973.
5 Masters, William H., and Virginia E. Johnson: *Human Sexual Response,* Boston: Little, Brown, 1970.
6 Masters, William H., and Virginia E. Johnson: *Human Sexual Inadequacy,* Boston: Little, Brown, 1970.
7 Kaplan, Helen: *The New Sex Therapy,* New York: Brunner/Mazel, 1974.
8 Berne, Eric: *Principles of Group Treatment,* New York: Oxford University Press, 1966.
9 _____ :*Games People Play: The Psychology of Human Relationships,* New York: Grove Press, 1964.

BIBLIOGRAPHY

Individual Psychotherapy

Balint, M., P.H. Ornstein, and E. Balint: *Focal Psychotherapy,* Philadelphia: J.B. Lippincott, 1972.

Brenner, C.: *An Elementary Textbook of Psychoanalysis* (rev.), New York: International Universities Press, 1973.

Chessick, Richard D.: *Techniques and Practice of Intensive Psychotherapy,* New York: Jason Aronson, 1974.

Dewald, P.A.: *Psychotherapy,* New York: Basic Books, 1972.

Halleck, S.L.: *The Treatment of Emotional Disorders,* New York: Jason Aronson, 1978.

Usdin, Gene: *Overview of the Psychotherapies,* New York: Brunner/Mazel, 1975.

Gestalt Therapy

Fagan, Joen, and Irma Lee Shepherd (eds.): *What Is Gestalt Therapy?* New York: Harper & Row, 1973.

Himelstein, Philip, and Chris Hatcher (eds.): *The Handbook of Gestalt Therapy,* New York: Jason Aronson, 1976.

Polster, Erving, and Miriam Polster: *Gestalt Therapy Integrated,* New York: Brunner/Mazel, 1973.

Zinker, Joseph C.: *Creative Processes in Gestalt Therapy,* New York: Brunner/Mazel, 1977.

Biofeedback

Basmajian, John V. (ed.): *Biofeedback: Principles and Practice for Clinicians,* Baltimore: Williams & Wilkins, 1978.

Beatty, Jackson, and Gray E. Schwartz (eds.): *Biofeedback: Theory and Research,* New York: Academic Press, 1977.

Brown, Barbara B.: *Stress and the Art of Biofeedback,* New York: Harper & Row, 1977.

Gaarder, Kenneth R., and Penelope S. Montgomery (eds.): *Clinical Biofeedback: A Procedural Manual,* Baltimore: Williams & Wilkins, 1977.

Psychodrama

American Society of Group Psychotherapy and Psychodrama: *Group Psychotherapy and Psychodrama,* (vols. 23–28), Beacon, New York: Beacon House, 1970–75.

American Society of Group Psychotherapy and Psychodrama: *Group Psychotherapy, Psychodrama & Sociometry,* (vol. 29), Beacon, New York: Beacon House, 1976.

Starr, Adaline: *Psychodrama: Illustrated Therapeutic Techniques,* Chicago: Nelson/Hall, 1977.

Yablonsky, Lewis: *Psychodrama: Resolving Emotional Problems through Role-Playing,* New York: Basic Books, 1976.

Group Therapy

Berne, E.: *Principles of Group Treatment,* New York: Grove Press, 1968.

Lieberman, Morton A.: "Group Therapies," in G. Usdin (ed.), *Overview of the Psychotherapies,* New York: Brunner/Mazel, 1975.

Rosenbaum, Max, and Milton Berger (eds.): *Group Psychotherapy and Group Function,* New York: Basic Books, 1975.

Slavson, S.R.: *Introduction to Group Therapy,* New York: International Universities Press, 1970.

Yalom, Irwin D.: *The Theory and Practice of Group Psychotherapy,* New York: Basic Books, 1975.

Hypnosis

Erickson, M.H. et al.: *Hypnotic Realities: The Induction of Clinical Hypnosis & Forms of Indirect Suggestion,* New York: Halsted Press, 1977.

Frankel, F.H. (ed.): *Hypnosis: Trance as a Coping Mechanism,* New York: Plenum Publishing, 1976.

Gill, M.M., and M. Brenman: *Hypnosis and Related States,* New York: International Universities Press, 1961.

Spiegel, H.: *A Manual for Hypnotic Induction Profile,* New York: Soni Medica, 1973.

Transactional Analysis

Berne, E.: *Transactional Analysis in Psychotherapy,* New York: Grove Press, 1964.

_____: *Games People Play,* New York: Grove Press, 1964.

Encounter Groups

Encounter Groups & Psychiatry: Task Force Report no. 1, Washington, D.C.: American Psychiatric Association, 1970.

Rogers, C.: *Carl Rogers on Encounter Groups,* Scranton, Pa.: Harper & Row, 1973.

Chapter 25

Psychopharmacology

Morris A. Lipton, M.D.
Kenneth O. Jobson, M.D.

EDITORS' INTRODUCTION

What is it like to be tense and frightened, and to feel that you are "going crazy," only to take the psychotropic drug prescribed by your physician and then feel much better? What is it like to be taking a drug that, if discontinued, may result in your losing contact with reality again? How must it feel to know that the voices may return, the visions may recur, or those frightening feelings of persecution may come back?

What about having to take one of the relatively new antipsychotic medications that bring on those troublesome side effects of dry mouth, lethargy, somnolence, flattened emotions, and psychomotor retardation, as well as the possibility of irreversible physical effects, including a neurologic state of grotesque facial grimacing?

What is it like to feel sad, hopeless, and to have neither energy nor appetite, and then, almost magically, begin to feel better 2 weeks after beginning a tricyclic antidepressant? To discover once again hope in the future, interest in work, beauty in the sunset?

How must it feel to have periodic "highs," during which decisions are made and money is spent, which can lead to later regrets? What is it like to be told that lithium can control these manic periods, and to discover that taking the medication does control the highs?

What is it like to feel dependent upon an antianxiety drug? To feel that you "must" take one before each party, two before your relatives arrive, and three in order to sleep soundly? How does it feel to read about the dangers of these drugs?

On the other hand, what is it like to be a physician, who knows that the newer psychotropic drugs are so effective with many depressed, manic, or schizophrenic patients, and then to have a patient who is unwilling to take the medication? The problem of noncompliance pertains not only to neuroleptic drugs, but also to medications used for hypertension, diabetes, and other physical conditions. Cannot the patient accept that he or she may need to be on psychotropic drugs indefinitely, just as diabetics may require medication all their lives? How frustrating it has to be for the physician to believe in doing what is best, and then to find that the patient will not cooperate.

The psychopharmacologic revolution has brought relief from suffering to many thousands. It has prompted new and exciting research into brain mechanisms. It has provided the physician with much-needed tools with which to help many patients. As with all scientific advances, however, psychopharmacology raises new questions to be answered. For the practicing physician, there is the realistic worry about side effects. The growing concern about tardive dyskinesia casts a shadow across the enthusiasm about major neuroleptics. There are other concerns, including the apprehension about the many patients who want and demand relief from all anxiety, as if life should not have troubled moments. Many patients clearly need the chemical relief drugs provide; others merely use drugs in their quest for oblivion. There are, however, those who fall between the two extremes. How easy it is to prescribe rather than to listen to these people. The physician can use the newer drugs to avoid encounter with such patients. How is the physician to decide whether or not to prescribe a neuroleptic for the individual patient?

Advances in psychopharmacology bring about increased complexity in clinical decision making. In this chapter, two authorities in the field, one of whom is a pharmacologist as well as a psychiatrist, present the reader with basic information, which can help the physician to be of greater assistance to patients in this complex, rapidly developing field.

INTRODUCTION AND HISTORY

Humans are unique among animals in their discovery and use of chemicals to enhance the quality of their lives. These chemicals have ranged from spices to improve the taste of food, to poisons used in hunting or warfare. We have found drugs that have relieved pain or fever, prevented the occurrence of or accelerated recovery from disease, altered mood and states of consciousness, and offered pleasure. Since humans are also social animals, they have used drugs to enhance their interpersonal relationships, and sometimes (to their misfortune) as substitutes for them.

The recorded art of medicine is replete with recommendations from folk medicine about the use of preparations derived from plants, insects, or different species of the animal kingdom. The conversion of folk medicine to a science followed the acquisition and utilization of the self-correcting method of thinking and inquiry called the *scientific method*. The generation of hypotheses and of methods for testing them began in the physical sciences during the Renaissance and moved to the natural or biological sciences about a century later. The development of powerful tools like the microscope and the techniques and concepts of biology and chemistry permitted the testing of hypotheses about the etiology and treatment of illness that had been in existence for more than a thousand years. Many were found to be incorrect or useless. Primitive theories about the etiology of disease were first replaced with infectious or toxic theories. The concept that illness might be caused by deficiencies rather than by toxins was developed at the turn of the twentieth century with the discovery of vitamins. Beginning about 100 years ago, the techniques of the chemist were applied to the ethnopharmacological preparations derived from folklore, and the specific therapeutic agents presented in these preparations were isolated, identified chemically, and often synthesized. New chemical preparations were then synthesized by the organic chemist.

Simultaneously, methods of clinical testing for diagnosis and treatment became more sophisticated. The art of diagnosis was converted to a science, with objective tests that often involved the use of the laboratory. These tests not only permitted more precise diagnosis, but also increased the capacity to measure clinical progress or deterioration as various treatments were employed. The power of the placebo was noted, and the need for controlled clinical trials in order to overcome the problems of nonspecific effects became evident. Although much of medicine remains an art and is likely to continue to be so, medically accepted horrors like tonsillectomy for children, thymic radiation, and the removal of teeth of young people to eliminate focal infection are much less likely to occur today than they did less than a half-century ago. A heightened sense of ethics and of caution, coupled with demands for harder evidence based on controlled clinical trials, must be given credit for this. It is a dramatic demonstration of the application of the scientific method to the solution of problems of human illness.

Involved as it is with the prevention and treatment of mental illness, psychiatry lagged behind many of the other medical specialties in the application of the scientific method. There were many reasons for this. High on the list of these reasons was the inability to fit mental illness into existing models of physical disease. Although the spirochete was discovered to be the cause of general paresis in the 1930s, and its elimination by antibiotics in the early 1940s clearly demonstrated the infectious nature of at least one type of mental illness, an infectious etiology for most other types of mental illness has not been demonstrated, despite many investigations over the years. This model has never been fully rejected, and currently there is ongoing research into slow viruses as a possible cause. Similarly, the dementia of pellagra was eliminated with the discovery that this illness was due to nutritional deficiency, and could be prevented or cured by the introduction of niacin or of niacin-containing foods into the diet. But this, too, represented only a small portion of existing mental illness, and despite efforts of practitioners of orthomolecular psychiatry and megavitamin therapy to demonstrate a nutritional basis for many types of mental illness, the weight of opinion remains that schizophrenia, depression, anxiety, learning disabilities, hyperkinesis and so forth are not associated with nutritional deficiencies.

Most forms of mental illness fall instead into that area of disease where a specific etiology has not been found, and where multiple etiologies are likely. Mental illness, therefore, more closely resembles hypertension, diabetes, and various gastrointestinal disorders in which the illness is apparently a consequence of environmental stress imposed upon a susceptible organism. The environmental stress is usually psychological, and the specific emotional vulnerability of an individual to it may depend upon previous life experiences. The biological vulnerability, on the other hand, may be genetic or may also be a consequence of biological insults during gestation, birth, and postnatal development. It even remains possible that multiple biological susceptibilities exist, and that these find an expressive final common path in the only forms in which the brain can express itself, that is, in changes of consciousness, mood, perception, and thinking. These changes and their behavioral and social manifestations are the symptoms with which the patient comes to the physician.

Medicine has a tendency to forget that treatment of the sick patient has multiple goals. These can be rank-ordered in a hierarchy that ranges from total reversal of the illness and its future prevention, with no residual defect as the highest goal, to symptom relief but no arrest of the illness as a lower but still acceptable goal. The term *cure* is not defined precisely, but it usually involves a total reversal of the illness, preferably with future prevention and no residual damage. But cures are even considered to occur when there is total reversal, no future prevention, but some residue. The highest form of treatment of which the physician is capable is employed in immunization techniques, in which a minor illness is created so that it may result in the production of sufficient antibodies to protect the host organism for long periods of time. This is common practice with polio, diphtheria, tetanus, pertussis, and smallpox. The infectious diseases that are treated effectively with chemotherapy or antibiotics, and the nutritional illnesses that are treated with appropriate vitamins, minerals, or other nutrients can also be cured, even though they may occasionally leave some residual scars or malfunction after the cause is eliminated. Furthermore, many of these illnesses may recur.

When delivery of health services is effective, the curable diseases are no longer a problem. The etiology is usually univalent and is understood. Elimination of etiologic agents leads to cure. On the other hand, the illnesses that the physician and patient face in modern medicine frequently have multiple etiologies and are chronic. Illnesses such as hypertension, arthritis, diabetes, the degenerative diseases, and cancer are treated for relief of symptoms and to slow or block the progress of the illness. In some illnesses, such as the common cold, treatment is aimed at relief of symptoms and avoidance of complications while the illness runs its course and remits spontaneously. In others, slowing the progress of the illness or even palliation during its course are highly desirable forms of treatment, although research continues to generate more effective forms.

The drugs used for the treatment of mental illness do not cure in the sense described above. Instead, they attentuate symptoms, slow the progress of the illness, and diminish the personal and social consequences of the illness. In this sense they are generally as effective as drugs used in the treatment of most chronic physical illness. When used in conjunction with psychological treatments and adequate family and social support systems, they are sufficiently effective to have generated what has been called a psychiatric revolution.

The discovery of treatments for the chronic illnesses has frequently been accidental, and their use is usually empirical. Frequently, the investigation of the mode of action of an effective empirical treatment has led to insights about pathogenesis and, occasionally, about the etiology of the illness it treats. But typically such investigations do not aim at the elimination of the etiologic agent, if for no other reason than that the etiologic agent is unknown.

Although the use of ethnopharmacological agents like marijuana, opium, cocaine, alcohol, caffeine, and other central nervous stimulants, and even psychotomimetic drugs, is as old as recorded history, the science of psychopharmacology is less than 30 years old. In a period of less than a dozen years, we discovered drugs that had relatively specific properties in reversing the symptoms of different forms of psychiatric illness, and other drugs that produced symptoms mimicking psychosis. In 1949, the antimanic properties of lithium were reported, and shortly thereafter the powerful psychotomimetic LSD-25 was discovered. Three years later, reserpine, which had been isolated chemically from the snake root that had been used in India for centuries, was found to have antipsychotic properties. At about the same time, the search for chemotherapeutic supplements to improve existing treatments for tuberculosis serendipitously revealed the antidepressant properties of a new class of chemicals, the monoamine oxidase inhibitors. The search for hypothermic agents to assist the surgeon in conducting long and complex surgical procedures led to the discovery of the unique antipsychotic properties of chlorpromazine in 1952. Shortly thereafter, meprobamate was found to have the property of relieving anxiety, and about 5 years later better antianxiety agents like chlordiazepoxide became available.

The discovery of agents that help in the treatment of psychosis, affective disorders, and anxiety states has been called a scientific revolution, and indeed in many ways it was. Prior to the discovery of such agents, *psychogenesis,* or the psychological etiology of all forms of mental illness, was the dominant ideology, and psychological treatment was considered to be the highest form of treatment for the mentally ill. Drugs that had been available for the treatment of mental illness prior to the late 1940s were such blunderbusses as the barbiturates, chloral hydrate and paraldehyde, which were usually given in large doses during the night and frequently during the day to assure a quiet ward. These same three drugs were used on an outpatient basis for the management of anxiety. They were effective only to the extent that they were sedative, and they produced all the side effects common to sedatives.

The new drugs were entirely different. First and foremost, they did not alter the state of the patient's consciousness radically, nor did they cloud perceptions. Thus patients could remain alert and responsive to their physical, social, and interpersonal environment while the troublesome symptoms associated with their illnesses diminished. Second, there was relative specificity of action on target symptoms so that the physician's armamentarium increased considerably.

Revolutions have their own consequences. At least four are worthy of mention. First, as indicated previously, was the erosion of the established position, which held that etiology was psychogenic and that psychological treatment was the best kind. Drugs presenting contrary evidence to this established theoretical position were not accepted readily, and were initially considered to offer mere symptom relief at best, and to be chemical straitjackets at worst. Symptom relief was not only considered to be a poor form of treatment, but was also felt to be frequently disadvantageous, since it removed the patient's motivation for working on the psychological resolutions of problems. A consequence of this was that psychotropic drugs were, and continue to be, used more by nonpsychiatrists than by psychiatrists.

A second consequence of the revolution was that nonpsychiatrists and organically oriented psychiatrists began to feel that drugs were the complete answer (for example, penicillin for infectious disease) and that psychosocial interventions were unnecessary. Physicians employing this approach had apparently forgotten that when dealing with chronic illness, in which cure is not possible, psychosocial intervention is mandatory, even in illnesses that are considered clearly medical. Thus, the treatment of the hypertensive patient involves not only the use of antihypertensive medication, but frequently an alteration in dietary habits so that fewer calories and less salt are ingested daily, the establishment of an exercise program, and assistance in the alteration of lifelong habits of work and of recreation. Frequently, assistance must also be given in the resolution of interpersonal conflicts with spouses, children, peers, colleagues, and employers. No less is required for the management by means of drugs of the patient with psychiatric problems. Research with schizophrenics has shown that the relapse rate with drugs is highly dependent upon the personal and social support systems offered to the patient along with the drugs. Research with depressed patients has shown that the effects of drugs and of psychological treatment aimed at resolving interpersonal conflicts are additive. Work with neurotic patients has shown that drugs are a powerful tactical weapon in attenuating the emotional upheavals associated with crisis, but that the resolution of internal and external conflicts by psychological means permits the development of new coping styles and new adaptations that no longer require the use of drugs. To use drugs without the sensitivity and time required to establish a therapeutic alliance with the patient is to invite disaster in the form of drug dependency, drug habituation, polypharmacy, and all the unfortunate consequences of these.

A third consequence of the revolution was the growth of knowledge about pathogenesis of mental illness, which stemmed from studying the mode of action of the new psychotropic drugs. The rationale was that if one could understand how a therapeutically effective drug acted at a cellular or molecular level, one could infer from its mode of action something about the underlying defect during the illness. It is research of this type, interacting with other basic science research in neurobiology, which has led to the various biological theories of mental illness that exist today. A less fortunate consequence of this type of thinking has been a tendency to seek new and more powerful structural analogs of existing effective drugs rather than to strike out in new directions. The somewhat stereotyped nature of drug development has led to the curious phenomenon that remarkably few new kinds of psychotherapeutic agents have been developed in the past decade. Recent developments in neuroendocrinology have led to what may become a new revolution in which naturally occurring centrally active polypeptides or synthetic analogs of these may be introduced as therapeutic agents. Still other major consequences of drug development have been its effects upon health delivery systems and its effectiveness in returning psychiatry to its proper place as a discipline within medicine.

There can be little doubt that the development of effective psychotropic drugs has had major consequences upon the mental health delivery systems. Drugs that accelerate the recovery of florid psychosis or suicidal depressions have reduced hospital stays and have permitted the reentry of patients into their families, their communities, and their jobs. In less florid psychiatric illness, hospitalization can be avoided entirely. The proliferation of community mental health centers has been correlated temporally with the psychopharmacology revolution, although it would be an exaggeration to attribute such centers entirely to this revolution. The destruction of exclusively psychogenetic theories of mental illness, which were rapidly moving psychiatry away from the remainder of medicine, has been accompanied by the return of psychiatry to what is usually called the medical model. This medical model should not be construed as an infectious disease model with univalent causality, but rather as resembling a broader model that physicians today employ in their concepts of most serious chronic illnesses. These include psychological, social, and occupational interactions with biological vulnerability. Thus, broader definitions of the nature of illness, both by psychiatrists and by other physicians, have brought them closer together. Recognition of the difficulties in changing the smoking, eating, and occupational habits of patients with physical illness should not discourage the primary physician's attempts to intervene in the direction of improving such habits. Recognition of these difficulties in what are usually considered emotionally normal patients should make physicians all the more sympathetic to the even greater difficulties in altering the defensive strategies and the frequently self-destructive habits and coping maneuvers of the patient with emotional illness. In neither case are drugs by themselves enough. If the problems are beyond the scope of the available time, the primary physician should properly refer the patient to a psychiatrist or, alternatively, work in collaboration with those who have the skills, motivation, and time to handle these types of interventions.

Although there has been relatively little in the development of totally new types of drugs in the past 10 years, there have been major developments in the sophistication with which these drugs are used. Perhaps the most important of these has been the development and utilization of methods for measuring levels of these drugs in the blood of patients. This, too, has followed a trend in medicine in which measuring levels of phenytoin sodium, digoxin, some anticoagulants, and barbiturates in plasma has become routine to ensure maximum clinical efficacy and to minimize toxic effects of overdosage. Plasma levels are also available in monitoring compliance, a frequently troublesome problem with psychiatric patients.

Revolutions invariably generate a vast literature. In the case of psychopharmacology, more than 20,000 papers have appeared in the past 20 years. Several new journals devoted exclusively to this subject have appeared. Several excellent textbooks have been written in the past few years. Because the topic area is so large and so active, we shall not attempt to offer a comprehensive bibliography. Instead, selected readings are suggested for each topic under consideration.

PHARMACOKINETICS AND PHARMACODYNAMICS

The proper use of psychotropic drugs requires knowledge of their pharmacokinetics and pharmacodynamics. *Pharmacokinetics* deals with drug absorption, distribution, metabolism, and excretion. These factors, coupled with the administered dose, determine the concentration of the drug at its site of action, hence both its therapeutic and its adverse effects. *Pharmacodynamics* refers to the biochemical mechanism of action, and attempts to relate the chemical structure of the drug to its action and effects. The voluminous literature about the psychotropic drugs that has accumulated in both of these areas is much too large to review adequately. Only general principles and a few pertinent details will be discussed.

Pharmacokinetics

Orally administered drugs are absorbed primarily by passive diffusion through the membranes of the gastrointestinal tract. With the exception of lithium, psychotropic drugs are all strongly lipid soluble, weakly ionized, and are absorbed mainly in the unionized state. Consequently, their absorption will be influenced mainly by gastric pH, interstitial surface area, gastrointestinal activity, and above all, blood flow in the gastrointestinal tract. This latter fact is especially important for the elderly, whose blood flow may be diminished by 50 percent. Oral administration is usually not so rapid as, nor does it yield blood levels so high as, parenteral administration. A notable exception is with the benzodiazepines, which are absorbed better by oral than by intramuscular administration. Following absorption, psychotropic drugs are not distributed evenly throughout the body. Largely because of their lipid solubility, they tend to concentrate in the body fat, red cells, liver, and brain. They are also bound to plasma proteins. The clinical implications are manifold. Significantly lowered plasma proteins, which may occur in the aged, can elevate the concentration of free drug. Alterations in the quantity of body fat can also alter their volume of distribution. The metabolism of the psychotropic drugs occurs mainly in the liver. The high liver-to-body-weight ratio that occurs in children results in different dose requirements. Drug catabolism in the liver involves demethylation, particularly on the side chain, and hydroxylation, especially of the aromatic ring. This is followed by esterification as the glucuronide or the sulfate to yield water-soluble substances, which are then excreted by the kidney.

These multiple reactions occur to different degrees and at different rates in heterogeneous patient populations, and this may account for variability in patient response. Probably much of the metabolic variability is genetic. But it is worth noting that the liver enzymes that perform these transformations can be altered significantly by other drugs. Barbiturates notoriously induce liver enzymes and increase the catabolism of other drugs. Other hypnotics, caffeine, and smoking do the same. Liver disease, like hepatitis and cirrhosis, diminishes drug catabolism.

Given the many factors, such as absorption, distribution, metabolism, and excretion, that can affect the concentration of active drug that reaches the desired sites in the nervous system, it is not surprising that all the psychotropic drugs show wide variations in blood levels among patients receiving identical doses. There is, therefore, no way to predict accurately the doses that will produce maximum therapeutic response with minimum adverse reactions without measurement of blood levels. Blood-level measurements have become routine in many fields of medicine. Lithium levels are readily monitored, and always should be. As the technology for measurement of the organic psychotropic drugs becomes simpler, it is desirable that other measurements should be too.

Pharmacodynamics

Current neurobiological theory proposes that communication between neurons across synapses is chemical. Presynaptic neurons discharge quanta of neurotransmitters, which cross the synaptic cleft and react with receptors of the postsynaptic neuron activating it. Specific neurons contain and discharge specific neurotransmitters. Similarly, receptors have a high degree of specificity for individual neurotransmitters. The best-recognized neurotransmitters of the CNS are norepinephrine (NE), dopamine (DA), serotonin (5HT), and acetylcholine (ACh). Neurons employing these neurotransmitters account for only a small fraction of the total CNS neurons, and other neurotransmitters undoubtedly exist. Gamma amino butyric acid (GABA) and other amino acids, such as glycine and glutamic acid, may have such a role. A variety of polypeptides like substance P, thyrotropin-releasing hormone, endorphin, and enkephalin may also have roles.

The investigation of the function of these neurotransmitters and of the changes induced in them by drugs has led to hypotheses about their therapeutic mode of action, and has also generated hypotheses about the nature of the biochemical pathogenesis of mental illness. Thus, there is the catecholamine hypothesis of affective disorder and the dopamine hypothesis of schizophrenia.

All the psychotropic drugs have been shown to affect one or another neurotransmitter function, and their pharmacodynamic properties are generally attributed to their capacity to influence neurotransmitters.

Tricyclic antidepressants have peripheral anticholinergic effects. These effects are related to the common symptoms, such as dry mouth, but are not currently considered to be related to their antidepressant activity. Instead, the most currently favored hypothesis as to their mode of action deals with their effects upon the reuptake of NE and 5HT from the synaptic cleft into the presynaptic neuron. When synaptic vesicles discharge their neurotransmitter contents into the synaptic cleft following stimulation of the presynaptic neuron, the released neurotransmitter may have three simultaneous fates. Some will react with the postsynaptic neuron receptor; others will be washed away into extracellular fluid, where they will be metabolized by monoamine oxidase; and still others will be inactivated by reuptake into the presynaptic neuron. The tricyclic antidepressants inhibit this last mechanism, in which the neurotransmitter is reactivated by reuptake. As a consequence, more of the neurotransmitter is available for the postsynaptic receptor. This is the most favored hypothesis for the mode of action of the tricyclics. Recently, there has been some evidence that some depressions are associated with low NE synthesis and release, and some with low 5HT. There is accumulating evidence that the tertiary amine tricyclics, such as amitriptyline, are more potent inhibitors of 5HT reuptake, while secondary amines like desipramine and nortriptyline are more potent in blocking NE reuptake. Active research is underway currently to determine whether there are indeed pure serotonergic and pure noradrenergic depressions, and also whether new compounds that are either pure serotonergic uptake blockers or pure noradrenergic blockers will be effective therapeutically. At present, the answer is still unknown.

The benzodiazepines, which are among the most commonly prescribed drugs, have the most elusive molecular mode of action. Behaviorally, they generally reduce both anxiety and aggression. They do not depress behavior, but instead cause an increment in behavior when the behavior has already been suppressed or inhibited by factors that are present in the environment or have been imposed by the experimenter. Thus, behavior that has been reduced by punishment, fear, aversion, novelty, and reduction of reward can be regained with the antianxiety drugs. Studies of the mode of action at the pharmacological level have demonstrated that, like the barbiturates, benzodiazepines decrease turnover rates of DA and 5HT and can block stress-induced acceleration of NE turnover. However, these effects are shared by barbiturates; furthermore, the benzodiazepines seem to exert these effects indirectly, because they do not affect the metabolic enzymes, the receptors, nor the uptake mechanism for these neurotransmitters. Recent work has shown that the action of the benzodiazepines may be upon neurons containing gamma amino butyric acid (GABA). GABA is present in the brain at concentrations 10 to 15 times that of NE or 5HT. Neurons containing GABA seem to be primarily inhibitory in nature. Such neurons interconnect with monoaminergic and cholinergic neurons and seem to regulate their firing rate. By means of mechanisms that are not yet understood, the benzodiazepines facilitate GABA transmission. Facilitating the activity of an inhibitory system diminishes the activity of noradrenergic, serotonergic, and cholinergic neurons, and this may underlie the antianxiety and sedative actions.

The antipsychotic or neuroleptic drugs are highly reactive compounds that affect many biological systems. Prominent among these are the anticholinergic as well as the antidopaminergic effects. Data accumulated from a large body of research in many laboratories suggest strongly that their primary mode of action is by inhibition of the dopaminergic system. Carlsson has put it very succinctly:

> These various drugs have only one basic pharmacological property in common. Namely an inhibitory action on dopaminergic neurotransmission. In fact, not only do all antipsychotic agents appear to possess antidopaminergic activity but it also appears that all antidopaminergic agents possess antipsychotic activity.[1]

The finding that all neuroleptics have antidopaminergic activity has led to the development of the dopamine hypothesis, which postulates dopaminergic overactivity in schizophrenia. However, there is no direct confirmation that the unmedicated patient with schizophrenia has heightened dopaminergic activity. Possibly, DA is involved in compensating for some as-yet-unknown fundamental defect, and manipulation of dopaminergic activity is effective only when the underlying defect exists. The nature of the primary defect is not yet known, but the suggestion has been made that it may involve an intrinsic defect in the inhibitory GABA system.

DEPRESSION

Introduction

Most patients who are experiencing sadness do not require psychopharmacologic treatment. Of those needing drugs for relief of their depression, almost all simultaneously need "other aid." This "other aid" may be supportive, reassuring, educational, or aimed at the acquisition of insight. It should always include a trustworthy and hope-instilling therapeutic relationship. Patients whose sadness is brief, clearly related to external events, and not life threatening should be treated without drugs. Such treatment can be offered by a primary care physician or by referral to a psychiatrist. Complicating the physician's decision-making process is the fact that depressions that need psychopharmacologic treatment often seem to begin as grief or short-term sadness following demoralizing experiences. Such reactions in themselves do not require drugs, but they may become prolonged, take on their own autonomy, and become true depressions. One must consider severity of the functional limitation, duration of illness, and type of depressive syndrome, the family history of affective illness, and the premorbid psychological status of the patient in deciding whether to institute drug treatment.

Depressions may be classified in various ways. In this chapter we have chosen to classify them according to the nature of the medication to which they respond.

Classification of Depressions

1 Schizophrenia-related depressions include schizophrenia with depression and schizoaffective illness. This is discussed under the heading of schizophrenia because when the schizophrenic component is treated successfully, the depression usually lifts.

2 Manic-depressive illness—the patient with a depressive phase of manic-depressive or bipolar-type illness usually shows:

   a Psychomotor retardation and/or hypersomnia

   b A history of previous manic or hypomanic episodes

   c A history of manic-depressive illness in the family

   d A rapid onset of depression, with a tendency toward frequent or rapid cycling into and out of depression

   e An age of onset for first depression early in adulthood; any patient below age 35 with depression and vegetative symptoms should be considered carefully for the diagnosis of bipolar depression

   f A particularly saltatory or discontinuous clinical course, with periods of full remission, normal function, or hypomania interspersed with sudden or severe depressions

   g A history of postpartum depression or extreme premenstrual sadness (although these can be seen in other forms of depression)

3 Unipolar depression is the most diverse of the three categories. It may include:

   a Situational or reactive depressions, which generally do not require antidepressant drugs, and in which drugs may be harmful. Grief constitutes this kind of depression, as does the sadness following the loss of home, job, face, or fortune. Situational depressions are generally responsive to environmental change, and are not so monochromatic in mood as are depressions that require antidepressant drugs. Occasional mild sedatives may be helpful. These depressions usually remit within a month, or when the loss is corrected. The chronic equivalent of such a situational depression may be called demoralization or an attitude of despair. When this is not accompanied by the "criteria of tricyclic responsiveness" (see following section), it seldom responds to such antidepressants. When a situational depression progresses into an autonomous and prolonged depression with biological features, antidepressants may be required.

   b Chronic characterological depression involves a lifelong pattern of maladaptation and unhappiness. This subgroup of depressive patients is heterogeneous, and includes many patients whose depression is unaltered by chemotherapy. Typically, such patients lack the somatic signs of biological depressions.

   c Tricyclic responsive unipolar depressions lack a personal or family history of manic behavior. They are frequently recurrent, and their recurrences are not clearly related to specific life events. Within this class of depression are the involutional depressions. They are more likely to be flavored with agitation, paranoid thinking, chronicity, somatic complaints, and psychosis. To the extent that they meet the criteria for tricyclic responsiveness, they should be so treated.

The patient who is experiencing depression should have assessment of the suicidal intent on the first visit, and regularly thereafter. If at any time the patient is judged to be suicidal, prompt referral to a psychiatrist and hospitalization must be considered seriously. The assessment of suicidal intent is not simple, and must be approached from several vantage points. The physician should ask directly whether the patient's depression has reached the point where he or she thinks of self-harm, and whether there is a plan for this. Relatives and friends should also be asked. Expressions of helplessness, hopelessness, and lack of self-esteem are correlated with increased suicidal risk, as are alcoholism, social isolation, divorce, and prior suicidal attempts. When there is any significant depression, firearms and drugs should be removed from the home. The patient and family should be alerted to signs of impending suicide, so that access to help may be instituted. One-third of all the patients who commit suicide have given direct notice of their intent, one-third have stated their intent indirectly, and one-third have committed suicide without giving notice.

Factors militating toward referral of the depressed patient to a psychiatrist include: significant risk for suicide, a history suggestive of manic-depressive illness, multiple recurrent depressions, depression that is unresponsive to the primary physician's attempts, psychotic depression, and schizophrenia-related depression. The patient should also be referred when the diagnosis is unclear, or when the primary physician is unfamiliar with the use of required methods of treatment. Factors that militate toward the primary physician's treating the depression include: the patient's being neither suicidal nor psychotic, the patient's having clear criteria for responsiveness to tricyclic medication, a depression secondary to disease or drug use when treatment of the disease or removal of the drug brings relief of the depression, and a grief- or stress-related depression of less than 1 month's duration.

Tricyclic-Responsive Depressions

Among the patients who classically respond to tricyclics, 80 percent respond to adequate dosage by mouth, without blood-level monitoring to ensure an effective range. Over 90 percent respond when adequate blood levels are ensured by measurement.

Most tricyclic-responding patients have unipolar depression, that is, the absence of mania or hypomania in the present and past. Factors predictive of response to the tricyclics are: insidious onset, duration of more than 1 month but less than several years, anorexia, weight loss, middle and late insomnia, psychomotor disturbances (agitation or slowing), and an upper socioeconomic class. Factors predictive of poor response to tricyclics include neurotic, hypochondriacal, and hysterical traits; multiple prior episodes of depression; somatic or paranoid delusions; or consistent depression that has lasted for years and has not responded to drugs previously.

The above tricyclic-response-criteria approach cannot be fully equated with the *American Psychiatric Association Diagnostic and Statistical Manual III* classification of major depressive disorders, which calls for the depression to be present for 1 month, and for five of the following nine factors to be present:

1 Anorexia or weight loss
2 Sleep difficulty
3 Loss of energy
4 Agitation or retardation
5 Loss of interest in usual activities
6 Decrease in libido

7 Self-reproach or guilt
8 Trouble in thinking
9 Recurrent thoughts of death or suicide

The following factors are not well established statistically, but nevertheless are clinically useful in estimating the probability of response to tricyclics:

1 The patient who will respond to a tricyclic antidepressant typically has a guilt-ridden or intrapunitive view of self. Both men and women respond adequately, although some reports indicate a more rapid and satisfactory response among men.

2 In depressed patients below 35 years of age, the full criteria are often unmet. If the criteria are met by a patient in that age category, closer examination of the patient's past and family history often reveals manic-depressive illness, which may also require lithium. There seems to be a lower frequency of response to tricyclics if the patient's mother has been chronically depressed or chronically psychotic.

3 Patients who experience depressions in the setting of physical disease, such as hepatitis, pneumonitis, infectious hepatitis, peptic ulcer disease, or similar ills usually remit when the underlying illness is treated. Those who have been exposed to depressogenic medications, such as reserpine, methyldopa, high doses of lecithin, or birth control pills usually improve when the offending drugs are discontinued. At other times, the classic symptoms and signs of tricyclic response, such as early morning awakening and weight loss, remain even after medication is stopped. In such patients, tricyclics are effective. When reserpine-induced depression which meets the criteria for tricyclic response 1 month after discontinuation of the reserpine is noted, tricyclics should then be started.

4 The patient who in the past has had a clearly satisfactory response to tricyclics, and who then lapses into a *forme fruste* of the depression with some "tricyclic criteria" is also often responsive to restarting tricyclics. Such patients typically present with insomnia, multiple somatic complaints, and decreased energy, but do not feel guilty nor have they lost weight. This group characteristically "doctor-shops" in an attempt to relieve their "unexplained" malaise.

5 Several groups of masked depressions are tricyclic responsive. The first group is typified by the elderly patient with single or multiple somatic complaints that do not have a physical explanation. Such patients may appear withdrawn, with motor and verbal slowing or with anxiety and motor restlessness. Inquiries should also be made with family members to explore for incidence of early morning insomnia, weight loss, and other tricyclic-responsive criteria. What may appear like dementias in the elderly may be masked depression or a depression superimposed on a mild organic brain syndrome. One of the most difficult psychopharmacologic decisions to make is whether or not to withhold a trial of tricyclic medication from a patient whose dementia workup has not shown a medical basis. Some patients who have the "pseudodementia" of a masked depression often appear, even after a thorough examination and history, to lack the criteria for tricyclic response; yet many such patients respond impressively emotionally, cognitively, and socially. The exclusion of the diagnosis of a masked depression in such patients is most difficult without a trial of tricyclic antidepressant in the therapeutic blood level range. The elderly, especially if they also have organic brain symptoms, are more sensitive to the central anticholinergic effects of the tricyclics. Such patients may develop a "central anticholinergic syndrome," with increased agitation and confusion. This group of patients should have careful monitoring of their responses to medication (see section on Geropsychopharmacology).

A second form of frequently missed tricyclic-responsive depression is that of the patient whose chief complaint is anxiety but who, after a careful history and examination, shows the "criteria for tricyclic response." Many of these patients will have their levels of anxiety improved if the physician chooses a tricyclic that is also a sedative, such as amitriptyline. Occasionally, such a patient may require the short-term use of benzodiazipines in addition to the tricyclic to attenuate the anxiety for the several weeks required for alleviation of the depression by the tricyclic. Treatment of the patient who is experiencing anxiety and depression and who has agoraphobia will be discussed under the section dealing with monoamine oxidase inhibitors.

A third group of masked depression includes the patients for whom chronic pain is the chief complaint. If upon examination the patient exhibits a depressed mood, and a thorough medical evaluation does not reveal an organic cause of pain, the patient may be found to be responsive to antidepressant medication. These patients are discussed under the section dealing with pain.

A fourth group, and one that is not generally considered to be experiencing a masked depression, includes patients with psychotic depressions that may have such prominent psychotic features that the depressive aspects of the illness may be overlooked. Some patients with tricyclic-responsive criteria have as a part of their symptomatology psychotic thought, often called affective delusions, which may be somatic or paranoid. These delusions may be as simple as the unaltered belief in their own personal guilt for some personal or family misfortune. Other presentations of these affective delusions include the beliefs that they are rotting inside, that their bowels are turning to stone, that the family is being punished for the patient's misdeeds, and that misfortune of some indescribable nature is about to befall them or their families. Even when such delusions are present in the patient's presentation, tricyclic criteria should be sought. The more closely that patients meet the strict tricyclic-response criteria, the more likely they will be to respond to tricyclics. The more the presentation lacks such tricyclic-responsive criteria, and the more all-inclusive the psychosis, the less likely it is that the patient will be tricyclic-responsive. Complicating the diagnosis of these patients may be their inability or unwillingness to give an accurate history of such matters as weight loss, sleep problems, and past personal or family history of similar episodes.

Electroshock Responders   The patient whose depression has responded to electroconvulsive therapy (ECT) is approximately one-half as likely to relapse into depression if he or she is maintained on a therapeutic level of tricyclics for 6 months after the ECT. In a patient who has met the criteria for tricyclic responsiveness, but was initially unresponsive to tricyclics and then responds to ECT, it would still probably be a good idea to continue on a tricyclic antidepressant for 6 months after the ECT. When the patient on tricyclics comes to ECT, one should be cognizant of the fact that the mortality of ECT is essentially that of the anesthesia, and that the anesthetic risk is influenced by the blood level of tricyclic. The urgency of the need for ECT is to be weighed against the time required to lower the tricyclic blood level and the additional anesthetic risk if the patient has low pAO_2 or anemia. Modern ECT, with unilateral electrode placement on the nondominant hemisphere, reduces postshock amnesia markedly and hence reduces morbidity.

The place of tricyclic medication in the treatment of "schizophrenia-related depression" is unsettled. It is clinical experience that at times tricyclics worsen the psychotic process of the patient with true schizophrenia, especially in doses over 150 mg per day. There is also clinical evidence that at times the patient with schizophrenia and depression experiences a lifting of the depression that correlates with the institution of tricyclic medication use. Within this schizophrenia-related depression group are several groups. One group, in fact, has manic-depressive illness that may be misdiagnosed as schizophrenia, and will respond to tricyclics in the therapeutic range. There are several problems if the clinician does not recognize such a patient. The unrecognized manic-depressive patient may initially respond with resolution of the schizophrenia-related depression, only to have his or her mania switched on by the tricyclic. This may happen acutely in the patient who is simply considered to have schizophrenia and whose state has been worsened by the tricyclic. Alternatively, it may occur after the patient leaves the hospital and has returned to a customary level of function. Thus, the tricyclic appears clinically to be able to treat the depression of manic depressive illness on the one hand, and on the other hand to be capable of both switching the patient to a manic state and to be able to treat the depression of manic-depressive illness on the one hand and, on the other hand, to be capable of both switching the patient to a manic state and accelerating the cycle of manic-depressive illness. The resolution of this paradox is first to recognize the manic-depressive, and, second, to treat such a depression only long enough to establish a response, and then to discontinue the tricyclic and substitute lithium instead. Generally, this tricyclic withdrawal can be gone after days or a few weeks of response. The timing should consider both the past history of being tripped into mania by a tricyclic and the depth of the depression. It is often preferable to withdraw the tricyclic too early than to risk tripping the patient into a manic episode by prolonged tricyclic exposure.

Starting a Tricyclic Antidepressant

When a patient has been found to meet the tricyclic-response criteria, a decision should be made as to whether to begin the tricyclic immediately or to "try something else first." If suicide risk is not especially evident, it is at times clinically wise to try something else first. This might even be a few days of environmental manipulation, such as hospitalization without medication. At times, new and useful information comes into the picture during this waiting period. In general, the harder the signs and symptoms of tricyclic responsiveness, the more quickly the clinician should utilize a tricyclic.

Every person who starts on a tricyclic should have a history, physical exam, and laboratory evaluations prior to being given the medication.

The History There should be a thorough medical and psychological history. Inquiry as to allergy, current or planned pregnancy, and breast feeding is mandatory. A history of current and past drug exposure is most important. This should include any over-the-counter or prescription anticholinergics. Clinicians will do well generally to avoid the simultaneous administration of two or more drugs with strong anticholinergic effects, because of their additive effects. The neuroleptic thioridazine and amitriptyline are both strong anticholinergics, and they should not be used concurrently. The patient's past drug responsiveness or nonresponsiveness to particular antidepressants is helpful in deciding the drug of choice and the dosage. The dosage, blood levels achieved, and duration of therapy in previous treatments are helpful, as is the history of other medications that have been used. The patient's family history of drug response is also helpful because of the approximately fortyfold variance seen in plasma levels of tricyclics on a fixed dose. Some of this variance may be on a genetic basis. The cardiovascular history should be through, with inquiry made as to arteriosclerotic cardiovascular disease, hypertensive cardiovascular disease, and any tachydysrhythmias.

The Physical Examination and Laboratory Evaluations The cardiopulmonary system, including standing and reclining blood pressure and pulse, the central nervous system, and the endocrine system must be evaluated by physical examination. The patient with unrecognized thyroid disease may not need tricyclics, and may be sensitive to the side effects. The physical exam often reveals reasons either to omit the tricyclics or to amend the dosage schedule.

The thoroughness of the laboratory work needed for instituting the tricyclics safely is unsettled. The following list provides a point of departure, based on clinical judgment.

1 ECG
2 Chest x-ray
3 Electrolytes
4 CBC
5 BUN and creatinine
6 Bilirubin, SGOT, ALK phos
7 Thyroid profile
8 Urinalysis
9 Albumin

Some special comments about the laboratory studies of a person being considered for a tricyclic are warranted. Disturbances in the internal milieu predispose to tricyclic toxicity. Abnormal electrolytes and hemoglobin should be explained and corrected prior to initiating a tricyclic. The patient with low potassium or anemia is more likely to develop a cardiac dysrhythmia while on a tricyclic. A decision should be made as to whether or not to investigate by means of laboratory studies the unusual causes of depression, such as porphyria. The patient with low serum albumin will have shorter tricyclic half-life and higher peaks of free plasma tricyclic, and thus should probably be given the drug in a multiple daily dosage schedule. Although it is not yet demonstrated, this may mean that the time for the monitoring of plasma tricyclic will have to be amended. The patient with a cardiac dysrhythmia may need to have a cardiologist involved in the decision as to the safety of a tricyclic.

Choosing a Particular Tricyclic

With the current state of knowledge, this is largely a clinical decision. Some characteristics of the tricyclics are given in Table 25-1. The clinician's familiarity with the particular drug is, of course, crucial. There is variance in the sedative versus arousal side effects of these drugs. Amitriptyline and doxepin are the more sedative drugs. Imipramine, desipramine, and nortriptyline are less sedative, and protriptyline tends to be activating. In the depressed patient with insomnia or anxiety, the sedative side effect can be used to an advantage. The patient whose schedule calls for full alertness may tolerate a less sedating drug better. There is also a continuum of anticholinergic effects that is helpful in choosing the drug for a particular patient. Amitriptyline is the most anticholinergic, and desipramine the least anticholinergic. Thus, one would probably not start with amitriptyline in a patient who was predisposed to peripheral or central anticholinergic toxicity. The definitive studies as to comparative efficacy of the various tricyclics, utilizing blood levels, have yet to be done. There are data showing a therapeutic window below which and above which one does not get the antidepressant effect with the secondary amine tricyclics, such as nortriptyline. In a setting where blood levels are not available, it is thus possible to be either above or below the therapeutic plasma level of these drugs. With the tertiary tricyclics, such as amitriptyline and imipramine, this window of efficacy has not been reported, and the curve of response is more sigmoidal. Because of this therapeutic window, a case can be made for avoiding the secondary tricyclic when blood levels are not available, unless there are special reasons for their use.

In the near future, there are likely to be further aids for selecting the most efficacious antidepressant for a particular patient. In some recent research, a low 24-hour urinary MHPG and a short-term lifting of mood in response to dexedrine administered in low dosages indicates a more likely response to imipramine,[2] while a high 3 methoxy-4-hydroxyphenol glycol favors amitriptyline.[3] It is likely that further access to patients' central serotonergic, cholinergic, dopaminergic, and

Table 25-1   Tricyclic Properties and Effective Blood Levels*

	Sedating	Anticholinergic	Effective plasma level ng/ml
Amitriptyline	+4	+4	(95–200)[‡]
Imipramine	+2	+3	(125–225)[§]
Doxepin	+4	+3	(100)[¶]
Nortriptyline	+2	+3	(50–150)
Desipramine	+2	+2	100 ng/ml
Protriptyline	+1	[†]	(70–225)

*Toxicity of all tricyclics is common at plasma levels above 500 ng/ml. Coma and death are not unusual at 1000 ng/ml.
[†]Not ascertained
[‡]Reported as total of amitriptyline and nortriptyline
[§]Reported as total of imipramine and desipramine
[¶]Reported as total of doxepin and desmethyldoxepin

adrenergic status will assist the clinician in this choice. In preliminary stages there are also nomograms for predicting dosage requirements based on 12- or 24-hour blood levels. These may be limited for usefulness by dose-dependent pharmacokinetics. Thus, despite a nomogram prediction of dosage required, the blood level may need to be rechecked. Hopefully, as the relative toxicity of the various metabolic products of the antidepressants are identified, the profile of 24-hour drug levels will help the clinician to avoid particularly dangerous drug-patient combinations.

The groups that should be started on low dosages of tricyclics include the aged, the young female, those low in body weight, those with a personal or family history of response to low dosages, and those on other agents that tend to potentiate the effect of or to elevate the blood level of tricyclics. Also needing initial low dosage are patients with low serum albumin, anyone predisposed to the side effects of the tricyclics, and those who would be endangered by sedation because of their activity schedule. Among those who are predisposed to the central anticholinergic syndrome are the chronically anxious, those with organic brain syndromes, and probably those with decreased cerebral oxygenation from cardiac tachydysrhythmias, low pAO_2, increased blood viscosity, or postural hypotension.

The first day's dosage of the tricyclics (excluding protriptyline) should be in the range of 25 to 75 mg, based on the patient's predisposition to toxicity and the urgency of treatment. The early appearance of postural hypotension, increased anxiety, or the sudden appearance of nocturnal confusion are evidence to either omit or amend the planned schedule of tricyclic dosage.

Typically, if there is no predisposition to toxicity, the dosage is brought to 150 mg per day by the end of the first week of treatment with imipramine, amitriptyline, and doxepin. Desipramine and nortriptyline generally are brought to a dosage of 75 to 125 mg by the end of the first week. Protriptyline may be started on a daily dosage of 30 mg, and should generally not be given in dosages of greater than 60 mg per day.

The tricyclics should be administered in a dosage schedule to take advantage of their side effects of sedation or stimulation. The more sedative tricyclics, such as amitriptyline and doxepin, should be administered at bedtime or divided between the hour before the evening meal and at bedtime. If the patients are agitated throughout the day and they would not be endangered by the possible sedation, they may be placed on a three doses per day schedule. Clinical experience, reports of postural hypotension and cardiac dysrhythmia, and our personal experiences using a halter monitor on patients who were on tricyclics suggest that dosages above 150 mg of amitriptyline, imipramine, and doxepin should be divided.

The traditional method of increasing a tricyclic by 25 to 50 mg per day when increases are warranted is reasonable. The tricyclics take from 1 to 6 weeks to reach a blood level plateau, depending upon the patient's age, liver function, thyroid status, weight, and the specific drug. With amitriptyline, imipramine, and doxepin, the plateau is generally reached by the end of the second week. With protriptyline and especially in the elderly, the blood level may still be rising during the third and fourth week.

What to Tell the Patient Who Is Starting on a Tricyclic

The physician should give the patient realistic hope, and use his or her position to educate and to improve compliance. The patient should be told to expect certain side effects, such as dry mouth and some somnolence at first. There may be constipation and mild blurring of vision. One might typically say, "Although I do not expect it, if you have any rapid or irregular beating of your heart, increased nervousness, or dizziness upon standing, I want to be notified. If there is any question about your medication, phone me." The physician should give the patient a contingency plan such as the physician's phone number and initially, weekly appointment dates for follow-up. The patient should be instructed to notify any other physician who might see the patient of his or her tricyclic use. The patient should be told not to start other medication without notifying the physician. Generally, the constipating effects of the tricyclics are such that it is a good idea to have a dietary plan on the first visit to offset part of this. It is often encouraging for the patient to hear something such as the following: "You will experience the side effects of the medication first, and later the benefits of improved sleep, increased strength, and resolution of your depression. The medication is not habit forming. The dosage required to treat your depression fully we will learn by your response, and so you should expect that we may have to adjust your prescription."

The Prescription   Tricyclics should be prescribed in child-resistant containers. The amount to be dispensed should initially not exceed 500 mg, or approximately the first week's supply. There should generally be a sedation warning on the prescription.

Monitoring the Patient on a Tricyclic

The patient starting on a tricyclic should have standing and reclining blood pressure and pulse recorded with each visit. The patient who shows signs or symptoms of postural hypotension or postural tachycardia can be instructed about how to avoid rapid standing, prolonged standing still, and extremes of environmental heat. This same patient may be instructed to use the gastrocnemius muscle to aid venous return or to buy support stockings to minimize venous pooling. The status of the patient's hydration and serum potassium should be checked. The patient on a tricyclic typically has a pulse increase of approximately 10 beats. The patient should be asked about other medications and about dryness of the mouth. The patient without some degree of dry mouth from the tricyclic is probably noncompliant. Any irregularity of pulse first noted after tricyclics are begun should be evaluated by physical exam and ECG, and consideration should be given to having a consultation and either reducing or withholding the medication. With severe urinary hesitancy from the tricyclic, the clinician may discontinue the medication, add urecholine in dosages of 10 mg three times a day, or switch to a less anticholinergic tricyclic such as desipramine. Clinically, the patient who is on amitriptyline and who cannot void often also has difficulty with voiding on desipramine. Constipation from the tricyclics can be severe, and when it is unrecognized it can lead to bleeding hemorrhoids, rectal prolapse, or obstipation, with its attendant medical and surgical morbidity. Weight should be monitored regularly. The patient on a tricyclic typically gains weight. Sudden weight gains can, at times, first suggest a *forme fruste* of congestive heart failure. Progressive weight loss in a depressed patient who is on a tricyclic suggests either an underlying medical problem that should be investigated or lack of efficacy at the maintenance dosage.

With each visit, the patient should be evaluated for suicidal potential. The depression may be graded on a four-point scale and plotted over time. Inquiry should be made as to sleep and energy. Worsening insomnia may indicate increasing suicidal danger and/or anticholinergic excess. The physician should be watchful for dilated pupils that are minimally responsive to light, or for an inordinate rise in resting pulse rate as a sign of anticholinergic excess. Typically, the patient first experiences an improved pattern of sleep, next an increase in energy, and finally a resolution of the depression. For example, the patient who at 2 weeks reports improved sleep and strength but no change in depression may be served best by having his or her dose unchanged for another week.

Laboratory monitoring of the patient on a tricyclic may be needed occasionally to evaluate toxicity. The patient who is started on a thiazide diuretic should have potassium checked, because low potassium predisposes to tachydysrhythmias form the tricyclics. The patient with reports of irregular pulse may need an ECG or, in unusual circumstances, may need Holter monitoring.

Routine laboratory monitoring of the blood level of the tricyclics is recommended for several reasons. There is a fortyfold variance in the plasma levels of tricyclics among patients on any given dose. Both the efficacy and the toxicity of the tricyclics are related to their blood level. Among the group of people who respond well initially to a tricyclic, only to relapse, a number have a decrease in the plasma blood level of the tricyclic, which is correctable. Problems with compliance are often discovered by the blood-level monitoring.

Currently, most laboratories measure total plasma tricyclic levels by gas chromatography, and this has been shown to be useful clinically. Research is under way to refine the methods even further. For example, it may be useful to measure both free and albumin-bound tricyclic, but this is still unresolved. The total of free and bound tricyclic correlates well with cerebrospinal fluid levels. It will be recalled that the tricyclics are metabolized to both inactive and psychoactive metabolites, measurements of the latter being of the greatest value. For example, when a patient receives imipramine, a blood level of at least 50 ng/ml of imipramine and 75 ng/ml of desmethylimipramine should be sought. The best goal is probably to maintain a total of imipramine plus desipramine of not less than 150 ng/ml and not more than 250 ng/ml. In the near future, the clinician will have available nomogram data using blood levels 24 hours after the first dose to assist in predicting the proper dosage. Such a nomogram is now available for lithium. The blood should be drawn at 8 to 15 hours from the last dosage. When the medication is given in the evening, a sample drawn 12 hours later is convenient. Properly collected and prepared, the plasma can be stored at room temperature and measured within 5 days. As a general rule, the first useful sample may be from 9 to 14 days after initiating the drug. This time frame is a compromise that approximates the plateau level but may well be below it, since occasionally that level is not reached for an additional 1 to 3 weeks. In a patient with predisposition to tricyclic toxicity, it may be prudent to get a 3- to 5-day level, and then extrapolate to the plateau to avoid overshooting the minimal effective dose.

If the first blood level is inordinately high, a total tricyclic of 350 ng/ml for example, but a beginning resolution of the depression is evident, the clinician can usually lower the dosage of tricyclic by a modest amount without causing a recrudescence of the depression and without waiting for the development of subtle signs of the central anticholinergic syndrome. If the initial blood level shows a total plasma tricyclic level of less than 20 ng/ml, there is almost certainly noncompliance. If the initial total plasma tricyclic is between 15 ng/ml and 100 ng/ml at 9 to 17 days and the patient's depression, including lack of energy, is unaltered, then the clinician should generally increase the dose of the tricyclic, barring any signs or symptoms of toxicity. There are two common mistakes in interpreting tricyclic blood levels. The first is to consider any level the plateau level. The second is to look only at the blood level and not at the patient. Occasionally, patients can have cardiac or central nervous system or gastrointestinal toxicity, even with low blood levels. Sometimes the variance may be in the laboratory and not the patient.

Most patients should have a plateau blood level, which is measured at 2 to 6 weeks, and this should be correlated with clinical state. At times, this knowledge avoids excess dosage; at other times, it illustrates the need to change drugs. Prior to the use of blood levels, it was often recommended to continue the trial of a given tricyclic at a fixed dose for 4 weeks to wait for a response. This time can be shortened considerably by blood-level measurement.

In monitoring the patient on a tricyclic antidepressant, it is important to consider the factors that may influence the blood level. Table 25-2 lists substances and states that have been reported to affect these levels. This list is based on clinical reports, and not all of them have been subjected to rigorous investigation. Those with the asterisks have been proven more definitely. Benzodiazepines do not seem to influence plasma levels of tricyclics. Special diets and antacids may slow the absorption of a single dose, but not the total quantity absorbed.

Maintenance Medication

Once resolution of the depression is achieved by the tricyclic, the next decision is how long to maintain the dosage. In patients without a personal or family history of mania, a general rule is to maintain the patient on the drug for 6 months. The patient with a history of mania should generally not be maintained on a tricyclic for longer than 1 month after resolution of the depression without attempts at tapering it off. This is to avoid increasing the rate of cycling in manic-depressive illness or triggering the patient into a manic state. Generally, the patient with a

Table 25-2 Drugs and Other Factors Influencing Tricyclic Plasma Levels

Decrease	Increase	
*Barbiturates—induce liver demethylation	*Neuroleptics—block ring hydroxylation	
*Alcohol—depends upon enzyme induction and liver mass	*Methylphenidate—blocks demethylation	
*Food–slows single dose absorption mainly	*IM route—bypasses the substantial first phase of demethylation	
*Antacids	Aspirin	Morphine
Estrogen	Amphetamines	Demerol
Cigarettes—possible stimulation of liver enzymes	Chloramphenicol	Adrenal steroids
	Haloperidol	
Chloral hydrate		
Diphenylhydantoin	*Influence of age*	
Pesticides (hydrocarbons)	*Children have higher levels with given dose/kg	
Glutethimide		
Meprobamate	*The elderly get higher peaks because of lowered protein binding	
Resins—Cholestyramine	*Desipramine and imipramine have higher levels with given dose/kg in the elderly	
Oral contraceptives	*Tricyclics have a longer half-life in the elderly	

*Strong supporting evidence.

longer history of depression should be maintained on the tricyclic for a longer period, and vice versa. There is the rare patient who appears to need long-term tricyclic medication, but this is the exception.

The patient who has been maintained on a tricyclic for 6 months can have medication decreased at the rate of 50 mg per week. Abrupt discontinuation of tricyclics, as with any markedly anticholinergic substance, can cause a syndrome of dysphoria, fatigue, myalgia, and insomnia that can be misinterpreted as the need for continuing medication.

The follow-up of a patient who has been on a tricyclic should include return appointments at 1 and 6 months. A contingency plan should include flagging of such symptoms as early morning awakening, which would herald a need for earlier return to the physician. The clinician is cautioned against missing a *forme fruste* of the "tricyclic-response depression" in the patient who has previously responded to a tricyclic. This is often seen as loss of energy, multiple somatic complaints, and insomnia.

Tricyclic Antidepressant Side Effects

At times it is difficult to decide which side effects are drug induced, which are placebo effects, and which are related to the depression. Most side effects of the tricyclics are related to their effect on the autonomic nervous system. These anticholinergic effects are dry mouth, constipation, urinary hesitancy, and mydriasis. Chewing gum, eating candy, or frequent sips of water have been recommended for the dry mouth, but the candy can precipitate monilial infections, and the water, if severely overused, can cause water intoxication. These methods are not very successful, but some degree of tolerance to the dry mouth usually develops. The elderly are more frequently bothered by the constipation and difficulty with initiating urination. A diet high in fiber and moderate quantities of fruit juice are often sufficient to counteract the constipation. In the hospitalized patient whose mentation limits his or her ability to report obstipation, the rectal exam and abdominal palpation should be performed periodically. Ten mg of urecholine three or four times a day is helpful to the patient who is having voiding difficulty that is secondary to the tricyclics. Tricyclics may cause a patient to be somnolent. The fully developed central anticholinergic syndrome is accurately described as follows: "mad as a hatter," "dry as a bone," "red as a lobster," and "blind as a stone." The patient is agitated and organic in the mental status exam, and experiences severe problems with memory and orientation. This is treated effectively with physostigmine.

Other autonomic side effects of the tricyclics include postural hypotension, occasional hypertension, and sweating that may be profuse and in a pattern limited to above the waist. The tricyclic antidepressants decrease a patient's tolerance to high environmental temperature because of their peripheral and central anticholinergic effects. The tricyclic antidepressants can precipitate narrow-angle glaucoma. Eye pain while on a tricyclic should be considered emergent glaucoma until proven otherwise.

The skin evidences tricyclic toxicity rarely by jaundice, occasionally by a pinpoint pruritic exanthem, and rarely by purpura. Agranulocytosis has been reported, but is very rare. Patients on tricyclics usually gain weight, and occasionally this is a problem that requires a moderate reduction of calories. The cardiac toxicity of tricyclics involves both anticholinergic and a quinidine-like effect. The heart rate usually increases. The QT interval and QRS interval may be prolonged. There may be flattening of the T-wave. Virtually every type of dysrhythmia reported in humans can be induced by tricyclics. In the patient with marginal cardiac compensation, the tricyclic may precipitate congestive heart failure. The patient with a recent myocardial infarction is particularly prone to serious arrhythmias when given a tricyclic.

Interaction of Tricyclics with Other Drugs   The drugs and states that influence the tricyclic blood level have been listed in Table 25-2. The sedative nature of the tricyclics is additive with all central nervous system sedatives, including alcohol and benzodiazepines. The anticholinergic side effects of the tricyclics are additive with other anticholinergic drugs. The list of substances with anticholinergic effects is legion, and the clinical problem is frequent. Because of the strength of its anticholinergic effects, amitriptyline should probably not be prescribed together in full therapeutic doses with thioridazine, chlorpromazine, atropine, scopolamine, or antiparkinsonism drugs.

The Monoamine Oxidase-Responsive Depressions

Monoamine oxidase inhibitors (MAOIs) are generally less effective than the tricyclic antidepressants, and are far more dangerous in the management of most depressions. The use of monoamine oxidase inhibitors (MAOIs) requires thorough familiarity with the medical and psychiatric aspects of their effects. In general, patients who require a MAOI should be referred to a specialist.

One use of MAOIs is for the severe tricyclic unresponsive depressions, when the patient or physician chooses to avoid ECT. A second category is a group of five syndromes that are responsive to MAOIs and are often resistant to tricyclics and to various forms of psychotherapy, education, or environmental manipulation. Some of these syndromes appear more as anxiety states. The five symptom clusters are as follows:

1 The hysteroid dysphorics, who are usually females with a history of repeated major mood swings that are often associated with environmental loss, sensitivity to rejection, and becoming overwhelmed when they fail to meet their own goals. These people are extroverted, often flamboyant, and seek to be "somebody's girl." When administered a tricyclic, they often develop insomnia, agitation, or depersonalization. Here the MAOI is a stabilizer of mood, with prophylactic value in modulating their repeated, often self-destructive "crashes."

2 The second syndrome is seen in people with multiple somatic complaints without evident organic pathology. At times, they develop hyperventilation and, at other times, tachycardia, tremor, and agitation. They are typically of ectomorphic build.

3 Phobic anxiety neurosis with panic attacks, which have their onset between ages 15 and 30 years, are heralded by sudden fear, sweating, and a feeling of impending doom. The first attack is often after an accident or death in the family. Patients may become agoraphobic, even to the point of being homebound. They may eat more and gain weight. Typically, they are concerned with "how far it is from home" or from their car, seeking safety with family, friends, and home. A subcategory of patients with phobic anxiety neurosis responds to low doses of certain tricyclics. Some who are unresponsive to tricyclics respond to MAOIs.

4 Chronic "free-floating anxiety neurosis" is often confused with schizophrenia. Patients may report pseudohallucinatory experiences, but do not have a thought disorder or protracted hallucinations. They often have diaphoresis, palpitations, and insomnia. The onset of this chronic anxiety state is between 15 and 30 years of age.

5 Certain focal psychogenic pain states respond best to MAOIs. These will be discussed under the section dealing with pain.

The features associated with good MAOI responses are hypochondriasis, somatic anxiety, irritability, and agoraphobia.

Limitations to MAOI Use   Patients who should not be given a monoamine oxidase inhibitor include: (1) anyone with a medical contraindication; (2) those with psychiatric conditions that may be worsened by the MAOI, which include most patients with manic-depressive illness, schizophrenia, many of those with substance abuse problems, and those with histories of certain types of impulse control disorders; (3) those without the intelligence, education, or stability in their lives to attend to the required limitations of diet and medication restrictions.

The monoamine oxidase inhibitors are a heterogeneous group of drugs that block the oxidative deamination of certain naturally occurring monoamines. Since catecholamines and serotonin are metabolized by monoamine oxidase, their levels rise when this enzyme is blocked. The therapeutic effects are related to such elevation, but so is the toxicity. At least 75 percent inhibition of the enzyme is required for the effects. The potential toxicities of MAOIs can be divided into direct effects, drug-drug interactions and drug-diet interactions. Because of their far-reaching potential for interaction with many disease states and with drugs and diet, a complete medical and psychiatric evaluation is required prior to their prescription.

Direct toxic reactions of MAOIs include rare hepatotoxicity, mainly with hydrazine-type MAOIs, such as phenelzine. Orthostatic hypotension can occur with any MAOI. It can be countered acutely by recumbence and chronically by dosage reduction and the measures already discussed in the treatment of tricyclic-induced orthostatic hypotension. Mild constipation is not unusual. Skin rashes, inhibition of ejaculation, and blurred vision have been reported. Excessive central nervous system stimulation is occasionally manifested by insomnia, tremor, or agitation. The disinhibiting, activating, and confidence-instilling qualities of these drugs occasionally cause patients to act on impulse in a manner that may be damaging in consequence.

MAOIs can have toxic interactions with many drugs and foods. Among the most dangerous are the indirectly acting amines, for example, tyramine in food, amphetamines, and to a lesser extent, the direct sympathomimetic amines, such as epinephrine. The stores of endogenous amines are increased by the MAOIs. The ingestion of indirect-acting exogenous amines releases these increased stores, which results in a profound sympathomimetic discharge manifested as hypertension. In its extreme form, the result may be a lethal cerebral hemorrhage.

Hyperpyrexia may result from the concurrent use of demerol and an MAOI. The mechanism appears to be a central release of serotonin. MAOIs interfere with the metabolism of certain other drugs. They increase the half-life and intensify the effects of barbiturates, alcohol, morphine, and many anticholinergic agents. They are synergistic with tricyclic antidepressants, and while this may be beneficial in very expert hands, it is more likely to lead to very serious adverse reactions. An MAOI should not be given within 2 weeks if a patient has had another, separate MAOI or a tricyclic, except by experts in very select cases.

Medicines to be avoided generally while on MAOIs include:

Amphetamines
Antihistamines
Insulin and other hypoglycemics
Meperidine
Opiates and other narcotics, including pentazocine hydrochloride
Reserpine
Cocaine
Anticholinergics
Barbiturates

L-dopa
Aldomet-methyldopa
Sympathomimetic agents
Tricyclic antidepressants
Procaine

Relative medical contradictions to the use of MAOIs include:

Cardiovascular disease
Hepatic disease (phenylzine sulfate to be avoided here)
Pheochromocytoma
Asthma
Cerebrovascular disease
Renal disease
Carcinoid syndrome

Foods to be avoided while on an MAOI (because of tyramine content, dopa content, vanillin content, or other amine content) include:

*Cheese (ripened or aged)	Chocolate
*Chianti wine	Pickled herring
Other alcohol, especially red wine and beer	Smoked salmon
Liver	Raisins
Coffee (more than 4 cups)	Ripe bananas
Lox	Bologna, sausage (stored or aged)
Pods of broad beans	Meats
Sour cream	Sauerkraut
Yogurt	Caviar
Canned figs	Avocados
Marmite	Bovril
Soy sauce	Game
	Lobster

The following list is useful for starting a patient on an MAOI after a medical and psychiatric evaluation.

Information regarding the use and type of MAOI should be given to:

The patient (orally and in the form of a card to carry and a diet sheet)
The patient's family or cook
The patient's primary physician
The staff (if the patient is hospitalized)
The patient's dentist prior to dental consultations (dental work requires amendment of the anesthetic and avoidance of the usual dosage of epinephrine)
The patient's druggist if the patient uses that individual as a source of other medications

*The most dangerous

The information given contains instructions as to permissible and prohibited (1) diet and beverages, and (2) medicines. A contingency plan should be available for complications, and the patient is told to phone the physician if there are any questions. Using the above obsessive approach avoids dangerous side effects and increases the efficacy of the drugs.

Choice of Individual MAOI and Dosage   Phenelzine is generally considered the safest MAOI, but should not be used if there is a history of liver disease. Phenelzine is begun at a dosage of 30 mg, and is increased in increments of 15 mg every 2 to 3 weeks. Most patients respond to doses of 45 or 60 mg, which usually inhibits monoamine oxidase (MAO) by about 85 percent. Occasionally, higher doses are needed. Tranylcypromine acts quickly, often within 1 week, is more potent, and is more activating to the unmotivated, the anergic, and the hypersomniac, but probably carries a higher risk of toxicity than does phenelzine. It is a reasonable choice for the patient with a history of liver disease who needs an MAOI. Phenelzine is started at doses of 20 mg per day, and has an average maintenance dose of 30 mg per day in divided doses. With each visit, the patient on an MAOI should have a standing and reclining blood pressure and pulse rate check, and an inquiry should be made as to the understanding and adherence to dietary and drug restrictions. Blood levels of the MAOI can be measured by studying the degree of MAO inhibition in the chemical laboratory. This monitoring parameter allows the psychopharmacologist to be confident that the patient has had an adequate trial, and may help avoid excessive dosage.

Lithium as an Antidepressant

A strong case can be made for suggesting that patients who require lithium should have their management partially or totally orchestrated by an expert in the use of lithium. This is true in part because of the behavior dilemmas associated with the care of both the manic and the severely depressed patient.

The prophylactic value of lithium in the management of manic-depressive illness is well established. It decreases the rate of cycling and modulates the severity of cycling into both mania and depression. The use of lithium in the treatment of recurrent unipolar depressions with vegetative symptoms and without a history of mania is more controversial. Its efficacy is reported to be correlated with presenting complaints of hypersomnia, weight gain, and severe motoric slowing, a fact often seen in the depressions of classic manic-depressive illness. A family history suggestive of a *forme fruste* manic-depressive state also suggests lithium responsiveness. The depressed alcoholic with a history of mood swings and a family history of manic-depressive illness may be responsive to lithium. Lithium given for prophylaxis against recurrent depression should be administered in a fashion similar to its use as a prophylaxis against mania.

Antipsychotic Medication in the Treatment of Depression

In general, neuroleptics are ineffective in the treatment of most depressions. However, the patient with a "psychotic depression" or with severely agitated depression with guilt and affectively laden delusions may have a resolution of psychosis or agitation when given an antipsychotic. The patient needing an antipsychotic medication for depression should have psychiatric consultation, because of the diagnostic issues involved in the question of "psychotic depression" and because of the high suicidal potential of depressed patients with psychosis or severe agitation.

Polypharmacy in the Treatment of Depression

The great majority of patients with depression who need psychopharmacologic care need only one drug, but occasional exceptions do occur. The patient on lithium who becomes depressed despite therapeutic lithium levels may also need a tricyclic antidepressant. A patient with an agitated depression who does not respond to a sedating tricyclic antidepressant will need the addition of benzodiazepine or of a neuroleptic to aid in the treatment of agitation or psychosis, respectively. Very rarely, in truly unresponsive severe depression, the careful and expert administration of a combination of tricyclic and an MAOI is warranted. This is a hazardous combination, and when used, the dosages, timing of administration, and monitoring must be rigidly controlled.

A Comment on ECT   Electroconvulsive therapy should neither be used frequently nor discarded totally. It is effective in treating many depressions, even when adequate trials of antidepressants have failed. Its mortality, when properly administered, is essentially that of the anesthetic. It is often the treatment of choice if the patient is in imminent danger of suicide. It is, at times, the treatment of choice when the patient has strong medical contraindications to the tricyclic antidepressants and MAOIs. It is the treatment of choice for the elderly and for the frail who cannot tolerate the adverse effects of drugs. The patient who responds to ECT should be maintained on a tricyclic antidepressant as discussed under that section.

MANIC-DEPRESSIVE ILLNESS

Introduction

Manic-depressive illness is generally episodic in nature. It may present as alternating cycles of depression and mania, recurrent depression, recurrent bouts of mania or hypomania, or psychosis that resembles schizophrenia. Mood swings may be as frequent as every 48 hours, or they may occur over intervals of many months. More subtle presentations include mania masked by spree drinking and more modulated forms of mood swings. Most people with moderate labile mood are neither manic-depressive nor lithium-responsive. On the other hand, many with manic-depressive illness are denied lithium and other effective psychopharmacologic treatments for this group of disorders because they are thought to have schizophrenia, grief reaction, or personality disorder. The illness most typically begins in the early thirties, but may begin in early adolescence or in the sixties. Women with manic-depressive illness are more likely to have episodes of depression or mania during puerperium. The differential diagnosis may at times be between manic-depressive illness and anxiety neurosis. The resulting course of manic-depressive illness and a family history of affective disorder often help to differentiate between schizophrenia and manic-depressive illness.

The manic patient is either euphoric or uncharacteristically irritable, and demonstrates both hyperactivity and flight of ideas. The manic state may be accompanied by bizarre dress, a sudden lessening of sleep, and an increase in the patient's expenditure of money. The manic patient may be recognized by the social disarray left in his or her wake. He or she is often expansive in writing, projects, and plans. The family history often contains the suggestion of such illness in previous generations, in the form of a high incidence of suicide, bankruptcy, and multiple divorces.

Treatment of Manic-Depressive Illness

This should generally be reserved for the psychiatrist because of such factors as the behavioral dilemmas and sudden suicidal potential of some of these patients.

Lithium is effective in slowing the cycling and modulating the intensity of the mood swings. It is effective prophylactically for both the mania and the depression of manic-depressive illness. It is the maintenance treatment of choice for mania. However, when the patient is hypomanic in a first episode, or because he or she has discontinued lithium, the addition of a neuroleptic that acts quickly until the lithium can bring control may be required. About 80 percent of patients with manic-depressive illness respond to lithium, but some do not, and others occasionally break through into manic episodes.

The patient with manic-depressive illness should have a discussion, and the family a list, of flag symptoms that often repeat as heralds of a recurrence of the depression or mania. There should also be a contingency plan for both depression and mania that involves behavioral and pharmacologic parameters.

Lithium

For a variety of reasons, lithium has been the most extensively and accurately measured of the psychotropic drugs. The technology for its measurement is relatively simple. Since it is an inorganic element, it is not metabolized. It is not bound by plasma proteins and it is not, therefore, subject to the sources of error of psychotropic organic compounds, which may be protein bound and, hence, may show a discrepancy between bound and unbound drugs. It is not stored in fat, but rather distributes intracellularly and extracellularly through body water. It is transported actively across cell membranes, and equilibrium is established actively in the liver, kidney, and spleen, but more slowly in muscle, bone, and brain. The plasma half-life of lithium ranges from 7 to 36 hours, but averages about 12 hours. Peak levels of lithium usually occur within a few hours, and after a single dose, 50 percent is excreted in 24 hours and 90 percent in 48 hours. Because of its short half-life, it has been administered in multiple daily doses, but recent work has suggested that its slower equilibration in the brain might permit a single daily dose. Lithium levels in patients are usually measured in the morning, and this seems adequate because of its rapid absorption and complete distribution within 6 to 10 hours. The dosage of lithium varies from patient to patient and is determined by monitoring blood levels. For many patients this will involve 300 mg three or four times per day.

Because lithium can be measured so readily and accurately, and because there is a therapeutic window below which there is no effectiveness and above which there may be considerable toxicity, it is the only psychotropic drug that is monitored routinely in standard clinical practice. Results of such monitoring have shown that in a large population there is marked individual variability in plasma level following a single dose, and even on maintenance medication at therapeutic doses taken orally. Despite many studies, there remains some disagreement as to what optimal plasma levels should be. Levels exceeding 1.5 milliequivalents per liter are generally toxic. Levels of 0.8 to 1.4 milliequivalents per liter are required for the treatment of acute mania. Disagreement exists for the maintenance management of unipolar and bipolar patients. Some investigators have recommended levels as low as 0.3 to 0.6 milliequivalents per liter, and others recommend maintenance of 0.8 to 1.4 milliequivalents per liter. Lithium carbonate package inserts recommend maintenance at levels of 0.6 to 1.2 milliequivalents per liter, and a multihospital collaborative study recommends lithium maintenance levels to 0.8 to 1.0 milliequivalents per liter. Although the variance in the recommended maintenance blood levels appears small, it should be recalled that lithium has a narrow therapeutic window and that acute toxicity can appear at levels about 1.5 milliequivalents per liter, while chronic toxicity may occur at lower levels. Clinical monitoring of symptoms must go along with laboratory monitoring of plasma lithium levels for optimum treatment. A priming dose of 600 mg lithium and a single blood sample collected 24 hours later correlate very highly with the steady state achieved during maintenance therapy. The use of this method may permit a more rapid establishment of adequate lithium levels.

The clinician should be thoroughly familiar with the use and toxicity of lithium. Acute lithium toxicity may be manifested by tremor, ataxia, somnolence, headache, coma, seizure, diarrhea, nausea, or enuresis. Subacutely, lithium can rarely cause sinus node dysfunction or premature ventricular contractions. The ECG should be intermittently observed in those on Li+ with known heart disease. The sinus changes and PVCs are important, and should not be confused with the 20 percent incidence of benign T-wave flattening on the ECG in those at therapeutic range. Among the chronic reported changes associated with lithium use are: hypothyroidism, with or without goiter, and nephrogenic diabetes insipidis. There are a few reports of nephritis in a subgroup of chronic lithium patients who have had prolonged evidence of renal-concentrating deficits or bouts of toxic serum lithium levels. A mild, fine tremor, mild nausea, or mild fatigue may occur when initiating lithium therapy. The primary physician should be certain that the patient who is being maintained on lithium has had evaluation of the renal function, the thyroid function (including TSH, FTI, and thyroid antibodies), and has had EEG, ECG, a CBC, and a monitoring of serum lithium.

The clinician should be aware of the fact that changes in water and sodium flux may produce changes in the lithium concentration. Thus, rigid dieting or fasting, salt restriction, diuretics, or any medical illness that changes water or salt balances should alert the physician to a need to either measure or at times withhold lithium. It is an unproven clinical impression that hypokalemia predisposes to lithium toxicity, and that variance in calcium intake may influence lithium metabolism. Lithium should not be given with supersaturated potassium iodide because of the reports of increased thyroid disease. Lithium should generally be avoided in pregnancy because of unconfirmed reports of an increased incidence of cardiac anomalies in the children of patients who took lithium throughout their pregnancies.

ANXIETY

Introduction

Fear and anxiety clearly resemble each other in their subjective feelings and objective manifestations. They differ in that fear has a manifest cause, while in anxiety the causes may seem trivial to the outside observer. Often, the underlying fear is repressed and is unconscious. Anxiety states may be separated into anticipatory anxiety and panic anxiety. Anticipatory anxiety is often chronic, and there is a dreadful feeling that there will be panic in the future, especially if a feared act is undertaken. In panic anxiety there is the attack itself, with all its dreadful subjective feelings and objective autonomic signs.

Anxiety in its milder form can increase coping and adapting mechanisms, but its capacity to result in diminished function is well known. In psychotherapy, anxiety may announce the breaking down of old defense mechanisms, and it may be elicited slowly and carefully by the therapist to facilitate psychological change. Overwhelming anxiety in psychotherapy may indicate an impending psychosis. In its severe forms, anxiety is so intolerable that the patient may attempt to blend it with a myriad of psychological defenses, or act to relieve it by fight or flight actions, which include self-medication or visits to a physician.

When clinicians see anxiety, they should look carefully for depression and anger, because they are often present in the same patient. The patient with anxiety is often restless, and may complain of difficulty in falling asleep, fatigue, short temper, and distractibility. Physical complaints include palpitations, muscular tension most commonly in the back or neck, headache, tremor, change in the frequency or caliber of stool, dizziness, shooting pains in the chest, and abdominal discomfort. A simple diagnosis of anxiety is usually incomplete. It should be made with both inclusion and exclusion criteria. The origin of the anxiety should be sought. Many psychiatric states present with manifest anxiety. Depression, the onset of schizophrenia, mania, neurotic conflict, more specific phobic anxiety states, and situational stress reactions may all present with anxiety. The observant physician can often diagnose early alcohol or sedative withdrawal in the hospitalized patient by the onset of anxiety or insomnia. Exogenous stimulants and anticholinergics may cause anxiety. Almost any medical illness can present with anxiety; hyperthyroidism is perhaps the prototype. The physician must guard against missing changes in the internal physiologic milieu as causes of anxiety. Hypoxia, hypoglycemia, carboxyhemoglobinemia, hypoperfusion, or anatomic changes in the central nervous system must be recognized.

Drug Treatment of Anxiety

Drug treatment of anxiety should generally be started after a diagnosis of its cause, and only if the anxiety has not responded to simple medical or psychological treatment. Even then, it should be instituted only if the level of anxiety is interfering with the patient's function. Antianxiety agents are more appropriate for acute anxiety, and are less so for chronic anxiety. Tolerance to them develops, and escalating dosage increases the risk. Antianxiety agents should generally only be prescribed when, in parallel, there is a plan for a more specific or permanent attenuation of the underlying causes. This may take the form of environmental change, treatment of medical illness, solution of problems through psychotherapy, or the acquisition of less stressful life-styles. Most prescriptions for antianxiety agents should be for short term, and only for "as needed" use. The physician should use the role of healer to enhance the placebo effect of these drugs.

Side Effects

All antianxiety agents have dose-dependent side effects. All of them may cause mild sedation and slowed reaction time. Thus, the potential hazards of driving or operating machinery must always be kept in mind. Some depressions, which are associated with an awareness and fear of diminished performance, are made worse by antianxiety agents that diminish performance even further. All antianxiety agents are at least additive with alcohol in their sedative properties, and many are more than additive. Ataxia, confusion, and postural hypotension are common with mild to moderate overuse. Teratogenic effects are rare, but some have been reported with several of these agents. Their use during the last trimester of pregnancy may result in a somnolent newborn who later goes through withdrawal symptoms. Almost all these agents are excreted in breast milk.

Specific Antianxiety Agents

The Benzodiazepines Some of the clinically important features of the different benzodiazepines are given in Table 25-3. The benzodiazepines have two main advantages. The first is the wide margin between lethal and effective dosage. Oral benzodiazepines are rarely, if ever, lethal unless they are combined with alcohol or other drugs. The second advantage is that tolerance and dependence are usually slow to develop. Barbiturates, meprobamate, and glutethimide have a much higher abuse potential. Still another advantage to benzodiazepines over most other currently marketed antianxiety agents is the minimal extent to which they induce hepatic microsomal enzymes. Thus, they can be used more easily with other medications. For example, they do not markedly alter the plasma levels of tricyclics, the dose of coumadin required, or the blood level of neuroleptics, as is the case with such notorious enzyme inducers as the barbiturates.

Table 25-3   Characteristics of Commercial Benzodiazepines

Generic name	Trade name	Half-life (hrs)	Major Psychoactive Metabolites	Influenced by Capacity to Demethylate	Requires Stomach Acid to Reach Psychoactive State
Diazepam	Valium	20–50*	Desmethyl-diazepam	Yes	No
Chlordiaze-poxide	Librium	30–50	Desmethylchlor-diazepoxide Demoxepam		
			Desmethyldia-zepam	Yes	No
Oxazepam	Serax	5–18	None	No	No
Clorazepate	Tranxene	30–60	Desmethyldia-zepam	No (probably)	Yes.
Lorazepam	Ativan	10–15	None	No	No

*As rough guide, 20 + years of age past 30.

    The differences in response to the various benzodiazepines are influenced by many factors. These include the rate of their absorption after oral or intramuscular administration, the conditions necessary for their absorption, their half-life, and whether the parent compound, its metabolites, or both are psychoactive. Most benzodiazepines should not be given intramuscularly, because they are absorbed more rapidly and predictably when given orally. The rate of absorption from the GI tract appears to influence substantially the acquisition of subjective feelings of calm, and this probably influences their popularity as drugs of abuse. There is a wide variance in the plasma level achieved among patients on a given dosage. Benzodiazepine plasma levels correlate with efficacy and toxicity, and such levels will probably be available routinely in the near future. Very high blood levels may suppress cough and gag reflexes, although this is not well established. Antianxiety efficacy correlates with steady-state plasma diazepam levels of 400 ng/ml or more. Desmethyldiazepam is present at lower levels, and levels exceeding 300 ng/ml are associated with increasing side effects. Chlordiazepoxide plasma levels above 700 ng/ml are associated in some studies with greater therapeutic benefit. Desmethylchlordiazepoxide plasma levels resulting from chlordiazepoxide administration are the best chemical correlates of efficacy. When a benzodiazepine is given in a fashion that results in very rapid rise of plasma levels, the incidence of anterograde amnesia increases. Lorazepam, whose absorption from the intramuscular injection is rapid, is associated with a high incidence of anterograde amnesia. The elimination half-life of these drugs varies markedly from person to person and among the various benzodiazepines. Oxazepam has a short half-life, and this may be employed to advantage in the elderly and in others who are particularly subject to the cumulative effect of sedatives and hypnotics. Since this drug does not undergo demethylation, its metabolism is more predictable in the myriad of conditions when demethylation is altered, as in drug-induced microsomal enzyme states, alcoholism, and in the aged.

Benzodiazepines are metabolized by demethylation, hydroxylation, and esterification. They should be differentiated clinically by whether the parent compound, its metabolic products, or both are psychoactive. First, the "pro-drugs," which must be metabolized before becoming psychoactive, include (in this country) chlorazepate and prazepam. Chlorazepate requires acid hydrolysis in the stomach in order to achieve its psychoactive state. When given with antacids or in achlorhydric states, it may not achieve effective blood levels. The transformation of prazepam to its more psychoactive forms happens after absorption. Chlordiazepoxide and diazepam start as active drugs, and are quickly metabolized to active metabolites, and more slowly to inactive ones. Oxazepam is already demethylated, and its metabolic products are inactive. With chronic administration of benzodiazepines, there is some pharmacokinetic tolerance that is related to changes in the ratios of psychoactive and inactive metabolites present.

The dosage of benzodiazepine used for a particular patient should generally be titrated individually because of the great effects of biological variance on absorption, tolerance, and side effects. The danger of fixed dosage schedules may be evidenced by ataxia, somnolence, or confusion from too high a plasma level. The probability of side effects is also related to the half-life, since drugs with long half-lives will achieve higher plasma levels on a fixed dose schedule than those with short half-lives. The elderly patient who metabolizes slowly on a fixed dose of diazepam may show toxicity as soon as 4 to 10 days after initiation of treatment. The effects of other drugs on the plasma level of benzodiazepines are only now being investigated.

All benzodiazepines can produce symptoms of withdrawal that are similar to those of withdrawal from other sedatives and alcohol. However, because of their long half-lives and the slower development of psychologic dependence, acute withdrawals with benzodiazepines are not as commonly a life-threatening condition. With severe or chronic overuse, with multiple substance abuse, and in the occasional idiosyncratic case, benzodiazepine withdrawal should be carried out after hospitalization by a physician who is familiar with withdrawal techniques.

Barbiturates   The barbiturates are rarely indicated as antianxiety drugs. The anxiolytic effect is probably because of their hypnosedative effect. There is a small margin of safety between effective and toxic dosage range. Tolerance and dependency usually occur with their chronic use. They stimulate liver enzymes, thus modifying the metabolism of many other drugs, such as tricyclic antidepressants, many neuroleptics, and coumadin. Withdrawal symptoms after chronic use are frequently severe, may be lethal, and hospitalization is generally needed.

Propranolol   The hyper-β-adrenergic state is a "flag" syndrome that may perpetuate anxiety. The patient who develops such symptoms of sympathetic discharge as sinus tachycardia or tremor, originally from fear of an actual, pending, or recalled traumatic event, may become classically conditioned. Such a patient then develops periodic anxiety and tachycardia, through a series of feedback mechanisms that are as yet incompletely understood. Such symptoms may be blocked with β-adrenergic blockers. There is marked variance in the blood levels of propranolol in different individuals with a given dose. Currently, the clinician uses evidence of mild β-blockade as evidence of adequate dosage. Propranolol's adverse effects include slowing of the pulse, negative inotropic cardiac effects, the occasional precipitation of asthma in susceptible individuals, feelings of coldness, and occasionally vivid, "colorful" nightmares. the abuse potential seems very low.

Sedative Antihistamines   These agents are less often chosen for use, and have little potential for abuse. They may ameliorate both urticaria and pruritis associated with anxiety. Otherwise, they have little to recommend them in the treatment of anxiety. There are isolated, unproven reports of tardive dyskinesia with the chronic use of these agents. They can cause paradoxical excitement or delirium, especially in children and in the aged.

The Propanediol Family   There are at least fifteen generic drugs and drug combinations containing the propanediols. Meprobamate once was regarded highly, but current data suggest that the efficacy of these compounds is comparable at best to the barbiturates, and at worst to placebo. They have a narrow range between therapeutic effects and toxicity. Physical dependence, tolerance, and severe withdrawals are not uncommon.

Antidepressants   The tricyclic antidepressants are useful in treating the anxiety or agitation commonly found in tricyclic-responsive depression, as described in a previous section. Thus, the patient with anxiety, early morning awakening, and weight loss should be evaluated as a possible candidate for tricyclic antidepressant.

Panic Attacks and Agoraphobia   Patients whose anxiety comes in terrifying bursts of panic and those with severe anxiety associated with incapacitating agoraphobia have both panic anxiety and anticipatory anxiety. The panic may be helped by judicious use of certain antidepressants (see the section about depression). The anticipatory anxiety is usually managed by some form of psychological treatment. Although benzodiazepines may also help to alleviate the anticipatory and chronic base of anxiety, they do not eliminate the panic attacks of agoraphobia, which respond better to certain antidepressants.

SCHIZOPHRENIA

Introduction

Schizophrenia may be viewed as a chronic illness of varying severity, with remissions and relapses. It is a psychotic disorder characterized by disturbances in thinking, feeling, and behavior. Affecting about 1 percent of the population, schizophrenia is the most common, but not the only, psychotic disorder. Psychoses may be related to alcohol, drugs, brain damage, metabolic disorders, and overwhelming emotional trauma. They may also be present in severe depressions and in manic states. Even though the drugs to be discussed are not specific for schizophrenia, but rather are broadly antipsychotic, diagnosis is imperative for initial treatment and especially for maintenance. This is so because some psychoses that resemble schizophrenia can be treated by removing the offending agent, whether it be drugs or a highly noxious environment, or by correcting the underlying medical disorder. The functional psychoses other than schizophrenia are better treated with agents that are more specific for the underlying illness. Thus, affective illness may be treated with lithium or antidepressants, while severe anxiety states with dissociative features may be treated as described in the section on anxiety.

Although the specific etiology of schizophrenia is not known, there is substantial evidence from consanguinity, both twin and adoptive studies, that there is a genetic diathesis in schizophrenia. Genetic vulnerability is probably a necessary condition for the development of the disorder. The same data, however, reveal that genetics alone is not a sufficient explanation. For example, the concordance of schizophrenia in those identical twins who develop this illness is about 40 percent, rather than the 100 percent that would be predicted from a purely genetic mechanism. Thus, the environmental contribution must be at least as great as the genetic. But the nature of the environment that contributes to the development of the schizophrenic phenotype is uncertain. Intrauterine and early postnatal damage have been considered as contributory factors. Traumatic early childhood emotional experiences, especially within the context of the family, may also be involved. The individual expression of schizophrenic symptoms shows a great range of variability, as might be expected from a complex illness that is a product of genetic loading, possible early psychological insult, and the complex psychological and social experiences of the developing human.

The diagnosis of schizophrenia, especially as it relates to drug treatment, should be made by both exclusive and inclusive criteria. Organic brain syndromes with psychoses (such as may be found in brain tumors, vascular disease, encephalitis, temporal lobe epilepsy, metabolic disorders, or drug- and alcohol-induced psychotic states), and severe functional disorders (such as obsessive compulsive neurosis or a definite manic or depressive syndrome) should be ruled out by history and appropriate clinical and laboratory examination. Since there are no laboratory tests for schizophrenia, the inclusive criteria are entirely behavioral and psychological, and since these criteria are affected significantly by past psychological and cultural experience, the diagnosis is not simple. For example, the diagnosis is made more frequently in the United States than in Europe.

Diagnostic criteria should include at least two from the following partial list of possible symptoms. In general, these symptoms should be present for at least 2 weeks.

1 Disorders of thought, which make communication difficult because of a lack of understandable or logical connections
2 Delusions of external control of one's thoughts or actions
3 Bizarre delusions, especially those of a paranoid nature

4   The feeling that one's thoughts are broadcast, and others may hear
5   The feeling that one can receive others' thoughts
6   Auditory hallucinations that provide a running commentary on the subject's thoughts or behavior
7   Hallucinations of any sort throughout the day for several days or intermittently for a month
8   Catatonic motor behavior

A family history of schizophrenia; an age of onset between the ages of 15 and 35; and a history from relatives or friends of gradual withdrawal from school, work, church, and family, with increasing isolation and atypical or bizarre behavior and profound mood swings, are helpful in establishing the diagnosis.

Treatment of Acute Schizophrenia

The nonpsychiatric physician is most likely to encounter schizophrenic patients early in the course of their illness, before a psychotic break has actually occurred. Since schizophrenics are by no means immune from medical and surgical ills, the primary physician may also be called upon to treat such conditions. Whenever possible, the general physician should refer schizophrenic patients to a specialist. Such patients may be at high risk for suicide, they are difficult to manage, and the consequences of their behavior are usually devastating to job, school, and family adjustment. All physicians who are responsible for continued treatment should work with other mental health workers because schizophrenics usually require assistance not only in symptom reduction, but also in stabilization and in adjustment to school, jobs, family living arrangements, and in the development of interpersonal skills. Even with proper medication relapse rates are inversely related to the adequacy of the psychosocial support systems available to schizophrenics. Furthermore, the suspiciousness, ambivalence, and irrational fears that are so common in schizophrenia combine to work against proper drug management. Failure to comply with the drug prescription is the most common cause of relapse. Fears of external control and oversedation are among the prominent reasons for compliance failure. The support systems are usually very helpful in diminishing such concerns and in securing compliance. Compliance is also improved by employing the patient in a drug management partnership as early as possible.

Commonly, patients with incipient schizophrenia first visit their family physicians when they are coping with the anguish, anxiety, apathy, hypochondriasis, sleep disturbances, and social withdrawal that so frequently precede an overt psychotic episode. At this time, a careful history and physical and neurological examinations should be accomplished to rule out the myriad of medical conditions that can produce similar subjective states. Simultaneously, a record of external stresses should be obtained, together with a mental status examination. If psychosis is suspected, referral to a psychiatrist should be made, but frequently this is refused initially by the patient. Brief symptomatic treatment with hypnotics, sedatives, or antianxiety drugs may be instituted in the prepsychotic patient, who should be followed closely. Antidepressant medications should be used cautiously, since they may precipitate a psychosis. The use of neuroleptics is seldom justified in patients who are not overtly psychotic. There are better anxiolytics and hypnotics. The neuroleptics have significant side effects, and compliance is poor. The danger of retrospective labeling of the patient as schizophrenic because he or she has responded to a neuroleptic drug can be avoided, and the neurological risks associated with long-term use of neuroleptics are eliminated. If symptomatic treatment without neuroleptics fails, referral to a psychiatrist is urgently needed.

Once a diagnosis of schizophrenia is made, the neuroleptic drugs are the cornerstone of treatment. However, exceptions to this exist. It has been found that about 30 percent of young patients with good premorbid histories who become acutely psychotic and whose presenting symptoms satisfy the criteria for schizophrenia may respond to hospitalization in specialized treatment centers that have experienced personnel and an excellent milieu, without requiring drugs.

Many patients with acute schizophrenia are pathologically excited, anxious, and disruptive. They are difficult to manage, and are a risk to themselves and to others. Such patients are a medical emergency, and should be treated with a sedative-type neuroleptic like the aliphatic phenothiazines or the very potent butyrophenones. Although there is great variance in the type of drugs and dose that is optimally effective for pathological excitement, 5 to 10 mg of haloperidol every 2 to 4 hours (not to exceed 40 mg daily) is usually effective. Intramuscular haloperidol is less painful and less hypotensive than chlorpromazine, and 5 mg may be given intramuscularly as needed. Maximal effects can be noted in less than 2 hours orally and in about a half-hour parenterally. If medication should be needed prior to transporting the exceptionally excited patient, haloperidol is the drug of choice. For catatonic excitement, it may be given intramuscularly every hour. Pathological excitement is a medical emergency, and the physician or the physician's team should be in constant physical and verbal contact until it is over. When the excitement has subsided, drug dosage should be diminished to a maintenance level.

Occasionally, the acute schizophrenic patient presents with apathy and withdrawal. For such patients, the neuroleptics with less sedative action may be employed. Ten mg fluphenazine hydrochloride twice daily by mouth, for example, can be employed initially, and this may be increased as necessary to 20 mg twice daily.

Important side effects from the emergency use of neuroleptics include hypotension and extrapyramidal signs. The former can usually be treated posturally, but may occasionally require administration of volume replacers and rarely of a pressor substance. If this is required, a pure alpha adrenergic stimulant like norepinephrine should be used because beta stimulants like isoproterenol or adrenaline can make the hypotension worse. Extrapyramidal symptoms like acute dystonia are not dangerous, but can be very frightening. These symptoms can be attenuated with antiparkinson agents, such as 1 to 2 mg benztropine orally, or the dopamine agonist, amantadine. It should always be remembered that the neuroleptics, while remarkably safe, can potentiate the depressant action of alcohol, narcotics, and barbiturates. Since most of them have anticholinergic activity, they can act additively with other anticholinergic agents. Thus, they should be avoided in a toxic psychosis, such as the central anticholinergic syndrome.

The acute schizophrenic who is treated in a conventional manner with the usual oral dose of phenothiazines usually requires treatment for 2 to 3 weeks before arousal symptoms like psychomotor excitement and insomnia are controlled. An additional, equally long period is usually required before there is remission of the affective symptoms. The symptoms related to perceptual and cognitive aspects of cerebration last even longer. Thus, delusions, hallucinations, and the formal thought disorder may persist for 6 to 8 weeks. The choice of neuroleptic during this time should be based upon the physician's and patient's past experience, and the dose should be determined by the patient's clinical response. There is a vast clinical literature on more than 20 individual neuroleptics, and details may be found in several textbooks of psychopharmacology. Suffice it to say that, although they vary more than fiftyfold in potency, as measured by the number of milligrams required daily and in the spectrum of their side effects, clinical efficacy is approximately equal in all of them when they are given in adequate dosage. However, individual variations in the rate of metabolism of the drugs may, for a particular patient, make one drug more effective than another.

Maintenance Medication

Neuroleptics do not cure schizophrenia, but are effective in attentuating or eliminating primary and secondary symptoms. If medication is not maintained, up to 70 percent of patients will relapse within a year, whereas less than 30 percent of those on medication will relapse. Among those who do not relapse, there frequently remain traces of symptoms that have an associated stigma, which makes family, job, and social adjustment difficult. As a result, schizophrenic patients rarely fulfill their full potential as students, workers, or parents. The crucial factors in preventing relapse are simultaneously adequate medication and an appropriate social support system. Vigorous efforts should be made to ensure these because the consequences of relapse and rehospitalization are devastating. Families, schools, and employers have learned to tolerate a single psychotic episode, but if this is repeated, the patient may be stigmatized permanently.

It is a safe general rule that the patient who has had a schizophrenic episode should be maintained on neuroleptics for a year. If this rule is followed, about 30 percent of the patients may be medicated for an unnecessarily long period. But aside from a good premorbid personality and excellent family resources and relationships, there is no way of predicting who these low-risk patients will be. Furthermore, the consequences of relapse, as indicated previously, are enormous. Hence, it is prudent to medicate all patients for a year, and then to diminish medication gradually or to introduce drug holidays. If the patient has had a relapse, medication should be maintained for 2 or 3 years. If there have been three relapses, it should be maintained indefinitely, perhaps for life.

Maintenance is not simple, because patients generally dislike neuroleptics and tend not to comply. The prospects for compliance can be increased in three ways. First, regular visits to the helping mental health workers can enhance motivation.

Second, blood levels of the phenothiazines should be taken to ensure optimum dosage. Third, long-acting phenothiazines may be used. These must be given parenterally, and are generally reserved for the chronic schizophrenic. A biweekly dosage of 12.5 to 25 mg fluphenazine decanoate is commonly used for some patients. Although it has been suggested by some that this medication can be given monthly, clinical experience and the blood-level data suggest that this is tantamount to giving frequent drug holidays.

For the less chronically disabled schizophrenics, oral medication suffices. For appropriate management of such patients, consideration must be given to pharmacokinetics and measurement of blood levels.

Blood levels of the phenothiazines can be correlated with efficacy and toxicity. This correlation is not so satisfactory as it is with lithium, the benzodiazepines, or the tricyclic antidepressants because of the very complex metabolic pathways and the large number of metabolites from phenothiazines. Nonetheless, there is interesting information of high clinical relevance.

First, there may be as much as twentyfold variance in blood levels among different patients receiving the same dose of phenothiazine orally. Blood levels after oral medication can be affected by other drugs. Alcoholics tend to absorb less effectively from the gastrointestinal tract. Antiparkinson drugs decrease plasma levels, perhaps because their anticholinergic properties may inhibit gastrointestinal absorption. Older patients tend to achieve higher plasma levels and to have slower elimination times than do younger patients at the same dosage per kilogram, and this may account, in part, for the greater sensitivity of older patients to the usual therapeutic doses of neuroleptics. Yet all these factors fail to account fully for the variability in blood levels among patients who receive the same dose. Parenteral administration of phenothiazines is more effective than oral administration. With chlorpromazine, for example, the parenteral dose averages about one-third of the oral dose, and there is both a more rapid rise and a higher peak. Yet, even with parenteral administration, there is great variance in steady-state levels.

Most of the phenothiazines have not been studied so thoroughly as chlorpromazine, which may be used as an example of the metabolic fate of this class of compounds. Chlorpromazine in the plasma is 95 to 98 percent bound. Its half-life varies from 2 to 31 hours in different patients. Its metabolism includes sulfoxidation, demethylation, N-oxidation, and ring hydroxylation. Esterifications as the sulfate or the glucuronide are the end stages of metabolism, and these products are excreted by the kidney. Metabolism occurs mainly in the liver and in the intestine, and more than 100 metabolites have been found. Many of these lack psychotropic activity, but they may not be devoid of toxicity. The cardiotoxic effects of thioridazine can be correlated with elevations of its sulfoxide, rather than with the plasma levels of the parent compound.

Again, even with optimum drug treatment, relapse rates of 30 percent occur in the first year. This does not result from compliance failures, but rather from interpersonal stresses in the psychosocial environment. Drugs are not enough, and management should involve a team approach that may include family therapy or helping the patient to disengage from highly conflicted families. It may also require job training and the acquisition of new social skills. Since the general physician can rarely afford the time and emotional investment required, referral to a psychiatrist or the assistance of psychologists, social workers, or other mental health personnel is helpful.

TARDIVE DYSKINESIA AND OTHER NEUROLOGIC COMPLICATIONS

Although a few cases were reported in the late 1950s, almost 20 years elapsed between the introduction of neuroleptic drugs for the treatment of psychoses and the common recognition that they were capable of producing tardive dyskinesia (TD), a serious neurological illness. The failure to recognize this hazard earlier can be attributed to the insidious onset of the iatrogenic syndrome in seriously psychotic patients whose spontaneous behavior often included grimacing, posturing, and unusual stereotyped behavior that resembles TD superficially. When the choreoathetoid movements of the tongue, face, mouth, and upper trunk muscles that are characteristic of TD began to be noticed slowly and gradually in schizophrenic patients maintained on neuroleptics, they received scant attention, even though in retrospect it is recognized that these dyskinetic and athetoid movements are quite different from the usual movements of drug-free schizophrenics. Occasionally syndromes resembling TD have been reported to appear idiopathically, and also to appear with such drugs as L-dopa diphenydramine, estrogen amphetamines, and anticholinergics used in parkinsonism; they are most unequivocally and most commonly related to neuroleptics. TD is found most commonly in elderly institutionalized patients, but is being reported increasingly in outpatients and in institutionalized children. Generally, TD is recognized after a year or more of neuroleptic treatment, but occasionally, persistent dyskinesia has followed exposure to moderate doses for periods as brief as a few months.

There are several uncertainties regarding the relationship of neuroleptics to tardive dyskinesia. The evidence suggests that the presence of organic brain disease, like that found in the elderly, makes TD more likely, but it also occurs in patients with no past history, nor evidence, of preexisting brain damage. Is the psychotic state a necessary condition for the development of TD? Since most patients receiving these drugs have chronic schizophrenia or dementia, it is found most frequently in these groups. But TD has also been found to occur in patients given neuroleptics chronically for psychosomatic syndromes, pain, severe psychoneuroses, and personality disorders. Is TD a consequence of total dosage of phenothiazines over a prolonged period, or does it relate more specifically to high dosage for briefer and perhaps more critical periods of time? As yet, these questions are not answered definitely. Does the route of administration or the choice of drug influence the development of TD? Again, it is difficult to be sure, because most chronic patients have, over the years, received many different drugs.

Neuroleptic drugs and some neurological illnesses produce neurological symptoms that must be differentiated from TD. Two to ten percent of patients have acute dystonia, with distressing clonic contractions of the tongue, mouth, and neck occurring within a few days after neuroleptic administration. This is especially true for younger patients, and when the more potent drugs are given intramuscularly. It may be sufficiently severe to cause opisthotonos or oculogyric crises. It is reversible, and can be treated rapidly and effectively with antiparkinson agents. Akathesia or motor restlessness occurs in 20 to 45 percent of patients within the first 2 months of neuroleptic treatment. It is frequently unresponsive to antiparkinson therapy and may require a change to a different neuroleptic. Drug-induced parkinsonism, with akinesia, rigidity, masklike facies, and bradykinesia, commonly appears during the first month of neuroleptic treatment and usually diminishes spontaneously over several months. When necessary, this problem can be treated with anticholinergic antiparkinson agents, but these should be used cautiously, and generally not for long periods. Not only are such agents generally unnecessary because the parkinsonism usually diminishes spontaneously, but they can produce an anticholinergic toxic brain syndrome. They may also make it more difficult to achieve adequate blood levels because they can diminish intestinal absorption of the neuroleptic. Potent anticholinergics can worsen symptoms of tardive dyskinesia. L-dopa, which is useful in the treatment of idiopathic parkinsonism, unfortunately increases agitation and exacerbates psychosis and is not used in neuroleptic-induced parkinsonism. Amantadine is antiparkinson and has little anticholinergic activity, but clinical experience with this drug is limited.

Wilson's disease, hypoparathyroidism, and dystonia musculorum deformans may have associated orofacial grimacing. Huntington's chorea has involuntary movements, but they are more commonly in the trunk and gait than in the face and mouth. Giles de la Tourette syndrome resembles TD in its facial grimacing, but differs in its coprolalia and vocal expression and in the fact that it occurs in the young age group. All these conditions are rare, but they must be considered in the differential diagnosis.

The anatomical or chemical etiology of TD is not known. The prolonged and frequently irreversible clinical picture suggests that structural damage occurs, but attempts to specify the lesion have not been successful. Pharmacological studies suggest that there is heightened activity or supersensitivity of the striatal dopaminergic system in TD. This may be a consequence of chronic dopaminergic blockade by the neuroleptics, which causes a condition resembling denervation supersensitivity of the dopamine receptors.

The treatment of TD is far from satisfactory. As mentioned previously, the most effective treatment involves reduction of functional dopamine activity, and this can best be achieved with additional neuroleptics. Since these same drugs are involved in the production of the illness, the tendency to escalate to higher doses of the drug to suppress the symptoms of the illness that it produces cannot be recommended. Diminution of dosage may make symptoms more prominent, but this may be transient, and symptoms may be reduced later. Diminution of dosage should always be attempted, unless the large doses are needed for the management of the psychosis, or unless the existing neurological symptoms are disabling or are totally unacceptable socially. Cessation of neuroleptic drugs completely shows the high degree of irreversibility of TD. Approximately one-half of the patients show no diminution of symptoms in 1 year.

Because treatment of TD is so unsatisfactory, emphasis should be placed on prevention. Neuroleptics should be used on a long-term basis only for psychotic patients, and not for the myriad of conditions for which they are sometimes employed. When they are used, the minimally effective dose should be employed, and this is especially true for patients over age 50, or for those with underlying brain disease. Repeated blood-level monitoring and careful examination for early signs is important because of the widespread clinical impression that the earlier TD is recognized and drugs are diminished or withdrawn, the greater are the chances for reversal. In this regard, it should be noted that in children and young adults, the earliest signs may be in fingers that make involuntary piano-playing motions, while in the elderly it appears in the involuntary movements of the protruded tongue. It should also be noted that few patients show all the signs of full-blown TD. When truncal involvement is prominent, there is a clinical impression that the TD is irreversible. Drug holidays are advocated to diminish the toxic load and to unmask suppressed neurologic signs. Withdrawal dyskinesia is a valuable sign of early TD. The capacity of patients to tolerate drug holidays without psychotic exacerbation varies from days to months, and during such holidays the patient and the family should be alerted to look for the emergence or intensification of psychotic symptoms. Drugs like amphetamines, L-dopa, and anticholinergic agents, which worsen TD, should be avoided. There is a serious dilemma created for the physician, patient, and patient's family when the patient requires neuroleptics for management of psychotic symptoms, and yet is developing TD. Some physicians have suggested that, when faced with this difficult choice, the patient and family should be brought in for a full discussion of the implications of this course of action, and that written, informed consent should be obtained if neuroleptics are to be continued. Although this is not general practice, it is especially worth considering when dealing with children and those adults who are likely to attempt to reenter the family and society fully.

There is active research aimed at finding antipsychotic drugs with fewer extrapyramidal symptoms and a lesser tendency to cause TD, and research directed both at predicting those who are susceptible and at improving the treatment. Since it is impossible to predict the degree or rate at which these goals will be achieved, the physician should be alert to prevention by the aforementioned means.

ALCOHOLISM

Alcoholism will not be defined here, nor will there be a detailed discussion of clinical methods of treating it or of orchestrating alcohol withdrawal. For these, the reader may employ detailed references. Most alcoholics can be managed by their interested primary physician, but all alcoholics should probably have a psychiatric consultation, to rule out psychiatric states that may be primary to the alcoholism and to explore treatment options for the alcoholism.

There is no drug that treats alcoholism. But drugs have an effective role in treating alcoholic withdrawal, the complications of alcoholism, and the treatment of underlying psychiatric states that predispose to alcohol abuse. Any drug treatment of alcoholism should be evaluated with the recognition that with some patients it is an episodic illness with a spontaneous 33 percent remission rate. Drug usage in alcoholism should be instituted only as part of an overall approach, with the patient's active participation in its planning and monitoring. Family therapy, behavior modification, environmental manipulation, and Alcoholics Anonymous are successful at times. The relationship between the patient and the physician or therapist must be practical, and must be sustained with the understanding that alterations and not cure may be the result. The use of benzodiazepine or other sedatives is rarely indicated in alcoholism, except during acute withdrawal.

The Wernicke-Korsakoff syndrome may present with a confusional state and severe disorientation, delirium, confabulation, and deficits in short-term memory. In some cases, the most prominent symptom is ataxia, nystagmus, or lateral rectus palsy. The Wernicke-Korsakoff syndrome is a result of alcohol-induced primary thiamine deficiency, although other deficiencies may also exist. It is treated through the replacement of thiamine. Thiamine should be given parenterally in the syndrome and during the first days of alcoholic withdrawal. Patients who have had the Wernicke-Korsakoff syndrome should probably be maintained permanently on large doses of thiamine orally because of the relapsing nature of the underlying alcoholism and because recent work has shown that they may have a higher requirement genetically for thiamine. Eighty percent of these patients have a polyneuropathy that should also be treated with pyridoxine (B_6).

Disulfiram

Disulfiram blocks aldehyde dehydrogenase, one of the two enzyme systems that metabolize alcohol. The chemical result is rapid accumulation of acetaldehyde after ethanol ingestion. The patient experiences 15 to 40 minutes of diaphoresis, palpitations, hyperpnea, facial flushing, throbbing in the head and neck areas, vertigo, hypotension, and blurred vision. This violent reaction is reasonably safe if the patient has been evaluated properly to exclude medical contraindications to disulfiram use. The drug is efficacious only in the motivated patient who will comply in taking it. Most patients can be maintained on 250 mg per day. A reasonable duration for such treatment is 6 months, but this must be individualized. The overuse of disulfiram results in a toxic organic brain syndrome with delirium. The patient with schizophrenia or manic-depressive illness should not be given disulfiram because it can precipitate psychosis in these states. This is probably through its inhibitory effect on dopamine beta hydroxylase.

Psychiatric States Underlying Alcoholism

Depression is frequently coincident with alcoholism. Suicide is frequent among alcoholics, and especially so with advancing age and in the setting of divorce or separation from family. Depression often lifts with withdrawal of the alcohol. Tricyclic-responsive depression should be sought, and is most often found in the subgroups of alcoholics who begin drinking after age 40. Tricyclics may be used in such patients when there is reasonable liver function, but alcohol-induced enzyme induction may make it difficult to get the tricyclic blood level into an effective range. Measurement of blood levels is especially important in such patients. The patient with manic-depressive illness may present as a spree drinker who drinks to dampen mania. Schizophrenics seem to use alcohol more commonly than the population at large, for a variety of reasons. Any patient on a neuroleptic who takes alcohol may experience dystonia or akathesia.

The patient with severe anxiety neurosis and panic attacks often increases alcohol consumption when the underlying problem is untreated. Conversely, when the underlying psychologic problem is treated, drinking diminishes spontaneously.

PAIN

Patients who suffer chronic pain without medical explanation can be divided into several categories. Some have as-yet-undiagnosed medical illnesses that surface months or years later. For others, the pain may be fully delusional. In most, the pain is real, but its psychologic elaborations place the problem properly in the realm of psychiatry. Depression is the most common psychiatric diagnosis in this group. A number of these depressions respond to tricyclic or MAOI treatment, with resolution of the depression and either disappearance of the pain or its tolerance. Tricyclic blood levels or MAOI levels are especially helpful in establishing the adequacy of the drug trial.

The patient with chronic pain of undetermined etiology is often served best by either the simultaneous care of his or her primary physician and a psychiatrist who is familiar with both behavioral and chemical approaches to pain, or by referral to a "pain center" (see Chapter 15). Less common among the psychiatric diagnoses of such patients are hysteria, schizophrenia, or neurosis associated with trauma. Malingering in this group is unusual. The clinician should not forget porphyria and Munchausen syndrome. Acute intermittent porphyria may present with colicky abdominal pain, whether of organic or psychogenic origin, show some tolerance or lessening with time, and some fluctuation from time to time. A positive response to a placebo does not establish a psychologic basis for pain; organic syndromes such as angina or cholecystitis may respond. Placebo responders constitute approximately one-third of the pain population. The "MADISON" score appears to correlate directly with a strong emotional component of pain:

M—Multiplicity. There is more than one pain, or a "major" and a "minor" pain.

A—Authenticity. The individual is most interested in the physician's believing in the authenticity of the pain.

D—Denial. "Nothing is wrong in my life but the pain."

I—Interpersonal variation. The pain comes mainly when "Aunt Minnie" comes to dinner.

S—Singularity. There is no other, or there has never been, pain like this.

O—"Only you can save me, doctor."

N—Nothing helps; that is, there is no fluctuation.

Chronic pain from obvious medical illness, such as progressive malignancy, is a topic that will not be covered here. It should be noted that in progressive medical pain states, the psychopharmacologist may assist the physician by such methods as the use of potentiators of the specific pain medication. Promethazine HCl, oxazepam, chlorpromazine, and dextroamphetamine have been reported to be useful. There is no known specificity, since these compounds represent antihistaminic, benzodiazepine, phenothiazine, and CNS stimulant classes. Polypharmacy is unfortunately very common, and leads to difficulties in management because drug-drug interaction occurs.

After proper medical evaluation and treatment, the chronic pain patient usually gets pain relief. There is a tendency for the more complaining patient to get less analgesic relief whatever the level of illness. Each patient complaining of pain should be considered to be in pain until there is conclusive proof that he or she is the rare malingerer. When acute pain requires analgesics, the physician should be prepared to use peripheral analgesics, such as aspirin and/or narcotics, in doses sufficient to ameliorate the pain. In such acute cases, the "usual" dose may be too low.

PEDIATRIC PSYCHOPHARMACOLOGY

Introduction

There is an unfortunate tendency to consider children as small adults with the same illnesses and with responsiveness to the same drugs as adults, but in doses prorated on a weight basis. Children are not merely small adults. Biologically, they differ in their capacity to absorb, detoxify, and excrete drugs. The capacity for enzyme induction differs in the young. Biological changes associated with adolescence alter drug metabolism. The ratio of liver and brain mass to total body mass differs considerably between children and adults. This is especially important for the use of psychotropic drugs whose site of action is in the brain and whose detoxification occurs mainly in the liver.

Children also differ from adults psychologically and socially. They are not autonomous, but are dependent upon their families and schools and are unable to escape from stress, as adults do so frequently, by means of an environmental change. Furthermore, they are not so stable as adults, biologically or psychologically. Rather, they are developing and changing at a rapid rate, biologically, emotionally, cognitively, and socially. Consequently, their diagnostic entities are usually less clear than those of adults.

All these factors have converged to make pediatric psychopharmacology less developed than its adult counterpart. Psychopharmacologic research in children compared to adults has also been impeded by less rigorous diagnostic criteria for childhood mental illness, greater ethical problems involved in controlled clinical research, and the problems of informed consent. Nevertheless, drug usage in children is common, and is usually aimed at symptom relief. Symptom relief can, however, also be achieved frequently by psychological means, such as the elimination of external stress. The evaluation of behavior disorders and of neurotic symptoms in children must always be made in the context of the child in relation to the family and social environment, and attempts should be made to improve these factors. Drugs should be employed only on the recommendation of specialists, and always with concomitant psychological interventions.

Neurotic Problems and Behavioral Disorders

Most children who are seen by child psychiatrists present with behavioral disorders that may include aggressive behavior, school problems, enuresis, or other types of behavior disturbing to those in their environment. In contrast to adults, they do not typically present with subjective complaints of nervousness, fearfulness, discomfort, or tenseness while still retaining otherwise appropriate role functions. Frequently, the disorder is reactive to stresses in the environment, rather than being intrapsychic and unconscious as in the typical adult neurosis.

For those behavior disorders in prepubetal children and adolescents in which anxiety is manifest or inferred, benzodiazepines have been employed. The results have not been impressive. Thus, in open clinical trials diazepam and chlordiazepoxide have often been noted to be effective in children with mixed diagnoses in which anxiety is a symptom. Chlordiazepoxide in doses of 10 to 50 mg per day has been reported to yield rapid symptomatic improvement in children with school phobia. Diazepam has been reported to be effective in children presenting symptoms of mild aggression, impulsivity, and temper tantrums. Mentally retarded children with behavioral difficulties are reported to respond with diminished anxiety to benzodiazepines used for 2 months in doses up to 60 mg per day. However, in contrast to these open clinical studies, the results of double blind placebo controlled studies have not been so favorable. One study compared diazepam and placebo for children who were in full or part-time residential care for severe behavior disorders with high degrees of anxiety. Neither ratings of anxiety nor of tension revealed any significant drug effects. Studies of children with manifest or inferred anxiety that compared psychotherapy alone with psychotherapy plus antianxiety agents in children have shown no beneficial effects, nor any advantage from the added psychotropic drug. Some believe that the benzodiazepines have no role in the pharmacology of psychoses or in the treatment of emotional disorders in children. However, the finding that benzodiazepines are useful preanesthetic compounds in children suggests that they may have specific utility in reducing situational anxiety. Nonetheless, their general and protracted use is not advocated because the side effects are similar to those of adults. Drowsiness and mild ataxia are not uncommon, and may interfere with school, work, and play.

Hyperkinesis

Probably the most common use of drugs in children is for that syndrome which is known by a variety of synonyms, such as hyperkinesis, hyperactivity, hyperkinetic syndrome in children, minimal brain damage, or minimal brain dysfunction. The syndrome is characterized by impulsivity, distractability, excitability, and hyperactivity. Such children also show frequent problems in learning. Because they are aggressive and frequently antisocial, they are unpopular with their peers and with their teachers. The diagnosis has been made more frequently in the past decade, and it is estimated that some 60,000 children are being treated with central nervous system stimulants for hyperkinesis.

Hyperactivity and learning problems can be associated with excessive anxiety, boredom, undernutrition, mental retardation, psychosis, and minimal brain dysfunction. Conditions other than minimal brain dysfunction should be ruled out by careful physical, neurological, and psychological examination before drugs are employed. Hyperactivity is often in the eye of the beholder, and increases in class size and its associated disciplinary problems can occasionally lead a teacher to remove a "pesty" child from the classroom by diagnosing hyperkinesis and sending him or her to a special education class. The diagnosis of minimal brain dysfunction should be made on the basis of inclusive criteria as well as the exclusive criteria mentioned above. The inclusion criteria should involve a careful history of the child's behavior since birth. Problems in sleeping, colic, fussy eating patterns, irritable disposition, difficulties in modifying behavior either with punishment or with positive reinforcement, and hyperaggressivity with siblings or peers are not uncommon preludes to the school problems. During physical examination, hearing, speech, and language evaluations should be carried out, and a careful neurological examination should be performed. Evidence of choreoathetoid movements, disorders of fine motor coordination, of laterality, and of spatial orientation should be sought. Several batteries of psychological tests are available to evaluate a child's attention span, motor activity, and behavior. Rating scales of behavior by parents and school teachers are also available.

More than 30 years ago, it was discovered that the central nervous system stimulant, amphetamine, exerted a paradoxical calming effect upon the behavior of hyperactive children. Research since that time has demonstrated that, by EEG criteria, some severely hyperactive children have low levels of central nervous system arousal. Low central nervous system arousal can be associated with deficiencies in central inhibition of both motor and sensory functions. The diminished inhibition can cause excessive and inappropriate motor activity, as well as easy distractability and an inability to discriminate between relevant and irrelevant stimuli. The action of central nervous system stimulants in these children is to stimulate their inhibitory control systems, and thereby achieve the paradoxical calming effects. Although the precise mechanism of action of the central nervous system stimulants is not fully known, it seems clear that stimulants are therapeutic for such children. Studies with diazepam, for example, reveal no significant effects on the hyperactivity syndrome, and sedative drugs can cause a great increase in hyperactivity. The doses employed for dextroamphetamine have been reported to range from 5 to 40 mg per day. Clinical experience suggests that doses of dextroamphetamine above 20 mg per day and of methylphenidate above 50 mg per day are rarely needed, and produce undesirable side effects. Improvement in behavior occurs in 70 to 80 percent of patients, and deterioration in 5 to 10 percent. Doses usually begin at low levels twice daily after meals, and are doubled weekly until an apparent optimum level, as measured by symptom relief, is reached. Side effects such as insomnia, anorexia, or severe depressive reactions may develop, and these call for dosage reduction. Drug levels can be monitored in the blood, but usually doses are estimated on the basis of parent and teacher reports of ongoing behavior.

Magnesium pemoline has an action similar to that of methylphenidate, and also has a longer half-life. Although it is less potent on a milligram-per-kilo basis, it can be administered once daily rather than twice daily, as is the case with dextroamphetamine and methylphenidate.

Children who are placed on stimulant medication for hyperkinesis often receive it for several years. During this time, some children may develop tolerance, and larger doses may be required. The appetite-suppressant qualities of these stimulants may lead to growth retardation. In order to minimize tolerance and the adverse effects of these compounds, drug holidays are frequently recommended. If the parents are able to tolerate the child's behavior at home, there is no need to administer it on weekends, holidays, or during summer vacations, when the disciplined control required for school is less important. The need for central nervous system stimulants usually disappears with the onset of puberty, but the behavior of hyperactive children as they become adults is only now beginning to come under scrutiny. There is some reason to believe that the hyperactive child carries some aspects of impulsivity and distractability throughout life.

Although there is no doubt that behavioral improvement of hyperactive children does occur with the central nervous system stimulants, it is disquieting to realize that recent studies have suggested that such children do not improve in their ability to learn. It would appear, therefore, that low doses that are less than optimum for behavior control may still be best, on balance, to achieve some behavioral control without diminution of the capacity to learn. It should be clear that stimulant-drug management of the hyperactive child is an imperfect form of treatment. Such treatment should be combined with psychological and educational approaches. Special education teachers and small classes with structured activities are useful in the school management. Reeducation of the parents to achieve more structure in the home, with well-defined tasks and limits, is useful. Behavior modification programs and individual psychotherapy may be required to alter maladaptive behavior patterns.

Enuresis

Prolonged enuresis, or bed-wetting, can be caused by medical illnesses like polyuria, urogenital pathology, urinary tract infections, or such endocrine or metabolic diseases as diabetes. It may also be a consequence of external stress or of intrapsychic conflict. Functional enuresis is reported to affect about 7 percent of children. Most of these have associated psychological problems, and will respond to behavior modification or treatment of the underlying depression or anxiety by psychotherapy. One type of enuresis noted primarily in males occurs during the period of sleep known as Stage-Four or non-REM (Rapid Eye Movement) sleep. This usually occurs during the first hours of sleep, during the transition between Stage-Four non-REM sleep and the first emerging REM period. It seems to be associated with autonomic arousal in the absence of elicitable mental activity. Children with this problem also have a higher incidence of night terrors, sleep talking, and sleepwalking. This type of enuresis has often been treated successfully with imipramine. A single daily dose of imipramine is usually administered before bedtime. Dosage variability is considerable, and it is usually selected on the basis of symptom disappearance. Demonstrable effects usually require a few weeks, and the low starting dose of 25 to 50 mg nightly should be elevated very slowly, and then only with continuous clinical assessment. Imipramine causes hypotension, and has been reported to induce ECG abnormalities in children. Monitoring of blood levels is highly desirable, especially if daily doses of about 100 mg are being considered. When tricyclic medication is employed for enuresis, it is usually administered for about 6 months and then should be tapered off gradually. Throughout this period, the child should be monitored medically. Since the symptoms seem to be associated with immaturity of autonomic bladder control, spontaneous remission usually occurs with maturation, and medication need not be employed unless the symptom itself leads to interpersonal problems with parents or siblings, or to a deterioration of school performance.

Psychoses

Psychotropic drugs have been used extensively for management of the behavior disorders that are associated with mental retardation, childhood autism, and childhood schizophrenia. The treatment of such problems is best left for the specialist. The diagnoses of these illnesses requires extensive experience, and the treatment is far from satisfactory. For autistic children, drug therapy is used to control explosive aggressive behavior and to minimize social withdrawal and apathy. The most common drugs are the antipsychotics, and these must be administered carefully because of their sedative properties, which may interfere with psychological treatment or education. Lithium and triiodothyronine have also been reported to be beneficial, but they are far from curative. The benzodiazepines, sedatives, anticonvulsants, and vitamins are all without evidence of therapeutic benefits. Barbiturates, hallucinogens, and amphetamines increase behavior disorganization, and may exacerbate psychotic symptoms.

Childhood schizophrenia is treated with drugs in the same fashion as childhood autism. Diminution of target symptoms with antipsychotics is usually the goal, and is designed to optimize psychotherapy and the educational environment. The long-term treatment of children with antipsychotic agents does not seem to interfere with growth or with sexual maturation. On the other hand, extrapyramidal symptoms such as salivation and dystonia are prominent. Children seem to have a high potential for developing neurological symptoms that appear upon discontinuation of long-term drug treatment. The neurological symptoms that appear have been called "withdrawal emergent symptoms," and are characterized by involuntary movements and ataxia affecting primarily the head, trunk, and extremities. These symptoms, which resemble those of tardive dyskinesia, usually appear within 2 weeks after drug withdrawal, and remit spontaneously within 2 weeks in about 35 percent of the children. Tardive dyskinesia may also occur, but its incidence is unknown. The psychosis of the schizophrenic child in contrast to adults reappears quickly when neuroleptic therapy is discontinued. Treatment with drugs, therefore, offers the unpleasant alternatives between floridly psychotic behavior or a rather high incidence of neurological symptoms when this behavior is controlled with neuroleptic drugs.

Mental Retardation

Mentally retarded children, particularly those who are institutionalized, commonly receive psychotropic drugs. Phenothiazines are the most frequently used of these drugs. A survey of 1,973 mental retardation institutions in 1966 showed that 51 percent of the residents were receiving such drugs, and that phenothiazines accounted for almost 60 percent of the psychotropic drugs employed.[4] Anticonvulsants are also commonly used, and polypharmacy seems to be the rule rather than the exception. Toxicity may be difficult to detect in the mentally retarded, and may be manifested by aggravation of behavioral disorganization. Thus, careful clinical and pharmacokinetic monitoring is essential.

No drugs are available to improve the intelligence of the retarded, and the available drugs are used only for improving the behavior of such children. Chlorpromazine in appropriate doses neither interferes with nor facilitates performance on intelligence tests, but in high doses the neuroleptic drugs used for long periods of time seem to interfere with learning, cognition, and performance. Furthermore, the mentally retarded are not immune from neuroleptic-induced tardive dyskinesia. While only 5 percent of the mentally retarded are institutionalized and 95 percent are not, there is a dearth of data from controlled clinical trials on the use of psychotropic drugs for the mentally retarded outpatient.

Depression in Children

Depression in children and adolescents, which has long been ignored, is now increasingly recognized. For those in late adolescence and early adulthood, suicide associated with depression is a leading cause of death. The use of antidepressants in children and early adolescents has not been approved by the FDA because of the potential cardiotoxicity. The available research data are very limited and, although some clinicians advocate the use of tricyclics in children whose age, height, and weight make them eligible for its use without violating governmental regulations, there is a general impression that psychotherapy is as effective and less hazardous. Antidepressant medications should be used rarely in this age group, and then only by specialists, and with concomitant psychological treatment. A possible exception to this is an anecdotal report that the few hyperkinetic children who become depressed from chronic amphetamines respond to treatment with imipramine.

GEROPSYCHOPHARMACOLOGY

Introduction

Elderly patients are subject to the same mental ills as younger adults, although in different proportions. Thus, depression and organic brain syndromes increase in frequency, while first episodes of schizophrenia diminish. Drug usage in the elderly is high. About one-third of adults beyond age 60 have used a psychotropic drug during the previous year, and 9 percent had received a high dosage.[3] A Veterans' Administration study of hospitalized patients showed that 61 percent were receiving psychoactive drugs.[4] Antipsychotic drugs are prescribed the most frequently, followed by antidepressants, antianxiety drugs, and cerebral vasodilators. Among patients receiving antipsychotic drugs, 20 percent received antiparkinson drugs as well.

In the elderly, the pharmacokinetics and pharmacodynamics of psychotropic drugs differ significantly from that of younger adults. Alterations may occur in absorption, distribution, metabolism, and excretion, as seen below.

Absorption

Absorption of diazepam and chlorpromazine have been demonstrated to be slower in the elderly, and other drugs, such as the tricyclics, are also thought to be absorbed more slowly.

Distribution

Since the percentage of body weight that is fat increases significantly with age, the volume of distribution of lipid-soluble drugs, such as diazepam, chlorpromazine, and the tricyclics, increases with age. With age there is a decrease in serum albumin and in total binding sites, which influences both the distribution and the kinetics of such highly protein bound drugs as the neuroleptics and tricyclics. Thus, the percentage of tricyclic bound to protein is significantly lower in the aged than in young adults. This means that it may be prudent to divide the dosages of the tricyclic to a t.i.d. or q.i.d. schedule to avoid high peaks of free drug. It may also mean that the blood for tricyclic levels should be drawn earlier than the usual 12-hour recommendation.

Metabolism

The aged often have a less efficient demethylation capacity. This influences their ability to metabolize those benzodiazepines and tricyclics that are demethylated to active products. Barbiturates are also metabolized less rapidly, hence the greater sensitivity of the elderly to this class of drugs; but they are still capable of inducing liver microsomal enzymes. Conjugation to sulfates and glucuronides is also diminished. Finally, it should be recognized that multiple drug use is common in the elderly. Some drugs, such as barbiturates, caffeine, and tobacco, increase psychotropic drug metabolism, while chloramphenicol, diphenylhydantoin, and disulfiram inhibit it.

Excretion

The reduced renal blood flow and concomitant decrease in glomerular filtration that are seen in the elderly probably account for many drug sensitivities in the aged. This would be compounded when they are on such agents as propranolol, which further reduces glomerular filtration. Lithium, which is handled almost exclusively by renal excretion, must be administered in lower doses in the elderly.

This concatenation of changes make it mandatory that psychoactive drugs be administered carefully to the elderly. A careful medical and psychiatric evaluation should be made prior to the use of any drug treatment. The dosage of psychoactive drugs will generally be lower by one-half to one-third, and the rate at which drug dosage is elevated should be slower. Toxicity at the usual dosages used for young adults is common in the elderly, and they should have blood-level monitoring whenever this is possible.

Organic Brain Syndrome

The primary physician is called upon to both diagnose and manage elderly patients. Psychiatric consultation may be helpful if the patient is thought to have a psychiatric illness that mimics or complicates an organic syndrome. Depression in the elderly often does this and appears as "pseudodementia." Organic brain syndrome may be defined as any mental disorder resulting from diffuse impairment of brain tissue function. Acute, often reversible, organic brain syndromes present with sudden onset of restlessness or somnolence, disorientation, and occasionally hallucinosis (especially visual). Chronic organic brain syndromes (that is, dementias) show deficiency of immediate recall, recent memory, and remote memory. There is also impairment of perception, orientation, intellectual functions of all sorts, deficient judgment, and lability or shallowness of affect. With both acute and chronic organic brain syndrome, the cause should be sought and eliminated when possible. Organic brain syndromes are common among the elderly, and may be superimposed upon major medical and psychiatric illness.

Organic Causes of Psychosis

The patient who presents with acute psychosis at over 40 years of age, or with a fever, tachycardia, or autonomic changes, should be considered to have an organic basis for the psychosis until it is proven otherwise. Signs and symptoms that are correlated with organic psychosis include blood behind the tympanic membrane or over the mastoid or other evidence of cerebral trauma, papilledema, nystagmus, pathologic reflexes, and tremor. The physician who is seeing the patient with a recent onset of organic brain syndrome must immediately consider meningitis, hypoglycemia, drug intoxication, poisonings, cerebral hypoperfusion, and cerebrovascular emergencies.

Management of Organic Brain Syndromes

The diagnosis of the underlying cause is basic. The patient with acute organic brain syndrome is frightened and disoriented. Psychologic interventions may be sufficient, and are always adjunctive. Orienting procedures, limit setting, environmental manipulation, a night light, and physical contact are helpful for the aged patient. Simultaneously, procedures to eliminate the underlying toxin, infection, metabolic disturbance, malnutrition, or drug overdose should be undertaken. If absolutely necessary, small doses of antipsychotics may be used. Two milligrams of haloperidol once or twice daily is usually sufficient.

The chronic organic brain syndromes frequently present as psychotic behavior. Senile dementia, Alzheimer's disease, and arteriosclerotic brain disease often show a mixed picture of organicity and psychosis. Late paraphrenia, characterized by paranoid delusions, thought disorders, hallucinations, and grandiosity without evidence of organicity, occurs occasionally. Schizophrenic symptoms may recur and exacerbate in patients who have had active symptoms earlier in life. A central anticholinergic syndrome is not uncommon because so many of the antipsychotics and antidepressants have anticholinergic properties and because antiparkinson agents are used so frequently. Treatment usually involves discontinuation of the offending agent, but the judicious use of physostigmine, when monitored properly, may be necessary in emergencies.

The treatment of psychotic behavior in the elderly follows the guidelines for treatment of psychosis in adults. However, the elderly are more susceptible to serious adverse reactions from administered drugs. Thus, hypotension may precipitate cardiovascular accidents, and often may decrease an already marginal cerebral blood flow. Fainting may cause fractures in the elderly. Tachycardias and arrhythmias may occur. Agranulocytosis and cholestatic jaundice may occur. Neurological side effects, such as akathesia and akinetic parkinsonism, increase with age. The tendency to develop tardive dyskinesia is also increased in the elderly. For these reasons, the dosage of antipsychotic medication should be kept low, usually at one-half to one-third of that employed in younger adults.

There is considerable ongoing research aimed at reversing or at least diminishing the manifestations of organicity by increasing blood flow or otherwise enhancing the metabolic activity of the brain. Hyperbaric oxygenation, cerebral vasodilators, vitamins, anticoagulants, CNS stimulants, and anabolic steroids have been tested. Most of these have not shown effectiveness. The dihydrogenated ergot alkaloids are used extensively, but remain controversial. Several double blind studies have demonstrated superiority over placebo for mood and cognitive impairment, but the effects are small.

The confusion and agitation following sedative withdrawal can usually be managed by replacement of a pharmacologic equivalent, such as a benzodiazepine.

Affective Illness in the Elderly

Depression is the most common psychiatric problem of the elderly. Elderly suicides account for at least 25 percent of all suicides. The causes of depression are multiple. In addition to biological changes in the nervous system with aging, which may predispose to depression, there are the additional problems of physical illness, bereavement, retirement, and loss of income. Depression in the elderly may present as hypochondriasis, dementia, or the more typical picture. Depressions of the elderly are usually drug responsive, but, as with all mental illness, the use of psychosocial treatments and supports systems is advocated. When tricyclics are used with the elderly, it should be remembered that they generally have a longer half-life and, thus, a longer time (3 to 5 weeks) to reach plateau. The aged are especially sensitive to the sedative, cardiac, hypotensive, and anticholinergic side effects of the tricyclics. Initially, the clinician should give a test dose, such as 10 to 25 mg of imipramine or doxepin, to observe for exceptional sensitivity. After this, the dose should be titrated. The aged generally require a lower dose to reach therapeutic blood levels. Octogenarians with tricyclic-responsive depression have responded to 30 to 75 mg per day of these drugs. A plateau plasma level of doxepin, plus desmethyldoxepin level of 110 to 150 ng/ml, may be achieved with such small doses. Alternatively, many of the "young old" require full doses. Doxepin and desipramine have been suggested as having less potential for cardiac toxicity in the elderly than other tricyclics, but this claim is currently inconclusive. Tricyclics can block the action of guanethidine, an antihypertensive that is often used in the elderly.

Mania that is first presenting in the elderly, although rare, may be confused with dementia. It is best treated with lithium at one-third to one-half of the usual doses. A measure of lithium clearance and frequent monitoring of blood levels is helpful. Lithium toxicity in the elderly may be subtle, and it develops at lower plasma levels in the elderly. In the aged person taking lithium, hypothyroidism that is secondary to the lithium may mimic dementia. Occasionally in the elderly, lithium toxicity presents as generalized neuromuscular irritability. Every "demented" aged patient should be examined carefully for an unrecognized depression of either a reactive or tricyclic-responsive type.

Insomnia

Insomnia is common in the elderly. The elderly tend to sleep less in general. Self-reports of the degree of insomnia are notoriously inaccurate, and may lead to excessive prescribing of sedatives and hypnotics. Chronic use of such agents should be discouraged. The experienced physician has seen many "dementias" and "deliriums" clear with discontinuation of the hypnotics. Insomnia that is secondary to pain, congestive heart failure, or the use of such stimulants as caffeine may be treated directly. Elderly demented patients may have their "days and nights mixed up," and this should be treated as indicated in the section on organic brain syndrome. Rarely, these people may need to have their sleep pattern interrupted by a single night of a short-acting benzodiazepine, such as oxazepam in moderate doses. The use of tryptophan and of dietary manipulations to treat insomnia in the elderly is still experimental.

REFERENCES

1 Carlsson, A.: "Antipsychotic Drugs, Neurotransmitters, and Schizophrenia," *Am. J. Psych.*, **135:**164–173, 1978.
2 Fawcett, J., J. W. Maas, and H. Dekirmenjian: "Depression and MHPG Excretion: Response to Dextroamphetamine and Tricyclic Antidepressants," *Arch. Gen. Psych.*, **26:**246–251, 1972.
3 Beckmann, H., and F. K. Goodwin: "Antidepressant Response to Tricyclics and Urinary MHPG in Unipolar Patients," *Arch. Gen. Psych.*, **32:**17–21, 1975.
4 Lipman, R. S.: in F. D. Menolascimo (ed.), *Psychiatric Approaches to Mental Retardation,* New York: Basic Books, pp. 387–398, 1970.
5 Mellinger, G. D. et al.: "Overview of Psychotherapeutic Drugs in the U.S.," in E. Josephson (ed.), *Drug Use: Epidemiological and Sociological Approaches,* Washington, D.C.: Hemisphere Publishing, 1974, pp. 333–366.
6 Prien, R. F.: "A Survey of Psychoactive Drug Use in the Aged in V.A. Hospitals,"*Psychopharmacology Bulletin,* **11:**50–51, 1975.

BIBLIOGRAPHY

General Textbooks

Baldessarini, R. J.: *Chemotherapy in Psychiatry,* Cambridge, Mass.: Harvard Univ. Press, 1977.
Barchas, J. D. et al. (eds.): *Psychopharmacology from Theory to Practice,* New York: Oxford Univ. Press, 1977.
Boissier, J. R. et al.: *Neuropsychopharmacology,* New York: American Elsevier, 1975.
Clark, W. G., and J. del Giudice (eds.): *Principles of Psychopharmacology,* New York: Academic Press, 1970.
Jarvik, M. E. (ed.): *Psychopharmacology in the Practice of Medicine,* New York: Appleton-Century-Crofts, 1977.
Klein, D. F., and J. M. Davis: *Diagnosis and Drug Treatment of Psychiatric Disorders,* Baltimore: Williams and Wilkins, 1969.
Klein, D. F., and R. Gittelman-Klein (eds.): *Progress in Psychiatric Drug Treatment,* vol. 2, New York: Brunner/Mazel, 1976.
Lipton, M. A. et al. (eds.): *Psychopharmacology—A Generation of Progress,* New York: Raven Press, 1978.
Seixas, Frank A. (ed.): *Currents in Alcoholism,* vol. 2, New York: Grune and Stratton, 1977.
Shader, R. I. (ed.): *Manual of Psychiatric Therapeutics,* New York: Little, Brown, 1975.
Usdin, G. L. (ed.): *Depression: Clinical, Biological, and Psychological Perspectives,* New York: Brunner/Mazel, 1977.
White, J. H.: *Pediatric Psychopharmacology: A Practical Guide to Clinical Application,* Baltimore: Williams and Wilkins, 1977.

Pharmacokinetics and Pharmacodynamics

Berger, P. A., and J. D. Barchas: "Biochemical Hypotheses of Affective Disorders", in J. D. Barchas et al., *Psychopharmacology from Theory to Practice,* New York: Oxford Univ. Press, 1977, pp. 151–173.
Carlsson, A.: "Mechanism of Action of Neuroleptic Drugs," in M. A. Lipton et al., *Psychopharmacology—A Generation of Progress,* New York: Raven Press, 1978.

Friedel, R. O.: "Pharmacokinetics in the Geropsychiatric Patient," in M. A. Lipton et al., *Psychopharmacology—A Generation of Progress,* New York: Raven Press, 1978.

Gottschalk, L. A.: "Pharmacokinetics of Minor Tranquilizers and Clinical Response," in M. A. Lipton et al., *Psychopharmacology—A Generation of Progress,* New York: Raven Press, 1978.

Gottschalk, L. A.: "Pharmacokinetics of Minor Tranquilizers and Clinical Response," in M. A. Lipton et al., *Psychopharmacology—A Generation of Progress,* New York: Raven Press, 1978.

Risch, S. C. et al.: "Plasma Levels of Psychotropic Drugs and Clinical Efficacy: A Review of the Literature 1967–1977," paper submitted to *American Journal of Psychiatry,* 1978.

Depression

Tricyclic Antidepressants

Asberg, M. et al.: "Relationship between Plasma Level and Therapeutic Effect of Nortriptyline," *Brit. Med. J.,* **3**:331–334, 1971.

Bielski, Robert J., and Robert O. Friedel: "Prediction of Tricyclic Antidepressant Response," *Arch. Gen. Psych.,* **33**:1479–1489, 1976.

Braithwaite, R. et al.: "Plasma Concentration: Amitriptyline and Clinical Response," *Lancet,* **1**:1297–1300, 1972.

Friedel, R. O., and M. A. Raskind: "Relationship of Blood Levels of Sinequan to Clinical Effects in the Treatment of Depression in Aged Patients," in J. Mendels (ed.), "Sinequan: A Monograph of Recent Clinical Studies," *Excerpta Medica,* New York:51–53, 1975.

Glassman, A. et al.: "Clinical Implications of Imipramine Plasma Levels for Depressive Illness," *Arch. Gen. Psych.,* **34**:197–204, 1977.

Goodwin, F. K.: "Drug Treatment of Affective Disorders," in M. Jarvik (ed.), *Psychopharmacology in the Practice of Medicine,* New York: Appleton-Century-Crofts, 1977.

Maas, James W.: "Biogenic Amines and Depression," *Arch. Gen. Psych.,* **32**:1357–1361, 1975.

Snyder, S. H., and H. I. Yamamura: "Antidepressants and the Muscarinic Acetylcholine Receptor," *Arch. Gen. Psych.,* **34**:236–239, 1977.

Monamine Oxidase Inhibitor Antidepressants

Klein, D. F. et al.: "Antidepressants, Anxiety, Panic, and Phobia," paper presented to A.C.N.P., December 1976.

Robinson, D. S. et al.: "The Monoamine Oxidase Inhibitor, Phenelzine, in the Treatment of Depressive-Anxiety States," *Arch. Gen. Psych.,* **29**:407–413, 1973.

Sargant, W.: "The Treatment of Anxiety States and Atypical Depressions by the MAOI Drugs," *J. Neuropsych.,* **3**(suppl.1):96–103, 1962.

Tyrer, P.: "Towards Rational Therapy with Monoamine Oxidase Inhibitors," *Brit. J. Psych.,* **128**:354–360, 1976.

Lithium

Cohen, I. M. et al.: "The Current Status of Lithium Therapy—Report of the APA Task Force," *Am. J. Psych.,* **132**:997–1000, 1975.

Sack, R. L., and E. DeFraites: "Lithium and the Treatment of Mania," in J. D. Barchas et al. (eds.), *Psychopharmacology from Treatment to Practice,* New York: Oxford Univ. Press, 1978, pp. 208–224.

Anxiety

Benzodiazepines

Dasberg, H. H. et al.: "Plasma Concentrations of Diazepam and of its Metabolite N-Desmethyl-Diazepam in Relation to Anxiolytic Effect," *Clin. Pharm. Ther.,* **15**(5): 473–483, 1974.

Gottschalk, L. A., and S. A. Kaplan: "Chlordiazepoxide Plasma Levels and Clinical Responses," *Compr. Psych.,* **13**:519–527, 1972.

Greenblatt, D. J. et al.: "Absorption Rate, Blood Concentrations and Early Response to Oral Chlordiazepoxide," *Am. J. Psych.,* **134**(5):559–562, 1977.

Shader, R. I., and D. J. Greenblatt: "Clinical Implications of Benzodiazepine Pharmacokinetics," *Am. J. Psych.,* **134**:652–656, 1977.

Propranolol

Tyrer, Peter: "Beta-Adrenoceptor Blockade and Its Relevance to the Study of Emotion," in *The Role of Bodily Feelings in Anxiety,* London: Oxford Univ. Press, 1976, pp. 10–23.

Schizophrenia

Antipsychotics

Davis, J. M. et al.: "Plasma Levels of Antipsychotic Drugs and Clinical Response," in M. A. Lipton et al., *Psychopharmacology—A Generation of Progress,* New York: Raven Press, 1978.

Garver, E. L. et al.: "Neuroleptic Drug Levels and Therapeutic Response: Preliminary Observations with Red Blood Cell Bound Butaperazine," *Am. J. Psych.,* **134**:304–307, 1977.

Lipton, M. A.: "Synthesis: Biological Contributions to the Theory and Treatment of Schizophrenia," in G. L. Usdin (ed.), *Schizophrenia: Biological and Psychological Perspectives,* New York: Brunner/Mazel, 1975.

Rivera-Calimlim, L. et al.: "Clinical Response and Plasma Levels: Effects of Dose, Dosage Schedules, and Drug Interactions on Plasma Chlorpromazine Levels," *Am. J. Psych.,* **133**(6):646–652, 1976.

Smith, R. C. et al.: "Plasma Butaperazine Levels in Long-Term Chronic, Non-Responding Schizophrenics," *Comm. in Psychopharm..* **1**:319–324, 1977.

Alcoholism

Greenblatt, D. J., and R. I. Shader: "Treatment of Alcohol Withdrawal Syndrome," in R. I. Shader (ed.), *Manual of Psychiatric Therapeutics,* New York: Little, Brown, 1975, pp. 211–235.

Kaim, Samuel C. et al.: "Criteria for the Diagnosis of Alcoholism," *Ann. Intern. Med.,* **77**:249–258, 1972.

Pain

Forrest, William H. et al.: "Dextroamphetamine with Morphine for the Treatment of Postoperative Pain," *New Engl. J. Med.,* **296**:712–715, 1977.

Hackett, Thomas P.: "Pain and Its Treatment," presented at the 1977 Harvard Psychopharmacology Conference, Boston, 1977.

Hackett, T. P.: "Pain and Prejudice, Why Do We Doubt that the Patient Is in Pain?"
Medtimes, **99**(2):130–138, 1971.

Pediatric Psychopharmacology

Campbell, M.: "Use of Drug Treatment in Infantile Autism and Childhood Schizophrenia: A Review," in M. A. Lipton et al. (eds.), *Psychopharmacology—A Generation
of Progress,* New York: Raven Press, 1978, pp. 1451–1461.

Lipman, R. S. et al.: "Psychotropic Drugs and Mentally Retarded Children," in M. A.
Lipton et al. (eds.), *Psychopharmacology—A Generation of Progress,* New York:
Raven Press, 1978, pp. 1437–1449.

Safer, D. S., and R. Allen: *Hyperactive Children,* Baltimore: University Park Press, 1976.

Wender, P. H.: "Minimal Brain Dysfunction: An Overview," in M. A. Lipton et al. (eds.),
Psychopharmacology—A Generation of Progress, New York: Raven Press, 1978,
pp. 1429–1435.

Geriatric Psychopharmacology

Eisdorfer, C., and R. O. Friedel: "Psychotherapeutic Drugs in Aging," in M. Jarvik (ed.),
Psychopharmacology in the Practice of Medicine, New York: Appleton-Century-
Crofts, 1977.

Lipton, M. A., and C. B. Nemeroff: "The Biology of Aging and Its Relation to
Depression," in G. L. Usdin and C. K. Hofling (eds.), *Aging: The Process and the
People,* New York: Brunner/Mazel, 1978.

Rowe, John W.: "Clinical Research on Aging: Strategies and Directions," *New Engl. J.
Med.,* **297**(24):1332–1336, 1977.

Wells, Charles E.: "Dementia: Definition and Description," in *Dementia,* 2d ed., Philadelphia: F. A. Davis, 1977, pp. 1–14.

Chapter 26

The Physician as a Marital Therapist

Peter A. Martin, M.D.

EDITORS' INTRODUCTION

The physician may be called upon to help patients who are caught up in serious marital problems, either as a result of their direct request or because the conflict interferes with the treatment of a family member's illness. In either case, often the physician is presented with situations involving strong feelings, widely differing viewpoints of the "cause" of the marital conflict, and competing overtures to take sides in the struggle.

For the marital partners, turning to the physician may be experienced as embarrassing, humiliating, or hope-inducing. They may come to an initial interview with feelings of fear, anger, or sadness. Sharing the details of a private relationship is difficult under most circumstances, but anticipating that one's often angry spouse may tell the physician something of one's intimate habits and reactions to stress may seem overwhelming. "Doctor, he's 37 years old and still masturbates." "She doesn't take care of herself—hardly ever takes a shower." "He may be president of the largest corporation in town, but when he's not at work he only seems interested in drinking and going to pornographic movies." "She does nothing during the day but watch television serials—hasn't read a book in 20 years."

The anticipation of disclosure of such behavior by one's spouse, often in ways that are distorted by the intense conflict, can make the reaching out for help a very painful procedure. It is important for the physician to keep in mind how painful it is for many couples to turn to a doctor for help with marital problems.

There is, however, the equally important issue of the doctor's inner response to the marital conflict. His or her own marriage may be distressed, or the physician may have grown up with parents who had a badly conflicted relationship. Either circumstance may impact upon the physician's response to the couple. This can occur in many ways. A physician with a spouse who is uninterested in sex may feel that a husband complaining about his wife's strong sexual needs is out of his mind. A physician who is strongly dominant in his or her own marriage may feel immediately that a patient who is unhappy with a submissive marital role just does not understand what marriage is all about. A physician who cannot tolerate oral sex personally may feel anxious if presented with that issue by a conflicted couple. In sum, the ways in which the physician experiences the marital couple and their problems can influence decisively the response of the physician, and therefore the physician's capacity to be helpful.

As the physician turns to what an expert in the field of marital therapy has to say about the role of the physician as marital counselor, it is important to keep in mind both what it may be like for patients to have some of life's private aspects exposed, and the ways in which those disclosures may impinge upon the physician's own uncertainties, vulnerabilities, and rigidities.

INTRODUCTION

A 1972 survey revealed that family physicians spend one-fifth of their working time counseling patients for emotional disturbances, which range from premarital and marital problems to drug or alcohol abuse to individual adjustment difficulties.[1] The greatest proportion of time was spent in marital counseling. One might anticipate that obstetricians and gynecologists might also be consulted by their patients, albeit casually, regarding marital problems. For that matter, all physicians convey by their relationships with their patients their willingness or lack of willingness to aid patients in problems not necessarily specific to the patients' physical complaints.

Nonpsychiatric physicians do not have the luxury of subspecialization, and may be called upon to handle individual, marital, sexual, and family problems as they arise. Some of these problems do not need referral to a specialist and, even when such referral is indicated, some patients refuse to accept it. Some physicians do not wish to lose their patients to specialists, and make referrals only to gain the consultant's recommendations as to the proper treatment approach. The physician might, for example, seek psychiatric consultation regarding whether or not a couple has a viable marriage. In this way, he or she may use the psychiatric consultant as a supervisor of the management of the patient, couple, or family. In so doing, skills and confidence will be gained by the physician.

The family physician, by virtue of knowledge of a patient's family and community, is often able to place a presenting problem in its proper perspective leading, therefore, to earlier diagnosis and allowing for better recognition and use of available treatment resources.

Psychotherapy is still a compartmentalized science and art. Individual, group, marital, family, and sexual therapy are not yet part of a thoroughly integrated system, and few therapists are trained and comfortable in doing all types of psychotherapy. However, as research and training continue to progress, future psychotherapists will be able to select the most appropriate psychotherapeutic technique for the needs of the patient, rather than trying to fit the patient to the technique with which the therapist is familiar.

Until the late 1950s, American psychiatrists generally saw only the identified patient, and deliberately excluded input from other members of the family. In the last two decades, however, a decided change has occurred, and now spouses, children, grandparents, and friends may be utilized not only for diagnostic purposes, but also to derive therapeutic advantages from a network of supportive systems. Although each individual should theoretically be able to handle many environmental stresses, some are unable to do so, which makes marital and family therapy a significant aid in maintaining homeostasis for such individuals.

The advantages that have accrued to the family physician have largely been abdicated, and many such physicians quickly refer individuals, couples, and families to other professionals. In particular, physicians have often felt uncomfortable in the area of marital and sexual therapy, because their training in the twentieth-century scientific tradition has often led them to focus on disease processes in organ systems (see Chapter 1) rather than on patients with illnesses or difficulties. Despite the advantage the physician has in performing premarital examinations, treating physical illnesses in parents and children, and even treating three generations of the same family, it is the nonmedical therapists who, to a large degree, have taken over the handling of sexual, marital, and family problems.

The functioning of the family in promoting mental health and preventing mental illness is of utmost importance, and physicians who deal with marital discord are, therefore, in the front line of defense against mental illness. They are concerned with how to help young parents establish and maintain a good marriage, and with helping older patients stabilize worthwhile marriages. This is done by developing a nurturing environment that can facilitate the mutual and individual growth of different generations. The fallacy behind separate treatment of individual, marital, and family problems is that they are indivisible in vivo.

Although the role of the family physician is strategic in promoting a healthy family atmosphere, many avoid this responsibility and are loath to think of themselves as marital therapists. It is not surprising that, in one survey, 7 percent of physicians stated unequivocally that they will not discuss marriage problems, even in response to patient requests.[2] What is not understood is that even without specific marital therapy training, the intensive medical school curriculum, internship, and daily experiences in the doctor-patient relationship may be the foundation upon which one builds specific psychotherapeutic skills.

Masters stated that even the treatment of sexual problems between marital partners has been taken away from physicians by eager nonmedical personnel.[3] Masters deplored the abandonment of this area by physicians, pointing out that, simply by completing a diagnostic physical examination of a patient, they have an immediate advantage in overcoming the patient's natural hesitance to discuss intimate matters. Not only may the physician's performance of a complete initial physical examination uncover physical factors contributing to marital and sexual difficulties, but it also adds a personal element of trust and confidence. The family physician is, then, in the advantageous position of combining the physical examination with marital and sexual therapy in a unified or holistic approach to the patient's or couple's needs. It can be a rewarding experience for physician and patient to discover the relationship between functional complaints and marital or sexual problems.

Physicians are psychotherapists, whether or not they acknowledge it. This position is based upon the observation that psychotherapy occurs whenever a therapeutic triad is present: (1) the patient's hopes and expectations are reinforced by (2) the practitioner's therapeutic motivations and faith in the ability to help, and (3) the hopes, beliefs, and expectations held by the social group in which both patient and physician are immersed.[4] Psychotherapy occurs when these forces interact, rather than occurring in accordance with whether the therapist is a psychiatrist or a family physician. Whether one chooses to call it counseling or psychotherapy, it is the same process.

This position may be illustrated by describing the marital and family therapy seminar and clinic operating in the Department of Psychiatry at the University of Michigan Medical School. This unit trains psychiatric residents, psychiatric social workers, clinical psychologists, pastoral counselors, interested residents in other medical specialties, medical students, and practicing physicians. In this clinic, the participants have the opportunity to observe and conduct marital therapy under supervision. No attempt is made to train nonpsychiatric physicians as psychiatrists, but rather to assist them in becoming comfortable with the handling of marital problems as physicians.

The emphasis in this type of training is that there are key skills that must be learned. These include empathic observation, empathic listening, and introspective self-awareness. The development of these skills enables the physician to serve as a therapeutic instrument.[5]

Although this chapter will highlight some of the specific aspects of marital therapy, the basic principles, including the importance of the attitude of the physician, are more important than pragmatic details. The eagerness and enthusiasm of inexperienced therapists who lack broad knowledge of behavioral science often lead to better results than those achieved by more experienced but less enthusiastic therapists. Nonpsychiatric physicians should allow their interest in learning to outweigh their fears of attempting treatment with which they have not had earlier experience.

MARITAL PROBLEMS

There are several ways to present marital problems. Perhaps, one of the most useful approaches is to present problems as they are experienced by the individuals who come to the physician for help. Included in this approach will be anger, love, adultery, secrets, sex, and jealousy.

Anger

The most frequently encountered emotional response in individuals having marital problems is anger, which in itself may lead to aggression and violence. The most commonly recognized overt manifestation of anger is verbal anger. Its often deafening sound in patients with marital problems can hardly be missed. What is often overlooked by the physician, however, is overt physical aggression as expressed in physical abuse, most commonly of wives and children. The failure to handle anger effectively may be a basic cause of the widespread breakdown of marriage today.

Anger is experienced frequently and intensely by marital partners because the intimacy of the relationship encourages the emergence of the individual's deepest wishes and needs. Lack of gratification of those needs, or disappointment of unrealized expectations, may lead to the response of hostility, anger, and primitive rage. Even when the anger is suppressed by the individuals involved, the physician may find the presence of vague, difficult-to-understand symptoms involving multiple body systems.[6] In other instances, psychological symptoms (for example, phobias, anxieties, obsessions, compulsions, and depression) appear to result from the individual's defensive management of underlying anger.

Surveys indicate that in 15 to 16 percent of intact families, physical abuse is a problem. Of couples who come for help with marital problems, 20 percent report physical abuse, although the actual incidence may remain hidden because physical abuse is considered a taboo subject or because the criminal justice system reacts and reports inconsistently when the physical abuse is called to its attention.[7] A study of a group of battered women, for example, developed six principal conclusions: (1) Battered women are a very common phenomenon (3.8 percent of emergency room visits). (2) Wife beating is connected with depression in women and sociopathy in their husbands. (3) Battered women face many realistic obstacles in taking effective action about their problem. (4) Psychiatric intervention is essential for many. (5) Battered women show a high early dropout rate in regard to psychiatric treatment. (6) There are multiple forces that entrap these women in the marital relationship.[8]

The physician's role in the battered wife syndrome is complicated. Often the patient is terrified and feels helpless. The physician must not go along with the patient if she lies about how she received the injury; rather, it is necessary to be aware of the possibility of battering with any injury. A complete history and physical must be performed, and telltale scuff marks, burns, or bruises must be looked for. Treatment should not be limited to caring for the physical injury; there may be emotional and socioeconomic problems as well. Perhaps of major concern is the patient's physical safety, and the physician must explore with the battered wife the question of whether or not she wishes police protection. Social agencies may help, and the physician should have some knowledge of which agencies are most appropriate in this type of syndrome. When the husband is a patient of the physician, that relationship may offer leverage in treatment. Conjoint and family therapy may be indicated, and an understanding of the roles that both the battered wife and her husband have played is essential. At times, divorce may be the only viable solution, but this step is often too devastating for some couples to consider, and they may remain together for years, occasionally until the wife is beaten to death.

Another syndrome that appears to be related to anger is the so-called *dyscontrol syndrome.* This phrase is used for symptoms arising from poor impulse control, whether the cause is organic or functional.[9] Often, medical students are not trained to take careful histories, with such questions as, "Do you have difficulty in controlling your temper?" "Has there been physical abuse in your home?" "Is there loss of control of sexual impulses?" "Have you been charged with traffic violations or drunken driving?" Many patients are reluctant to admit uncontrollable temper, out of a sense of shame or a fear of the consequences. Many families, although victimized by the loss of control, aid in the denial.

There are sharply different views regarding the treatment of anger. One influential approach is to accept the fact that aggression is an inborn tendency, which cannot be bottled up and needs to be drained off periodically to avoid a much larger outburst in the future. This is the *catharsis theory,* and some therapists, using this reasoning, teach their patients how to "fight fairly."[10] Generally, a set of rules is presented, within which the fighting is deemed to be constructive. The physician is a commonly chosen authority figure with whom the couple can ventilate angry feelings and have a cathartic experience. The difficulty is that, though the individual may feel better temporarily, the "catharsis" avoids the need for facing and resolving conflicts, and encourages repetition of the same sequence. This can act as a powerful reinforcer, which may actually increase future acts of aggression. Thus, the long-term effects of catharsis are negative, and research has failed to support its value in the treatment of anger and aggression.[7] The encouragement of indiscriminate emotional release may, in some patients, lead to a further breakdown in their precarious psychological functioning.

Another approach to the treatment of anger recommends supportive techniques, including logical discussion, advice, guidance, and setting realistic limits.[11] The physician must assess each couple separately when anger and aggression are the predominant features. No simple recurring pattern emerges from such case material and, as in all branches of medicine, a good history often allows for better understanding of the underlying causes. Often, however, physicians tend to avoid treating patients with symptoms of anger and violent behavior. Their inner feelings of anxiety or distaste must somehow be dealt with in order to offer patients early intervention into what may become a progressively escalating pattern of anger and aggression.

At times, anger has a certain adaptive function, and serves as an energizing, expressive, discriminative response to stress.[12] For example, anger may energize one's behavior by increasing the vigor with which the individual acts in response to stress. Often, however, the anger may have a disruptive effect by interfering with functioning. In working with patients with marital problems, anger may serve important expressive or communicative functions. It may encourage the start of communication and the discussion of previously unexpressed problems. It can either be constructive or destructive, depending upon the way in which people express their anger or what they do when they become angry. Individuals involved in intimate relations may need help in expressing negative feelings in order to resolve conflict rather than merely to escalate a sequence of mutual antagonism.

For other individuals, to feel anger is less distressing than to feel anxious, apathetic, fearful, depressed, or helpless. Psychotherapy of marital partners who are manifesting inadequate control of anger must impart to the couple skills for coping with the provocation of anger. Novaco has recently advocated a set of cognitive self-control procedures designed specifically to regulate the arousal of anger.[13] These include: (1) education about personal anger patterns, (2) self-monitoring of anger arousal, (3) the ability to understand provocations from a different viewpoint, (4) self-instruction to guide one's appraisal of events and to cue nonantagonistic responses, and (5) the ability to remain task oriented when provoked. Such interventions are designed to impart a sense of personal control in the management of provocation. It would not be difficult for an interested physician to learn to utilize these skills.

Mace has devised another method of managing anger that involves training couples to deal with anger in three successive steps.[14] These steps involve the following:

1 Acknowledge the anger. This means simply learning to say, "I'm getting angry with you."
2 Renounce the anger as inappropriate. This does not mean that one does not have the right to become angry. Anger, at times, is appropriate. However, in a loving marriage the expression of anger should not be a challenge to fight, but rather an invitation to negotiate.
3 Ask one's partner for help. This is a request for a joint investigation into the discovery of causes and solutions.

Love

Closely related to the anger seen in marital disharmony are complaints about the lack of love from a mate. This complaint, which predominantly came from wives in the past, is now being heard from husbands also. The wife often explained her medical and psychiatric symptoms on the basis that her husband did not love her. Now one hears of husbands contemplating leaving home because "there must be more to life than this"—generally meaning that he feels overworked and without gratitude or love from wife and children. It is interesting to note that this emphasis on love is a late twentieth-century phenomenon, accompanying the development of what has been called the companionship marriage. People presumably did not complain about lack of love during earlier times, in marriages where the expectation was not that affection would be a central part of the relationship.

Often in the practice of marital therapy, counselors find that individuals complain of being unloved. Further investigation frequently reveals that many such individuals are not really talking about love, but are talking about a desperate demand for attention which, if the attention is not forthcoming, may lead to intense anger. Often such individuals need to use almost every person they meet to prove their own worth. They may have multiple short-lived involvements with a wide variety of individuals. This pseudo-love is too self-centered to be thought of as love. It is pseudo-love that is closely related to hate. These primitive reactions are not related to mature love, which, in contrast, would be experienced as something that makes the recipient feel good, and is an underlying and fairly constant base of the relationship, rather than a short-lived phenomenon. Anne Lindbergh considers mature love to be the motivating power that enables the giver to offer strength, power, and peace to another person. She states, "It is not a result; it is a cause. It is not a product; it produces. It's a power like money or steam or electricity. It is valueless unless you can give something else by means of it."[15] Fromm writes:

> Nonproductive or irrational love can be . . . any kind of masochistic or sadistic symbiosis, where the relationship is not based upon mutual respect and integrity but where two people depend on each other because they are incapable of depending on themselves. This love, like all other irrational strivings, is based on scarcity, on the lack of productiveness and inner security.[16]

It is important to emphasize that in true or productive love, the closest form of relatedness between two people, the integrity of each individual is preserved. Although conflict and tension are occasionally present, the underlying base is joy and happiness, not hurt and hate. This distinction between pseudo-love and mature love is important inasmuch as the rage that the physician sees in some marital couples is often related to pseudo-love. My clinical experience suggests that encouraging the abreactions of hatred, and assisting couples to fight, rarely contributes to maturation either of the individual or of the marriage. In fact, for some, the frequent eruptions of hatred in marriage have destructive impact upon the integrity of the ego functions of one or both individuals.

Adultery

The problem of adultery is one that is likely to be encountered by physicians who see couples. It may be uncovered as the underlying cause of various physical complaints, or as the immediate precipitating cause of a suicide gesture. Often, by means of such a gesture, one individual attempts to avoid the loss of love implied in a mate's extramarital affair. Often the discovery of the infidelity is experienced as a severe injury, with resultant feelings of helplessness, guilt, rage, and disintegration of coping mechanisms.

Although physicians often choose to ignore adultery, the fact that one-third of couples engaging in extramarital sex divorce and two-thirds remain married suggests that it is an important issue. What appears to matter to the couple is the meaning of the extramarital affair, the motive behind the man's or woman's liaison, and how that liaison is interpreted by the spouse.

A physician may be called into the picture with male cardiac patients who, while engaging in extramarital sexual activity, undergo profound physiologic changes, including severe elevation of pulse and blood pressure. The incidence of sudden death during sexual intercourse apparently is higher under these conditions than during marital intercourse.[17]

Often, the problem of extramarital sex is presented to the physician in a disguised way, as a complaint from the partner of the unfaithful mate regarding sexual performance. The individual having an affair may experience symptoms of impotence, frigidity, inability to complete intercourse, premature ejaculation, or others. The sexual difficulty in the spouse often leads to suspicions and accusations of infidelity, which often are denied. The physician must inquire tactfully about such a possibility, in order to diagnose correctly the cause of the sexual disturbance.

Secrets

The preceding section on infidelity leads naturally to the problem of secrets in a marriage. The management of secret material from one's spouse differs from one school of marital therapy to another. Some feel that if the physician is told in strict confidence by one of the spouses of any secret, the confidence must be kept. The physician cannot inform the partner, who is also a patient. Sending one partner to another physician may alleviate the difficulties, but it is likely to increase suspicion and disturb the one who is sent away. It is possible to handle the secret judiciously until the problem is solved, but to accomplish this the physician must be careful not to become involved as one partner's ally at the expense of the relationship with the other. Occasionally, one spouse wants help in exposing the secret, and the physician must utilize a high level of judgment in deciding whether or not knowledge of the secret will be helpful or harmful to the spouse.

Other marital therapists deal with the issue of secrets in a different way. These therapists announce to the couple during the initial diagnostic interviews that the therapist does not want to hear any individual secrets and that, if presented with confidential material, he or she will feel that it should be shared in the joint interviews.

Sex

The treatment of sexual problems is covered in another section of this book (see Chapter 28). However, at this point it is good to emphasize the existence of a clinical entity known as the happy but sexless marriage.[8] Couples involved in happy and productive marriages vary tremendously in the frequency of their sexual relationships. Some have very little sexual activity and yet, at the same time, appear to have happy, productive marriages. Under certain conditions (debilitating cancer, paraplegia, diabetes with impotence, etc.), the marriage continues to be a happy one, even though sexual relations are not present. It appears that when the bond between marriage partners is secure and stable in other ways, the loss of sex does not necessarily make the relationship an unhappy one.

Another issue is the unconsummated marriage. Occasionally the primary physician may see women who have never had intercourse with their husbands, even after years of marriage. Interestingly, most of these marriages do not end in annulment or divorce, but continue until the wives decide to do something about their underlying problems that lead to avoidance of sex. At this time, the physician often discovers that the husbands of these women may be gentle, timid, sexually naive men. They love their wives, however, and are able to become sexually active without treatment once the wife's psychological problems leading to avoidance of sexuality are resolved.

Jealousy

Jealousy is an outstanding feature in two different kinds of marriages. One is the marriage described as the "love-sick wife, cold-sick husband."[19] Here jealousy is experienced often by the possessive, dependent wife. The other clinical entity wherein jealousy is common is the paranoid marriage. Conjugal paranoia is a classic example. Early in many of these marriages, the husband may be considered as simply jealous or "mean." Later, the delusional system often involves pathological jealousy and delusions of infidelity. The physician must be careful not to be misled by the paranoid partner. Because the delusions are well systematized and the patient appears mentally lucid, it is easy to believe the story to be true. Interviewing the patient's spouse is essential for the correct diagnosis of the disorder, and knowing the spouse as a patient allows the family physician to recognize the distorted nature of the paranoid patient's projections.

PATTERNS OF MARITAL RELATIONSHIPS

Another approach to understanding marital problems is the recognition of the most common patterns of disturbed relationships in treating marital problems. There are four marriage patterns that are in striking contrast to the healthy, smoothly functioning marriage. These will be described briefly and include: (1) the "love-sick" wife and "cold-sick" husband,[19] (2) the "in-search-of-a-mother marriage,"[20] (3) the "double-parasite" marriage,[22] and (4) the paranoid marriage.[22]

The "love-sick" wife and the "cold-sick" husband is the most common, and in many ways, most difficult marital problem encountered. Often called the hysterical-compulsive match, this pattern occurs at all socioeconomic levels, and demonstrates clearly the role of the unconscious factors involved in the choice of mates. Generally, the wife comes for treatment first with complaints of anxiety, depression, or physical symptoms. She reveals evidence of considerable emotional decompensation, and blames her distress entirely on her husband. She insists that she has the ability to love, but that her husband is cold, unresponsive, and significantly distressed. Often, such wives complain that the husband is either oversexed or undersexed. The solution is seen as a complete change in the husband's personality. When considered individually, the wives often seem to have hysterical personalities, or even deeper disturbances, such as borderline psychotic condition. Of importance, however, is the fact that their relationships to their husbands are symbiotic and parasitic. Central to their dilemma is the issue of low self-esteem and their subsequent need to search desperately for constant and overwhelming approval from others.

The husbands are often intelligent, responsible individuals who have established areas of competence outside their marriages and family. They show little evidence of emotional decompensation, but differ radically from their spouses in their lack of emotionality. In treatment, these men do not seem at all like their wife's presentation. They are closer to "normal," although beneath the surface many are found to experience great deprivation and significant need to distance themselves from others. A major disturbance is their inability to achieve emotional intimacy.

The major difficulty in such relationships is that the partners are unable to develop and integrate a viable pattern of intimacy, and then each begins to see the problems as solely that of the mate.

The "in-search-of-a-mother" marriage most often reveals a dependent and often passive husband, with an obsessive and strong-appearing wife. Frequently, the couple seeks marital therapy when the husband's extramarital affair has surfaced or terminated. These men seem to search unconsciously for a mother figure to take care of them, to protect and to love them. They are often irresponsible, and frequently have difficulty with alcoholism. A less common pattern is a more active one, in which the men are successful in many of their activities, but from an interpersonal viewpoint relationships are shallow.

The wives are characteristically mothering individuals who are reliable and dependable. Most show an unusual ability to endure traumatic marriages, and they often accept their husbands as "bad boys." Closer observation of these women often reveals their need to organize, dominate, and control others.

This type of pattern is not uncommon, and may often be complementary until the husband enters a liaison with an "even better mother."

The "double-parasite" marriage is a pattern in which two people cling desperately to each other because neither feels that he or she can make it independently. Most commonly, one sees a passive-dependent husband married to a passive-dependent wife. Alcoholism, drugs, depression, and vocational failure are common. Each expects the other to do most of the giving, and when these expectations are not met, anger and panic often ensue. This type of disturbed marital pattern is often seen at an earlier stage in the marriage than the other two types.

The paranoid marriage may present in several different ways. One extreme form is called *folie a deux,* in which the marriage is maintained by both individuals, sharing the same delusion. Another form of paranoid marriage (conjugal paranoia) is characterized by the focusing of one partners' delusional system entirely on the behavior of the spouse. Often in these marriages, the two partners' identities are lost in their fusion. Rarely do they come spontaneously seeking help with their relationship, but are more often seen when one of them gets into difficulty at work or in the neighborhood.

In conjugal paranoia, the more active spouse characteristically finds fault, humiliates, and degrades the less active spouse. This often proceeds to a frankly delusional state involving pathological jealousy and delusions of infidelity.

These four types or patterns of marital dysfunction account for a large number of the couples who present themselves to the physician for help. The recognition of the basic patterns will assist the family physician in the treatment of the couple.

PSYCHOTHERAPY OF MARITAL DISORDERS

The treatment of marital disorders starts with taking a good history. Although the fact that two people are involved may seem to make history taking more difficult, it can lead to many helpful diagnostic clues. Often, for example, the spouses' descriptions of the same events will be completely different. For example, one couple being seen conjointly were describing their sexual experience of the previous evening: the wife complained that during sex, just as she was about to reach an orgasm, the husband pulled away from her, so that she could not climax. The husband vehemently denied that this took place. Finally, in frustration he stated, "This is an old complaint of yours. A long time ago you were told to hold me closely so I couldn't pull away. Why didn't you hold me closely last night?" To this she replied, "I did hold you to me last night. You pulled away, anyhow." The husband was disbelieving, because he had experienced the wife as unemotional and uninvolved in the lovemaking. The therapist, who has not been an observer of the event, is often confused as to the precise sequence of events, and must rely on repeated observations of the couple as they interact with each other in the therapist's office. By so doing, each individual's characteristic style of relating and use of particular psychological defenses will become apparent. Through these observations, which are often made during the course of taking a history, the physician can come to a conclusion about the role playing by both spouses. An example involving the couple above was that the husband became increasingly involved in a close working relationship with the physician. The wife, however, could not form such a helpful working relationship, objected to any solutions offered, and at the point of some degree of intimacy in communication, withdrew to protect herself from being hurt. She appeared to use the mechanism of *projective identification*—accusing others of doing what she was doing. The accumulation of evidence and the clarification by the physician of this evidence are, of course, sequences followed in all fields of medicine.

Psychotherapy of marital partners starts with taking a history. Here it is helpful to focus on three different areas. When one sees the couple together initially (and this is strongly advised), it is helpful to take a detailed history of the marriage itself, as well as the history of each of the spouses. One should understand the chief complaints of each mate about the marriage, as well as what each sees as positive about the relationship. A history of the current difficulties can be followed by a longitudinal account of the marriage, and then the exploration of each spouse's individual development. In this way, a psychodynamic understanding of each individual becomes available, as well as an understanding of their relationship.

History taking is important insofar as it leads to the answers to four basic questions. These are: (1) Who is this person who entered into this type of relationship with this specific other person? (2) How did this relationship promote, impede, or prevent the continuing growth and development of the individual? (3) What areas need correction? (4) What is the best method of accomplishing this?

It is helpful to focus on the early period of the couple's relationship, inquiring specifically for those factors that attracted each to the other, and attempting to get at what each partner hoped would come out of their relationship. It is also important to obtain information about the nature of each spouse's parental marriage. There may often be a tendency to repeat patterns from the earlier generation.

It is important to take a thorough sexual history from the couple. To do so the physician must be comfortable dealing with the details and specifics of the couple's sexual relationship.

At the end of a diagnostic interview(s), the physician would have data about each spouse individually, and about the nature of their relationship. In regard to each spouse individually, one needs to know the following: (1) the capacity for independence, (2) the capacity for offering support, (3) the capacity to accept support, (4) the capacity for lust, (5) the capacity for sensuousness, and (6) the capacity for love.

In regard to the marital relationship itself, it is helpful to understand the relationship in terms of both conscious and unconscious contracts.[23] In this regard, a couple is aware of some of what the contract includes—that is, what they consciously expect from the other, and that which the other may expect from them. In addition, however, there are unconscious aspects of marital contracts, and the sensitive physician may infer from the historical material significant aspects of the unconscious expectations that each partner had of the other.

Following the diagnostic work involved in taking an adequate history, the physician needs to decide which of a variety of techniques would seem most appropriate for a given couple. There is some preliminary evidence that, under most circumstances, seeing the couple conjointly may be the most effective treatment approach.[21] However, under certain circumstances the physician may wish to see one or both spouses separately, or to see one spouse and refer the other to a colleague. It is at this point also that the physician needs to determine whether or not the marital pathology is of sufficient intensity or of an uncomfortable enough quality so that referral to a psychiatrist might be considered.

The major thesis of this chapter, however, is that physicians should be actively involved as marital therapists. There is a wide variety of available techniques, and training opportunities are present in the form of continuing education in many sections of the country. However, as Skynner suggests in regard to family therapy (see Chapter 27), often the physician must do some reading about marital therapy, and then have the courage to venture out and try to be of help to his or her patients. The techniques themselves are many, and in another publication I have outlined the major approaches currently available.[22] However, unless there are specific reasons for not doing so, the family physician should increase his or her experience with conjoint interviewing. In particular, it will be helpful in working with couples under such circumstances to focus on the various aspects and levels of the marital contract.[23] Clarification of previously repressed aspects of their expectations of each other can often result in striking changes in the quality of the relationship and in the individual symptoms experienced by one or both of the individuals.

This focus really underscores the importance of the physician's clarifying the dynamics of the relationship involved in the marriage. As one part of that, the physician must become confident in using his or her own emotional reactions to the material presented in the joint interviews. If the physician, for example, experiences an intense reaction, in either a positive or a negative way, to either of the participants, this is often a clue that can lead to important insights about the nature of the marital problem.

However, it is important in using one's own responses to be keenly aware of the ways in which one's own feelings and values may influence both what one hears in the interviews and what one assumes is normal in marriage. Perhaps more than in any other situation, the clinical situation that provokes male physicians to potentially destructive feelings is the love-sick wife, cold-sick husband syndrome. Women in such circumstances occasionally come to feel that the male physician would be a desirable substitute for the "nonloving" husband, and may attempt seductively to engage the physician in an erotic relationship. Occasionally physicians participate in such destructive relationships, or find a way to terminate the doctor-patient relationship. What is advised here is that the male physician may use his inner responses to better understand the patient's style and its contribution to the presenting marital disturbances. The more fragile such a woman's ego structure, the more intense her emotional needs, and the more ready she may be to endow the physician with superior powers. For such women, the open seductiveness may be an attempt to establish a life-saving attachment to a helping figure.

In this same marital relationship syndrome, the physician may respond in a negative way to the husband who is not needy, not clinging, and does not value the physician highly, thereby reinforcing the wife's problem by agreeing with her.

A related problem is the interface between the marriage problems of the physician's patients and his or her own marital situation. For example, if the physician is listening sympathetically to a patient complain about a spouse who never calls to indicate whether he or she will be on time for dinner, the physician may experience guilt in regard to the same personal offense. Traditionally, physician's marriages have been described as frequently troubled, with spouses usually considered to be neglected and martyred. However, some studies reveal that male physicians are considerably less prone to marital failure than others of comparable age in the general population.[24] In contrast, however, other studies show that women physicians are at least 40 percent more prone to marital instability. The traditionally jaundiced viewpoint of physicians' marriages is often based on clinical experience with disturbed physicians' marriages. Emotionally ill physicians often do not seek help early enough for themselves, and if there is a marital problem, the male physician often tends to designate his wife as the patient.

A new marital syndrome among physicians has recently been described. This is related to the increasing number of women medical students. The female medical student may feel inferior, and may unconsciously assume a depreciated female role. However, as she becomes a professional and gains a sense of competence, her self-image alters, which may lead to marital disharmony that, without help, can result in divorce.[25]

The physician who is working with marital problems can often enhance the growth and development of his or her own marriage. Conversely, physicians who are courageous enough to work at optimal growth and development in their own marriages often are better able to serve their patients as marital therapists.

PREMARITAL EXAMINATION

The premarital examination is an aspect of preventive medicine that has been sadly neglected by many members of the medical profession. Traditionally, the physician has occupied a position that offered great opportunity for the recognition and handling of existing interpersonal problems, with all the position's implications for prevention of future problems and promotion of health. However, the primary physician's lack of time, training, and interest in marital counseling has forced patients to go elsewhere for premarital assistance.

The premarital examination is conducted by some physicians by merely completing the laboratory work necessary to rule out venereal disease. The patient may not be examined, let alone counseled. A thorough medical, reproductive, and social history, as well as a complete physical and pelvic examination, should accompany the laboratory tests. Contraceptive and sexual counseling complete the premarital examination, which can be an important event in the life of the involved young couple. Sexual counseling to such a couple has been an area in which physicians have been considered to be persons of authority. This is related to the fact that physicians are licensed to examine the body and its "private parts." However, the failure of many medical schools to give sufficient attention to the teaching of sexual counseling leads to the production of physicians who are not knowledgeable in this area and, indeed, may have considerable resistance to learning about sexual therapy.

DIVORCE

The family physician is often the first to be asked for advice when marital discord occurs. Often there is a crisis, and the physician's intervention can contribute to prevention of a future contested divorce. Even in situations, however, wherein the marital relationship is finished and divorce is imminent, the physician can be of help. An experienced legal authority has written guidelines for physicians to follow in these situations, based upon the common-law written statutes, Supreme Court legal decisions, and moral codes of all major religions.[26] This approach stresses, whenever possible, the preservation of the family unit and the protection of the children. The current human rights movement, however, takes the opposite approach. Here the individual is supreme, and divorce follows easily from this viewpoint.

Certainly children can be seriously damaged by dissolution of the family. How best to help the children and the parents becomes the crucial issue. As a consequence of this, "divorce therapy" is now considered a special technique to assist individuals and families through this difficult period.

CONCLUSION

Underlying this chapter is the ideal of the complete family physician—a wise, mature human being who is well trained medically. In practice, many factors prevent our full development as physicians. Yet if physicians take advantage of the opportunities for growth and development to be found in the practice of medicine, they may overcome to some extent their fear of areas such as marital therapy in which they have not received specific training. By tackling problems in these areas, the physician will be rewarded by personal growth and find considerable gratification in being of greater help to patients.

REFERENCES

1 Stanford, Betty J.: "Counseling a Prime Area for Family Doctors," *Am. Fam. Phys.,* **5:**183–185, May 1972.
2 Herndon, C. M., and E. C. Nash: "Marital Counseling," *JAMA,* **180:**395, May 1962.
3 Masters, William H., and Virginia E. Johnson: *Human Sexual Inadequacy,* Boston: Little, Brown, 1970.
4 Ehrenwald, Jan (ed.): *The History of Psychotherapy,* New York: Jason Aronson, 1976.
5 Ornstein, Paul H.: "The Family Physician as a Therapeutic Instrument," *J. Fam. Prac.,* **4:**659–661, April 1977.
6 Wittkower, Eric, and Eva P. Lester: "Marital Stress in Psychosomatic Disorders," in D. W. Abse et al. (eds.), *Marital & Sexual Counseling in Medical Practice,* 2d ed., Hagerstown, Md.: Harper & Row, 1974, pp. 218–230.
7 Saunders, Daniel G.: "Marital Violence: Dimensions of the Problem and Modes of Intervention," *J. Marr. Fam. Couns.,* **3:**43–49, January 1977.
8 Rounsaville, Bruce J. (moderator): *Battered Wives: Dynamics and Treatment Strategies,* panel at Annual Meeting of the American Psychiatric Association, Toronto, Canada, May 1977.
9 Elliott, Frank A.: "Neurological Causes and Cures of Explosive Rage," *Med. Opinion,* **2:**33–46, February 1977.
10 Charney, Israel: *Marital Love and Hate,* New York: Macmillan, 1972.
11 Reynolds, R., and E. Siegle: "A Study of Casework with Sadomasochistic Marriage Partners," *Soc. Casework,* **40:**545–551, 1959.
12 Novaco, Raymond W.: "The Functions and Regulation of the Arousal of Anger," *Am. Psyciat.,* **133:**1124–1127, October 1976.
13 _____: *Anger Control,* Lexington, Mass.: Lexington Books, 1975.

14 Mace, David R.: "Marital Intimacy and the Deadly Love-Anger Cycle," *J. Marr. Fam. Couns.,* **2:**131–139, April 1976.

15 Lindbergh, Anne M.: *Locked Rooms and Open Doors,* New York: Harcourt-Brace, 1974.

16 Fromm, Eric: *Man For Himself,* Greenwich, Conn.: Fawcett Publications, 1947.

17 Wolfe, Walter G., and Don E. Detmar: "Disease, Surgery, and Family Relationships," in D. W. Abse et al. (eds.), *Marital & Sexual Counseling in Medical Practice,* 2d ed., Hagerstown, Md.: Harper & Row, 1974, pp. 206–217.

18 Martin, Peter A.: "The Happy Sexless Marriage," *Med. Aspects Human Sexuality,* **2:**75–84, May 1977.

19 Martin, Peter A., and H. Waldo Bird: "The Love-Sick Wife and the Cold-Sick Husband," *Psychiatry,* **22:**246–249, 1959.

20 _____: "One Type of the In-Search-of-a-Mother Marital Pattern," *Psychiat. Quart.,* **36:**283–293, 1962.

21 Berman, Ellen, and Harold I. Lief: "Marital Therapy from a Psychiatry Perspective: An Overview," *Am. J. Psychiat.,* **132:**583–592, June 1975.

22 Martin, Peter A.: *A Marital Therapy Manual,* New York: Brunner/Mazel, 1976.

23 Sager, C. J. et al.: "The Marriage Contract," *Fam. Process,* **10**(3):311–326, 1971.

24 Rose, K. Daniel, and Irving Rosow: "Marital Stability among Physicians," *Calif. Med.,* **166:**95–99, March 1972.

25 Berman, Ellen et al.: "The Two-Professional Marriage: A New Conflict Syndrome," *J. Sex & Marital Ther.,* **1:**242–253, 1975.

26 Pearlman, Thomas W.: "Domestic Relations—Advice for the Physician," *Rhode Island Med. J.,* **57:**108–109, March 1974.

Chapter 27

The Physician
as Family Therapist

A. C. Robin Skynner, F.R.C. Psych.

EDITORS' INTRODUCTION

How does it feel to be the "head of the family" in a physician's office, to be subject to critical scrutiny, overt demands, and complaints by one's mate and children? How does it feel for an executive in a physician's office to tolerate unjust, previously unspoken, criticisms from one's young adolescent child, who already has demonstrated an inability to make an adequate social and emotional adjustment? How does a sibling feel as a brother and sister attack him or her or their parents verbally in the confines of a physician's office—in the guise of family therapy? Then, too, what does the treating physician think and feel when, by his or her own standard, unjust accusations or flattery come forth in family therapy? What does the physician think when a previously poised parent becomes unwilling to discuss a problem further or becomes violently angry with a member of the family?

Central to this chapter, however, is the belief that many physicians who are interested and willing to recognize their potential effectiveness in dealing with the family as a whole may learn some basic concepts of family therapy. Hopefully, such physicians may consider seeking ways to enlarge their knowledge and skills in an area where they can accomplish so much.

Chapter 4 discussed in detail what it can be like both for family and physician to meet and to explore a family problem. In that instance, the context was essentially diagnostic—the goal was to obtain information with which to understand the family of the patient, in order to appreciate the family's strengths and conflicts better and to evaluate their impact upon the patient. This chapter encourages the physician to take another step: to become a family counselor. For those who are willing to try, this step is often associated with considerable anxiety. For most, it will be a new experience and, as such, raises the issue of the physician's competence. Skynner encourages the physician to get his or her feet wet. If courses in family counseling are not available, one is encouraged to read and make a start. For those who do so, an important issue will soon surface.

The issue is the use and/or misuse of the physician's personal experiences in families. Most physicians experience, intimately, only two families. This is a small data base and, if not amplified by reading, training, or clinical work, it may lead to uncertainty about the appropriateness of certain family transactions and, consequently, uncertainty about how to be helpful. The physician who has been raised in a family dominated by a patriarchal father, and who dominates his or her own family, may be asked to help a family in which a submissive wife has entered with the children into a coalition against an authoritarian father. As one part of this family drama, a son is involved in early delinquency, which embarrasses the father. Does the physician see the family pathology as the father's authoritarianism, as the angry coalition of mother and children, or as both? If the physician's orientation about family power reflects only his or her experiences in two families, the physician is apt to be of little assistance to this particular family.

Limited though the physician's experience in families may be, it can be put to positive use. For example, the female physician who recalls her own pain at the death of her mother when she was 15 may use personal insights to be of help to the father and teenage daughters who come to her following a similar loss. Recalling both the pain and that which helped ease it can provide a base from which to understand and be helpful.

The physician's capacity to be helpful to families—the therapeutic use of self—should not be underestimated. The use of one's own experience can be crucial but, as with all powerful therapeutic agents, there is always the potential of misuse. The thoughtful physician will minimize the risks of misusing personal experience and, with courage, will find that efforts to help families will succeed frequently, and may lead to increased understanding of the physician's own past, present, and future.

Family therapy is a relatively new treatment modality, and one that lends itself especially to the practice of the primary physician. Understanding the relatively simple techniques involved and demonstrating an adventurous spirit can help the physician to produce gratifying results with many of the patients seen in everyday practice. Although seeing whole families may seem strange, there are striking parallels between this type of treatment and other forms of medical practice.

Communication is at the core of medical practice. All forms of medical practice involve the gathering of information by a series of questions and answers, according to a set of concepts in the physician's mind about the structure of disease processes and about possible links between symptoms or signs and the underlying disorder that would explain them. Physicians start with the assumption that the patient's complaint is meaningful, and that inquiry about an abdominal pain, an inflamed joint, or the wasting of some muscles will lead, if the questioning is persistent and the physical examination thorough, to a coherent and rational pattern of physical processes. This pattern accounts for all our observations, predicts other consequences that we may search for and find (then or at a later date in the development of the disease), and suggests actions we may take to arrest the pattern or change its course.

This process requires that, in the time interval between hearing the initial complaint and the final reaching of a secure diagnosis, we tolerate a period of uncertainty and puzzlement. We try one hypothesis after another, with each of them failing to fit, and to test them we widen the search into history and bodily signs. The process is like attempting to solve a crossword puzzle; both the process and the puzzle are made possible by our fundamental confidence that each does have an answer, if we are sufficiently persistent and thoughtful—that all the words in the puzzle, or the functioning of all the systems in the body, can be assumed to fit together in a patterned, coherent, meaningful way.

All this is, of course, too obvious to need stating in the case of ordinary medical practice with physical disorders, and the simple but fundamental point is that family counseling applies these basic principles to the family as a system of individuals, just as psychiatry extends such principles from the study of organic systems, as in internal medicine, to the study of the whole person as a social-psychological-physical system.

This is important to realize at the outset, because the practitioner without previous experience in the family approach will at first feel very uncertain of its value, much as all medical students need time and practice before they have confidence that the painstaking accumulation of facts through history taking and physical examination will lead to effective diagnosis and treatment. Just as unsophisticated individual patients may object to examination of their blood pressure or testing of patellar reflexes, and insist that they have come for treatment of a headache and not of their legs or arms, so the nonsymptomatic members of families will often make the physician feel that it is quite unreasonable to ask them to attend therapy when the "problems" so clearly lie in the referred patient, not in themselves. In the same way that the medical student learns to ignore irrelevant objections by becoming convinced through experience that a systematic approach is best, so will the physician discover that regarding the whole family as an interlocking system may produce far more effective understanding of, and results in treating, the problems about which they are complaining.

In medical schools, this conviction regarding physical illness is attained by working at first under the supervision and guidance of experienced physicians and being helped to see, over and over again, that the part (symptom) is understood and altered most effectively in the context of the whole (the anatomy and physiology of the whole body). Many general practitioners in North America, if they are working near universities or large cities, may be able to take part in family therapy training courses. Here they can observe experienced family therapists at work through one-way screens or on videotape, or see families themselves while under supervision, thereby observing the value of a family approach. Despite the greater availability of training programs in the United States, for a considerable number of physicians working in more rural areas the situation will be similar to that in Europe, where many professionals who were armed only with courage and a textbook of family therapy began to use the technique.

Where this is the case, the physician should begin by adding an occasional family session to the customary way of working, without any expectation of "results" beyond perhaps gaining a better view of the total family situation. The physician can also convey a similar attitude to the family by saying that, though nothing may come of the sessions, perhaps some fresh viewpoint and approach may emerge. The physician can relax, avoid feeling pressured by any expectations, and use the situation as a learning experience. Doing so will provide a totally different perspective of the family interaction and of the function that the illness of the referred patient serves in its "psychic economy." At the next contact, striking improvements may have occurred, even though no attempt has been made to alter the situation directly.

ARRANGEMENTS AND INTERVIEWING TECHNIQUES

Getting the family to attend as a group is not usually a problem, provided one has confidence in the value of family therapy and conveys this confidence in one's voice and manner. It should be a problem least of all for the general practitioner, who has gained the family's confidence and trust through past involvement. In the psychiatric department of the Queen Elizabeth Hospital for Children in London, where most referrals were from pediatricians or family practitioners, it was so rare for a father not to attend that his absence was a source of animated discussion, and usually proved to be the most important fact explaining the presenting problem. Yet this hospital was located in the poorest part of London's East End, where most fathers had to change a shift or lose a half-day's pay to come.

However, if doubts or objections are raised—usually by a parent who says that there are no problems in the family apart from the symptoms of the identified patient—it usually suffices to say that the latter does indeed need help, but that there is more hope of success if other members of the family can be involved. The practitioner is helped both by obtaining information about the problem (parents readily appreciate the fact that siblings may have received confidences or noticed events or coincidences that did not come to their own attention) and by encouraging the collaboration of both parents in a treatment plan that they have worked out and agreed upon together. Few mothers disagree when told that fathers are important too, and that mother will be able to seek the children's welfare and health even more effectively if she has the father's understanding and cooperation through sharing in the discussion.

Once the family is assembled, members are invited to sit in a rough circle, perhaps with some play material in the center for younger children (these should be such as to avoid too much noise or mess, as well as to give some opportunity for nonverbal communication—crayons and paper, or a doll's house and flexible family figures are ideal). My technique is to indicate that the discussion is a collaborative effort by sitting in the circle rather than behind a desk, and to direct all activity toward encouraging a "collaborative" rather than a "directive" interview (see Chapter 1) in the early stages. And I usually shake hands with each member of the family, ask to be introduced to everyone, which not only gives an opportunity to record names, ages, and other items of the family structure, but demonstrates my interest in all family members. I indicate my understanding that there is a problem affecting some member of the family, and ask whether the family will tell me something about it. It is important to look with curiosity from one member to another, and to take care not to catch any one person's gaze for too long. In this way, the individual who takes the lead will be determined by the family power structure, rather than by a signal from oneself. The pattern of interaction that follows will often say more than the actual words spoken, and is noted attentively. For example, the mother may control the interview and put words into everyone's mouth, while the father looks resignedly out the window or at his watch. The referred child who is alleged to have the "behavior disorder" may behave well, though looking depressed, while the allegedly "good" one behaves abominably and "gets away with murder."

In the early stages, attempts will usually be made to get the doctor to change to a more directive form of interviewing by keeping the identified patient in the limelight and by keeping exploration away from more general family relationships: "Why does she do these things, doctor?". . . . "We just want some advice". . . . "Do you think some drugs would help her?". . . . "Everything's fine at home except for her; couldn't you just arrange some therapy for her?". . . etc., etc.! All this is best dealt with by explaining patiently that one needs more information from everyone before understanding of the problem is achieved and decisions about diagnosis and treatment are made. Though there are many approaches, the quickest, easiest, and least anxiety-arousing route into the more general family dynamics, in my experience, is to ask for a recent example of the problem complained of, and then get the family to give a play-by-play account of events preceding and following it by insisting on detail. Asking about the *effects* of the problem on other members of the family and about their *management* of it brings everyone into the discussion in a completely natural, nonthreatening way. The family relationships and emotional undercurrents quickly begin to become apparent. Mother may say that father leaves it all to her, and that she wishes he would take more part. Father may answer that whenever he does, she interferes, so he has given up trying. Mother may reply that this is the whole trouble—he should stand his ground with her and with the children and be more of a man. Father may hint darkly that he might play a more active role in the daytime if he were encouraged to be more of a man when alone with her at night. And so on.

Once the discussion is underway, the doctor can be less active, while making sure that everyone is having a chance to contribute, while drawing out feelings people may be too anxious to voice at first, and while checking each person's idea about how the others feel, against the reality of the actual feelings expressed. The physician chairs the discussion in a relaxed, encouraging, fair, and sympathetic way, asking questions to clarify that which is being said, and constantly confronting the family with the fundamental principle that *it is their task to make the problem meaningful to the physician if they are to be helped.*

In a later part of the interview, the nonverbal aspects of the interaction can be made explicit, especially those that contradict the verbal statements. Though the parents may protest that there is never any form of aggression or violence in the family, the children may be enacting scenes of extreme violence in their drawings. Or the parents may both focus on the referred child, and the fact that their eyes never meet may say everything about the unhappy nature of the marital sexual bond.

In a later part of the interview, the siblings too, if tactfully encouraged and supported, will begin to "spill the beans" and provide the key information that helps explain the mystery and confusion experienced by the doctor when vital facts were being withheld earlier. Indeed, the siblings may do most of the work if they are given firm and fair direction from the physician. They are not only close enough to be aware of the real problem, but are often disengaged enough from the interaction of the parents and referred patient to see this interaction more objectively. Just to ask the siblings what they think about the problem, and what would be necessary to solve it, leads frequently to answers that are awesome in their appropriateness, wisdom, and simplicity.

However a solution is reached, the element of simplicity is usually striking. All physicians have had the experience of being thanked by patients for helping them to solve problems, when all that was done was to listen patiently and to help them sustain their thought past the point where it usually turned back into the same circle. Once people are helped to clarify their attitudes and aims, they often see contradictions that were invisible to them before, and find more satisfactory compromises. The same process occurs in family counseling, as family members become aware, perhaps for the first time in their lives, of agreements and conflicts between their different desires, and then negotiate compromises that are more satisfactory to all. These simple procedures frequently result in profound and rapid positive changes in the functioning of the family, as well as changes in the symptoms that the referred patient had presented. The physician may think that nothing grand or clever enough to account for such improvement has been done, but improvement occurs even after interviews that leave both the physician and the family feeling confused and disappointed. The following is a clear example; changes of this extent and rapidity are quite common, even with seemingly hopeless cases that have undergone years of conventional treatments.

CASE A: Ann, aged 27, was referred to me from a mental hospital in a neighboring city, where she was being compulsorily detained for her own safety, because of severe depression and wrist cutting. The wrist cutting had occurred repeatedly since the age of 11, and together with other self-destructive behavior such as drug overdose and refusal to eat, had led to many admissions. Though she had completed training as a secretary, she was unable to work and was living on welfare. She claimed, and her family agreed, that she had suffered lifelong depression and incapacitating social anxiety, was unable to make and keep friends, spent long periods sitting alone in darkened rooms, and wanted only to die.

Besides medication and other routine hospital treatments, she had undergone $2\frac{1}{2}$ years of psychotherapy with a psychologist at the hospital at the time of referral. Change had been very limited.

In view of the limited progress, the psychiatrist who had been responsible for the case requested a family consultation, and put strong pressure on the family to accept. His insistence was vital, since the parents, brother (2 years younger), and patient lived a long way away, and since the father, a rigid, cold, remote man, was known to be intensely hostile to psychiatrists, claiming, "If they get their hands on you, they drive you mad," and insisting that there were no problems in the family except those displayed by Ann.

Through the consultant's ultimatum, the whole family was soon assembled for consultation. As expected, the father took over and gave a long and detailed account of Ann's "illness," assuring me there was nothing wrong with anyone else. I heard him out patiently, nodded and accepted all he said, and then asked for Ann's account.

She agreed with her father's description of her as inexplicably disordered from birth, and attributed her self-destructive episodes to despair at her social inadequacy, which resulted from overwhelming feelings of anxiety and fears of further failure.

I next brought in the brother who, to the surprise of both parents, reported that he had always suffered from similar, but less severe, social anxiety. Following this, the mother said that she had always shared this problem too, but had not wanted to divulge this, for fear the children would lose confidence in her. Ann was quite incredulous, protesting that this could not possibly be true. Her amazement was only matched by that of her mother, as the father next reported that he had always felt similar anxiety in social situations as well, and coped only with great difficulty and constant struggle.

This was the essence of the interview. The remainder of the time was used to look at the reasons why Ann had volunteered for the role of scapegoat. This was explained partly by her feeling that males were favored, so that this role compensated and gave her an important place in the family. This was really the whole treatment, though the parents and Ann came once more to report subsequent changes a month later.

A few days after the first interview, the father wrote to say that "Following our recent consultation we had the most relaxed family discussion that we had had for years, and would like to make arrangements for our further meetings." At the second (and last) session, Ann looked lively and attractive, had changed her drab appearance with a striking "Afro" hair style, played a leading part in the session, and insisted on seeing my secretary afterwards to pay the fee herself, instead of letting her father do so. She confirmed her father's initial statement that "She hasn't looked back from the moment we left this room. . ." by saying: "Everything is just better. I am working, planning for the future, have taken on a 3-year course of training. I know it's going to be difficult, but I still want to do it. . . . Before, I had no other aim but the grave . . . but now I want to make a success of it." The urge to cut her wrists had "absolutely gone." Mother confirmed these improvements, saying it was "just wonderful."

In this case it was possible to have an unusually detailed follow-up through the assessments of the consultant and of the other professionals who continued to have contact with her, and they reported that these improvements have been sustained and increased, despite some variations in mood, reported in the following 30 months.

An extract from a letter Ann wrote to me after the second consultation conveys vividly the chain-reaction of improvement even one such discussion can lead to by opening up communication in the family.

> It is really quite amazing how things have changed in so short a time. I must say I was terribly skeptical to begin with, and my father was too; we really didn't believe that by just talking to someone, anything could really change at all, but obviously we were wrong, because somehow absolutely everything has changed, and our attitudes now, seem to be having a snowballing effect, which is making everything better . . . I have a picture in mind of each of us ploughing through life up until now, completely enclosed within a brick wall, and although we were a "family" to the outside world, we were *never* a family at all. It was always a ghastly criss-cross combination of two-vs.-two in some form or other. Now it seems just as though all the brick walls have been broken down, and we can reach each other.

At the end of the letter, Ann enclosed a diagram of the change as she saw it (see Fig. 27-1).

Differentiation

This example shows with striking clarity the way in which members of a family may assign fixed and limited roles to each other, thus restricting their ability to grow toward balanced, independent functioning. Instead, members are tied together in a state of partial fusion and are unable to operate autonomously because they need other family members to contain or express some psychological functions for them. This need is most obvious in the case where there is a scapegoat who is assigned the task of containing a particular set of feelings that the family as a whole are excessively fearful of, and so cannot cope with. By Ann's carrying the burden for everyone, the rest of the family was enabled to function effectively. The scapegoat role is determined by many factors, not the least of which is a dim awareness on the part of the person filling it that playing this role is vital to the psychic balance of the family, and has its rewards and importance as well as its pains and handicaps. The scapegoat is always as much volunteer as victim, and the role is fulfilled out of love as well as fear.

Family members who are assigned to carry the "strong" and seemingly positive roles are equally bound within the system, because they are threatened with symptoms of disequilibrium unless the "weak" member carries the fears and failings of all. These weaknesses may in fact be no more than a normal sensitivity or tenderness, which is essential to a full life and is experienced as a defect only because it is condemned and rejected. Thus, clearer differentiation, with each family member taking responsibility for his or her own strengths and failings, is ultimately of benefit to everyone.

Collaborative discussions of the kind described, where the doctor assists all family members to express their feelings clearly and helps each to see the others as real persons, obviously help this differentiation to take place progressively.

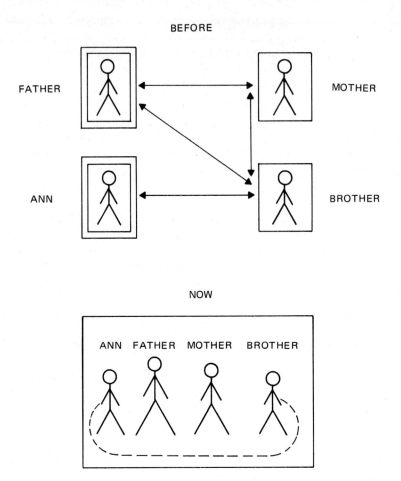

Figure 27-1

Awareness of this principle can enhance the psychological benefits of the general practitioner's interventions, even when seeing individual patients alone or seeing a couple without their children. Helping one family member to differentiate and define himself or herself more clearly may lead other family members to clarify their own identities, just as drawing the frontier of the United States draws part of Canada's as well. Bowen, a distinguished pioneer in the field of family therapy, has developed this type of approach with particular clarity and sophistication.[1] He concentrates much of his work on helping a key figure in the family (usually not the referred patient), or the parental couple, to achieve a higher degree of "differentiation of self." Bowen's principle is that therapists best help patients to gain clearer identities and boundaries when the therapists define *themselves* as real persons, and are not open to manipulation or willing to control the patients' lives to an inappropriate degree. This forces patients to take responsibility for their lives in increasing measure, and should prove especially fruitful in general practice. Hatfield, a British general practitioner, has attempted to modify Bowen's methods to suit the general-practice setting.[2]

A family whose members have ill-defined boundaries and are low in degree of "differentiation of self" will be more vulnerable to both internal and external stresses, and disturbances will tend to spread not only through the nuclear family but also through the extended family system, so that a stress initially impinging on one member may lead to dysfunction in several members. Many other individuals in the network may then present to the family physician, not only with obviously nervous or psychosomatic symptoms, but with injuries, infections, and other more obviously "physical" disorders. Kellner has demonstrated a "clustering" of different types of illness in members of families at times of stress, illnesses that are seemingly related to emotional contagion.[3] Particularly in rural areas, where the family practitioner is intimately acquainted with large interrelated family networks, knowledge about the spread of such ripples of disturbance not only makes the work more meaningful, but allows the physician to concentrate attention at the source of the disturbance, which may greatly reduce the need for prolonged intervention.

DEVELOPMENTAL STAGES

Raising a family can be viewed as a process in which the parents help the children to master a series of developmental challenges by giving the children difficulties they must struggle to overcome and by giving support and information to help them do so. At the simplest level, for example, the mother no longer ties her children's shoelaces, but patiently helps them to do this for themselves. At the more complex level of learning to form relationships and to fit into society, the response of the parent similarly has to be tailored to the level of social development that the child has reached. During the first year or so, the child is learning to love, trust, and internalize a secure and comforting image of the mother; at this stage, the latter must be readily available and must provide consistent care and comfort, while demands for conformity and self-control are at a minimum. Over the next couple of years, the child becomes more active, independent, and assertive, so that the parents must provide increasing control and discipline to help the child develop adequate inner controls and find compromises between personal impulses and the demands of society. Later still, at about age 4 or 5, the precursors of what one day will be mature sexuality and marriage make their appearance in a developing curiosity about sexual differences and a romantic attachment to the parent of the opposite sex. Next comes school, and the need to fit into the larger social group in the classroom and in the playground or "gang"; then adolescence, the first budding of real sexuality as well as social pressures for greater independence from the family; and so on.

The family interview will focus around rather different issues, depending upon the amount of difficulty the family experiences when passing through this developmental sequence. In addition, the interview will have to provide a different kind of "input," depending upon the developmental challenge with which the parents cannot cope, and which the physician has to help them provide or must provide personally when the family cannot do so even with advice and support. With one family, this role may be more to act as a model of a nurturing, accepting parent, particularly where the mother has received no adequate model of love and nurturance from her own mother and so cannot meet her child's needs. In another family where no adequate models of firm and kindly control have existed in the parents' early histories, the model for this may have to be provided first by the doctor. And if parents are anxious and inhibited about sexuality and any display of physical affection, the doctor may have to provide an example of relaxed acceptance of such matters by the comfortable and open way in which he or she talks about them.

Some examples will convey the essential principles involved.

CASE B: Jean, who was referred to the Child Guidance Clinic at the age of 12 for soiling, had a long history of disturbance, accidents, and physical illness. She had always craved affection, saying that she would not stop soiling until her mother displayed her love. She was showing increasingly violent tempers and outbursts of violence, and would lock herself in the toilet. She had no friends, believed that everyone was against her, and in fact provoked much bullying.

The mother was a thin, withdrawn, apathetic woman who had had a similar history of deprivation and difficult relationships in her own childhood, and wanted to get rid of Jean by placing her in a boarding school. Jean's father had deserted the mother soon after Jean was born.

At the first interview, Jean behaved like a very young child, clinging to her mother and refusing to leave her. I, therefore, saw them for a joint interview where Jean sat close up against her mother, holding her hand and gazing at her silently. She expressed great relief when she was able to reveal, with encouragement and support, that she did indeed feel that her mother did not love her and might leave her, and that she clung to her for this reason. She was then able to admit that she hated her mother, sometimes wished that she were dead, and that her greatest terror was that her mother might find this out, for then she would surely abandon her. Asked what she would choose if she could have "three magic wishes," her replies were: (1) "Stop messing my drawers," (2) "Mother not to be so angry," and (3) "Not to be so angry myself."

Following this, it was possible for the mother to express in Jean's presence her feelings of unhappiness and despair over the present situation, especially her own feelings of worthlessness and incompetence as a mother, to a point where she hated Jean for making her feel so inadequate. With encouragement, the mother was then able to speak of her own early deprivation, and to say how difficult she found it to give her child what she had never received herself.

This 45-minute interview comprised the main treatment needed, and succeeding 15-minute visits at increasing intervals were primarily for follow-up. Two weeks after the first interview, both looked happier and more relaxed. Jean sat farther away from her mother and no longer needed to touch her. Both agreed that they were less angry with each other and were able to show affection more easily. A month later, Jean was sleeping well, and the temper tantrums had largely ceased. She had lost her fears that accidents would befall her mother or that the house would catch fire (which were present at her first session), and said she now felt sure her mother loved her, and was not worried that her bad feelings would drive mother away. Eighteen months later, this improvement had not only been maintained, but Jean had completely lost her paranoid feelings at school, was making friends, and had become able to stand up for herself.

The most striking aspect of this case is the deprivation of maternal love and care, perpetuating itself over generations—a vicious circle in which the pain of rejection bred hostility and withdrawal, which in turn heightened the feelings of rejection and inadequacy. The role of the physician in these interviews was that of a good, nurturing "mother," providing the affection, acceptance, support, and containment that had been lacking in the mother's childhood, and that could not, therefore, be supplied to Jean. Provided there is real acceptance by the doctor of parts of the personality seen as "bad" and destructive by the family, little is sometimes needed to effect a profound change, since a limited intervention can change a vicious circle of this kind into an ascending spiral.

CASE C: Roger, aged 11 when first seen, had been treated unsuccessfully at two clinics over 4 years for nocturnal enuresis, anxiety, and behavior problems. For him, treatment had included a pad and buzzer, various forms of medication, and psychotherapy, while prolonged casework had been done with the mother, through separate interviews that did not include other members of the family. A family interview was arranged, and was attended by both parents, Roger, and his 4-year-old sister.

Detailed exploration of the family interaction and parental management of the problems yielded a picture of parents who grumbled and nagged, but were never really firm. The father acknowledged that he would argue with Roger for up to a half-hour to get him to get some coal, but would end by getting it himself "for the sake of peace." I pointed out that Roger, who was behaving at the interview like a caricature of passive resistance, doing nothing to contribute to the discussion and leaving everything to the adults, was clearly in control of the family. This was because the parents needed to see themselves as kind, loving, and loved by the children, and always put the latter first and their own needs, including the marriage, last. The parents were encouraged to reverse this order, and to put the marriage first and Roger last.

As the marital relationship began to be discussed, the mother burst into tears and acknowledged that she felt unsupported by the father, who left all the discipline to her. The father tried to evade the issue, and I deliberately "stung" him by criticizing him sharply, hoping that he would be able to identify with the more active and critical role I was playing, and so be provoked into playing a strong part in the family.

At the second interview, which was arranged 3 months after the first (note the interval), Roger had improved remarkably in behavior and was more cheerful, cooperative, and confident. The parents also reported that they were getting along better. The bed-wetting, however, was unchanged, and I considered this to be related to the fact that the parental control was still relatively weak and vacillating. I expressed this openly, pointing out how the parents (by appearing so helpless and apathetic) were trying to manipulate me into taking over their responsibility for solving the problem. I pointed out in a blunt, provocative way the resemblance between their behavior and Roger's, suggesting they were demanding that I should "wash out the sheets for them," as they felt obliged to wash his. The hope, again, was to stimulate them and strengthen their resolve by making them so angry with me (though within a sufficiently supportive context) that they would be determined not to give me further cause to provoke them.

At the third interview, 4 months later (7 months after the first), all the improvements in the boy and in the marital situation had continued, and also Roger's enuresis had ceased, except for an occasional wet bed. The whole family appeared happy and satisfied. Asked what had made the change, the mother said: "Your approach. You brought it out into the open so that we could talk about it, and you were firm with Roger. Other doctors spoke very quietly to Roger and made us feel that it was our fault and Roger that it wasn't his fault. In these family interviews there has been talk in which the whole problem has come into the open."

Note that she does not mention the fact that I not only was firm with Roger, but also placed both parents in the role of naughty children, and scolded them too. They had repressed this fact, and remembered only that I scolded the boy, but they seemed to have forgiven me, as I find people usually do when one inflicts pain deliberately in their interests.

In this case, there was adequate maternal affection and care (if anything, overindulgence), and the missing function to be supplied was related more to the traditional role of the father—to make the demand that the child give up his infantile demands and self-indulgence, and discipline his impulses in a way that would make him a more acceptable member of society. A certain measure of sternness, abrasiveness, and insistent demand for compliance is often required. Psychiatrists who have been trained in analytic techniques often find this very difficult, even repugnant, but the family practitioner who has not moved so far away from the authoritarian aspect of the medical role may well learn these skills more easily.

> CASE D: Alan, aged 12 at the time of his referral for complaints of abdominal pain and loose stools, was seen in the company of his clergyman father, his mother, and his elder sister, aged 14. Exploration of the problem and the family interaction around it revealed that the boy had considerable anxieties about falling short of the high standards he had set. The father said that he also developed abdominal pain and changes in bowel habits under stress, while the father's mother had recently undergone a colectomy for "ulcerative colitis."
>
> Though facts about the family were accumulated, neither my cotherapist nor I felt any real progress was being made toward an understanding of the problem. We seemed stuck with a static picture of two overconscientious and inhibited parents who were doing all they could to please the children and to avoid arguments, and were also trying to please us by being "good patients." In expressing this openly, we saw that the latter was the essential problem, and pointed out that though the family functioned in a loving and constructive way generally, they seemed overconscientious, and there did not seem to be much room for "fun." This comment was taken up vigorously by the children, who confirmed that this was exactly what was wrong. In particular, Alan obviously missed the company of his father, who tended to withdraw into his study, and gave so much time to his parishioners that there was little left for his family. These exchanges seemed to have considerable meaning for everyone, and they went away thoughtful.
>
> At the second interview a month later, considerable change had occurred. The

mother appeared very lively, with her eyes twinkling, and I was struck by a sexual attractiveness not noticed before. Even the father spoke with more lightness and humor, as if he might be beginning to enjoy himself. Both parents reported that the whole family was indeed having more "fun," and that the children had used the previous interview to insist that the family should go out together every Saturday, which everyone was enjoying.

The parents commented on the improvement in the boy's symptoms and general confidence, but he still looked glum and wistful. I commented on this facial expression, which puzzled me, and my social worker colleague, who was irritated by the father's lack of involvement, suggested that the boy must feel angry with him for his lack of emotional commitment and contact at home, as in the interview.

Supported by this, the children took a more active role, complaining that the parents never expressed their real feelings, but instead tried to consider everyone else to a point where there was so much self-sacrifice that the wrong decision was made for everybody, and all felt resentful. At this, the father said: "This is charity gone mad!" and all agreed they should speak their minds more directly.

Still puzzled by the boy's continuing wistful sadness, I asked whether he had been separated from his mother in babyhood, but it was then reported that the father had been away studying at a university for a whole year when the boy was five, and had seen the family for only a short time each week. The boy's expression now made sense to me, and I suggested that he had never forgiven his father for coming back, or his mother for transferring her affection back to the father. After thinking for a moment, the boy agreed, saying that for some strange reason he could remember the year he had with his mother alone in the clearest detail, and had felt a happy intimacy with her as they went about together. He could not remember his sister during this period, nor could he remember anything about, or after, his father's return.

At this point, the father said that the boy would have an opportunity to make up for this, as the mother and children were going off together for a holiday shortly, while he was obliged to stay at home to continue his work as a minister.

We pointed out sharply that this was quite the opposite of what was necessary. It might be more important for the parents to clarify their own marital and sexual relationship, so that Alan would have to face the issue of their attachment to each other, rather than to him. This would give Alan the opportunity to confront and overcome his jealousy. At this point, Alan said how difficult it was to be a vicar's son, and I suggested that, since clergymen were often thought by most people to be above ordinary human vices, including sex, it might be harder to imagine that the parents still had a loving physical relationship, and that he could thereby fantasize more easily that he had the closer tie to his mother. Alan said enthusiastically, "That really hits the nail on the head!"

Another appointment was arranged for a month later, but shortly before the month was up, the mother phoned to say that the improvements were by then so marked that the family all felt they no longer needed to come (they lived far away from the hospital). It was our impression that this was a consequence of genuine improvement rather than resistance, and it was left for the family to contact us if further problems occurred. Nothing further has been heard.

In this case, there had certainly been no deficiency in nurturance, since the mother had had a warm and enjoyable experience with this boy in his infancy, while the father was very much respected. Control, indeed, was too rigid and restrictive, rather than the reverse.

Though it is true that some of the family problem arose through the father's failure to involve himself actively enough in family affairs, the main problem seemed to have more to do with the parents' difficulty about feeling comfortable in their relationship as a sexual couple, so that the children had not been confronted with a clear situation in which to face and overcome problems of exclusion, jealousy, and sharing.

RELATING PRESENT PROBLEMS TO THE FAMILY HISTORY

A variety of family therapy techniques exists. Some focus on present interaction, and others on past history and previous generations. Time-consuming methods are obviously impracticable for the family practitioner, but they are fortunately not necessary in the majority of cases. Of those families referred to me, two-thirds or more either respond adequately (as judged by the happiness and satisfaction of the family members themselves) to the simple principles and methods presented, or can be seen as unmotivated or as best left alone for some other reason.

Nevertheless, it is usually illuminating, even with these simple methods, to have some idea of the family backgrounds. A brief inquiry into these backgrounds often relieves the parental guilt, since parents see that problems did not originate with them but were passed on through them from previous generations. Much can be learned in 10 minutes or so. One can say, "It would be helpful to see each of you against your family backgrounds, so that one can understand what kinds of experience, and hopes, and fears you brought with you into raising a family together. Could you tell—very briefly—what your fathers and mothers were like in their personalities—how you got on with them—your brothers and sisters—that sort of thing?"

Very often, the source of the presenting difficulties soon becomes apparent. The wife may have more difficulty with her sons than her daughters because she resented the fact that her brothers were favored and given better educational opportunities, while girls were not valued so highly. Or perhaps the husband's own father was away at the war in his early years, and he both lacked a satisfactory masculine model and also resented his father's return. Now he cannot be a satisfactory model for his sons, since he not only has never internalized this role, but also fears his own sons' jealousy if he plays it. Or the wife's father may have felt too great an emotional attachment to her as compared with his feelings for her mother, so that the wife reproduces this intense attachment with a son by spoiling him and arousing the jealousy of her husband, who then rejects the son and has an affair because he is angry with his wife, thus driving her and the son even closer.

Such information frequently makes everything more understandable to the doctor and to the family, though in other cases it may be no more than a routine inquiry that yields no additional help. Perhaps the simplest and most common way in which it proves of value is in demonstrating an "oscillation" of the child-rearing attitudes running through the generations. The children are un-manageable because the parents are overindulgent, because they are reacting against the fact that the grandparents were strict and punitive, because. . . . Parents can change their approach more readily once they see that their attitudes to child rearing are natural responses to, but overcompensations for, mistakes that were made with them.

Some cases, however, prove resistant unless one uses such a "three-genera-tional" approach in a more systematic way. No doubt these are among the cases the general practitioner will refer to an expert family therapist, after having reached an impasse with the simpler "two-generational" methods described. Nevertheless, the family practitioner needs to know something about these more difficult situations and techniques, just as he or she needs to have some awareness of physical conditions that require the attention of a specialist in order to know when to seek help. It will be easier to grasp some of the general principles in-volved from an example.

CASE E: John, aged 14, was referred by the family practitioner because of incessant conflict with parents and teachers, with a vicious circle whereby increasing stubborn-ness and laziness on the boy's part led to escalating pressure and recriminations from the adults. This in turn stimulated greater resistance and argument.

He was seen together with both his parents and his elder sister, June, aged 17. The eldest, Richard, aged 20, was studying at a distant university and was unable to attend.

A picture soon emerged of two likable and decent parents, if anything, overat-tached to the children and with too great an investment in their success, making up for the disappointments of their own early lives by trying to give to their children what they wished they had received themselves. To the parents, this felt like loving and car-ing, but to the children, both of whom shouted angrily at the parents to "get off their backs and leave them alone," it clearly felt like intrusion into their developing autonomy and interference with their own identities, since the parents were trying to live their lives for them.

They later realized that this long-standing conflict had reached a crisis point because John, the youngest, was about to "leave the nest," and the accusations of his childishness and irresponsibility were in part expressions of the parents' desire to keep him a child. Similarly, his provocative, immature behavior displayed his wish to re-main the idolized baby, despite his complaints of the parents' overconcern.

I was struck, also, not only by the way John's behavior kept his parents' atten-tion focused on him, but by the way his provocativeness intensified whenever I tried to get them talking to each other, especially when we discussed the marital relation-ship.

I pointed all this out at this and at a second, similar family session (all interviews were spaced a month apart), but met with much resistance from the parents, par-ticularly from the father. They could see that they were creating the problem and making it worse by all they did, but still wanted advice about how to make John work harder and behave better. In fact, John was improving, they admitted, but the pre-senting complaint about school work at the first session was replaced by concern at the second that he might be taking drugs, and at the third that he might be stealing.

As this simpler approach was blocked by the parents' resistance to looking at themselves, and particularly at their deprivation and the unfulfilled desires for nurturance that they projected onto the children (and then envied when they gratified them vicariously), the third and fourth sessions were held with the parents alone to study the family backgrounds and marital relationship in the absence of the children's disruptions.

The family histories were explored and summarized in a "genogram" (see Figure 27-2), a simple means of portraying a family tree. As this was drawn, the couple became thoughtful when they realized that the youngest siblings in their own families of origin were also a focus of overprotection by their own parents, and were dependent, demanding, and irresponsible—"just like John." Also, the mother's stepfather (the children's maternal step-grandfather), who was deeply loved by all, had died 3 months after John's birth. In addition, John's arrival, at a time when the father had returned to college following service in the army and when the mother then had three children to bring up with little financial or emotional support, had been a "last straw" in the most unhappy period of their marriage. She said, "Having two was bad enough, but three was awful. If his course had taken 5 years rather than 3, he would have found himself divorced with three children hanging on him. . . I'd have left!" Both agreed that the sexual relationship had been unsatisfactory at this period.

At the second marital session (fourth interview), following this exploration, the parents had begun to accept their own part in John's problems. Mother was aware that, though she had struggled to escape her own mother's clutches, she had been jealous of the attention her youngest sister managed to provoke and felt similarly envious toward John. The father was able for the first time to discuss his own weaknesses—such as lack of ambition, procrastination, day-dreaming—"many of the things John shows. . . I drove my own mother crazy with it!" Both began to look at their pain at losing their children as they were growing up, and the need to restructure their lives. Mother said she would like to take a job again, and I ended by prescribing "more pleasure, several times a day" for the couple, urging them to think more of themselves and less of the children.

At the final (fifth) interview, the whole family was seen together, including the eldest, Richard, who was on vacation from the university. The parents sat together on the sofa, looking happy and united as a couple, the mother no longer tense and anxious but relaxed and glowing, both gracefully resisting any effort by John to provoke and involve them. With the parents' permission, I showed the children the genogram, and told them of the painful circumstances and marital difficulties surrounding John's birth; to this they added the interesting fact, which was confirmed by the parents, that the youngest child of the previous generation (mother's youngest uncle) had been regarded as a problem by his mother (the maternal great-grandmother), and the same overprotective/regressive relationship had existed there too.

The session ended on a cheerful and optimistic note, with the father saying: "As far as problems go, things are a lot better. . . we all seem to be happier. . . the school problems have improved considerably." They felt they could now cope themselves, and no further appointments were made.

STRUCTURE; HIERARCHY

Like all groups, families need some decision-making procedure whereby conflict between members can be resolved, and activities can be coordinated for the

GENOGRAM

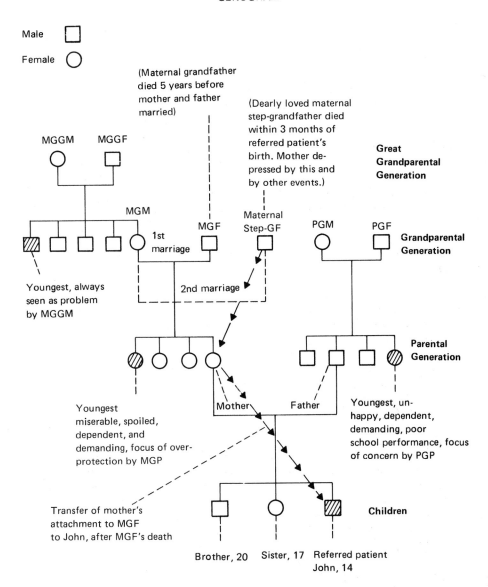

Figure 27-2

welfare of all. The Timberlawn Psychiatric Research Foundation's research confirmed objectively (see Chapter 4) the impression of most family therapists that a *firm parental coalition* is a vital factor in the functioning of healthy families.[4] Ideally, decisions are reached after negotiation in which the children's views are heard and carefully considered, but even a rigid yet definite structure is less harm-ful than a chaotic, overpermissive situation where no consistent control is pro-vided and self-control, therefore, cannot be learned. The main requirement is col-laboration and mutual support between mother and father in the management of the children, so that they form a strong "government" and are able to make un-popular decisions when these are necessary for the well-being of individuals or of the family as a whole and so that the children are not able to "divide and conquer."

Diagrams similar to that spontaneously drawn by Ann (Case A) are often used by family therapists to represent family alliances and hierarchies (see Fig. 27-3). The normal family shows the most important bond lying between the parental couple, with lesser bonds among other members (A). Some examples of potentially pathological patterns include a strong coalition between mother and son with father excluded (B); same-sex pairings between parents and children (C); and excessive preoccupation of the parents with each other, thus excluding the children (D).

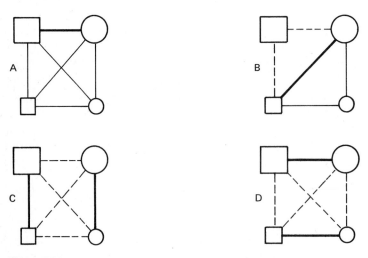

Figure 27-3

As the last diagram suggests, there is an appropriate measure of parental dominance and agreement. Seeing parents who disagree yet are able to resolve differences amicably for the welfare of the family is a far more valuable model for learning to cope with the outside world than a rigidly united parental relation-ship in public, with arguments behind closed doors.

The case histories already given illustrate many of the points clearly, as well as illustrating my impression that, in the course of a child's growth, at first the mother, then the father, and after that the parents as a couple need to take the central place in order for specific developmental issues to be faced. This impres-sion is not necessarily shared by all family therapists.

WHEN IS FAMILY THERAPY APPROPRIATE?

In my experience, this is one of the first questions general practitioners ask when one speaks about the family therapy method, and naturally they hope for a list of conditions or criteria that will enable them to come to a reasonably straightforward and clear-cut decision, as with decisions about other forms of medical treatment. Unfortunately, a satisfactory answer cannot be given in this form. To decide in advance whether family therapy (or indeed any other kind of psychotherapy) is likely to succeed and, if so, whether the problem needs a specialist's help or can be coped with by someone less expert, is unfortunately a judgment that requires the highest level of expertise. A fair level of competence as a psychotherapist may be attained within 5 years, in the sense of being able to carry out effective treatment with a wide variety of cases; it is the following 10 to 20 years that provide the more difficult knowledge of when to leave well enough alone—how to limit one's intervention to fit the patient's desires and strengths, rather than to fit one's own skills and life values. This leaves us with the impossible situation that only the specialist can safely decide who should not be referred to him!

We have, therefore, to find another approach to the problem, and one possible approach is that already used by the general practitioner for many of the physical ailments that come to his or her attention—that simple remedies be tried before more complicated and time-consuming ones, and that the specialist's help should be requested when one's own efforts have not brought about the hoped-for improvement. However, we need to consider the different uses of the family interview for diagnosis, for counseling or therapy, and for support.

Diagnosis

In child psychiatric or child guidance practice, I made it a routine many years ago to ask the whole family to attend the initial diagnostic interview, and have never encountered any contraindication to this practice. If a private discussion is indicated at some point, the joint interview can be interrupted and others can be asked to wait outside while one talks with the couple or with one or more individuals separately, and then later brings the whole family together for the final summing up and to thank them all for coming.

The family practitioner is, of course, in a different situation, since the first encounter with a problem will usually take the form of one member's coming to see him, and a family interview will be a special arrangement rather than a routine one. If the physician follows usual practice, many problems will respond to counseling of the individual alone. Even an obvious family disturbance may be no more than a temporary disequilibrium that is in response to some unusual stress (such as a bereavement, a child's leaving home for college, a promotion to a post of greater responsibility, and so on) for which adequate support systems already exist within the extended family or community, and which will right itself given a little time.

But where the existing psychological forces of healing and growth do not restore the balance, and repeated visits are made to the physician with the same or different complaints, or where a number of different members of the same family seem to be attending with unusual frequency, a diagnostic family interview is indicated and may save much time in the long run. This is best proposed along the lines already suggested, as a family conference where everyone, with the guidance of the physician, will put their heads together to try to see whether some stress or unresolved conflict might be causing disturbance or delaying improvement. By making it clear that this possibility is being eliminated as one might perform a routine blood test to make sure that certain diagnoses are eliminated safely, the family interview can be relaxed and unhurried, without any sense of pressure upon the physician to justify it by producing some dramatic conclusion at the end. If the joint interview is unproductive, that in itself is valuable information, like any other investigation that produces a negative result.

If the joint interview yields some positive result, either directly at the time or indirectly after an interval, which affords an opportunity for further interaction and working out of what has emerged in the home situation, then further joint interviews or family counseling is indicated.

Any problems of *relationship* that persist, as well as most *neurotic* symptoms and *habit* or *psychosomatic* disorders, are almost always treated more rapidly by further conjoint interviews. Where the problems appear to stem from a mother's difficulty in fulfilling her nurturing function, treatment of the mother and child may suffice. However, even here the father's ability to support the mother in this task may make all the difference and may relieve the physician of the need to perform this supportive role personally for more than a brief period. Indeed, one great advantage of family therapy is its focus on mobilizing the great supportive and therapeutic potential of the family itself.

In problems centering around control (for example, soiling, wetting, stuttering, behavior problems, tics, and other obsessional or compulsive phenomena), the presence of the father is particularly vital, and his failure to participate in discipline and in the setting of limits is most commonly the crucial issue. Problems of jealousy and sharing in the children usually have a counterpart in the parent's difficulty in sharing and cooperating with each other. This is demonstrated most readily in a joint family interview, even if its expression in the sexual relationship requires further interviews for the parents as a couple. Psychosomatic disorders also frequently yield more readily to joint family sessions; they so often express, or are triggered by, emotions that are denied and suppressed in the family system as a whole until the physician gives sanction and a sense of safety for them to be discussed openly. Irrational fears of the harmful effect of anger, jealousy, or sexual excitement are often prominent in such disorders.

Most problems that are amenable to other forms of psychotherapy are, in general, responsive to conjoint therapy as well, and the greater information provided by direct observation of the family and marital interaction, together with the therapeutic potential of the family itself, usually speeds the process.

Most therapists agree that the discussion of marital problems in general terms with children present is not only harmless, but is often reassuring to the latter, who are relieved to discover that their feelings of responsibility for their parents' unhappiness are unfounded, and that the doctor is going to help. The usual practice, however, is to exclude the children from discussion of the details of the parents' sexual relationship. This explicit exclusion of the children by the doctor is often beneficial in giving insecure parents sanction to "shut the bedroom door" and avoid excessive sacrifice of their personal and sexual relationship to the demands of child rearing.

Such marital therapy may be carried out by joint interviews, but if one of the partners is unwilling, some fruitful work with the more cooperative partner may be worthwhile nevertheless. Individual counseling may also be the only recourse, even when the main problem resides in the family as a whole, if the family cannot be assembled because of the death, geographical separation, or resistance of important members.

Also, in adolescence the developmental task of weakening family bonds indicates separate treatment; referring the teenager for therapy in a small "artificial" group is particularly effective and in accord with the course of normal development. However, a few family sessions may help to reveal and loosen pathological degrees of attachment.

Support

After the general practitioner and the specialists who have been brought in to help with a case have exhausted their resources in efforts to cure or substantially improve a disorder, the task of long-term comfort and amelioration of suffering will often remain with the former. This is as true for psychological problems as for physical disease and dysfunction. Less complex psychological problems can be helped by the general practitioner; those of moderate severity are often responsive to the psychotherapist (whether the approach is individual or conjoint); but the most severe types of disturbance may remain intractable to all approaches, and will need indefinite periodic support together with more active treatments, such as medication and admission to the hospital, at times of crisis and decompensation.

In such cases, the conjoint family approach greatly facilitates supportive work, enabling it to be carried out both more effectively and with less expenditure of time. Through the physician's support for the whole family, the family members learn to support one another. The memory of the last visit to the doctor and of the emotional warmth and reassurance received can be kept alive by the family group as a whole far longer than by any one individual. When one member is in temporary despair, others will remember and repeat the encouragement and reassurance they all heard together. Because of this, effective support can be provided, even through very widely spaced interviews. With many of the deprived, inadequate, multiproblem families, adequate support can be provided by interviews every 3 months or more, though even monthly visits would have been inadequate for the individuals seen alone. The family visits would be looked forward to eagerly and recollected as happy; small improvements would be recounted with pride, and advice and praise would be absorbed attentively.

Similar considerations regarding frequency of interviews also apply, however, to counseling. Whereas, in individual work, interviews once a week are generally regarded as the minimum frequency if substantial progress is to be made (and even this, of course, is very little compared with most analyses), family sessions are, in my experience, more effective when the interval between them is longer. When I tried to find the optimum frequency 14 years ago, most families said that 3 weeks seemed about right; if they came sooner they had not finished working out the implications of the previous session and putting these implications into practice, while a longer interval led them to forget and to lose the impetus. In practice, I have found an interval of a month usually equally satisfactory and more convenient administratively. This possibility, that less frequent intervention is not only as effective but is in fact *more* effective, has been curiously overlooked by most family therapists, though Bowen has recently reported a similar finding.[5] It is obviously of even greater importance to the pressured general practitioner than to the psychiatrist.

Though conducting sessions every 3 weeks or monthly is suitable in most cases, it should be emphasized that more frequent interviews are necessary in times of crisis, or when depression is a prominent feature. The same is true when feelings of depression and loss are not apparent at first but are likely to be uncovered through the family discussions. Such families can often be recognized by histories of loss and deprivation (for example, the death of grandparents during the early life of the parents) and by a clinging, "babes-in-the-wood" quality about the family relationships.

Unlike most conventional forms of psychotherapy, one striking advantage of family therapy is its effectiveness across a wide range of socioeconomic, educational, and intelligence levels. In my experience, it works as well with the deprived and disadvantaged as with the middle-class. However, a more directive, active, managing approach is often more effective with the former, when the parents have lacked the necessary learning experiences in their families of origin to enable them to be adequate parents themselves. The physician must, therefore, provide some of these experiences through personal example, encouragement, and advice. Minuchin and his colleagues have made a special study of disadvantaged families, and have described special techniques suited to their difficulties and limitations.[6] With intelligent, better-educated, less disturbed families, it is often more productive to help them to understand the cause of the problem, but to leave it to them to work out their own solution, as in conventional analytic work.

Results, Research

Gurman and Kniskern have recently reviewed over 200 outcome studies of conjoint family and marital work, and those interested in scientific appraisal of the effectiveness of this type of approach should begin with their excellent overview. Two of their conclusions are pertinent:

Family therapy appears to be at least as effective and possibly more effective than individual therapy for a wide variety of problems, both apparent 'individual' difficulties as well as more obvious family conflicts. . . . For certain clinical goals and problems, e.g. decreasing hospitalization rates for some chronic and acute inpatients, treating anorexia, many childhood behavior problems, juvenile delinquency, and sexual dysfunction, systems therapies offer the treatments of choice.[7]

A clinical study of the outcome of referrals to the psychiatric department of a children's hospital throughout 1 year, after the referrals had been treated by the family techniques described here, reported that about one-fifth improved satisfactorily after one interview, about one-third within two interviews, and almost one-half within five. One-third were clearly demonstrated, within one or two interviews, to be either unwilling to make the changes and effort required for improvement to be possible, or to contain fragile, "borderline" individuals who needed support rather than exploratory psychotherapy.[8] The accuracy of this rapid screening-out, and the time it saved, can be judged from the fact that almost all of the two-thirds who remained were helped adequately either by the family interviews or by other methods that were based on the diagnostic information provided.

Ideally, some form of training, either through an ongoing seminar or through a few days' full-time experience, whereby expert therapists can be witnessed via videotape or through one-way screens, and where the "feel" of family interviewing can be obtained through participating as a family member or as a therapist in role-plays of simulated families, is desirable. But general practitioners who lack such opportunities can safely, and with benefit, begin looking more closely at the family systems of their patients.

REFERENCES

1   Bowen, M.: "The Use of Family Therapy in Clinical Practice," *Comp. Psychiat.*, 7:354, 1966.
2   Hatfield, F. E. S.: *Understanding the Family and Its Illnesses,* unpublished.
3   Kellner, R.: *Family Ill Health,* London: Tavistock, 1963.
4   Lewis, J. M. et al.: *No Single Thread: Psychological Health in Family Systems,* New York: Brunner/Mazel, 1976.
5   Bowen, M.: "Principles and Techniques of Multiple Family Therapy," in J. O. Brandt and O. J. Moynihan (eds.), *Systems Therapy—Selected Papers; Theory, Technique and Research,* Washington: Groome Child Guidance Center, 1971.
6   Minuchin, S. et al.: *Families of the Slums,* New York: Basic Books, 1967.
7   Gurman, A.S., and D. P. Kniskern: "Research on Family and Marital Therapy," in S. L. Garfield and A. E. Bergin (eds.), *Handbook of Psychotherapy and Behavior Change: An Empirical Analysis,* 2d ed., New York: Wiley, 1978.
8   Skynner, A. C. R.: *Systems of Family and Marital Psychotherapy,* New York: Brunner/Mazel, 1976. (British edition entitled *One Flesh, Separate Persons; Principles of Family and Marital Psychotherapy,* London: Constable, 1976.)

BIBLIOGRAPHY

General textbooks are limited in number, but one by the present author, which is referred to in reference 8, attempts to give an outline for the field, and includes clinical examples. A highly recommended textbook is:

Glick, I. D., and D. R. Kessler: *Marital and Family Therapy,* New York and London: Grune and Stratton, 1974.

These are well complemented by another introductory text, which includes descriptions of such "action" techniques as "family sculpting."

Bloch, D. A. (ed.): *Techniques of Family Therapy: A Primer,* New York: Grune and Stratton, 1973.

An excellent paper that summarizes the differences among the different schools of family therapy, by authors who have actually witnessed the practice of different experts as well as reading their accounts, is:

Beels, C. C., and A. Ferber: "Family Therapy: A View," *Family Process,* 9:280, 1969.

The following includes transcripts of actual interviews by different experts; the interviews are of various styles:

Haley, J., and L. Hoffman: *Techniques of Family Therapy,* New York: Basic Books, 1967.

Among more specialized approaches to family therapy, the following describes a technique that is particularly suited to the less educated and disadvantaged:

Minuchin, S.: *Families and Family Therapy,* Cambridge, Mass.: Harvard Univ. Press, 1974.

And for a description of more intensive, long-term work with severely disturbed psychotic families, the following is an excellent guide for those who may become involved in more complex situations:

Boszormenyi-Nagy, Ivan, and James L. Framo (eds.): *Intensive Family Therapy,* New York and London: Harper and Row, 1965.

Chapter 28

The Physician and the Treatment of Sexual Dysfunctions

Helen Singer Kaplan, M.D.
Michael A. Perelman, Ph.D.

EDITORS' INTRODUCTION

What is it like for a woman to be unable to reach a climax, or even to enjoy sexual intercourse? How does it feel to have a heritage of guilt about sexual self-play, and then be told by one's physician that masturbation to orgasm may be a step in achieving sexual gratification with one's spouse? Then, too, how must it feel to be able to masturbate to orgasm, but be unable to have an orgasm through intercourse? What is it like to marshal one's courage to talk about a sexual problem to one's physician, only to find that the physician then becomes obviously uncomfortable? How must it be to undergo repeated pelvic examinations and endocrine studies that are searching for a "cause"? All these experiences have to affect self-esteem, the capacity for overall relationships, feelings about the future, and outlook on life in general.

What is it like for a man to be impotent or to have premature ejaculations? What emotional sacrifices are involved in discussing such symptoms with one's personal physician or with a specialist, a stranger? What does it do to a marriage when a man finds that symptoms of dysfunction are absent during a casual sexual encounter with another woman? How do the sexual failures affect the marital relationship, a person's self-esteem, joy in living, productivity at work? How embarrassed are men about the secret of their sexual impotency, knowing their talk of potency is fraudulent?

How do physicians deal with their own sexual difficulties? Do they avoid professional help, or develop rationalizations about why they have no sexual desire? How does the presence of such personal difficulties influence the physician's attitude toward patients who have similar symptoms? Could envy or vicarious curiosity enter into the attitude? Does treatment of patients with common sexual problems have to be influenced by the physician's personal sexual problems? Then, too, if the physician is aroused sexually by the patient and by his or her account of sexual problems or activities, how will that influence the doctor-patient relationship?

The evaluation and treatment of patients with common sexual problems presents the physician with a remarkable opportunity to be of help to patients in ways that may influence the subsequent quality of patients' lives profoundly. Newer concepts in the sexual therapies offer the physician valuable pragmatic approaches. As with other helpful treatment agents, however, there is also the possibility of a damaging outcome. In this chapter, two outstanding experts in the field of sexual dysfunction present a concise overview of the field. They emphasize the interrelationship of biologic and psychologic factors in the etiology of sexual dysfunction, and suggest to the physician both a conceptual approach and the specific techniques that may be helpful.

The last quarter-century has brought remarkable advances in our knowledge of human sexuality. These data are in the process of being assimilated into the main body of medicine; the increased understanding is being translated into innovative new approaches to the treatment of sexual difficulties. These developments promise relief to many people with distressing sexual problems, people who were previously thought to be beyond help.

In the past, sexual dysfunctions were regarded as manifestations of serious psychopathology, and were considered with therapeutic pessimism. Evidence now suggests that sexual problems, while they may be manifestations of profound emotional disturbances, mental illness, or serious marital problems, are not invariably so. They also occur commonly in people who function well in other areas, have no other psychological symptoms, and enjoy good marital relationships. In many cases, the sexual dysfunctions have their roots in more immediate problems, which were ignored until recently, such as the anticipation of failure to function, real or imagined demands for performance, and fear of rejection and humiliation by the partner.

Many patients who suffer from sexual problems respond rapidly and favorably to treatment methods that are designed to modify immediate obstacles to sexual functioning. In fact, it appears that for many patients the new sex therapy is far more effective than the traditional psychiatric approaches.

Apart from this difference in the focus of intervention, sex therapy differs from traditional forms of treatment in two respects: first, the objectives of sex therapy are essentially limited to relief of the patient's sexual dysfunction; second, sex therapy is distinguished by its use of specially structured sexual and communicative experiences as an integral part of treatment.

The objectives of the two traditional forms of treatment for sexual disorders, psychotherapy and marital therapy, are comprehensive. Psychoanalytic treatment attempts to reconstruct the patient's personality by fostering resolution of unconscious conflicts. Similarly, marital therapy tries to improve the quality of the couple's total relationship by helping them to resolve previously unrecognized destructive transactions. Within the context of psychotherapy or marital therapy, sexual symptoms are seen as reflections of underlying conflicts and problems, and their relief is viewed as a product of the resolution of these more basic issues.

On the other hand, the aim of sex therapy is much more limited, and is concerned primarily with improving sexual functioning. Nevertheless, in the course of sex therapy, intrapsychic and transactional conflicts are almost invariably dealt with to some extent. However, therapeutic maneuvers are mainly at the service of the primary objective of sex therapy: the relief of the sexual symptom. Sex therapy relies heavily for its therapeutic impact on erotic tasks that the couple conduct at home. The main innovation and distinctive feature of sex therapy is the integrated use of systematically structured sexual experiences with conjoint therapeutic sessions.

Sex therapy in one form or another is being employed by a rapidly increasing number of clinicians. The explosive popularity has resulted in new methodological techniques and claims of effectiveness. This chapter, however, will reflect a view of sex therapy as a specialized branch of psychotherapy. The sexual dysfunctions may be conceptualized as psychosomatic symptoms.[1] Our orientation is multicausal and eclectic, based on the concepts that sexual dysfunctions are the product of multiple etiologic factors, and that the treatment armamentarium should comprise an amalgam of experiential, behavioral, and dynamically oriented modalities. The specific approach to sex therapy described in this chapter is being employed, developed further, and more importantly, evaluated systematically.

BACKGROUND

Until recently, the clinician attempting to treat sexual disorders was at a serious disadvantage in not having reliable basic data. Sexual behavior had never been studied directly and systematically in the laboratory, and accurate, basic data were virtually nonexistent. In contrast to the extensive available information regarding other bodily functions, sexuality was terra incognita. Therapists in this field had to work empirically, and essentially in the dark.

The assumptions about sexuality that formed the basis of treatment of sexual disorders in the past were often incomplete and inaccurate. Conclusions based on such inadequate data were confused further because they were interpreted within the framework of the highly emotionally charged and biased sexual attitudes of our time. Not surprisingly, many of the traditional beliefs that guided sexual treatment until recently have proved to be false and even misleading in the light of recent studies. A prime example of the confusing influence of such inaccurate concepts was the long-cherished proposition that "vaginal" orgasms express normal and healthy female functioning, while a preference for clitoral stimulation reflects a deep-seated neurosis. Until Masters and Johnson demonstrated in the laboratory that there is essentially only one kind of female orgasm (which, incidentally, always has both vaginal and clitoral components), the dual orgasm belief was universally accepted in psychiatry.[2] This misconception impaired effective treatment of female sexual inadequacy. In addition, it led to unnecessary feelings of frustration and shame for many women and couples, and usually to interminable and disappointing psychoanalyses which, not surprisingly, never succeeded in the mythical goal of eradicating clitoral eroticism.

Despite tremendous recent advances, sexuality still remains a mystery in many respects. Basic data, especially in the area of female sexuality, are incomplete; the physiologic determinants of the sexual disorders have not yet been identified fully, and critical questions regarding clinical management remain to be answered.

However, significant progress has been made in recent years. The first major contribution was that of Kinsey and his group, who openly gathered data on human sexuality.[3] Basic knowledge about the biologic determinants of sexuality was advanced by MacLean (among others), who investigated the relationship between brain functions and sexuality and pleasure.[4] Money and Ehrhardt contributed new insights into the hitherto unsuspected but powerful effects of prenatal androgen on later adult sexual behavior.[5] The studies of Harlow and his group yielded data on the role of early experiential peer and mothering variables in primate sexual behavior.[6] Money not only studied the complexities of gender identity, but also produced a conceptual integration of the interaction between experiential and organic, that is, hormonal, determinants of sexuality.[7]

Perhaps the greatest contribution to the long-overdue termination of the "dark ages" in human sexuality came from the pioneering studies of Masters and Johnson.[2] Their monumental efforts have finally made basic data on the long-neglected physiology of the human sexual response available to the clinician. For two decades, Masters and Johnson studied the sexual behavior of men and women during approximately 14,000 sexual acts. Their observations included a wide spectrum of sexual behavior under every imaginable condition. They studied coitus in many positions, between strangers, between happily married couples, and between couples who had had various sexual and interpersonal difficulties. Different techniques of erotic stimulation, including self-stimulation, were explored. The sexual behavior of men and women with a wide range of ages was studied. Sex was observed during menstruation. Sexual responses of men who were circumcised were compared with those of men who were not circumcised. The effects of various contraceptive devices on sexual behavior were studied. In addition, sexual responses were investigated in the presence of various pathological conditions, including the artificial vagina. These studies finally yielded an accurate picture of the basic psychophysiology of human reproductive functioning.

This information has had a tremendous impact on the field, by opening up the possibility for the development of rational and effective treatment of sexual disorders. The recently accumulated data on the physiology, neurology, and endocrinology of male and female sexual responses that are basic to the understanding of human sexuality provide the conceptual foundations for the rational practice of sex therapy.

The Triphasic Concept of Sexuality and Sexual Dysfunctions

The human sexual response is a highly rational and orderly sequence of physiological events, the object of which is to prepare the bodies of two mates for reproductive union. There is evidence to suggest that the sexual response is comprised of three discrete but interrelated phases, and that sexual dysfunctions can be conceptualized as disruptions of one or more of these. Both clinical and physiologic evidence suggests that the sexual response of both genders does not actually comprise a single entity, but may be divided into three components: desire, excitement, and orgasm. Desire is an appetite that has its locus in specific centers and circuits in the limbic brain. Excitement and orgasm involve autonomic reflexes in the genital organs. Excitement is an autonomically mediated genital vasocongestive reaction, which produces penile erection in the male and vaginal lubrication and swelling in the female. Reflex clonic muscular contractions of certain genital muscles produce orgasm in both genders. Each of the three responses is governed by a separate neurophysiologic apparatus, and therefore is subject to separate impairment by emotional inhibitants. These specific inhibitory patterns produce the various sexual dysfunction syndromes.

In addition to *hypoactive sexual desire,* which can occur in either gender, there are six sexual dysfunctions; three of them are male and three are female. The planned American Psychiatric Association Diagnostic and Statistical Manual III defines inhibited sexual desire as "Persistent inhibition of desire for engaging in a particular form of sexual activity. The basis for the judgment of inhibition is made by the clinician taking into account age, sex, occupation, and the context of the patient's life."[8] This diagnosis is often used in conjunction with other dysfunctional categories, but may occur in individuals who can respond with excitement and orgasm when stimulated physically.

Inhibition of the excitement phase is manifested by incomplete genital vasocongestion, which in the male results in partial or total failure to attain or maintain an erection (*impotence*). In the female, there is an inability to maintain or attain the characteristic lubrication-swelling of the genitalia (*frigidity* or general unresponsiveness). Impotence can occur in males who ejaculate and experience full sexual desire.

Impairment of the orgastic component of the sexual response may result in either *premature ejaculation* or *retarded ejaculation* in the male, and orgastic dysfunction in the female. The premature ejaculator fails to acquire adequate voluntary control over his orgastic reflex, which results in rapid climax. In contrast, the patient with retarded ejaculation suffers from involuntary overcontrol. There is an absence or delay of emission and/or ejaculation, even though he receives adequate stimulation. In some few cases, inhibition is confined to the ejaculatory phase only, while emission remains intact. This disorder, *partial retarded ejaculation,* is characterized by a seepage of semen during climax, which presumably is produced by the emission response. The patient does not experience perineal muscle contractions, nor does he feel the orgastic pleasure or satisfaction.[1]

The term *orgastic dysfunction* is used here to designate a specific inhibition of the orgastic component of the sexual response. This may occur in the presence of adequate erotic desire and excitement. The woman suffers from primary orgastic dysfunction if she has never experienced an orgasm; if, on the other hand, the disorder developed after a period of being able to reach orgasm, it is considered a secondary orgastic dysfunction. The orgastic dysfunction may be absolute or situational. If it is absolute, the patient is unable to achieve either a coital or clitorally induced orgasm under any circumstances; if she suffers from situational orgastic dysfunction, she can reach a climax, but only under specific circumstances.

The final disorder is a uniquely female complaint that has no analog in the male. *Vaginismus* is due to an involuntary spasm of the muscles surrounding the vaginal entrance, specifically of the sphincter vaginae and levator ani muscles, which occurs whenever an attempt is made to introduce an object into the vaginal orifice. Anatomically, the genitalia of vaginismic women are normal. However, whenever penetration is attempted, the vaginal introitus literally snaps shut, so tightly that intercourse is impossible, and even vaginal examinations frequently must be conducted under anesthesia. In addition to the primary spasm of the vaginal inlet, patients with vaginismus are also usually phobic of coitus and vaginal penetration. This phobic avoidance makes attempts at coitus frustrating and painful. Vaginismus may be associated with disturbances of any of the sexual phases, but it is not necessarily so. Many women who seek treatment for vaginismus have a normal desire for sex, and are sexually responsive and orgastic.

ETIOLOGY

The delicate and complex sexual responses of men and women depend upon the integrity of multiple determinants. The first requirement for a successful sexual response, is, of course, that the sexual organs be physically sound. Therefore, organic factors should always be evaluated when a patient presents sexual complaints. However, given physical health, the sexual responses are highly vulnerable to the effects of emotional stress, and are subject to disruption by adverse conditioning.

Anxiety about sexual performance and specific learned inhibitions of the sexual response are usually the immediate and specific causes of the sexual dysfunctions, but sexual problems may also have a deeper structure. The superficial causes or immediate anxieties that operate at the moment of lovemaking are the common, final pathways by which a complex of multiple, deeper, or more remote causes may do their damage. The concept of immediate and remote causes is not unique to sex therapy, but is a central principle in psychosomatic medicine, and has important implications for treatment.

A Psychosomatic Concept of Sexual Dysfunction

Successful sexual intercourse depends upon a complex sequence of hormonal and physiologic events that are highly vulnerable to the effects of both acute and chronic emotional arousal. Acute fear or anger is accompanied by profound physiological reactions that can interfere directly with the autonomically mediated vascular reflexes that produce erection in the male and lubrication-swelling in the female. Such emotions may also inhibit the higher centers that mediate sexual appetite. Also, the sexual responses of both genders depend upon a proper hormonal balance and, especially, upon an adequate supply of androgen. Chronic stress, depression, defeat, or conflict can produce significant endocrine changes, which may entail a depression of circulating androgen via the hypothalamic-pituitary axis. It is not surprising, therefore, that such long-standing, adverse emotional states may be accompanied by various psychosomatic disorders, including sexual difficulties.

In addition, the sexual responses are readily conditionable. The orgastic reflexes, in particular, are highly subject to learned inhibition if sexual arousal is associated with negative feelings of fear, guilt, or threat of injury of any kind. Thus the negative contingencies, both subjective and objective, which are likely to follow erotic impulses and expressions in our culture are often damaging to the sexual response.

The acute and chronic emotional problems that may impair the sexual response and the negative contingencies that can produce inhibition of orgasm do not seem to be specific. Any problem that upsets a man sufficiently to disrupt his visceral genital responses physically, or to depress that individual's testosterone level, can cause a sexual dysfunction. In this manner, a stressful sexual ambience, anticipation of failure, the destructive and critical demands from a hostile wife, or more subtle forces that are seldom recognized consciously (such as the anxiety mobilized by the wife's resemblance to his "taboo" mother, guilt about sexual pleasure that echoes from early religious injunctions, and threats to a fragile self-esteem should "performance" fall below some inappropriate standard) can all "cause" a man's erective response to fail. These deeper causes are often related directly to sex. It is equally true, however, that forms of anxiety and depression that are not even remotely related to sexuality may also, by upsetting the patient, result in erectile failure. A man whose job is in jeopardy and a woman who feels trapped and exploited may simply not be able to summon the abandonment that is necessary for sexual functioning.

Seen in this light, sexual symptoms are not defenses against anxiety in the same sense that hysterical symptoms are. Like all psychophysiologic symptoms, they appear where psychic defenses *fail* to protect the individual from being flooded with emotion. The actual symptom is a manifestation of the damaging physiologic concomitants of painful emotion, which interferes with the delicate sexual reflexes.[1]

The origin and nature of the vulnerability of the sexual apparatus to stress in people who develop sexual dysfunctions are not presently understood. It may be speculated, however, that some sexual dysfunctions are analogous to such functional psychophysiologic conditions as spastic colon, constipation, tension headache, and essential hypertension—disorders that are characterized by individual tendencies, observed from early childhood on, to respond to any kind of stress with specific hyperactivity of the vulnerable organ systems. As will be elaborated in the section on treatment, the essential strategy of sexual therapy consists of obtaining symptom relief by modifying the immediately operating sources of sexual stress, by altering the "here and now" negative contingencies that impair the couple's sexual responses. Relief of sexual symptoms, like relief of psychosomatic symptoms in general, can often be accomplished by limiting therapeutic intervention to the removal of specific obstacles, that is, the specific sources of anxiety.

However, deeper and more remote causes, such as unconscious conflict or marital disharmony, may frequently underlie the stressful transactions that have caused the specific sexual problem and continue to evoke anxiety when the patient tries to make love. If the clinician who treats sexual difficulties is to transcend the role of a technician who dispenses remedies in a mechanical fashion, is not to be limited to removal of immediate stress, and is to go beyond "sensate focus" and "squeeze," then the clinician must understand the structure of the dysfunctions on all levels. In addition to understanding and developing technical skills to modify the immediate causes of sexual dysfunctions, the clinician must also gain insight into the dynamics of the many deeper causes from which sexual difficulties may spring, and develop the therapeutic skills to modify the deeper roots of the difficulty if necessary.

BIOLOGICAL DETERMINANTS OF SEXUAL DYSFUNCTIONS

The successful act of intercourse ultimately rests on the physical integrity of the sexual organs and of their supporting vascular, neurological, and endocrine systems. Many physical illnesses and drugs may cause impotence or lowered sexual interest. Moreover, sexual dysfunctions that result from medical disorders may be indistinguishable clinically from purely psychogenic problems. Although by far the most prevalent causes of sexual dysfunctions are psychological, physical factors must always be ruled out before sexual therapy is commenced.

Estimates regarding the number of sexually dysfunctional patients who demonstrate some organic component range from 3 to 20 percent. In our experience, about 15 percent of the patients seeking relief from sexual dysfunctions were found to have early diabetes, use narcotics, abuse alcohol, or suffer from previously undiscovered local pathology of the genital organs, neurological disease, and other physical contributory causes. Obviously, the clinician must remain alert to those physical factors that may play a role in the sexual complaints of many patients.

Diagnosing Organic Pathology

A clearly situational pattern of dysfunction establishes physical integrity of the sexual organs and indicates that the etiology of the disorder is most probably psychogenic. If, for example, a man has nocturnal emissions and morning erections that are clearly undiminished in frequency, firmness, and duration from his previous level, the chances are that the impotence he experiences when he tries to have intercourse with his wife has psychological roots. Even under such circumstances, however, one must be careful not to place excessive reliance on a situational pattern to establish pure psychogenicity because some organic conditions fluctuate in their effect. Thus, the man's impotence may result from the ingestion of certain short-acting drugs or medications.

Illness and such psychophysiologic states as drug ingestion, depression, and fatigue all may affect sexual functioning adversely. However, organic factors do not affect men and women in the same way, nor do they have identical effects on the different components of the sexual response. Libido, erection, and ejaculation in males; and desire, lubrication-swelling, and orgasm in females differ in their vulnerability to various physical agents and conditions, and the various dysfunctions have different differential diagnoses. Therefore, patients suffering from the different dysfunctions require specific types of medical evaluations, while in certain clinical situations organicity can be ruled out fairly safely on the basis of the interview and history alone.

Interactions Between Organic and Psychic Factors

The interaction between physical disorders and sexual behavior is complex, and depends upon the physical effects of the illness or drug as well as upon the psychological characteristics of the "host." The same physical impairment can have vastly different effects on different individuals, depending upon their prior sexual histories, their relationships with their partners, and their ego integration. In general, if a man has had an active and successful sex life prior to illness, a secure and open and loving relationship with his wife, and sufficient psychic strengths to deal constructively with frustration, his incapacity will be limited strictly to that imposed by his illness. In patients who are vulnerable in various ways, however, the disability and disruption may proliferate.

Few organic disorders destroy the sexual response completely. More commonly, sexual functioning is impaired only partially by diabetes, neurological disease, antihypertensive medication, or advanced age. However, the patient's alarmed or discouraged response to partial impairment and/or the partner's partial impairment may then produce complete dysfunction by virtue of these emotional reactions. This is similar to the sequence of events that may follow a transient episode of psychogenic impotence that escalates into a chronic problem because it leads the patient to anticipate failure in subsequent attempts at lovemaking.

While sex therapy obviously cannot alter the underlying illness, it is highly effective in dispelling reactive performance anxiety. Therefore, when a man's impotence is due to a combination of physical and psychic factors, that is, when he has a partial impairment of erectile capacity that has been exacerbated by his fear and distress about the problem, he is amenable to sexual therapy. For this reason, a medical diagnosis of a disease that impairs the sexual response, such as diabetes, does not rule out sexual therapy for the patient, unless it is established that the physical incapacity is complete. Many of the couples in which one spouse is partially handicapped can be helped to function adequately sexually. Thus, for example, when the male is impotent on the basis of diabetes but has a desire and orgastic phases that are intact, the couple can often learn to enjoy sexual experiences that do not include penetration. It is the aim of the therapist to help sexually disabled persons realize their maximum capacity.

THE EFFECT OF ILLNESS AND DRUGS ON SEXUALITY

Depression, stress, and fatigue can damage sexuality profoundly, and masked depression and anxiety states are frequently involved in the etiology of sexual dysfunctions. Physical illness may affect sexual functioning adversely. When a person feels ill and debilitated or is in pain, he or she is not usually interested in pursuing erotic matters. Some diseases depress libido, while others have damaging effects by virtue of pathogenic mechanisms that specifically injure the sex organs or their nervous or vascular supply. A disease may have endocrine effects on the sex centers of the brain, or the process of the disease may diminish androgen or damage the genital organs directly. Any physical disorder, surgical procedure, or medication prescribed for a medical illness that reduces the effective androgen level may be expected to depress libido in both genders and to impair the erectile responses of males. Endocrine diseases that affect either pituitary or gonadal functioning, or both, may thus produce sexual problems. Finally, any condition that either causes pain during intercourse or interferes with intromission or stimulation may affect the sexual response adversely.

In 1974, Kaplan presented a detailed analysis of all the medical and surgical disorders that may cause or contribute to the sexual dysfunction.[1] Drugs may affect various aspects of sexual behavior. Some alter libido or the intensity of sexual interest and pleasure, while other substances affect only the physiological response of the genitals.

There are several different mechanisms by which drugs can influence sexuality. Essentially, this involves a chemical alteration of the nerves that regulate the sexual response. Some drugs act primarily on the brain and, presumably by altering the functioning of the sex centers, can enhance or diminish libido. Narcotics appear to inhibit sexuality in this manner. Other types of medication influence the peripheral nerves that regulate the functioning of the sex organs. Certain types of antihypertensive medication act in this manner, while still another mechanism of action for these drugs involves altering the response of the genital blood vessels. In 1974, Kaplan summarized the effects of drugs on sexual functioning.[1]

PSYCHOLOGICAL DETERMINANTS OF SEXUAL DYSFUNCTION

It is generally agreed that the great majority of sexual difficulties are created by psychological factors. There is, however, no agreement regarding the nature of these factors, and considerable controversy and confusion exist in the field because many different and even contradictory "specific" psychological causes have been advanced by various authorities.

Anxiety is the predominant emotion that impairs sexual functioning. Anxiety can disrupt the excitement and orgasm reflexes, and may also inhibit sexual desire. Sexually disruptive anxiety does not seem to originate from one specific base; rather it appears to originate in a wide spectrum of causes, both immediate and remote. These two sets of causes operate on different levels, but they are not incompatible and do not comprise a true dichotomy. In fact, they exist in dynamic equilibrium with each other. In the past, traditional psychiatry has concerned itself with the understanding and resolution of the remote causes, while essentially ignoring the immediate obstacles. In contrast, the new therapeutic approaches attempt mainly to modify the immediate antecedents of the sexual dysfunctions, and tend to ignore the more remote causes. Yet both seem important, and concomitant intervention on the two levels seems the most rational approach, one which promises to be effective with a wide variety of patients.

The immediate causes of sexual dysfunctions operate in the "here and now" to ruin the sexual response at the moment in which the individual is engaging in sexual behavior. In a general sense, we see the immediate causes of sexual dysfunctions as arising from an antierotic environment that the couple has created, which is destructive to the sexuality of one or both. An ambience of openness and trust and a pattern of genuine communication allow the partners to abandon themselves fully to the erotic experience.

Apart from these generalities, the specific sources of anxiety, defenses against sexual abandonment, and obstacles to full sexual enjoyment that emerge repeatedly in the course of sex therapy include:

1 The couple's avoidance of, or at any rate their failure to engage in, sexual behavior that is exciting and stimulating to both. This can result from mere ignorance and misinformation, but in more difficult cases it is a product of unconscious fear and guilt about sexuality.

2 Fear of failure, which is often exacerbated by pressure to perform (performance anxiety), is an extremely common source of anxiety, which impairs the sexual response of many men and women. Overconcern about pleasing one's partner, which is rooted in a fear of rejection, is a related and also highly prevalent source of anxiety.

3 The tendency to erect perceptual and intellectual defenses against erotic pleasure. People who are anxious about sexuality may keep control by presiding as judge over their lovemaking. Masters and Johnson have labeled this destructive tendency "spectatoring."[9]

4 Failure of the couple to communicate openly and without guilt and defensiveness about their genuine feelings, wishes, and responses.

5 Anger of the spouses with one another, which is commonly not perceived clearly.

These immediate sources of anxiety and specific defense mechanisms against sexual feelings all may result in the inability to abandon oneself fully to the erotic experience, and in this way may produce sexual dysfunctions.

The more remote etiologic factors that are cited most often as forming the underlying substrate of sexual difficulties are unconscious intrapsychic conflicts deriving from early family experiences, marital disharmony, and the sexually restrictive attitudes of our society. These factors have emerged from the conceptual frameworks of psychoanalysis, systems theory, and learning theory.

Unfortunately, at this time there is no single satisfactory theory for the etiology of the psychopathology of the sexual dysfunctions. Numerous formulations have been proposed, each having real merit, yet none explains etiology comprehensively, in a unified conceptual framework.[1]

SEX THERAPY

Sex therapy differs from other forms of treatment for sexual dysfunctions in two respects: first, its goals are essentially limited to the relief of the patient's sexual symptom, and second, it departs from traditional techniques by employing a combination of prescribed sexual experiences and psychotherapy.

Limited Goals

Sex therapists differ somewhat in how they define their therapeutic goals. All focus on improving sexual functioning; however, some espouse somewhat broader objectives, and therefore include improvement of the couple's communication and general relationship in the therapeutic endpoint. However, the primary objective of all sex therapy is to relieve the patient's sexual dysfunction. All therapeutic interventions, the tasks, psychotherapy, couples therapy, etc., are ultimately at the service of this goal. This admittedly limited objective distinguishes the new sex therapy from other modalities of treatment, such as psychoanalysis and marital therapy. Psychoanalysts and marital therapists also treat patients whose chief complaint is sexual dysfunction. However, their theory is based on the concept that sexual problems are invariably expressions of underlying conflicts and/or destructive interpersonal transactions.

The main aim of psychoanalytic and marital therapy extends beyond relief of the patient's sexual problems, and includes the resolution of broader intrapsychic and interpersonal difficulties. The therapeutic emphasis is on resolving the sexually distressed patient's deeper intrapsychic or interpersonal difficulties. The improvement of sexual symptoms that may occur during the course of therapy is regarded as a product of the resolution of more basic personality problems and/or changes in pathological marital dynamics. For those engaging in such therapy, the psychotherapist does not terminate treatment when the patient's impotence improves or the woman experiences orgasm. Treatment is concluded only when therapist and patient feel that basic unconscious conflicts, which derive from childhood and/or the fundamental sources of marital discord, have been resolved.

In contrast, while the many remote and deeper intrapsychic and interpersonal influences that may underlie some sexual symptoms are recognized and respected, the initial site of therapeutic intervention for sex therapy is the modification of the immediate causes and defenses against sexuality. The remote aspect of the problem is dealt with only to the extent that it is necessary to relieve the sexual target symptom, and also to ensure that the disability will not recur. Psychodynamic and transactional material is interpreted and neurotic behavior is modified, but only if they are directly operative in impairing the patient's sexual functioning, or if they offer obstacles to the progress of treatment.

Sex therapy is considered completed when the couple's sexual difficulty is relieved. This is not to say, of course, that treatment is terminated as soon as the patient manages to have intercourse on one or two occasions. However, treatment is ended when the dysfunction is relieved, and when the factors that were directly responsible for the problem have been identified and resolved sufficiently to warrant the assumption that the patient's sexual functioning is reasonably permanent and stable.

Treatment Format and Therapeutic Tasks

Treatment formats used by various sex therapy clinics and therapists have one feature in common—they all provide for both the prescribed use of sexual experiences and psychotherapeutic sessions. The use of behavioral prescriptions within a treatment context is not unique to sex therapy. Recently, family and group therapists have also been experimenting with the therapeutic application of "family tasks" and other types of specifically structured interactions. These developments reflect the recent, growing trend in psychiatry toward greater respect for and utilization of experiential factors in modifying human behavior. This trend represents the beginnings of a departure from the traditional treatment strategies, which tended to rely exclusively on insight to produce change. However, while the incorporation of experiential behavior modification is being explored in some other therapeutic contexts, it finds its fullest expression in the new sex therapy, where the sexual tasks constitute a major and essential treatment tool.

While all sex therapists make use of prescribed sexual tasks, workers in this field differ considerably with respect to the specific formats they employ. Therapists who follow the Masters and Johnson format see patients daily for a period of 2 weeks. Other programs see couples once or twice per week for as long as necessary to restore and stabilize sexual functioning. Some sex therapists follow Masters and Johnson in employing mixed gender co-therapy teams.[9] Others have found this unnecessary, and appear to attain comparable results with well-trained solo therapists of either gender. Some programs insist that one member of the therapy team be a physician; others have no such requirements.

Since a crucial ingredient of successful therapy is the participation of two individuals in the sexual exercises that are required to improve the previously destructive sexual system, the use of couples is important. However, flexibility is needed with respect to the extent to which both partners are required to participate in each of the psychotherapeutic sessions. Usually, the couple is seen together during the initial evaluation and in most subsequent sessions. But the therapist remains alert to situations that require the spouses to be seen individually, for example, evidence that sexual "secrets" exist, or material that must be dealt with and that may have a deleterious effect on one of the partners or on their relationship. In addition, some disorders require that treatment focus primarily on one or the other partner. When such a situation exists, it is not necessary to insist on the couple's joint attendance at therapeutic sessions, nor on the participation of both in the sexual exercises. For instance, in orgasm-phase disorders, individual sessions for the dysfunctional partner may be the treatment of choice. These treatments initially emphasize masturbatory reconditioning, so that the partner's participation would be unnecessary or even contraindicated.

Recent attempts to combine erotic experiences with group process for preorgasmic women and for premature ejaculators constitute a further modification in format. These programs provide treatment for single individuals as well, a population that had previously been unattended to by sex therapy.[10] Couples groups for mixed sexual dysfunction have also been attempted, but it is too early to evaluate this and similar experiments conducted by clinicians. The combined use of group modalities with sex therapy holds considerable promise.

It is important to experiment with new forms and variations in order to improve our clinical techniques and to identify the "active ingredients" (that is, the essential change-producing factors of sex therapy). Unfortunately, because of the great needs in this area, some "therapists" seem to be exploiting the current interest in sexual therapy by initiating poorly conceived and sensational quasi-orgy "therapeutic" procedures.

A variety of tasks with different goals and effects has been developed by sex therapists. For example, Masters and Johnson use a systematic sequence of tasks, which begins with "sensate focus."[9] This consists essentially of a period of coital and orgastic abstinence for both partners. During this time, they take turns in gently caressing each other, thereby substituting the goal of giving and receiving pleasure in sexual contact for the destructive goal of feeling one must give a sexual performance. Another technique used in sex therapy is the stop-start penile stimulation prescribed for the couple in the premature ejaculation case that will be presented later in the chapter. This method is specifically indicated to teach orgastic control to those experiencing this disorder. Other sex therapists use a variety of erotic films and literature, masturbation, vibrators, and various techniques of erotic stimulation as part of their treatment procedures. In general, it is the aim of the therapeutic tasks to dispel performance anxiety, fear of rejection by the partner, and guilt and shame. These factors seem to be highly prevalent deterrants to the sexual abandonment that is a prerequisite for adequate sexual functioning.

The apparently simplistic tasks referred to above often have a profound impact on the patient, and appear to be instrumental in modifying chronically destructive sexual behavior and difficulties rapidly. Unfortunately, the mechanisms by which they exert their therapeutic power and influence are not clearly understood. Some hypotheses suggest themselves when these phenomena are viewed from the perspective of psychiatric theory. It may be speculated that three factors (possibly among many others) contribute to the improvement in sexual functioning that seems to be produced by the prescribed sexual experiences: (1) they alter the previously destructive sexual system—the secure ambience created by sex therapy provides the couple with an opportunity to learn to make love in freer and more enjoyable ways; (2) the resolution of sexual conflict is facilitated when the couple engages in previously avoided sexual experiences; and (3) the tasks evoke the emergence of previously unconscious intrapsychic and dyadic conflicts, which then become available for psychotherapeutic intervention and resolution.

Programs differ as to the specific tasks that they employ in treatment and in their specific treatment format. However, the most significant differences among sex therapy programs arise from differences in the conceptualization of the therapeutic process, which are ultimately reflected in the conduct of the psychotherapeutic aspect of sexual treatment. Some of the clinicians who practice sex therapy have had no prior instruction in the theory of psychopathology, nor have they had clinical training in psychotherapy. They lack the theoretical conceptualization of the therapeutic process that is an essential prerequisite to clinical competence; consequently, they are forced to work empirically and to deal only with surface causes. They rely exclusively on sex education and counseling and on the prescription of erotic tasks to achieve therapeutic objectives. This approach can be effective with simple problems. However, most sexual problems need a more complex approach. Therefore, in sharp contrast, psychodynamically oriented approaches place heavy emphasis on psychotherapy. Although the sexual experiences are crucial to the success of treatment, they constitute only one aspect of the total therapeutic process. They are of value primarily when they are integrated within a psychodynamic framework during the therapeutic sessions.

The Psychotherapeutic Session

By itself, psychotherapy is a relatively ineffective or at best a slow method of treating the sexual dysfunctions. However, when sexual exercises are combined with psychotherapy that is conducted with skill and sensitivity, psychotherapy becomes immensely important and, in fact, is indispensable to the success of the new sex therapy.

The primary level of intervention of sex therapy is to modify the immediately operating obstacles to the couple's satisfactory sexual functioning. These obstacles generally yield, at least in part, to education and clarification of sexual misconceptions and, most importantly, to the experiences that expose the couple to new and previously avoided sexual interactions.

However, treatment is by no means limited to such "surface" interventions. Defenses and resistances are constantly being mobilized in the course of treatment, even when both spouses are essentially healthy, and the therapist must deal with these by means of psychotherapeutic techniques, which require a knowledge of the psychodynamics of human behavior.

The psychotherapeutic interventions that are conducted as part of sex therapy are shaped both by the couple's intrapsychic and dyadic problems and by the specific nature of their sexual difficulties. Therefore, the therapist should not proceed to conduct a therapeutic session until an adequate evaluation of the nature of the sexual problem has been made. This requires that the therapist have a precise mental picture of what actually happens when the couple makes love, of what each partner is doing to and with the other, and a clear idea of the reactions of each spouse to the sexual transactions that were prescribed at the previous session. To implement this objective, the therapeutic sessions begin with a detailed review of the couple's experiences as they conduct the prescribed sexual tasks. The therapist also needs insight into the nature of the couple's subjective experiences, so that he or she can formulate the problem clearly. What is the husband feeling when he begins to try to arouse his wife? Is he afraid that he may ejaculate too soon or be unable to perform? Is she afraid he will reject her if she is slow to climax? Not surprisingly, couples tend to be vague when questioned about intimate details of their sexual feelings and behavior. In order to understand the problem so as to formulate a treatment plan, the therapist must persist until the questions elicit a clear picture.

Therapist: How do you usually make love?

Man: Well, you know, we get into bed, and then we make out . . . and then we have intercourse.

Therapist: I need a more detailed picture than that. Can you tell me exactly what you both usually do and experience?

Woman: Well, he plays with my breasts, and kisses me and then we have intercourse.

Therapist: How long does foreplay usually last?

Man: Oh, 5 to 10 minutes—right?

Woman: Yes, that's right.

Therapist: (to woman) How do you feel about the way he caresses you?

Woman: I like it.

Therapist: Yes?

Woman: Yes, sure. Well, I would like it to last a little longer sometimes, but he's very good. It's not his fault. It's my problem.

Therapist: I'd like to hear more about that.

Woman: Well, he always starts to touch my breasts and it begins to feel very good. But then he stops very soon. And then I feel a little down, but he wants to go on. So we go on.

Therapist: Can you tell him that you'd like him to play with your breasts more?

Man: You encourage me to go on. How was I supposed to know I go too fast for you!

Therapist: Well, I think we might talk about this a little more. (to woman)

When do you start actual coitus—when you feel like starting, or when he is ready?

Man: Gee, I guess we start when I have a good erection—but she sort of lets me know when she's ready. (to woman) You let me know when you're ready, right?

Woman: Well, not when I really want to. I just think he's getting tired of fooling around, and then I let him know. I know I'm not going to have an orgasm anyhow—so what's the point? I just want him to have a good time. When he has a good erection and starts breathing fast, I give him the "go ahead."

If, at any stage in the course of the interview, the therapist is not quite certain about some points, clarity can be gained by sharing the confusion with the couple. During the sessions, one must persist in questioning and point out contradictions, evasions, and areas of vagueness in their replies until an accurate picture of their sexual transactions is obtained by the therapist as well, and until they feel comfortable about discussing the material.

Therapist: (to woman) What goes on in your mind during intercourse?

Woman: Well, I like it, and . . . I don't know . . . just nothing.

Therapist: Can you forget about him altogether and just lose yourself in pleasure?

Woman: No, of course not; that's selfish.

Therapist: (to man) How about you?

Man: Well, I think about her a lot, but then I get to a certain point, then I forget about everything. (to woman) It's not that I don't consider you, but I'm nowhere. I just come, and it's great!

Therapist: Sure, that's good. In fact that is necessary for good functioning.

Woman: I can never do that. I didn't know it was supposed to be that way. (to man) How can you just do that?

In this manner, the therapist was provided with an opportunity to introduce the crucial topic of the wife's defenses against sexual abandonment.[1]

It is essential to the couple's future sexual adjustment that they be encouraged to talk to each other in an open, authentic, and nondefensive way. They must continue to listen to and talk to each other until each understands what the other is feeling. Once this pattern of communication has been established, then each can learn to know exactly where the other is in his/her sexual response cycle, what each is feeling, and what is essential for a successful sexual relationship.

Levels of Psychotherapeutic Intervention

The therapist's decisions with respect to the nature and depth of psychotherapeutic interventions are dictated not only by the verbal material presented by the couple in the sessions, but also by their reactions to each prescribed sexual experience. As is true of the prescribed sexual exercises, every psychotherapeutic maneuver and interpretation must be based on a definite rationale, which can only be formulated on the basis of a clear understanding of the couple's sexual relationship, in terms of both their actual behavior and its dynamics. Insight may occur on many levels, ranging from a patient's recognition on a superficial level of the self-destructive effects of avoidance of sex, to the realization on a genetic level that previously unrecognized and unresolved childhood fears of a parent are responsible for the current anxieties that are impairing the sexual relationship with the spouse.

The conduct of the psychotherapeutic component of sex therapy is influenced by its limited objective, that is, to relieve the patient's sexual problem. Hence, interpretations are usually directed only to those aspects of the patient's behavior that are clearly defenses erected against sexuality and/or that constitute resistances to the treatment processes. A patient's unconscious Oedipal conflict, or the fact that the couple is engaged in a power struggle of which they are only dimly aware, may be perfectly apparent to the therapist. However, unless these issues present manifest obstacles to the cure of sexual symptoms, the therapist should not make the couple aware of them, and should refrain from interpreting the unconscious roots of these problems in an effort to foster their resolution. However, if such material presents obstacles to the couple's sexual adequacy, the psychodynamically oriented therapist intervenes actively on any level of depth that is indicated by the situation.

The fact that "deep" intervention is usually conducted in sex therapy only when it is directed to those issues that present manifest obstacles to the cure of sexual symptoms distinguishes this approach from other psychodynamic treatment modalities. Psychoanalytically oriented psychotherapists do not usually discriminate between symptoms by focusing on the resolution of specific difficulties presented by the patient while leaving other difficulties untouched. Rather, as noted earlier, an attempt is made to reconstruct the patient's neurotic personality and, in pursuit of that goal, to interpret unconscious material.

Although there are exceptions, in sex therapy, as a general rule, the therapist at first employs an educational and behavioral approach. This is followed with clarification of communication between the couple and the simplest kind of insight-producing tactics. The therapist proceeds to deeper levels of intervention only if and when that becomes necessary to deal with the patient's resistances and defenses. The way in which resistances are handled will perhaps serve to illustrate this principle.

The Management of Resistance   Resistances to the therapeutic process almost invariably arise in the course of treatment and, actually, their emergence and resolution are crucial to the success of sex therapy. Resistances that are mobilized in the course of treatment reveal the previously hidden causes of the couple's sexual problems, and in this manner create the opportunity for resolution and change. Resistance may arise either in the symptomatic patient or in the spouse. When the spouse obstructs the progress of treatment, this is usually an indication that the patient's sexual dysfunction serves some unconscious function for his or her mate. Often, spouse resistance emerges when it becomes clear that there has been an improvement in the patient's sexual functioning, and that the symptom will be cured shortly. On the other hand, when treatment mobilizes resistance, that is, anxiety in the symptomatic patient, this occurs just prior to remission of the symptom. In other words, resistance mobilized by the rapid changes in sexual functioning that occur in the course of sex therapy is often due to anticipatory anxiety. The spouse unconsciously anticipates that the mate's improved sexual adequacy will lead to abandonment or some other "calamity," while the symptomatic patient also anticipates some injury should his or her sexual functioning improve. Once the symptom has disappeared, the patient's anxiety usually abates.

Resistance in one or both partners frequently takes the form of an avoidance of, or a failure to respond to, the prescribed sexual task. Obviously, treatment cannot proceed unless the couple conducts the prescribed tasks. But apart from such considerations, avoidance of sexual tasks is also indicative of the presence of intrapsychic and dyadic problems that must be resolved, at least in part, before treatment can proceed to a successful conclusion.

Techniques used for handling resistance may range from repetition of the task in a way that produces lower levels of anxiety, to simple confrontation of a self-destructive behavior pattern, and to analytic work with highly threatening unconscious material. In cases refractory to the usual strategies of sex therapy, some therapists stop treatment, consider the case a treatment failure, and suggest such alternative types of therapy as psychoanalysis or marital therapy. However, in our experience, a substantial number of patients who suffer from sexual dysfunctions that are not amenable to sex therapy when it is limited to intervention on a primarily experiential level can be treated successfully, providing their deeper conflicts are resolved. Therapists have at their disposal a wide array of psychotherapeutic techniques with which to foster insight and resolution of the more fundamental roots of the sexual symptom. For example, the therapist may interpret unconscious material to foster the patient's insight into and resolution of the deeper issues that underlie resistances and defenses against sexuality. At other times, the techniques of conjoint therapy are useful in revealing and resolving malignant transactions of which the couple were unaware previously. In such cases, the therapist may interpret the unconscious roots of the pathogenic interactions that interfere with the development of a good sexual relationship between partners.

When brief sex therapy techniques are not effective in relieving a couple's sexual dysfunction, the therapist may then choose to intervene on a deeper level, that is, to attempt to modify the roots from which the problem springs. Sometimes this strategy proves to be successful. Other cases remain refractory even to deeper forms of interventions. The character of the psychotherapeutic process changes when it is conducted within a system that employs a dynamic interplay between experiential and insight-producing techniques. The process becomes more active, creative, and effective when both modalities are combined and used concomitantly.

In conventional psychotherapy, the patient can circumvent a sexual problem successfully for many years. This is impossible in the new sex therapy, where the patient is actually confronted with the experience that he or she is trying to avoid. The value and potency of such experientially induced confrontations seem to be enhanced considerably when these experiences are integrated into the eclectically oriented therapeutic process. Thus, the dynamic combination of experiential and psychotherapeutic techniques fosters more rapid resolution of the sexual conflict, and reaches a greater range of patients than does either psychotherapeutic intervention or an experiential method alone.

Treatment Strategies

The sexual tasks that are prescribed for a couple are designed to implement the basic treatment strategies of sex therapy. These differ for the various syndromes.

Premature Ejaculation and Vaginismus Premature ejaculation and vaginismus respond to specific treatment strategies. While all tasks must be tailored to the individual patient's needs, the essential change-producing tasks and experiences seem to have been clearly identified for these two syndromes; consequently, the behavioral prescriptions are relatively standard.

The essential maneuver in vaginismus is the gradual dilatation and desensitization of the conditioned spasticity of the vaginal inlet, and the concomitant resolution of the sexual phobias that often accompany that condition. The cure of premature ejaculation rests in repeated penile stimulation with a partner to the point of impending orgasm. Both of these strategies have proven highly effective for the vast majority of patients who suffer from these conditions. But even these simple behavioral maneuvers evoke material that can alter a patient's life beyond the improvement of genital functioning. The case presented below illustrates a positive modification of a relationship as a result of curing premature ejaculation.

Mr. A and Ms. B.: Relationship discord secondary to premature ejaculation.
Background information: Mr. A., a 25-year-old self-employed painter with a 7-year history of premature ejaculation, had been involved for the past 3 years in a relationship with Ms. B., a 20-year-old manager of a retail fabric shop. He was success oriented and had become involved with his career to the exclusion of Ms. B., who felt unappreciated and had considered terminating the relationship because of the poor quality of their sex life. Ms. B viewed sex with him as "unexciting," and avoided sex with him because she so often felt "cheated." Her sexual rejection of him exacerbated his sexual problem, and indirectly helped to maintain his focus on his career rather than on their relationship. Ms. B. had defensively increased her time commitment to her job, leaving only one evening a week for them to be together. They had developed an avoidance pattern that is typical of sexual dysfunction cases, with their sexual frequency diminishing from daily at the beginning of their relationship to less than once a month. Ms. B. summarized their relationship in response to the following questions:
Therapist: Do you still find your partner attractive?
Ms. B.: Yes, except when I'm frustrated (sexually), then I feel even hate . . . . We used to satisfy each other pretty well by other means, but as time went on and we both fully realized the problems, we just couldn't face it, so we didn't touch each other after a while.

Mr. A. was raised by "wonderful, but old-fashioned Italian Catholic" parents, with minimal discussion of sex in the home. He became aware of sexual impulses at age 10, and began masturbating in his early teens. During masturbation, he would usually bring himself to orgasm quickly. He experienced premature ejaculation in all of his sexual encounters, regardless of the partner or the duration time of stimulation.

Ms. B. also came from a middle-class Italian-American home, but her parents had married and divorced each other twice. She reported no discussion of sex in the home, but the importance of love was emphasized. She had never masturbated. She was orgasmic with manual stimulation from Mr. A., but anorgasmic during coitus. She was depressed about her present and past relationships. Her first lover had died of cancer, and she reported that her second partner had deceived her frequently. She had entered her present relationship with some of the defenses characterizing the result of unrequited love. She summarized her relationship history in the following manner:

The one who loved me—died
The one who didn't—lied
The one who couldn't—tried

Formulation: It became apparent that Mr. A. harbored considerable hostility toward Ms. B., yet he was also considerably concerned about pleasing her. In part, his career involvement grew out of a desire to impress her so that she would not abandon him. The effect of this was decidedly the opposite, since she was feeling abandoned and was close to terminating the relationship. It is possible that his conflicts had their roots in disturbances in his interactions with crucial members of his family in early childhood. It is also possible that these conflicts played a role in the genesis of his sexual problems. Certainly, it is safe to assume that a psychoanalyst confronted with this case would proceed on this premise. Accordingly, the therapist would attempt to help the patient resolve his residual Oedipal conflicts and gain insight into the unconscious sources of his anger with women and his fear of abandonment by maternal figures, with the expectation that he would thereby gain ejaculatory competence. The marital therapist, on the other hand, would try to identify and resolve the transactional causes of Mr. A.'s problem, that is, the hostilities between the couple, which very possibly might reinforce the man's prematurity. This approach would be no less valid, for it was obvious that this couple had serious problems in their relationship. As mentioned above, the quality of their relationship reflected Mr. A.'s ambivalent feelings toward his girlfriend. Moreover, her fears, on some level of awareness, that if her boyfriend were to function well sexually he would abandon her for a more attractive woman, had also had an adverse effect on their relationship. The interpersonally oriented therapist would, therefore, consider the resolution of this couple's destructive relationship interactions as the first order of business.

As noted above, in contrast to these approaches, the sex therapist's initial objective is to attempt to modify the immediate cause of prematurity, which presumably is the patient's anxiety at high and prolonged levels of sexual excitement, an anxiety that often results in a lack of awareness about his sensations prior to orgasm. Such awareness of the sensations premonitory to orgasm is essential to the acquisition of voluntary control over the ejaculatory reflex. Based on this hypothesis, during the second therapeutic session in such cases, the patient and his partner are instructed in the stop-start procedure, which enables the achievement of ejaculatory control without producing insight into the intrapsychic or interpersonal dynamics that may play a role in the genesis and perpetuation of the dysfunction. Essentially, the therapist instructs the woman to stimulate the man's penis intermittently, and instructs the patient to focus his attention on the premonitory cues to orgasm. This is not to imply that therapeutic interventions are limited to the prescription of such behavioral tasks. On the contrary, the sex therapist must be a skilled psychotherapist and couples therapist. However, those skills are employed in order to implement the top-priority objective, namely, the relief of the sexual target symptom. Once again, psychodynamic and/or transactional material, that is, the remote causes of the sexual symptom, are dealt with skillfully and effectively, but only insofar as these variables present immediate obstacles to the couple's sexual adequacy and/or give rise to resistances that interfere with the implementation of the essential therapeutic tasks.

Treatment: Obstacles to treatment began by the third session, when the couple managed to avoid the sexual tasks for a whole week. Mr. A. rationalized his behavior on the grounds that he was extremely involved with business, and could rarely find time for the exercises. Ms. B. felt irritable, and avoided doing the exercise at the one time when he was available. She reiterated her negative feelings about the relationship, and blamed the entire noncompliance on him. She stated, "I've decided to give this whole thing 'til February. If he doesn't live up to all his promises, or at least try to live up to them, this girl is leaving him." Such an ultimatum usually indicates a poor prognosis for sex therapy. When Mr. A. attempted to reassure Ms. B. that he would change his behavior, she became even more adamant that she saw the future as bleak. At this point, her resistance became the primary obstacle to treatment and had to be contended with. The therapist did this with two maneuvers. First, he joined her resistance, allowing that Mr. A. was probably the culprit she painted him as, but that it was in her best interest to have a functional sexual partner. Second, and most important for this couple, she was reassured that Mr. A.'s avoidance was due to anxiety about sex and fear of failure, not lack of caring. This reassurance allowed her to invest herself more fully in the therapy, which was successful from that moment on. Each responded very positively to the exercises, which allowed them to communicate more and to spend more time together sexually.

As they became aware of their insecurities, they were also able to love each other more deeply. They learned to care about each other's sexual and emotional needs. Their sex life became mutually fulfilling, and Mr. A.'s control improved greatly. Their sexual successes generalized to other aspects of their lives. Ms. B. reported, "My new knowledge and awareness made me a much more confident woman . . . never a raving maniac anymore." Mr. A. stated, "The program has made me a more tolerant, level-headed, and rational person . . . . I never thought it would be as awesome a turnaround as it was." Two-year follow-up indicated that Mr. A.'s ejaculatory control had remained stable, and Ms. B. was able to have orgasms during coitus. The couple felt deep love for one another, had married a few months earlier, and seemed reasonably content.

This case was highly gratifying, but somewhat atypical. Frequently, dysfunctional patients can be relieved of their symptoms, but changes in basic personality structure or in the fundamental dynamics of the marital relationship are not the norm. Typically, there is a specificity of outcome with sex therapy, which will be discussed in the section on outcome.

Erectile Dysfunction, Retarded Ejaculation, and the Excitement Phase and Orgasm Phase Dysfunctions of Females The behavioral prescriptions used in the treatment of the other sexual dysfunctions are more variable than those used in the treatment of premature ejaculation and vaginismus. As is evident from the preceding section, the sexual dysfunctions are associated with a great variety of deeper causes, and patients utilize a wide array of mechanisms to "turn themselves off." The therapist must be perceptive and flexible in order to identify accurately the factors that are operative in a given case, and to devise effective therapeutic tasks that fit the patient's specific requirements. However, treatment is governed by certain basic principles. The following appear to be useful.

The Initial Therapeutic Objective: During the initial phase of treatment, the therapeutic efforts are guided by one overriding aim—to get the dysfunctional patient to function adequately just once. The therapist attempts to implement this objective by maximizing the erotic factors and minimizing the inhibiting ones in the couple's sexual system.

A single successful experience often has a marvelous therapeutic effect on the discouraged patient who fears that sexuality is gone forever. It restores confidence, instills new optimism, and demonstrates dramatically that the problem is solvable. In addition, by virtue of the fact that the patient and/or partner had to overcome certain resistances in order to achieve this initial success, such an experience sets the stage for further exploration of the manner in which the patient's defenses and interactions with the partner have operated to impair past sexuality.

Obviously, one or even several successful sexual experiences cannot be considered a "cure." However, the therapist can use the leverage afforded by confronting the patient with the fact that good functioning is possible if conditions are right to shape the couple's behavior gradually toward the achievement of permanent sexual adequacy and confidence in their sexual capacity which, again, are the ultimate goals of sex therapy.

Relatively little intervention is required to arrange the conditions under which minimally conflicted patients can function sexually. The reassurance provided by the therapist in granting the couple permission to enjoy sex, the sensate focus exercises (with their emphasis on initial orgastic and coital abstinence, which removes the pressure to perform and the fear of failure), and the subsequent teasing, sensuous exercises that heighten erotic tension often suffice to enable the patient to function initially. When necessary, achievement of this goal can be facilitated further by the therapist's suggestion that the patient employ the temporary use of fantasy to distract from the momentary anxiety that may be experienced at crucial stages of excitement. The therapist may also recommend techniques that are designed to enhance clitoral stimulation for the woman who suffers from orgastic inhibition.

However, more complex interventions are required when the patient has deeper or more complex problems. Patients who suffer from severe sexual conflicts may be able to function initially only under exceptional conditions. And the therapist should be able emotionally to accept any nondestructive form of activity that enables them to function, no matter how bizarre and unnatural or "perverse" these activities appear. For example, if an impotent patient is able to produce good erections when he engages in sexual behavior while he is clothed, but loses his erections as soon as he undresses, he may be encouraged initially to proceed with lovemaking with his trousers on; and then gradually to accustom himself to freer sexual expression. Or, while she is alone, the anorgastic woman may require intense clitoral stimulation with a vibrator, accompanied by bondage fantasies, to achieve her first orgasm. The therapist should be comfortable with this method of functioning. After she has experienced her initial orgasm under these reassuring and intensely stimulating conditions, it is then often possible to get the patient to respond gradually to her partner, without the vibrator and with less intense stimulation if she so desires.

Outcome

Several factors affect the outcome of sexual therapy. Negative prognostic indicators include medical problems, drug and alcohol abuse, depression, phobic-anxiety syndromes, and marital disharmony. The prognosis in some instances is so poor that our practice is to evaluate carefully such problems as depression, high-anxiety states, substance-abuse problems, and serious anger within a relationship before accepting a couple for treatment.

One of the most important and interesting prognostic indicators relates to the phase that is inhibited. As a group, orgasm-phase disorders in both the male and the female have a favorable prognosis in as high as 90 percent of the cases. Various centers throughout the country report a cure rate for anorgasmic females that ranges from 90 to 95 percent. Similarly, the probability of learning ejaculatory control is usually reported to be about 90 percent, regardless of other factors. The data for retarded ejaculation are not clear, but this disorder is more resistant than premature ejaculation. Similarly, while the outcome for anorgastic women in terms of becoming orgastic on clitoral stimulation is excellent, it is poor for becoming orgastic on coitus.

By contrast, patients suffering from desire-phase problems have a relatively poor prognosis with sexual therapy (and for that matter with other kinds of therapy as well). In other words, the person who feels little desire for his or her spouse is seldom cured of this inhibition within the format of 12 to 14 sessions of brief sexual therapy. There are some exceptions, of course, but these are relatively few as compared with the strikingly good outcome sexual therapy enjoys with the orgasm-phase disorders. The prognosis for excitement-phase disorders falls midway between the approximately 90 percent cure rate of the orgasm-phase disorders and the approximately 10 percent cure rate of the desire-phase inhibitions. More specifically, some impotent patients improve rapidly, and relatively little resistance is mobilized in the course of therapy. Other patients suffering from excitement-phase problems seem psychodynamically more like desire-phase patients; they are resistant during the course of therapy, and do not respond well to sexual therapy. Depending upon the population treated, the cure rate for impotence with sexual therapy falls within the 50 percent range.

These striking differences in prognosis of the three phase disorders suggest the hypothesis that these syndromes are the product of different underlying causes.[8] Specifically, it may be speculated that, as a group, orgasm-phase disorders tend to be caused by the kinds of "superficial" anxiety that were described in the section on etiology and that yield easily to behavioral techniques. On the other hand, the kinds of anxiety that produce a loss of erotic desire are more apt to be of the "deep" kind, of which the patient is not likely to have conscious awareness and which are highly resistant to treatment. According to this view, impotence, the excitement-phase disorder, can be produced by either "deep" or "superficial" anxieties, and in fact this hypothesis seems to be borne out by clinical evidence.

Enhancement

This discussion has focused primarily on the mechanisms by which the sexual tasks diminish the negative forces that inhibit the patient's sexual responses. However, the sexual tasks have an effect that extends beyond the therapeutic—these experiences are also powerful instruments for positively enhancing sexual pleasure. The experiences teach couples to "get in touch" with their own previously avoided sensuous and erotic feelings, that is, the experiences sensitize them to their erotic wishes and free their potential for sexual pleasure. In the course of the sexual exercises, each spouse is given an opportunity to explore activities that are potential sources of heightened stimulation and pleasure for him- or herself and for the partner. The partners learn to be more sensitive to each other and more accepting of each other's eroticism. Both learn to recognize "where" they are, individually and together. Both develop more realistic and less judgmental attitudes about sex, which enables them to ask for and to give sexual pleasure without shame or fear. They learn to enhance their sexuality with fantasy and with more effective and imaginative modes of stimulation. If sex therapy is successful, they learn to be free of the compulsion to strive for coitus and orgasm, and to focus instead on sensual pleasure. At the same time, they also learn to explore and to be open to any procedure that enhances their own and their partner's pleasure. Finally, and perhaps most importantly, they learn to take responsibility for their own sexual pleasure, and to give themselves the "permission" for accepting their sexuality nonjudgmentally and for enjoying its expression without guilt.

REFERENCES

1 Kaplan, Helen S.: *The New Sex Therapy,* New York: Brunner/Mazel, 1974.

2 Masters, William, and Virginia Johnson: *Human Sexual Response,* Boston: Little, Brown, 1966.

3 Kinsey, A. C. et al.: *Sexual Behavior in the Human Male,* Philadelphia: W. B. Saunders, 1948.

4 MacLean, Paul: "New Findings Relevant to the Evolution of Psychosexual Functions of the Brain," *J. Nerv. Ment. Dis.,* **135**(4):289–301, 1962.

5 Money, John, and A. A. Ehrhardt: "Fetal Hormones and the Brain: Effect on Sexual Dimorphism of Behavior—A Review," *Arch. Sex. Behav.,* **1**(3):241–262, 1971.

6 Harlow, H. F., and M. K. Harlow: "The Affectional Systems," in A. M. Schrier et al. (eds.): *Behavior of Non-Human Primates,* vol. 2, New York: Academic Press, 1965, pp. 287–334.

7 Money, John: "The Determinants of Human Sexuality," in C. J. Sager and H. S. Kaplan (eds.), *Progress in Group and Family Therapy,* New York: Brunner/Mazel, 1972.

8 Spitzer, Robert et al.: "Sex in DSM III," paper presented at the meeting of the Eastern Association for Sex Therapy, New York, 1977.

9 Masters, William, and Virginia Johnson: *Human Sexual Inadequacy,* Boston: Little, Brown, 1971.

10 Perelman, Michael A.: "The Treatment of Premature Ejaculation by Time-Limited, Group Sex Therapy," doctoral dissertation, Columbia University, 1976, *Dissertation Abstracts International,* University Microfilms no. 73–29, **37**:395, 1977.

Chapter 29

Consultation from the Psychiatrist

John J. Schwab, M.D.

EDITORS' INTRODUCTION

What is it like to be told by your physician that a psychiatric consultation is indicated? What does it mean? Does your physician think that you are crazy? Has he or she given up on helping you, or even really understood what is wrong with you? Does the physician want to get rid of you?

Does the recommendation of a psychiatric consultation come as a shock or a relief? How well was it discussed by your physician? Were you even told? Was the psychiatrist called "another consultant," "a nerve specialist," or "a neurologist"?

What will the psychiatrist be like? Young or old? Male or female? Will the psychiatrist be odd? What type of questions will be asked? Will I have to talk about sex? Will he or she want to know about Dad's drinking? Will he or she think I'm crazy? What if electroshock is recommended?

For the patient, the recommendation of a psychiatric consultation may provoke strong feelings and a wide variety of concerns about the meaning and consequences of the consultation. It may also be seen as meaning something in terms of the relationship with the primary physician. The referring physician, however, also may have concerns about suggesting the consultation. What will really be gained? Will it alienate the patient? Will it complicate the already difficult treatment? What will the psychiatrist think about the referral, the patient's medical treatment, the close relationship between patient and referring physician?

To call in any consultant is an announcement of the physician's need for help. How comfortable is this for the physician? To request a psychiatric consultation, however, may for some physicians be different from requesting a surgical consultation. It may be because both patient and physician anticipate that what is to be explored by the psychiatrist is the intimate aspect of the patient's thoughts, feelings, and relationships.

In this chapter, Schwab, who became a psychiatrist after practicing and teaching as an internist, helps the reader to decide when a psychiatric consultation may be indicated, how to prepare patient and physician for the consultation, and how to make the best use of what the consultation may have to offer.

INTRODUCTION

A fascinating study shows that physicians who have had a particular psychosomatic disorder seldom refer patients with that same disorder for psychiatric consultation.[1] This finding brings into sharp focus the subjective, highly personal elements of psychiatric referral for medical and surgical patients. In this chapter, we will examine the general problems (real and symbolic) of psychiatric referral, as well as some specific ones. Then we will look at referral from the patient's point of view, present guidelines and indications for referral, and discuss what the doctor should expect from the psychiatrist. Finally, we will explore the therapeutic potential of the psychiatric consultation, and outline procedures that can be used to treat medical patients with emotional distress.

In the last few decades, psychiatry has developed from an esoteric medical specialty occupied mainly with supplying supervised custodial care for the mentally ill or counseling for middle- and upper-class patients, to a major medical discipline—a specialty concerned with the treatment of the mentally ill in a wide variety of office, hospital, and community settings. Prior to World War II, only a fraction of the medical schools in the United States had Departments of Psychiatry. However, during the war, psychiatrists, working closely with their medical and surgical colleagues, demonstrated their skills in treating service personnel who were suffering from combat fatigue and psychosomatic disturbances. For the first time in their professional careers, numerous physicians and surgeons saw that psychiatrists' efforts often helped patients, and also learned something about psychiatry. Then, during the 1950s and 1960s, with the growing belief that medical care was a basic right, psychiatry entered the general hospital. In the last 10 years, the growth of psychiatric consultation-liaison services has generated interest in psychiatric referral practices. These developments have led to concern about the number of medical and surgical patients with emotional illnesses.

The Need for Psychiatric Consultation

In England, Crombie and a panel of colleagues used the following classifications to assess the proportion of emotional illnesses in 100 consecutive new patients (the numbers in parentheses indicate percentages):

1 An illness all or nearly all organic (52)
2 An illness that was mainly organic, but with some abnormal emotional content (21)
3 An illness with emotional and organic components in equal proportion (13)
4 A mainly emotional illness, but with some organic content (6)
5 An illness all or nearly all emotional (8)

In all, 48 percent of the patients were suffering from illnesses that were mainly emotional or were severely complicated by emotional disturbances.[2] Lipowski reviewed numerous American studies, and concluded that about 50 to 80 percent of outpatients and 30 to 60 percent of inpatients in general hospitals "suffer from psychic disease or psychiatric illness of sufficient severity to create a problem for the health professions."[3] The University of Florida studies showed that about 30 percent of the total medical inpatient population was in need of psychiatric consultation.[4] Because these and similar estimates were obtained from psychiatrists' and researchers' assessments of psychiatric morbidity, we did a study in which we examined the need for psychiatric consultation solely from the patients' point of view.[5] The researchers questioned 50 general medical inpatients who had been referred for psychiatric consultation, and 50 matched inpatients who had not been referred, about *their* opinions of the need for psychiatric consultation. Almost four-fifths of those who had been referred stated definitely either that a consultation was needed or that it might have been indicated during hospitalization, and about one-third of the nonreferred group expressed similar opinions. In order to diminish the possible influence of hospitalization, both groups were reinterviewed 1 year later in their homes. The follow-up study confirmed the original findings. Thus, about 35 percent of all medical inpatients, referred and nonreferred, expressed the belief that a psychiatric consultation might have been helpful while they were hospitalized for a medical illness.[6]

INCREASING INTEREST IN PSYCHIATRIC CONSULTATION

Psychiatric consultation is receiving increasing attention for a number of reasons. First, large numbers of patients are seeking medical help for problems in living that may be attributed to the rapid sociocultural changes taking place throughout the nation. Some of these problems involve the "generation gap," changing sexual mores, and women's dissatisfactions with traditional roles and a subordinate status.

Sociocultural Changes Make Problems

Numerous medical patients breathe a sigh of relief during a consultation, as they state that finally they have an opportunity to talk freely about what is really bothering them—for example, tensions with their adolescent children and concerns about how to relate to young people who are clamoring for freedom, using marijuana, and developing different life-styles. Many patients are confused about changing sexual mores. Some middle-aged parents feel that their traditional attitudes toward sexual behavior are being challenged; others are resentful because they think they were deprived of the freedom of sexual expression that they observe about them; and still others are in conflict as a result of their attempts to compensate by engaging in "new" sexual activities and adventures. Many women admit to lack of satisfaction with the traditional mother-wife supportive roles. They know that they are educated and capable, and that the changing social situation provides opportunities for them to work or to be creative in many ways. They feel that they have been subordinated, and they are angry about it.

These tensions are stressful, and as a result people are turning to physicians and other health professionals for relief from the symptoms of anxiety and depression, which they attribute to such stress. They are looking for help with the everyday problems of living and their concomitant physical symptoms (medical side effects), and physicians are expected to provide solutions or psychiatric referral.

Greater Knowledge about Mental Illness

An associated reason for the increasing utilization of psychiatric consultation is the greater knowledge about mental illness. Not only do people feel the tension and pain of neuroses, but they are also keenly aware that emotional distress limits their effectiveness, undermines their happiness, and ultimately leads to more serious disturbances.

Many family practitioners, pediatricians, and doctors in other specialties are aware of their patients' emotional and mental distress, as well as the relative shortage of psychiatric services. Continuing education programs make them aware that they can supply much of the needed professional expertise to alleviate psychic anguish and psychophysiologic distress. But many of their patients manifest mental disorders of such complexity or severity that psychiatric consultation is needed for clarification, diagnosis, and treatment.

PROBLEMS WITH REFERRAL

Although psychiatric consultation is receiving greater attention and obtaining acceptance, there are problems—both general and specific—with referral.

General Problems

Stigma of Mental Illness   Some doctors fear that their patients will not accept psychiatric referral because of the stigma attached to mental illness. Undoubtedly some stigma still exists, and unfavorable attitudes toward psychiatry persist. However, studies of attitudes toward mental illness indicate that the general public accepts mental illness more readily and is much more inclined to view it as a medical problem than it did 30 years ago.[7,8,9,10,11] And in particular, general medical practice accepts psychiatric consultation more favorably than it accepts many other psychiatric services and endeavors. Physicians' fears of patients' adverse reactions to psychiatric consultations are usually groundless, as will be discussed later. In looking for factors related to patients' differential reactions to psychiatric consultations, we found that orientation of the hospital personnel was extremely important. When the staff and the referring doctor have generally favorable and accepting attitudes toward psychiatry, medical patients incline in that direction; unfortunately, the converse is also true.[12]

Doubts as to Effectiveness of Psychiatry   Another general problem is that many physicians are dubious about the results or even the value of psychiatry. It is true that some patients receive only minimal measurable benefits from psychiatric care; yet there have been significant changes in the last two decades, and recent outcome studies are encouraging.[13] Both the tranquilizers and the antidepressants have benefited large numbers of patients, and enabled these patients to return to productive life. And we should recall that general psychiatry, as a treatment specialty, is still young. Continuing research is opening up new therapeutic avenues.

The Psychiatrist Mystique   A third general problem is that some elements of mystery still surround the psychiatrist. Many physicians do not inform their patients in explicit terms how the psychiatrist works, or exactly what he or she will do. A gap between medicine and psychiatry exists because of divergent training, differing concepts of illness, and problems with communication. Too often, physicians feign ignorance of human behavior, and psychiatrists discard or even disavow their medical knowledge.

Specific Problems

Resistance   In addition to these general problems with psychiatric referral, there are some specific problems. For example, despite their doctor's skillful handling, a few patients will manage to block psychiatric referrals because of the need to maintain their neuroses; such resistance may be an integral part of a neurosis. Psychiatric referral is seen by such patients as a threat to their maladaptive patterns of behavior, a threat which jeopardizes the primary and secondary gains of illness. Often these are the very patients for whom psychiatric referral is a necessity. In fact, the patient's truly *obstinate* resistance, in the face of the physician's conviction that referral is necessary, usually identifies this type of patient. In such instances, the doctor will have to maintain a staunch position, and use the relationship with the patient as leverage to effect the referral. When this is not done, further work with the patient is invariably clouded by doubt and dissatisfaction.

Influence of Hospitalization   Patients' variable reactions to hospitalization are other factors that influence attitudes toward referral. Sometimes hospitalization diminishes or even suspends a patient's neurotic problems. A patient who has been grossly disturbed prior to entering the hospital may find that the hospital is a sanctuary; the symptoms may disappear temporarily, and the patient may be seen as not needing psychiatric referral. On the other hand, those who function reasonably well on the outside may not be able to adjust to the hospital routine and to the atmosphere of illness. Their behavior in the hospital may become disruptive or distinctly pathological, resulting in the need for psychiatric referral.

Diagnosis   The most fundamental consideration entering into the decision of whether to refer a particular patient is the specific problem of diagnosis. The two main factors bearing on diagnosis are the medical and social ones.

From the medical point of view, the greatest difficulties in diagnosis are presented by patients with concurrent physical illness and emotional distress. Medical students are taught to be parsimonious with diagnoses. In fact, they are too often expected to exercise diagnostic skills to subsume all the patient's symptomatology under one diagnosis—to come up with a single disease label. Such an approach was necessary originally in order to achieve precision in medicine, but that approach is highly unrealistic in real life. It implies that the presence of one type of illness precludes the possibility of other illnesses. In the last few years, the obvious shortcomings of this approach have become evident. A number of investigations show that patients with a higher frequency of somatic complaints and physical illnesses also have more psychiatric complaints and mental illnesses. Roessler and Greenfield state: "Psychiatric patients do visit medical clinics more frequently than controls, but they do so because they suffer a greater frequency of 'real illness.'"[14] And, in their definitive studies of healthy populations, Hinkle and Wolff found that illness was not distributed randomly; some had had many more illnesses than others, and those who had had the greatest number of bodily illnesses, regardless of their nature, were the same patients who "experienced the greater number of disturbances of mood, thought, and behavior."[15]

When a patient has concurrent mental and physical illness, there is always the danger that one of the two will be emphasized or seen as causative of both. Thus the patient may not receive comprehensive treatment. Also, both physicians and psychiatrists agonize over the fact that a psychiatric disorder may mask a medical one, which, if untreated, may have serious consequences (see Chapter 14).

In addition to the diagnostic difficulties centered about the concurrence of mental and physical illness, certain social factors, such as "social distance," are responsible for problems with diagnosis. Scott points out that, because physicians usually come from a higher social class, their social distance from the more disadvantaged may limit their ability to recognize any but the most clear-cut mental symptomatology in lower-class patients.[16] Some research has confirmed this statement. In a study of 153 general medical inpatients at a hospital where psychiatric consultations were freely available to all patients, only 17 percent of the lower-class depressed patients were referred, in contrast to 33 percent of the middle-class depressed and 100 percent of the upper-class depressed.[17] Other studies, such as Duff and Hollingshead's *Sickness and Society,* are corroborative.[18]

Difficulties in communication may be one factor responsible for failure to diagnose mental illness in lower-social-class medical patients. But there are a number of other factors. First, the lower-class patients may be intimidated by the hospital routine, and may be so fearful of revealing themselves to middle-class physicians and nurses that they conceal anxiety, depression, and other mental distress. Second, the physicians' and nurses' sympathetic countertransference may obscure their views of the patients' emotional illnesses. They may regard the poverty-stricken individual's symptoms as natural, saying to themselves: "If I were living with that much hardship, I, too, would be upset." With such feelings, they may miss the diagnosis of mental illness. Or they may defend themselves against such feelings by remaining aloof or detached, and thus miss a case of depression or other mental illness. Third, it is difficult to distinguish between the symptoms of lower-socioeconomic status and those of illness. The symptoms of some mental illnesses, particularly of depression, are class-related, and display some differences from class to class. Often depression is a reactive mode stemming from childhood experience. As a consequence, we can expect the manifestations to be partially shaped and often tinted by demographic and class-specific behavioral patterns. The effects of poverty, deprivation, and little education can produce a sense of despair and futility that is related either to class status or to depressive illness.

Referral from the Patient's Point of View   Because referral processes are frequently discussed but rarely studied, we obtained data on: (1) patients' attitudes toward referral, and (2) their reactions to their referring physicians. In one study of 50 consecutively referred medical patients and a matched group of 50 nonreferred patients, we found that prior to the consultation about 80 percent of both groups expressed favorable, or at least neutral, attitudes toward a prospective consultation (or a hypothetical one). At the end of the consultation, the percentage who voiced favorable or accepting attitudes was even higher. That shift, however, lacked stability and probably reflected the impact of the immediate encounter with the psychiatrist. Most of the patients reverted to their original attitudes when they were interviewed by an independent researcher 24 hours later. We searched for factors related to patients' differential reactions to referral and consultation. Neither sociocultural factors nor the extent of the patients' knowledge about psychiatry was significant. However, those who had obtained their knowledge of psychiatry from professional sources, advanced reading, or from previous therapy reacted much more favorably to referral than those whose knowledge had been gained only from the popular news media or hearsay. Also, patients who believed that their total life situations were adversely affected by, or associated with, their physical illnesses tended to react more favorably to referral than those who saw no such associations.[19]

In each group, about one patient in five displayed a rigid, unyielding attitude, and reacted unfavorably even to the mention of the word "psychiatry." These patients stated that their negative attitudes were the result of a previous disappointing personal or family experience with psychiatrists or mental hospitals.[19]

In another study, we asked a group of 30 consecutively referred patients, "What did you think of your doctor's decision to refer? Did it change your opinion of him or her? If so, how?" After the consultations, 66 percent evinced positive attitudes toward their referring physicians, 17 percent expressed ambivalent attitudes, and 17 percent were hostile and derogatory. Later, however, most of the patients (70 percent) stated that the referral had not changed their opinions of their referring physicians. Of significance, however, is the fact that most of those who expressed a changed opinion later (30 percent) felt that the referral had increased their respect for their doctor—"It showed that my doctor cared."[20]

Almost all medical patients have anxiety about referral and an impending consultation with a psychiatrist. But for the great majority, this heightened anxiety is tempered by a sense of relief, or at least by healthy curiosity. The anxiety stems from a number of sources. The major one is concern about the psychiatrist—not the referring doctor. The patient worries about what the psychiatrist will be like. "Will the psychiatrist be friendly, or aloof, strange, cold, odd? What will I be asked? Will I be able to give the right answers?" Thus, the psychiatric mystique and doubts about one's adequacy are primary concerns felt by medical patients facing psychiatric referral. The anxiety that sometimes appears as hostility may spring from other sources: "Will I be blamed? For what (fantasies)? What will my spouse, parent(s) think? Does this mean that I am going crazy?" Therefore, in addition to anxiety, we can see that the patient can also be worried about blame and shame.

Patients may also be concerned as to whether the referral is evidence of a changing relationship with the doctor. The patient thinks, "Is my doctor trying to get rid of me? Does this mean that my doctor doesn't trust me? What does my doctor know about me that I don't know?" Or the patient may fear that the referral will change the relationship: "Will my doctor look upon me differently—as a person who is confiding in another professional?"

GUIDELINES FOR REFERRAL

Doctors are aware of the problems that psychiatric referral can create, but often their concerns about patients' reactions are either excessive or unfounded. Some doctors have a basic mistrust of referral in general. They fear that it will mean the loss of patients, reveal inadequacies, or endanger established doctor-patient relationships. The doctor is concerned with such questions as, "Will my patient think

I regard him or her as troublesome? Unworthy? Or that I lack understanding?'' But the doctor's greatest fear is that the patient will not accept the referral. We have noted that the overwhelming majority of patients react favorably or neutrally to referral and, especially, that the doctor's and the staff's attitudes toward psychiatry are fundamental factors influencing not only the patient's reactions to the referral and the doctor, but also to the psychiatrist. A number of authorities in this field maintain steadfastly that the doctor should deal openly with the patient about the referral, answer the patient's objections directly, and also educate the patient.[20,21]

In working with medical patients, the following guidelines for referral are helpful:

1 Begin with an open, forthright discussion with the patient. This discussion should be candid, and should explain in simple terms why the referral is necessary. It is important at this time for the doctor not to rely on diagnosis by exclusion. Do not state: "You ought to see a psychiatrist because we can find nothing wrong with you." Instead, say: "The evidence indicates that there might be an emotional problem that is partially responsible for your symptoms. A psychiatric consultant can help us determine whether this is so."

2 Recognize the patient's feelings. The doctor should encourage the patient to ventilate feelings about the impending consultation. Ask: "How do you feel about it?" Even if fears and negative feelings emerge, this does not mean that the patient will refuse the consultation or react adversely. As Bartemeier has said, "When the fears are out in the open and the distortions are dealt with, the patient is better able to accept the consultation."[22]

3 Clarify the psychiatrist's role. The physician should explain that the psychiatrist is being called in only to ascertain the extent and meaning of the patient's emotional distress and that there is no prior intention to make a case for psychogenic etiology.

4 Set realistic expectations of the psychiatrist. The doctor should neither oversell psychiatry nor promise miracles to the point that the patient's expectations reach magical proportions. Resulting disappointment can affect the relationship with the referring physician as well as with the psychiatrist.

5 Inform the patient that referral is not a last-resort measure. Too frequently, the doctor tells the patient, implicitly or explicitly, that the consultation is a last-resort measure, thus loading the dice against the consultant, because the patient's anxieties and the possibilities of distortion are increased.

WHICH PATIENTS ARE REFERRED?

Manifest Psychopathology Not an Accurate Index

The degree of manifest psychopathology displayed by a patient would seem to be the most logical indication for referral. However, the experience of most psychiatric consultants reveals that the level of psychopathology does not really determine whether a given patient will be referred. One reason for this is that most physicians interpret their patient's disturbed behavior subjectively. A doctor may delay suggesting psychiatric referral for the patient whose severe depression is regarded as a natural reaction to a serious medical illness, or for the patient whose disruptive behavior is thought to be caused by a diagnosed central nervous system disease. Actually, the depression or disruptive behavior may be indicative of psychiatric illness that requires attention. However, that same physician, on that same day, may call for an immediate consultation for the patient who breaks into tears for no apparent reason. Doctors' frustrations about diagnoses, dissatisfactions with responses to treatment, and even their own personal conflicts also may determine whether a patient will be referred.

Causes for Referral Vary

Only a small percentage of medical and surgical patients with psychiatric disorders are referred for psychiatric consultation. Generally, these are patients who are mentally ill demonstrably, usually expressing psychotic symptomatology, or threatening suicide. Another group that is consistently referred is composed of patients who create obvious difficulties for the staff. Some are involved in litigation, and are threatening to sue the physician or hospital. Others are patients with serious medical or surgical illnesses who decide abruptly to sign out of the hospital against medical advice. And still others are the large number of "management problems"—patients who display abrasive behavior or refuse to follow the prescribed medical regimen, thereby upsetting the hospital staff. A major group consists of the medical and surgical patients who are neurotically ill and cry for help by openly discussing their emotional turmoil and even their intimate living problems with other patients as well as with the staff.

Patients with defined psychosomatic disorders, psychophysiologic illnesses, or personality disorders are referred for psychiatric consultation inconsistently. Recent advances in medicine and surgery have given physicians greater confidence in dealing with patients afflicted with peptic ulcers, rheumatoid arthritis, asthma, and other illnesses that are generally considered to be psychosomatic. But all too often, patients with psychophysiologic illnesses are referred for psychiatric consultation only after the doctor has spent an inordinate amount of time and effort on the diagnostic workup to ensure that a defined or treatable medical illness is not present. When these patients are referred for consultation, it is usually late in the period of hospitalization and is often used as a last-resort measure just prior to discharge. At that point, the physician, who may be frustrated by the failure of scientific medicine to find a discrete cause for the patient's complaints, usually expects the psychiatrist to assume some responsibility for the patient's care.

Most patients with personality disorders are not referred for psychiatric consultation. Usually the attending physician attempts to provide definitive medical care, and does not refer the patient unless the characterologic disturbance disrupts the therapeutic regimen, or the personality disorder has special significance because of the physician's own characterologic makeup and/or particular frustrations and conflicts on a given day. A physician who believes emphatically that alcoholism is solely a lack of will power may refer medical or surgical patients with alcohol problems as a punitive measure, without being fully aware of the dynamic factors involved in the decision to refer. Or an authoritarian physician who demands that patients be compliant and submissive may refer a hostile or irritating patient because that patient's attitude just does not fit the doctor's model of the correct doctor-patient relationship.

This brief description of the types of medical and surgical patients referred for psychiatric consultation only categorizes groups of patients; it does not portray their human distress. But the agonies and doubts felt by these patients can be grasped by working with their emotional problems as well as with their medical illnesses.

How to Get the Most from the Psychiatric Referral

To obtain optimum benefits from psychiatric referral for their patients and themselves, it is best for doctors to:

1 Attempt to develop as much mutual trust in the doctor-patient relationship as possible. Although this is almost every doctor's implicit or explicit modus operandi, studies of general medical inpatient populations have shown that patients with high levels of anxiety or other evidence of emotional distress (those most likely to be referred), hold much more negative and distrustful attitudes toward doctors, nurses, and the hospital than other medical patients.[12] Knowing this, the doctor should ask the patient about such attitudes, make every possible effort to promote trust, and strive to enhance communication between them. Open communication is the essence of the doctor-patient relationship.

2 Prepare the patient for referral by using the guidelines that have been presented. Binder urges the doctor to answer patients' objections to referral directly and truthfully, and emphasizes that the doctor's empathy with the patient is a decisive element.[23] Watters insists that the doctor should take an active role in making the referral, and that referral opens up many opportunities for the doctor to lend hope to the patient.[24]

3 Supply the psychiatrist with basic medical data, one's own opinion of the patient's emotional condition including possible factors contributing to the need for referral, and explicit reasons for referral. Referral requests that ask only, "Please evaluate," or "Does this patient need psychiatric treatment?" are not only relatively meaningless, but also may be indicative of lack of involvement with the patient. The "either-or" question—either real disease or emotional illness—usually cannot be answered by the psychiatrist; also it betrays a lack of sophistication on the part of the referring doctor. Instead, the doctor should note as explicitly as possible why there is concern about the patient, and what the problem appears to be. From the psychiatrist, the doctor should expect an assessment of the patient's mental status, personality, interpersonal relationships, and the environmental factors producing stress. The psychiatrist's formulation should point out both the psychodynamic and the environmental factors involved, including strengths and resources as well as weaknesses and problems, and should lead logically to a statement about diagnosis, prognosis, and recommendations for treatment.

4 Follow through by meeting with the psychiatrist to discuss the findings and recommendations, and to resolve problems that may have arisen between the patient and the referring doctor, between the patient and the psychiatrist, or between the two doctors. Furthermore, such follow-through can be educational for referring doctors by increasing their knowledge of psychiatry as well as their understanding of particular patients.

    5 Maintain a working relationship with one or two psychiatrists. This not only facilitates referral procedures, but more importantly, enables the doctor to become more knowledgeable about how the psychiatric consultant works, and to develop realistic expectations about referral.

THE THERAPEUTIC POTENTIAL
OF THE PSYCHIATRIC CONSULTATION

Too often, little attention is given to the therapeutic potential the consultation has for the patient or the principles of therapy that can be used by referring physicians as well as by psychiatrists. Medical patients' emotional reactions to physical illness can supply a model that illustrates therapeutic procedures.

Three-Stage Model of Reactions to Physical Illness

The first stage is coincident with the onset of physical symptoms, the diagnostic workup, and admission to the hospital. Patients respond to these stressors with anxiety, a basic psychobiologic reaction that is evoked when illness is perceived as a threat to life and values. Some research on medical patients during the first 48 hours of hospitalization showed that 50 percent had moderate or severe manifest anxiety as measured by standardized anxiety scales.[25] During this first stage, the treatment approach includes primarily supportive psychotherapy, sometimes medications, and often, the utilization of other resources.

    The psychotherapeutic principles consist of explanation, clarification, and reassurance. The physician's discussing the patient's concerns about the nature of the illness, the diagnostic plans, and the treatment program enables patients to employ their intellectual defenses against anxiety. The resulting clarification diminishes doubt and confusion and, in conjunction with reassurance, tends to allay anxiety. The reassurance should neither state nor imply that all will be well, but instead should indicate clearly that the patient's distress has been communicated, that it is understandable, and that some degree of anxiety is a normal response to the threat of physical illness. The reassurance is aimed at helping the patient to maintain a requisite level of self-esteem. This is a crucial factor at this time, since the loss of self-esteem early in hospitalization can be the forerunner of increasing emotional distress and interpersonal difficulties during the course of the illness. The goals of the psychotherapeutic approach are to: (1) assist the patient to employ intellectual defenses against anxiety, and (2) assist the patient to maintain self-esteem by assurance that fears and anxieties are not abnormal.

    Sometimes medications, particularly adequate nighttime sedation, are helpful, but usually, one should not place too much reliance on antianxiety medications unless the anxiety is so excessive that it appears the patient is undergoing some degree of ego disorganization. Small doses of an antianxiety drug can be helpful. When the patient's anxiety appears overwhelming, it may be best not to probe too deeply into its roots. Also, during this stage the doctor should attempt to enlist the aid of family members. Frequently they can provide the patient with enough support and reassurance to diminish the anxiety.

The second stage occurs later in hospitalization, usually after the diagnostic workup or surgical procedure has been carried out and the patient is on a treatment program. Emotional reactions to physical illness that appear at this time are usually syndromes reflecting defenses against anxiety, rather than manifest anxiety. Predominately, these involve such characterologic features as passive aggressiveness, compulsive attention to details of medical care, erratic emotional outbursts, or withdrawal.

Attempts to use a psychotherapeutic approach at this time are usually handicapped by the antitherapeutic milieu; the staff have differing perceptions of the patient and are off-balance. As a result, the patient is confronted by disparaging attitudes and inconsistencies. To work effectively with such management problems, the doctor should use a staff-oriented approach. After a brief interview with the patient, most of one's energies should be devoted to: (1) interpreting the patient's behavior to the staff, (2) offering to serve as a mediator between the patient and the staff, and (3) developing consistent approaches toward the patient. The psychotherapist's goals during the second stage are to function in the roles of interpreter and mediator.

During this second stage, defense mechanisms sometimes crumble, so that the patient overuses denial and projection, may threaten to sign out of the hospital against medical advice, may display paranoid ideation and behavior, or may become psychotic. These are psychiatric emergencies that require prompt, drastic action. In working with such a situation, the doctor should follow three principles: (1) persuade rather than confront, (2) get help from others, and (3) let the patient save face. At this time, the doctor needs allies; consequently, other family members, a minister, and/or staff workers should be called upon to solicit the patient's cooperation and to alleviate emotional distress without laying bare its roots and, always, without "putting the patient down."

The third stage in this model occurs during convalescence and recovery when a number of varied emotional reactions may appear. For example, mounting anxiety as the day of discharge nears is usually clear-cut evidence that the patient is threatened by problems at home or at work, and has a basic sense of inadequacy about the expected return to the healthy role. Continued physical complaints, or the appearance of new and unexpected medical symptoms, usually indicate that there are problems of secondary gain. After evaluating the patient, the doctor should not work with the patient individually, but in meetings with the patient and the family instead. During family conferences, the doctor has an opportunity to explore difficulties at home or at work, come to grips with conflicts, define mutual expectations, clarify attitudes, and, in conjunction with the recommendations from the consultee, outline a program for increasing rehabilitating activity that is understood and is agreed upon by all concerned.

Depression is often seen during this stage; but, like anxiety, it is a basic psychobiologic reaction that may precede, accompany, or follow physical illness.

However, when it appears during the third stage in this model, it may be evidence of a "giving up," a loss of hope, which in turn is associated with a poor prognosis. At such times, the doctor has to apply an intensive, comprehensive treatment program that includes individual psychotherapy focused on *eliciting* the meaning of the real or imagined loss, *evoking* the expression of feelings (usually ambivalent), *exploring* factors producing lowered self-esteem, *clarifying* environmental forces, and *providing* support.

Psychotherapy, Medications, Resocialization, and Rehabilitation

The comprehensive treatment approach includes a resocialization and rehabilitation program that calls for greater social interaction, increasing physical activity, and other activities to supply tangible evidence that the patient can do something. For the resocialization program to succeed, the doctor should enlist the aid of the family, other health professionals, such as occupational and physical therapists, and community resources, such as clergy and rehabilitation counselors. Antidepressant medications are also a fundamental part of this treatment program (see Chapter 25).

The goals for this third stage, therefore, are to: (1) obtain consensus among the patient's family and others about the extent of the patient's activities after returning home, (2) encourage more social and physical activities, and (3) increase self-esteem. Increased self-esteem is the fulcrum on which the success or failure of brief psychotherapeutic interventions balances.

REASONS FOR GREATER INTEREST IN CONSULTATION-LIAISON WORK

Finally, greater interest and involvement on the part of referring physicians, nurses, and psychiatrists in consultation-liaison work is important for four major reasons.

1   The immensity of the patient's needs is disclosed by epidemiologic studies showing that about 18 percent of the general population suffers from emotional distress of sufficient severity to require mental health care.[26] And it appears that about one-third of all medical inpatients and outpatients suffer primarily from mixtures of psychic and social distress, which are often compounded by physical ailments. Therefore, medicine needs new approaches, such as those supplied by physicians, nurses, and psychiatrists working together in consultation-liaison activities.

2   Consultation-liaison work has importance for nurses and other staff workers in general hospitals. Liaison activities are vitally needed efforts that enhance and support the work of staff personnel who are exposed to the extreme vicissitudes of the human condition when they are working in renal dialysis units, coronary care units, and other places in the general hospital with seriously ill patients and distressed families for many hours a day. These staff workers are in need of such supportive measures as "weekly debriefing sessions" or periodic group therapy sessions, as well as in-service education.

3 Consultation-liaison work has special significance for physicians and psychiatrists. Brosin has noted that technological medicine lacks the "emotional communication input so necessary to sustain the doctor as an altruistic professional worker. By giving him an overall view of the patient and his family, the consultation can revive the doctor's humanistic impulses and resist the dehumanizing process."[27]

4 We live in an era that is rightfully concerned with prevention. In consultation-liaison work, the referring doctor and the psychiatrist have an opportunity to see patients whose emotional illnesses are relatively acute, and are often not encumbered by a train of crystallized defenses and interpersonal complications. Therefore, this work can not only prevent the development of more serious and more chronic mental illnesses, but also, by prompt intervention, it can alter familial attitudes and reactions so that other family members do not become interpersonally impaired—coping can become a family endeavor that promotes mental health and deters illness.

REFERENCES

1 Abrahams, D., and J. S. Golden: "Psychiatric Consultations on a Medical Ward," *Arch. Intern. Med.,* **112**:766, 1963.

2 Crombie, D. L.: "The Procrustean Bed of Medical Nomenclature," *Lancet,* **1**:1205–1206, Jan.–June, 1963.

3 Lipowski, Z. J.: "Review of Consultation Psychiatry and Psychosomatic Medicine: II. Clinical Aspects," *Psychosom. Med.,* **28**:201–223, 1967.

4 Schwab, J. J. et al.: "Differential Characteristics of Medical Inpatients Referred for Psychiatric Consultation: A Controlled Study," *Psychosom. Med.,* **27**:112–118, March–April, 1965.

5 _____ et al.: "Medical Inpatients' Reactions to Psychiatric Consultations," *J. Nerv. Ment. Dis.,* **14**(3):215–222, 1966.

6 _____: "Evaluating Psychiatric Consultation Work," *Psychosomatics,* **8**:309–317, Nov.–Dec., 1967.

7 Star, S. A.: *A Study on the Public's Attitudes on Mental Illness,* Chicago: Univ. of Chicago, National Opinion Research Center, 1950.

8 Cumming, E., and J. Cumming: *Closed Ranks: An Experiment in Mental Health Education,* Cambridge, Mass.: Harvard Univ. Press, 1957.

9 The Joint Commission on Mental Illness and Health: *Action for Mental Health,* final report, New York: Basic Books, 1961.

10 Crocetti, G. M. et al.: "Are the Ranks Closed? Attitudinal Social Distance and Mental Illness," *Am. J. Psychiat.,* **127**(9):1121–1127, March 1971.

11 Rabkin, J.: "Public Attitudes Toward Mental Illness: A Review of the Literature," *Schizophren. Bull.,* **10**:9–33, Fall 1974.

12 Schwab, J. J. et al.: "Evaluating Anxiety in Medical Patients," *J. Chronic. Dis.,* **19**:1049–1057, 1966.

13 Meltzoff, J., and M. Kornreich: *Research in Psychotherapy,* New York: Aldine, 1970.

14 Roessler, R., and N. S. Greenfield: "Incidence of Somatic Disease in Psychiatric Patients," *Psychosom. Med.,* **23**:413, 1961.

15 Hinkle, L. E., and H. G. Wolff: "Health and the Social Environment: Experimental Investigations," in A. Leighton et al. (eds.), *Explorations in Social Psychiatry,* New York: Basic Books, 1957, pp. 105–137.

16 Scott, W. A.: "Social Psychological Correlates of Mental Illness and Mental Health," *Psychol. Bull.,* **55**(2):65, 1958.

17 Schwab, J. J. et al.: "Sociocultural Aspects of Depression in Medical Inpatients," *Arch. Gen. Psychiat.,* **17**:538, Nov. 1967.

18 Duff, R. S., and A. B. Hollingshead: *Sickness and Society,* New York: Harper and Row, 1968.

19 Schwab, J. J.: "Psychiatric Consultation: Problems with Referral," *Dis. Nerv. Sys.,* **32**:447–452, July 1971.

20 _____ et al.: "Medical Patients' Reactions to Referring Physicians After Psychiatric Consultation," *JAMA,* **195**:1120–1122, March 28, 1966.

21 Jaffee, M.: "Psychiatric Referral," *Rocky Mountain Med. J.,* **60**:26, 1963.

22 Bartemeier, L. H.: "On Referring Patients to Other Physicians," *Northwest Med.,* **56**:312, 1957.

23 Binder, H. J.: "Helping Your Patient Accept Psychiatric Referral," *J. Okla. Med. Assn.,* **45**:279, 1952.

24 Watters, T. A.: "Certain Pitfalls and Perils in Psychiatric Referral," *Am. Practit.,* **3**:198, 1952.

25 Schwab, J. J. et al.: "Anxiety in Medical Patients," in *Excerpta Medica International Congress Series No. 134,* Proceedings of the First International Congress of the Academy of Psychosomatic Medicine, Palma de Mallorca, Spain, September 1966.

26 Dohrenwend, B. P.: "Sociocultural and Social-Psychological Factors in the Genesis of Mental Disorders," *J. Health Soc. Behav.,* **16**:365–392, 1975.

27 Brosin, H.: "Communication Systems of the Consultation Process," in W. M. Mendel and P. Solomon (eds.), *The Psychiatric Consultation,* New York: Grune and Stratton, 1968.

BIBLIOGRAPHY

Pasnau, R. O.: *Consultation-Liaison Psychiatry,* New York: Grune and Stratton, 1975.

Schwab, J. J.: *Handbook of Psychiatric Consultation,* New York: Appleton-Century-Crofts, 1968.

Strain, J. J., and S. Grossman: *Psychological Care of the Medically Ill,* New York: Appleton-Century-Crofts, 1975.

Chapter 30

The Physician and the Dying Patient

Eric J. Cassell, M.D.

EDITORS' INTRODUCTION

What is it like to be dying and to have a detached individual as one's physician—how would this differ from dying when one has an empathic physician? How much does it help if the physician has come to grips with his or her mortality, and can deal with death rather than avoid thinking about it? Does it always help to be told all the truth? How important is it to be able to rely on the presence and support of one's physician? These issues are important for many dying patients. In this chapter, an internist and teacher who confronts this challenge takes the reader with him as he ministers to a dying patient.

Most physicians have three types of experiences with death and dying. The first is the direct involvement with dying patients. The second is the physician's involvement with the loss of parents, family members, and friends. This more personal and disruptive experience is only rarely without pain. The ability of the physician to be more simply human than professional in response to personal loss encourages the work of mourning to reach a successful conclusion. Often, however, the physician struggles to maintain a more detached and "objective" position and, in so doing, not only postpones or circumvents personal mourning, but makes it most difficult for other survivors either to be "with" the physician in his or her pain or to mourn appropriately themselves. The physician's unmourned losses may lead to such excessive distancing from death as to make the physician unavailable for the kind of sensitive involvement with dying patients outlined in this chapter.

A third type of experience with death is at a different level, and involves the expectations, fears, and fantasies of the physician's own death. Such concerns are often submerged, but ubiquitous. Awareness of one's finitude, coupled with the thoughtful individual's concern about the meaning of one's life, can lead to concern, anxiety, or despair. When this pain is avoided totally by the denial of personal death, the physician is more apt to respond to dying patients with detachment and distancing.

The challenge to the physician presented by this chapter is one of both maturity and wisdom. Perhaps some readers will react, as we did in reading it, with the hope that, as that final life chapter is experienced personally, there will be available to them the kind of physician-guide presented in the following pages.

INTRODUCTION

I am going to illustrate the care of the dying by following one patient from my first visit with her until her death. The details are drawn from her hospital chart and from my office records, and most of the dialogue comes verbatim from tape recordings of our visits. Try to imagine that we are seeing and discussing this woman together, through the course of her illness.

Sally Gordon is a sprightly, pleasant-appearing woman with light brown hair and a sparkle on her face that goes with her wry humor. Smooth skin and the suggestion of a double chin (she is somewhat plump—especially for her short stature) make you think she is younger than her 62 years. Her daughter or one of her sisters is almost always with her, and the bedside table has pictures of her grandchildren and other family objects.

The surgeon asked me to see Sally Gordon the second time she came to our hospital, in April 1975. She was admitted because of persistent back pain that had raised the possibility of metastatic cancer. In August 1974, when she had been 61, she had had vaginal bleeding, and after 10 days she had visited her gynecologist. He had found a pelvic mass that had not been felt by him 6 months earlier, and advised hospitalization. Mrs. Gordon said he told her, "I feel something there and I don't know just where it is, and you're in trouble." She had asked him whether it meant a hysterectomy, and she remembers him saying, "It's a lot more than that."

Originally from Boston, she was living in Alabama, where her husband, a highly specialized electronics engineer, was working. She preferred to come to a hospital in New York, where most of her family lived.

Examination under anesthesia confirmed the pelvic mass. Preoperative studies revealed no evidence of metastatic disease, although the barium enema showed a constricting lesion at the junction of the sigmoid and descending colon. At operation in September 1974, she was found to have adenocarcinoma of the colon extending into the serosal fat and metastatic to several mesenteric lymph nodes and the right ovary. A segmental sigmoid resection and bilateral salpingo-oophorectomy were done. The left ovary was not involved.

Postoperatively, she developed a right serosanguinous pleural effusion, at first thought to be from pulmonary infarction, but later believed to be a malignant infusion because a preoperative chest x-ray revealed a small effusion and ascites showed in the preoperative sonogram.

Before operation, the surgeon explained to her that she might require a temporary colostomy, which she dreaded. It was her understanding that "the tumor ate a hole in part of the colon and was working itself away from the colon." After surgery, she said she was relieved because, although "of course, it was malignant, they got everything, and all the radiologists and everybody said there was no concern for treatment and everything was fine. So that was that."

The surgeon was explicit to the family about her extremely poor prognosis.

She went home in 10 days, feeling fine and optimistic about her future. She was pleased about her weight loss (keeping her weight down had always been a problem), and pleased that her bowels were moving. She said later that she had "almost a phobia about bowel movements, something I never even thought about before. I interpreted somewhere that the movements were very important—after all, it was colon surgery." Her preoccupation with her bowels continued until her death in June 1977.

She came back to New York in April 1975 for a 6-month follow-up. There had been a 5-pound weight gain, which worried her because "Why should I gain weight when I'm eating so little, although I'm delighted to have so little appetite." The surgeon showed no concern, and told her how well she looked.

While she was in New York she decided to see an orthopedist about her back pain, which had been present for many years. The many other physicians who had seen her about her back always told her it was "nothing" or "a little arthritis," but it was a nagging concern to her. The orthopedist she consulted in New York found ascites during his examination and suggested a bone scan, thus raising for her the specter of recurrent cancer, and she was readmitted to the hospital.

The surgeon asked me to see her, rather than an oncologist, because I had cared for many patients who were dying of malignancy, and had become interested in the problem of the dying patient. In the surgeon's mind, in mine (and probably, in yours), she was already in the category "dying patient."

DEFINITION OF A DYING PATIENT

Why? She was not literally about to die. She did not think she was dying, nor did her husband. Indeed, she felt fine (except for her back). On the other hand, as every physician knows, she was going to die of her cancer no matter what was done. The dictionary definition "at the point of death" is certainly not how doctors use the word *dying*. A resident once said that a dying patient is someone for whom medical science has no more to offer. And a surgeon told me that "a dying patient is a patient whom I can't help." Those definitions are important to us because they describe the state of mind of the physician who sees a patient like Mrs. Gordon. That state of mind can be induced by a pathology report ("metastatic carcinoma to lymph node") or by a chest x-ray showing a large carcinoma of the lung. But, conversely, that mindset may not follow the diagnosis "Stage 1 Hodgkin's disease," whereas a few years back it would have. Malignancies are not the only diseases that elicit that reaction, because so will "multiple sclerosis" or almost any disease where we feel helpless. The point is the feeling of helplessness, not the fact behind the feeling. For example, when a patient is admitted to a coronary care unit with a heart attack and shock or congestive heart failure, doctors do not usually act or speak as though the person is "a dying patient." There is much they can do, and because of that they do not feel helpless.

The first point about the care of the dying, then, is that the definition of a dying patient is not at all precise.[1] It is not like other definitions of disease in medicine, but is based on the doctor's feelings—and the predominant feeling is, I believe, helplessness. For physicians (and for everybody else) feeling helpless is very uncomfortable. Because of that, the doctor who cares for the dying must deal not only with the patient but with personal feelings of helplessness. If you think your job is the cure, or even the care of disease, then you have nothing to offer the dying patient, for by definition your tools (and thus yourself, because we so often confuse ourselves with our tools) have failed. But if you believe your job is the care of the sick, then the dying patient represents a difficult and often painful challenge, but one that should not often make you feel helpless.

TOOLS FOR THE CARE OF THE DYING

The tools that are available in the care of patients with fatal illness are the same as elsewhere in medicine: diagnostic studies, drugs, technology and surgery for the control of symptoms and disease processes, command of support personnel and ancillary services, but above all, knowledge. Our knowledge is of several kinds: knowledge of the natural history of disease and of pathophysiology, knowledge of the psychology of illness, knowledge about the behavior of patients and their families, and knowledge about ourselves. Physicians do not usually include knowledge of the psychology of illness, the behavior of patients and their families, and knowledge of themselves in the list of their therapeutic tools, because they forget that they themselves are the primary agent in the care of the sick. Surgeons know how important is their judgment and the skill of their hands, and psychiatrists understand that it is they and their relationship with the patient that makes their knowledge work for the patient, but the rest of us have seemingly forgotten that. Antimicrobials are used for infection and antiarrhythmics for cardiac arrhythmia, but it is you, the physician who is using those drugs and working with your patient, who makes the patient better.

The second basic point about the care of the dying, then, is that it is physicians themselves, including their relationships with their patients, who are the primary agents of treatment. All the tools listed above are just that—tools in the service of the agent, or of the doctor and doctor-patient relationship. If learning to use yourself and the doctor-patient relationship consciously in the care of the dying is difficult, I promise you that it will increase your skill in the care of every other category of patient.

I suppose it is necessary to point out the difference between what I am speaking about and "hand holding" or "bedside manner." A hand holder is a doctor who sympathetically responds to patients' every whim, even while knowing that harm may be done to the patient—harm by not refusing some desire. Good doctor-patient relations can easily withstand the fact that sometimes pain, suffering, or even the painful truth are necessary for a long-term goal. Bedside manner is charm, and charm alone does not make patients better. On the other hand, neither does anticharm—the attitude of doctors who go out of their way to be gruff and tough so as not to seem soft. Optimally, then, everything that is done with the patient and the family is directed not only toward the patient's good, but also toward strengthening the doctor's relationship with the patient.[2,3,4]

Let us go back to Sally Gordon. (I usually ask patients, male or female, whether I can use their first name, because I am more comfortable that way. Other physicians are more comfortable always using last names. What is most comfortable for you and the patient is best.) As I said earlier, back pain precipitated the admission. Although I had reviewed the chart of the previous admission and had been briefed well by her surgeon, I listened and questioned her to get the story of the entire illness from her. Doing that not only gave me a review of the case, but told me what she considered important, both good and bad. Sometimes patients will ask, "Don't you have it in the records?" I say that I want to hear the story from *them*. In fact I do, but that also says that it is the person who is my interest, not just the disease or the record.

From her recitation, I learned that her back pain had gotten much worse after the orthopedist had pointed out the ascites and requested the bone scan. Although pain had been present for many years ("The doctors say my back is older than I am."), she had begun to connect back pain with the malignancy. I asked, "Had you had pain as bad as that in the past?" She said, "Just before the bleeding episode—not just before, about May [she bled in August], and it subsided after the surgery. I was hoping, foolishly, that that would take care of my back."

It is very common, once serious disease has been diagnosed, for patients to interpret everything that happens in the light of their illness. Even though the back pain had been around for years, it was now being connected, in her mind, to the malignancy. As you will see, the back pain, which was now connected by her to cancer (although the two are not related in this instance), was to be the key to establishing my relationship with Mrs. Gordon on a firm basis.

See also how she had begun to worry about her bowel movements. At this point I suspect, but do not know, that she is afraid of local recurrence and bowel obstruction because of the "dreaded colostomy." Later I discovered that her brother-in-law was dying of bowel cancer, and that it was his colostomy and her perception of his "awful state" that provided the spectre of her worries. Often we brush aside such fears as unrealistic, but we should not because they almost always have a basis in the patient's memories or associations. Thus even when we reassure someone because a worry is unfounded, we must keep the worry and its source in mind because it will probably return again. Worries are not random things; they are connected to one another and to what patients believe about the body, about causes of disease, and about what will happen to them. These fears often distort the sick person's perception of events and reporting of symptoms, and therefore our care. For optimum care in general, and especially with the dying, we need every clue and every bit of help we can get in managing the patient. With the dying, because there is often so little leverage against the disease, we must work as effectively as possible with the patient. For that we need to know all we can about the person. To understand the source of worries like Mrs. Gordon's, one has only to ask, "Why are you afraid of a colostomy? Do you know somebody who has had one?"

History also revealed some exertional dyspnea in the week or two prior to admission, which she dismissed as "nerves." When I was finished taking the history she said, "Of course, I'm terribly frightened and terribly nervous." I asked, "What are you frightened about?" She said, "Well, that it might be something serious." "Like what?" I questioned. She said, "Like an obstruction, or like another tumor, or like a malignancy." I replied, "Okay, then I guess we had better address ourselves to those things and make sure what is going on, so we know what to do and how to go about it."

The issue of truth telling had come up at a time when I was not ready to talk specifics. Discussions about what to tell the patient often neglect to point out that medical care is a process that takes place over time, and that patients ask questions or probe all through their care. Notice that I did not dismiss her concern or offer vague "reassurances" like "I'm sure everything will be okay." Rather, her worry was acknowledged and I declared my intent to go after the answers. By using "we," I suggested that we had mutual interests—she and I were becoming a "we" in her care.

Physical examination (in the presence of her daughter, which she seemed to wish) showed evidence of fluid in the right chest and obvious ascites. Also present was mottled red-brown skin on the right midback, the sign of overuse of a heating pad. There was a rash attributed to codeine allergy.

During the physical examination she said, "I'm awfully hard on myself. I always have been—I kind of whip myself. I've had a couple of nervous breakdowns, like." ("Crying, not eating," but no hospitalizations, and occurring at times of family stress.) I asked, "So far, how have you done, knowing that you had a cancer, being operated on, and all that?" "Great," she replied, "but this time I'm not as good as last time." "Why?" I asked. She said, "Because I have all those things to worry about that almost happened last time." "Like what?" I questioned. "Malignancy and going for tests and things like that and all those bad results," she replied.

The history and physical were over. I had obtained the story of her disease and its course, some idea of her background and her family (important to her consideration of the pleural effusion was her father's death from lung cancer), and some concept of what kind of a person she was. In addition, I knew what she had been told about her disease. It came up spontaneously, but if necessary I would have asked, "Can you tell me what your understanding of your disease is?" or "What have the other doctors told you about your illness?"

Such information will tell to what extent denial is operating, whether the patient has been told lies in the past, and is or is not aware of that. In addition, the depth of the patient's medical knowledge is made clear, so that I do not underestimate or overestimate her knowledge, or get out of step with the other physicians or care takers. All these facts enter into the decision about what and how she should be told.

GOALS OF TREATMENT

All this information is necessary to establish the goals of treatment.[4,5,6] In the care of patients with fatal illness, determining short- and long-term goals is as vital as in every other illness or treatment situation. Death is inevitable, but here, as elsewhere in medical care, the overriding goal is that the patient and physician remain as much in command of the situation as fate allows. Neither the patient nor the doctor should have the feeling that the disease is dragging them around the way a cat worries a cornered mouse, for that is the feeling of helplessness and loss of control. In the patient, such feelings lead to depression, despair, and suffering. Patients in that state can be almost unmanageable, and often will not do the simplest things to help themselves. A doctor who feels helpless and out of control generally avoids the patient and the situation that promote those feelings, which, though understandable, simply makes things worse.

To repeat: the overriding goal of treatment is to give patients a sense of control over their fate. It does not matter how short or restricted life may be. In the treatment process, the physician is the patient's agent. The other goals to be discussed are in the service of the primary aim of control. A patient should die the person he or she is. The subsidiary goals are (1) the control of the disease or disease manifestations to the extent feasible—not necessarily to prolong life, but to improve comfort or function, or to determine mode or place of death; (2) the control of symptoms, and teaching the patient how to manage symptoms; (3) when possible, to smooth and ease relations with other family members so that the family is able to deal better with the dying patient before death, as well as with their own feelings after the death; and (4) to achieve the best possible prognostication. This does not necessarily mean predicting the length of survival, which is often incorrect, but it does mean attempting to predict what symptoms will occur, their timing, and their response to treatment. Uncertainty in these matters is well known, but it should be remembered that no matter how uncertain the physician is, patients are more so—and it is their needs that are being met.

Often the first thing to do is to conduct studies that determine the extent of the disease. The care of terminal patients requires as much knowledge of disease and disease processes as the care of other patients. Knowing just where we stand prepares us best to meet all our goals. However, the choice of diagnostic studies and procedures should be only in the service of the goals described above. The best test of necessity for any procedure is whether the outcome will alter action, or alter what is told to the patient. In addition, the timing of procedures should take into account the patient's fears and concerns. Things are rarely so urgent for the patient with a fatal disease.

An extensive disease workup was carried out over the next 2 days with Mrs. Gordon. It included bone and liver scans, chest films, and blood studies. She refused a projected barium enema. On my next visit, I found almost a different person. Initially, although self-described as nervous, she was in command of herself, listened, and gave thoughtful answers to questions; she had an almost sprightly, but definitely self-determined, air. Now I found her to be groaning, "whiney," almost aggressively pitiful. Such patients have a quality that would frustrate a saint. It says, "Help me—but I know you cannot." What had brought about the change was fear. In the course of the tests and the paracentesis, her fear of malignancy and disability had been reawakened. Fear could have been enlarged by the fact of the test themselves, or even by someone's thoughtless comment. Such things often happen, and are beyond our control, although we must deal with the consequences. Fear is never made to go away by telling the patient not to be afraid, or "don't worry." Fear is controlled by exposing it and relieving it at its source. Sometimes that is as simple as correcting misinformation. One of my patients, who was not frightened about his metastatic disease to the liver, became very fearful that he had "cancer of the lymph nodes." A physician examining him had spent an inordinate time searching for cervical lymph nodes, and had then called a colleague to check something. Both left the bedside without a word to the patient, except that they had been "looking for lymph nodes."

In this instance, the back pain was the focus of Mrs. Gordon's distress and groaning. I knew that to return control to her, to establish the fact that she could be in control of pain, and to show her that I was going to help her, I would have to relieve the pain. It is not uncommon to find patients in that pitiful state when they have cancer or other diseases that they believe to be fatal. They whine or groan or just lie apathetically.[7] On other occasions, they are abusive to their family or to the staff. Whatever the behavior, it generally alienates the nurses and doctors; that makes the patient feel not only more helpless, but also abandoned. Almost invariably, there is one symptom on which the distress is focused. While anything may be considered intolerable—from impacted feces to dyspnea—pain is most commonly the key. Characteristically, the patient is suffering not merely the pain or dyspnea of the moment, but sees him- or herself as having to live that way forever—as never being free from the pain. That may also annoy and distance the physician, because the objective findings may not seem to warrant the suffering.

I started to discuss pain medications with Mrs. Gordon. As is characteristic of patients in this state, nothing would satisfy her. Codeine gave her a rash; propoxyphene was too weak; Percodan made her dizzy; meperidine was too strong; she was afraid of morphine. My dominant feelings became frustration and anger at trying to help out, but being told I was helpless. She said, "Maybe taking out the liquid [she had had a diagnostic paracentesis] did it, but if anything, don't you think it would relieve it a little?" I replied, "It has nothing to do with it. Your back is your back—you've had that back for 15 years. Your back is not cancer. Your back is not fluid. Your back is not any one of those things. Your back is not dying." She said, "But what is it? It's incapacitating me and my life and my husband and everything." I said that we had better solve it, and she said, "Yeah, but there may not be any solution. It's taking me over."

The back pain was the key. I found a trigger point[8] in the right infraspinatus, injected it with 10 ml of 2 percent xylocaine, and relieved the pain. I also gave her 50 mg meperidine and 25 mg IM chlorpromazine at the same time. I chose the small dose of meperidine because she was afraid of being "out of this world." If it had been insufficient, I would have increased the meperidine with every 3-hourly dose until pain control had been achieved. Had she not expressed fear of being too groggy, I would have started with 100 mg of meperidine. The order was written "every 3 hours unless patient refuses," rather than as needed (p.r.n.), because I did not want the patient to remain in pain or be at the mercy of a nurse who felt that the patient should avoid narcotics. The usual constraints on analgesics, narcotic or otherwise, have no place in the care of the dying patient. She received only two doses that day, and two the next day, and required none further. She refused the chlorpromazine after the first dose, because she felt it made her too sleepy. By the third day, the pain of 15 years was gone, and never returned in a meaningful way through the remainder of her illness.

How had that happened? For 15 years she had been told by physicians and her family that the pain was "arthritis" or "nerves." While emotional tension may produce pain (generally muscular), pain is not emotional. Pain is pain, and the physical source can generally be found and the symptom treated. If it has been present long enough, it will produce alteration in gait, habitus, or habits that help perpetuate the pain. But, if the patient is willing, a source of intervention can usually be found through careful questioning and physical examination. Too many of us have been so thoroughly trained to treat diseases, not symptoms, that we never learn how to treat symptoms. Yet most of our patients do not have "real diseases"; they have symptoms. In the dying patient, whose disease cannot be cured, successful management demands symptom relief.

Several things had been accomplished with Mrs. Gordon. I said I would help her, and I did; the basis for my relationship with her had been established. The doctor-patient relationship is complex, but trust is the cornerstone. Patients generally enter the relationship expecting to trust. There are instances where, because of previous experiences in life or with physicians, the patient is unable to trust. The job is very much more difficult then, because unless some element of trust can be developed, almost none of the goals I am describing can be met. The best way to encourage trust is to show that you care and will come through on a promise. The obverse is not to promise what you cannot do. But if the promises are kept small and honest enough—even a night's sleep for someone who has not slept, or the delay of a dreaded procedure—patients will begin to believe that you, the physician, care about them, are dependable, and are in control of the situation. I dwell on this because the patient's wants are often trivially simple from a technical standpoint, and yet are vital to him or her. Those who have not been seriously ill may not appreciate what even mild distress over a long period can mean, and what profound gratitude can follow relief. Furthermore, the symptom, as in this instance, may have nothing to do with the disease. What counts is not only what the doctor believes necessary, but what the patient thinks is important.

Diagnostic studies of Mrs. Gordon revealed a right pleural effusion, ascites, abnormal liver scan, normal liver chemistries, and normal bone scan. Barium enema, when she felt ready for it, was normal. Cytology of the ascites showed no malignant cells. A thoracentesis removed 2 liters of fluid, also with negative cytology. The normal findings were reported to her and to her husband. Her self-control had returned, and she was again the person I first met. She still had doubts about her back pain (how could she not—it had been present on and off for so long), but she could not dispute that, between the infiltration of xylocaine and the analgesics, the pain had been controlled. After discussing the negative findings, I said, "It is possible that fluid may reaccumulate in your chest and/or abdomen, even though we did not definitely tie it to the cancer. The question has not been resolved. There are ways of keeping the fluid from reaccumulating, and we are going to have Dr. Faber [an oncologist] come to see you to help make a decision about the best way to approach this." She said, "I hope it is not going to be surgery." The fear of surgery, and notably of a colostomy, reemerged. I could honestly reply, "No, it's not." There was further discussion about how thoracentesis could be managed as an outpatient, and how she could learn to manage her own medications. I reiterated, "What I'm telling you is that my expectation is that your problems will not be over when you get out of this hospital—that you may accumulate fluid in your chest or belly, even without a diagnosis of cancer. Some kinds of tumors leave that effect behind them." She became anxious and said, "Is there a question of a tumor?"

"You were operated on for one, weren't you?" I said.

"No, I mean now, presently," She answered.

"No," I told her.

"Oh," she said, obviously relieved.

"But," I went on, "there is a question in your mind, and everybody else's mind, as to whether this has anything to do with the cancer you had before, isn't there?"

"Right," she said, pointing to her abdomen. "But this doesn't bother me. It worried me and it worried my husband." Some further conversation ensued, and I said again that Dr. Faber would see her.

"He's the lung man?" she asked.

"No, he's not," I replied, "he's a cancer specialist, and we need his advice." She grimaced and groaned. I said, "I'll tell you what—we'll call him a dermatologist."

"Nope, you said it, and that's what he is." She smiled.

"Hiding the word won't make it go away," I said to her. "When the word is out in the open, it's just what the word is. When the word is back there in your head, it's hell and damnation."

TRUTH TELLING

With the completion of initial studies, the findings had to be discussed with the patient and her family. The question of "truth telling," around which there has been so much controversy, had arisen.[1,9,10,11]

Surveys of physicians' attitudes[1,11] have shown that a small percentage never tell their patients the diagnosis and prognosis, and a larger percentage always tell their patients, but the majority of physicians indicated a flexible attitude. This largest group discussed the diagnosis as depending upon the type of patient, patient attitude, personality, and so on. Things are changing, I believe, and truth telling is becoming the dominant mode. But, as the previous conspiracy of silence often produced great harm, so, too, can the unvarnished truth.

For example, a 36-year-old attractive, divorced mother of two had an unsightly small lesion on the skin of her chest. Her physician removed it in the office, and sent it to the pathologist. The lesion was reported as benign, but the pathologist called the physician and said that there were a few cells that suggested mycosis fungoides. The physician then described the disease and its course to the woman in detail, ending with, "but we will always be able to keep you comfortable." Discussing the visit, she said, "He told me more about mycosis fungoides than I ever wanted to know." It took 2 weeks to put the matter to rest. The slides were submitted to a nationally known skin pathologist, who dismissed the lesion as trivial. In those 2 weeks, every mark on her skin was seen by the woman as a portent of a dreadful death. And every fear and fantasy was related to her life situation as the sole caretaker of two young children and as one who was at the start of a new career.

That is an example of a kind of mindless truth telling that appears to be becoming more and more prevalent. But did her physician tell her the truth? Or did he unburden himself of his own anxieties? Seemingly more the latter.

What is the truth in these matters? Is the truth that Mrs. Gordon has metastatic carcinoma from the bowel to the ovary, with evidence of continued disease activity from which she will surely die? That would seem to be a true statement. But suppose I told you of a patient who fit that description, and asked what I should do for her tomorrow? Or next week? You would surely ask for more information. The true statement about Sally Gordon contains remarkably little information on which to *act* (nor do statements like "Hodgkin's disease, stage IIA," "oat cell carcinoma of the lung," or even "congestive heart failure"). Those are diagnostic statements, but one cannot act on them without more information, such as: who is the patient, what is the duration of illness, has it been treated or untreated, and so on. Those diagnostic terms are a shorthand that unlocks a mine of information about cause, course, pathophysiology, treatment, and more—information that is changing all the time, as the physician learns more. Because we, and patients, have become so used to those shorthand symbols, we confuse them with the thing for which they stand—information.

The real issue is, how much information does the patient require? What information does the patient want, and how much information is needed in order to make the patient an effective partner in his or her care?

The world is changing. Modern medical care requires a partnership between physician and patient. That may not have been so when treatment was exemplified by penicillin for pneumonia, because penicillin worked whether the patient cooperated or not. But in the case of chronic illness or long-term disease, patients themselves must do most of the things involved in their treatment, from taking potent medications correctly to following dietary or exercise regimens. And only an informed patient who feels like a partner in the process can be expected to participate fully.

Nowhere is that more true than in the patient with fatal disease who must do that most difficult but deeply rewarding thing: die well.

THE FUNCTION OF INFORMATION

The crucial issue to be resolved is the function of information. All animals, including humans, have a fundamental need to act. *The functions of information are to reduce uncertainty and to provide a basis for action.* The two functions are inextricably related. When this is understood, knowing what and how to inform patients becomes, if not easy, then easier. The basic problem faced in life is uncertainty about what to do. Moment to moment, week to week, and year after year, uncertainty exists at every turn. Wherever uncertainty exists, it is reduced by information. There are multiple sources of information. We generally think of the environment, the world around us, as the primary information source, but it is only one, because uncertainty is not only about facts. (Is diastole clear? Is the breast mass harder?, etc.) It is also about intent; the intent of an utterance, an act, or a person. And uncertainty also exists about causes and outcomes—why did this happen to me, and what will happen next? The world around will not necessarily, perhaps not usually, supply enough information, and consequently, other sources become important. Knowledge, from whatever source, stored in memory; unconscious or repressed needs, desires, fears, or fantasies; previous beliefs about how the world (and disease) works, including causes and outcomes, are sources of information. Other people are also important sources of information, and the most reliable others are not necessarily the most knowledgeable (from the physician's point of view), but rather those whom the person believes are most like him or her, or who have the same basic interests in the matter at hand. Which is why patients will often heed the advice of a neighbor in preference to that of a physician, despite the doctor's obviously greater factual knowledge.

There is one other way in which uncertainty is reduced, which is vitally important to the relation between doctor and patient. That source is faith or trust in another person—in our situation, the physician. A few moments reflection will show that in terribly important things like serious illness, there is never quite enough information to reduce uncertainty about the right thing to do, or about the future, completely. This is particularly true since those information sources listed above may produce conflicting answers—especially when the unconscious or repressed needs, desires, fears, or fantasies have been added (this is why, despite their knowledge, when physicians are sick, they are patients). In this setting of irreducible uncertainty, faith in the certainty of the doctor helps to solve the problem.

All of us have patients whose blind faith in our performance is disturbing, since we know how fallible we are. Attempts to dissuade such patients are useless, since their faith is not based on our performance alone, but on their need. Their need often arises from great fear and distrust of their body, which is seen as a mysterious source of danger. This is true in health or in minor illness, and doubly so in serious or fatal illness. Thus, the patient's incredible trust in the doctor's knowledge and certitude is virtually his or her only source of safety in a sea of uncertainty. The danger is that the physician may come to believe the patient's view, and may start to have the same faith in personal omniscience. But another danger is that the doctor may become so uncomfortable in occupying a role that is not and cannot be true, that he or she breaks the trust simply to be rid of the burden. This kind of trust in physicians explains why a patient may become very angry with a doctor when the doctor makes an error that is small in itself and in its consequences. The anger is not so much with the physician for being fallible (which is something everybody knows), but with oneself as the patient for being so dependent upon the doctor and so fearful of the body.

The basic point is, however, that physicians cannot disown the trust of their patients without destroying their effectiveness. They can only understand it as an aspect of the doctor-patient relationship that they must learn to use.

TRUTH TELLING REVISITED

Now that we understand that information reduces uncertainty and permits action, let us look again at the problem of truth telling. Did the physician who told the woman about mycosis fungoides reduce her uncertainty? No, he increased it markedly. Did he indicate, with his information, a direction of action? No action or decision was required, but he did put in doubt all the actions in which she was presently engaged—job, new life direction, child raising, and so on. Did he increase the patient's trust in him as a physician and promote the relationship? No, he destroyed it.

The question of truth telling remains, but now in a different form. Information is one of the therapeutic tools of the physician. The amount and degree of detail, the kind, its timing and truth content must depend upon the needs of the patient, the clinical situation, and the relation between doctor and patient. But each item must meet three tests.

1 Will it reduce the patient's uncertainty now or in the future?
2 Will it improve the patient's ability to act in his or her own best interest now or in the future?
3 Will it improve the doctor-patient relationship, the basic therapeutic modality, now or in the future?

And in all of this, the physician must remember that he or she is but one source of information, and that the other sources are generally not known to the physician.

Before returning to test this discussion against the case of Mrs. Gordon, let me venture the opinion that an outright lie will very rarely meet the tests outlined above. But in the case of fatal disease, or its possibility, the whole truth in all the detail the physician knows, now and into the future, without reference to the patient, will almost never meet those tests.

Any discussion of what to tell patients inevitably raises the question of denial. Denial does not have a very good reputation these days. In these times, everybody is supposed to know everything, and everything must be put into words, or so it seems to me. What a pity! Denial of the unpleasant is a universal psychological mechanism that can be extremely useful. It takes about 1 week of clinical experience to see patients successfully use denial to protect themselves from painful truths that are apparently so obvious that denial should be impossible. Some of the current objections to denial are a reaction of our public against the tendency of some physicians not to communicate with their patients. But that is not the whole story. The basic problem presented by denial is that a lie is involved—telling oneself an untruth. The classic instance is that of the patient with cancer on a cancer ward who tells the visitor how lucky the patient is to be well because, after all, everybody else on the ward has cancer. We stand in awe of such a belief in the face of a constantly assaulting reality. Unfortunately, for denial to remain intact, the onlookers must also lie—the family, the nurses, the doctors, and all others who know the truth. They must all watch their words, and be discreet, both in conversation and in chart notation. With the burden goes responsibility. The use of denial by a patient means that those around must share in the responsibility of protecting from pain. I believe that it is the attempt to avoid that difficult responsibility that has played a part in causing denial to be a disvalued mode for dealing with fatal illness or death. When we hear a physician simply telling the patient the "whole truth," we must wonder whether the doctor is not simply escaping responsibility and burdens, rather than doing something that is primarily in the interest of the patient.

Denial takes many forms: simply not hearing what has been said, avoiding all conversation by absence or by changing the subject, forgetting details in whole or in part, or interpreting in a benign manner what one would have believed could only have a terrible import. Even the word usage of a patient may indicate denial where the patient apparently knows the whole truth (see Chapter 3).

Such language usage by patients is very common, and because of that, it is very difficult to hear. It is an example of how partial denial can be maintained by a patient who knows the truth. Similarly, the patient may seem, like Sally Gordon, to know the whole story, yet selectively deny some features of the illness.

Since denial is a process occurring over time, patients may gradually remember what was told to them or ask for more information at a later date when they are better able to deal with it. Patients' right to deny is as basic as their right to be told the truth. The fundamental right of patients in such matters is to have their wishes respected, whether or not the doctor agrees. Understanding patients' wishes in this regard can only come about through give and take, through interaction occurring over time. For that reason, discussions should go slowly, with the doctor eliciting questions that can then be answered, rather than merely telling the facts. If there is doubt about whether the patient really wants the answer, the doctor can supply a partial but true answer, and elicit further questions to ensure what the patient wants. It is always possible to ask the patient, "What do you mean?" It has been amply demonstrated that when a patient really asks, he or she really wants to know.

While taking a history from Sally Gordon, I learned that she knew that the original lesion had been malignant ("Of course it was malignant . . ."), but also that she had been reassured that "they got everything and all the radiologists and everybody said there was no concern for treatment and everything was fine." But, let us suppose that I had been the physician who discussed things with her after the original surgery. Could I have lied to her at that time? To do so would have required explaining a bowel resection for a pelvic mass, perhaps on the basis of "inflammation." Two things would have put the lie in jeopardy. First, the original gynecologist had said, "I feel something . . . and you're in trouble," and, when asked if it meant a hysterectomy, replied, "It's a lot more than that." Secondly, the finding at operation so surely indicated future recurrence that I would want to avoid undermining her future trust in me.

By the time findings had to be reviewed, I had learned four important facts about Mrs. Gordon that had bearing on the discussion. First, that she had handled the news about malignancy well after her surgery. But this time, she was not doing so well because of her "fears of an obstruction, or, like another tumor, or like a malignancy." Those fears of another bowel tumor had been expressed repeatedly. The meaning and source of those fears were not known to me, and are an example of information coming from another source. Second, her father had died of lung cancer. Third, her brother-in-law, who had had a colostomy because of colon cancer, was doing poorly. Such previous experience with a disease provided information that patients may bring to bear on their own illnesses, and that may contradict what the physician says unless it is confronted. Fourth, she related a history of periods of depression that were related to family crises and required psychiatric care, but not hospitalization.

This last is of particular importance. The reason most often given by physicians for not telling the truth to patients is the fear that the patient will not be able to "take it." Included is the belief that some patients may commit suicide upon hearing that they have cancer. The evidence does not support this fear.[12] While patients' previous life adjustment unquestionably has an effect on the manner with which they deal with terminal illness,[13,14] previous emotional illness is not in itself a contraindication to imparting true information. Since information is always being transmitted, the question for the "unstable" just as for the stable individual is whether the information meets the goals described above. To protect someone from painful information in a manner that increases uncertainty and paralyzes action because it conflicts with other sources of information[10] hardly supports their personality or reduces stress.

In the actual discussion with the patient, I was quite frank. I discussed the negative findings, including the (surprisingly) negative pleural and ascitic fluid cytology. I asserted that no tumor recurrence was evident. Here the definition of tumor was hers, not mine. There was, indeed, no evidence of recurrent bowel tumor. But, as noted above, the point was important. While it may be, indeed often is, necessary to educate a patient to the meaning of a word as used by physicians, it is also necessary to remain within the patients' usage. Where a particular word is crucial to the discussion, it is essential to ensure that both physician and patient have the same understanding, which is best done by asking, "What do you mean by . . .?"

While denying the presence of recurrent tumor, I made no attempt to avoid the words "malignant" or "cancer." Nor did I hide the possible relationship of her present findings to the previous cancer. Indeed, I demonstrated that just such a fear already existed in her mind and in her husband's. Furthermore, I insisted that Dr. Faber be called a cancer specialist, because I knew that he does not conceal that fact himself. Furthermore, what I said about a word like "cancer" is true. In the open, it is just a word—unspoken, it operates as a symbol of dread.

In all this discussion, I not only told what I thought the future would bring, but discussed in detail what it would mean (in the short run) to her, and how she could be taught to manage the problem with the help of her physicians. Thus I reduced the uncertainty of the immediate future—even though unpleasant—and connected it to positive action on her part. Thus I emphasized her control.

One final word about relating information. The discussion with the patient avoided euphemisms—words like "active," "suspicious," "condition," "nasty," "mitosis," when what is meant is cancer. There are times when euphemisms are useful, but what they generally do is signal to the patient that the doctor is afraid to use the actual word, because in everyday speech euphemisms serve that function (for example, bathroom tissue). The conventions of everyday communication do not cease because serious matters are under discussion. In fact, doctors are often afraid to use such language. The doctor must learn that to tell someone he or she has cancer does not mean that the doctor gave it to them. In addition, the use of the actual word by the physician indicates that he or she is not afraid of the word and is larger than the word, and that is reassuring to patients.

The day following the frank discussion, Mrs. Gordon's spirits were excellent. Her back pain was not severe, she had been experimenting with medications, and she was finding it easier and less troublesome than she had expected. Doctors do not expect to find patients in good spirits after such conversations. The more usual instance is the following. A woman of 69 was operated on for carcinoma of the ascending colon. At surgery, extensive local and metastatic disease was present. Her husband had died of cancer a year and a half earlier, and had not been told the truth. That had been extremely distressing to her. Three days after surgery, I found her deeply distressed. At her urging, the surgeon had been truthful with her. Most of us are familiar with the scene and know its consequences. The patient wants honesty, but in its trail comes depression, long postoperative recovery, and more severe or prolonged pain than that following surgery for nonfatal disease. That sad picture is one of the reasons why physicians often try to avoid honesty.

But in that and similar instances, the truth does not reduce uncertainty or point to action, but rather the contrary. It raises questions. Will I have pain? Will I be able to take it? Will I be a burden to my son? Will I die slowly? Should I call my sister back from Ireland? And so on. *No piece of information should be imparted unless the physician is prepared to answer the questions raised by the information, and to teach the patient how to act against the consequences.* If no questions are asked by the patient when common sense or experience suggests that the information imparted should raise questions, then the doctor should elicit the questions or even suggest them, if necessary. The process of imparting information is not complete until the facts, possible consequences, and alternative actions have been specified.

Why, then, was Mrs. Gordon in better spirits after the conversation than before? Because the information *reduced* uncertainty. It did not raise it. The uncertainties already existed in her mind (and in her husband's). She was already worried. But her worries were focused on phantoms and fears arising from her imagination. Concrete reality is rarely worse than imagined fears. If you wonder what fears and uncertainties are raised by what has been told to the patient, you need only ask to find out. With experience, one finds that the same questions arise again and again.

I asked Mrs. Gordon, "Sally, what are you frightened of? What are you scared of when you're scared?"

"Well, if it's a malignancy, then I have maybe just so long to be around, and . . . " she hesitated.

"And?" I said. "Is that what you're frightened of, dying?"

"Yeah. I'd like to be around for a little while longer." Her voice was positive.

"Well, I can understand that," I said.

"And," she continued, "I also have seen people have treatment that have been miserable."

In common with many others, she was more afraid of the suffering and misery of treatment than she was of dying. But patients treated in the manner I am describing do not have the suffering and misery that worried Sally, because that suffering and misery comes more from the feeling of helplessness and hopelessness than from the treatment or the disease. I could and did offer positive reassurance on that point.

No attempt was made to conceal our uncertainty about her actual status, nor our belief that the underlying cause of recurrent serosal transudates was most probably the previous malignancy.

Toward the end of the discussion I said, "Let me tell you again—even if it turns out that you are dying, which doesn't seem to be the case now, even if that's the case, it still has to be managed, doesn't it? Even when you know you're dying, you don't just blow away. You have day by day to go, and you have to learn how to manage that."

Dr. Faber, the oncologist, agreed that, despite the negative cytology of pleural and ascitic fluid, she should be treated as someone with metastatic cancer from the bowel, given 5-fluorouracil 15 mg per kg intravenously for 3 days, and then continued on chronic chemotherapy every 10 days to 2 weeks.

A pneumothorax followed the thoracentesis. This did not clear, and by the fifth day the air had increased, suggesting a bronchopleural leak. A chest tube was inserted, which functioned poorly and had to be replaced. Sufficient quantities of fluid drained so that it was evident that the chest would probably refill promptly after the tube was withdrawn. Therefore 20 mg of nitrogen mustard was instilled through the tube, which was clamped for 6 hours and withdrawn the following day. Parenteral 5-fluorouracil was started. The patient tolerated all the considerable discomforts of the tube and the nitrogen mustard extremely well. Increasingly, she learned how to manage pain, what drugs to use, and how to time them. Thus, even though the experience was unpleasant, it served to reinforce how much control she had over her situation, and how competent she could be. Each event that occurs can be used by the doctor to make the same point. If nausea or vomiting is to be anticipated, then the patient is instructed in the control of them. In each instance, the patient's trust in the physician's reliability and prognostic accuracy is increased. Since the doctor is predicting small and short-run events that are usually quite familiar to him or her, the chance of accuracy is considerable. Where uncertainty is present or alternative possibilities exist, these too should be mentioned. Doing this calls on a phenomenon known to Hippocrates. To the patient, accurate prognostication of even unpleasant events shows the physician's mastery of events and disease almost to the same degree as the ability to cure. It is in the nature of the doctor-patient relationship that when the doctor is in control, so is the patient.

DEFINITIVE THERAPY IN TERMINAL ILLNESS

This phase of her illness brings up the question of definitive therapies in the patient with fatal disease or terminal illness. Here, as elsewhere in medical practice, one chooses therapies to achieve a set goal. I do not like to do things whose aim is solely "to do something," although occasionally, because of family or other pressures, that becomes necessary. With Mrs. Gordon, chronic chemotherapy was chosen because it occasionally slows the progress of disease, and its mode of administration and side effects usually do not create other problems. For advanced disease with widespread metastases and terminal illness, it would have had no advantage. On the contrary, even minimal slowing of the disease process might prolong the patient's dying and distress, although I will discuss that in greater detail later.

The nitrogen mustard offered a chance of stopping recurrent pleural effusion, and is an example of a treatment aimed at a specific symptom or manifestation that in itself causes major problems. Dyspnea is a difficult symptom to manage, since the fear of choking to death that it evokes is so primitive. Patients can be taught, with difficulty, how to avoid the almost automatic body responses (such as the "asthma position" of shoulders up and forward, with hands on knees), which increase anxiety and increase the severity of the symptom. Morphine, in small doses, is also useful, and can be easily self-administered subcutaneously. Oxygen in the home also provides comfort. Whatever reduces the anxiety also reduces the severity of the symptom. Where repeated thoracenteses become necessary, considerable ingenuity may be required to make them innocuous. Although they are to be avoided, problems of infection are of less importance than in patients with benign disease.

Persistent bleeding from the bowel or incipient intestinal obstruction may be reasons for bowel resection even in the face of metastatic disease. With these decisions the physician is, in essence, choosing one mode of death over another. Such choices must take into account many variables, from the suspected time of survival (usually longer than one thinks) to patients' fears—of surgery, costs, home situations—specific desires, and so on. Those many factors, which are almost always present in serious illness, are perhaps nowhere more important than in fatal illness.

Since the primary goal is to maintain maximum function and freedom from interference by the disease and by medical care, and to keep the patient in as much control of his or her circumstances as possible, some disease manifestations are more to be avoided than others. Metastatic disease to the spine, aside from causing pain, may lead to cord compressions and subsequent paraplegia. Thus, radiation therapy is often indicated, even if prospective survival time is quite short. Disease progression at such sites may be very rapid. Thus, alertness to any symptom indicative of spinal disease or neurological involvement is necessary. Other areas of bony involvement may also produce pain or predispose to pathologic fracture, and can often be radiated with benefit. Radiation to the upper lumbar spine will usually be accompanied by nausea, against which the patient should be forewarned and forearmed with enough medication and detailed instructions for its use. Antiemetics given before the nausea is expected are more effective than medication started after nausea or vomiting has started.

Alertness to symptoms poses a problem. Early in the course of the illness, patients may interpret any symptom, however remote or commonplace, as a sign of the return or progression of the disease—remember how Mrs. Gordon connected her long-standing back pain to her malignancy. Much of the physician's time with the patient will be spent in providing reassurance. Nonetheless, one wants to know what symptoms are present, and the interest of the doctor always gives a symptom more importance to the patient. Patients in bad situations, indeed all of us, always give the worst interpretation to every word or clue; therefore the physician may have to say specifically why certain questions have been asked. We do not want patients to feel that their lives are literally hanging on our words, or connected to a chest x-ray or blood count, for that is a terrible state. We are trying to focus on living, not merely by lectures, but by providing the tools to keep their illness at a minimum. Sometimes that can be very difficult. For example, a single woman in her forties had a mastectomy for comedo carcinoma. Within 2 years, she had developed asymptomatic pulmonary metastases. The nodules melted away after bilateral oophorectomy. (She asked, "Why do they call it castration when ovaries are taken out for this reason, but oophorectomy when done for other reasons?''—a good question.) During all this time she was well and functioning and her career burgeoned, but she was overwhelmed by fears. After each chest x-ray, she would break into tears when told it was negative. She always wanted to know ''her percentages'' (something I avoid), and even called the American Cancer Society to find the average length of remission after oophorectomy. Each visit to my office was agony. Two years after the oophorectomy, she was apparently free of disease. Meeting her surgeon, I told him how well she was doing. ''Is she enjoying these extra years of life,'' he asked, ''or are they more years of dying?'' ''More years of dying, I'm sad to say,'' I replied. I could not seem to teach her what I am describing in this chapter. But then something happened. The oncologist who had been our consultant, and for whom we all had affection and admiration, died suddenly of myocardial infarction. His death was sad to me, but it was to her the lesson that finally made the point that death may happen to anyone; it is living that counts. The pulmonary nodules returned about 6 months later, and she handled it well. She took an active part in the choice of appropriate therapy, and sought advice carefully. She has now been on calusterone for about 3 years, and is apparently free of disease. Her body fears are not gone, but the added years are years of life.

One is always balancing the benefit of diagnostic studies, doctors' visits, questions, and so forth, against the goals. Flexibility is the key.

PSYCHIATRIC ILLNESS IN FATAL DISEASE

Mrs. Gordon went home to Alabama and to her previous life. She did well, and had no difficulty with the chronic 5-fluorouracil. Psychiatric symptoms arose that were similar to those she had experienced in previous years. She consulted a psychiatrist near her home, who felt that she had every good reason to be depressed. She was, after all, dying. Her family physician and others shared that opinion. I did not. While depression may be common in patients with fatal disease, it is by no means inevitable. There has been considerable discussion about depression in the dying patient,[15,16,17] but it is important to distinguish symptoms that are a necessary part of the illness from those that come from its treatment. We believed previously that prolonged fatigability was a necessary sequela of myocardial infarction. It ceased to be common when patients were no longer maintained at bedrest for many weeks. Sadness, unhappiness, anger, or other emotions may all occupy the patient from time to time, as they do the rest of us. Depression may also be present, but in patients who have been treated in the manner I am describing, it is usually brief. When present, it is generally proximate to the original illness, to a recurrence, or to a particularly difficult aspect of the disease.

Why should Mrs. Gordon have become depressed when she did? She was functioning well and aside from poor appetite (which she liked), she was essentially free of symptoms. It appeared more likely that her depression was associated with emotional problems that were either unrelated to or only peripherally related to her malignancy. That turned out to be the case when she successfully sought other psychiatric care. The error is to see the dying patient as so totally occupied in the dying process that no other emotional stresses seem pertinent. Mrs. Gordon's depression was due to the same kind of emotional material that had precipitated it in years past when she did not have cancer. The patient with fatal disease, even when that disease is terminal, has as much right to relief of emotional pain as any other person, and much has been written on the subject.[5,18,19] Furthermore, the usual rules of privacy and confidentiality should be observed with dying patients as with others.[5]

Psychotropic agents such as the tricyclic antidepressants can improve these patients profoundly, just as phenothiazines or minor tranquilizers may help control anxiety.[2,17,20] However, one should be careful when using minor tranquilizers like the benzodiazepams, meprobamate, or barbiturates, which have a sedative effect. Sometimes the patient's anxiety or agitation comes from the physical confinement of the illness, if this was a previously active person. The sedatives slow the patient's activity further, and that slowing may increase depression, agitation, or anxiety. In such instances phenothiazines are better.

THE FAMILY

The family of the patient may also require considerable help in adjusting to the coming death. When one family member is seriously ill, family dynamics change.[21] Relationships may be so disrupted that the family unit does not recover, whether the sick person lives or dies. On occasion, long-standing conflicts disappear, and everyone seems closer and happier. During remissions the old battles can reemerge in those families, but because of the preceding peace the battles now seem worse than ever. The basic point is that when there is sickness in one member of the family, the family unit itself may become sick, and you may have to give thought to the others. All the psychological mechanisms that appear in the patient, from denial to anger, occur in the family and are frequently directed at the physician. Anger and suspiciousness can be difficult to deal with. The family sometimes views the doctor, hospital, nurses, or anybody caring for the relative as "them," the enemy from which the patient must be protected. They question every medication and decision. If the doctor is extremely open, they seize with hostility any expression of doubt or indecision. If the doctor is closed to them, they bombard him or her with unanswerable questions. Frequently, such families will play one physician against another, thereby placing considerable strain on staff relationships. Such behavior tends to personify all injury. If family members feel pain or distress, it is because some person has done it to them. The hurt and sadness of the impending death are often not seen for what they are, the reaction to the loss of a loved one, but rather what others are doing to them directly. The physician is the prime target. And they may use every wrong act of every physician all the way back to Hippocrates as current evidence—injury is timeless. In these situations, which fortunately are not common, I am extremely uncomfortable. When anger alone is the emotion, it has sometimes helped to point out that it is easier to be angry with me than with the real enemy, fate or disease. But in the face of the whole battery of anger and suspiciousness, inter-pretation is rarely useful. When that happens, then I must try doubly hard to re-main open to the patient, who rarely shares in the behavior. In these litigious times, there is no question that such family actions can impair the quality of care that the patient receives. It helps, however, to keep one's eyes focused on the pa-tient and the patient alone.

In the more usual instance, even though the sick person remains my primary responsibility, I try to meet family needs also. Direct conflict most often appears at the point of truth telling. The family may say that the patient "can't take it." But it is often not clear who cannot take what, and it is necessary to make delicate inquiries to find out where the problem lies. I try to explain to the family what my goals are, how information functions, and how I handle telling the patient. If conflict remains, I do what I think best for the patient.

On one occasion, the family flatly and adamantly refused permission for me to tell the sick mother what her state was. I went along with their wishes. Her disease, metastatic tumor to the brain, progressed and the patient, who appeared to know very well that she was dying, became more depressed. She was dis-charged from the hospital after radiation therapy, but returned a month or so later with acute bacterial pneumonia. Without the pneumonia she did not have many weeks to live, and this acute illness, untreated, would have been a kind end. Against my advice the children refused permission to leave the pneumonia un-treated. The infection cleared rapidly with antibiotics. One day as I saw her on my rounds, I was struck by what a sorry sight she was. Slumped down in the bed, with I.V. tubings and the other paraphernalia of acute disease connected, with her left hand restrained because she had attempted to remove the I.V., apathetic and watching me intently, she looked like most other dying patients in the modern hospital—what my patients used to look like before I began treating them as I am describing here. I had forgotten how awful it was. What a miserable way to end a human life: as an object. As I walked out of the room depressed, one of the sons stopped me to thank me effusively for the wonderful things I had done for his mother's pneumonia. I lost my temper and told him how un-necessary I thought it was for his mother to be in that state. My anger helped no one, not me, not the son, and certainly not the patient. But I resolved never to let that happen again. If patients choose denial, that is their right, which I will cheer-fully respect. But never again will I allow the family's denial to destroy the death of the patient.

Most often, however, even when they disagree initially, the family comes to see that honesty helps not only the patient, but the rest of the family also. It is in-herently a bad situation, it seems to me, when the family knows something the pa-tient does not. A conspiracy of silence develops, which may loosen family bonds at a time when closeness is most important. Perhaps the most painful situations are those in which the dying person knows the truth, but the rest of the family either thinks that the patient does not know or refuses to let the patient talk about his or her illness or fears. When that happens, to the distress of illness is added the loneliness of unburdened fears—not only fears about illness or death, but also fears and problems concerning the children's future, the spouse's life ahead, all the details in the lives of those who will be left after the person dies. Even if the family does not wish to discuss these things with the patient, the physician can do so by making it clear to the patient that he or she is available for open and direct conversation.

It is best when the family takes the opportunity of open knowledge to bring things to closure. Those old pictures of the dying parents giving their blessings and final directives to the remainder of the family are not merely romantic fantasy. When patients are aware and in control of their circumstances, a calmness is present in their rooms, even with a grieving family. Leavetaking becomes a desirable possibility. It may be necessary and useful to have other staff members work with the family. Social workers are increasingly skilled in working both with dying patients and with their families. In some institutions, a team approach has been successful for handling these problems, both before and after the death.[6,22]

While the emotional reactions to impending death in both patient and family can be handled by others, the dying person's doctor cannot remain aloof from them and hope to achieve the goals that I have described. No matter who else comes into the patient's room, there is usually only one identified by the patient as "my doctor." It is that relationship, I believe, that makes the goals achievable. One final word about the family. However well the terminal illness goes from the physician's point of view, the family will not be pleased at the time of death. In this respect, the care of the dying is different from returning others to better function or good health. The survivors have suffered an irremediable loss and tragedy. No parent is so old that it is "all right" when he or she dies. A mother or a father has died, and life will always be different for the survivors now. The family may be relieved that the suffering is over, but guilt seems inevitably to accompany that relief. No matter how aware the doctor is that suffering and distress were minimal, or could have been much worse, the survivors will have perceived suffering, if only because they are suffering. While the family may not appreciate what has been done at the time, they usually become aware eventually of how well things have been handled, and become grateful at the mode of death. The "death with dignity" movement of recent times has led to expectations that death can be almost beautiful, or at least dignified. That is patent nonsense, as physicians know only too well. Our desire is that patients die as much themselves and in command of their death as possible. Nothing can lessen the pain of loss. What we are trying to avoid is making the pain more. And, sadly, a life lived poorly cannot be remade on a deathbed.

THE TERMINAL PHASE

Mrs. Gordon visited her family in New York in the spring of 1976, about 1 year after discharge. I examined her when giving the 5-fluorouracil she still received every 2 weeks. She was cheerful and healthy-appearing, in keeping with the reports I had received. After her husband's retirement, they had moved to Florida. However, her liver was enlarged and nodular. There was no ascites. The extent of metastases had obviously increased. In response to her general question, I told her how well she was doing. If she had asked a direct question about her liver or its nodules (as have other patients), I would have answered equally directly. Her conversation suggested that she had chosen to deny the illness, and I saw no reason to interfere.

She remained well until March 1977, when I got a frightened telephone call that her abdomen was enlarging. Her local physician said he could find nothing. She was soon to come to New York to see her daughter and her just-born third grandchild (this daughter's first child), and I suggested she see me. Moderate ascites was present, the liver was larger, and there was tumor palpable in the old suprapubic incision. She was pessimistic about her future, and was sure "I'm just about finished." I said, "You believe that old tale, don't you? About when a grandchild is born a grandparent dies?" She nodded and said, "Well I know that happens." In our further conversation, I tried to reinforce my statement that her death was not inevitable at this time. I was attempting to reverse her mind-set that she was now dying. It was the only therapeutic tool that might still be useful. It can, within limits, be successful. No one who works with the dying can fail to be impressed by patients' occasional ability to die when they predict, or to stay alive until a predetermined event has occurred, such as a child's graduation, a birth, or a set of holidays. I was attempting to actuate the same phenomenon to restore her balance with her malignancy as I have with other patients. A similar instance is that of the patient with chronic urinary tract infection who remains well and asymptomatic until some other event, physical or emotional, changes the balance, and frank clinical illness ensues. Recovery merely means chronic asymptomatic infection again.

Mrs. Gordon's chemotherapy was advanced to every 10 days. The ascites increased, and she became uncomfortable. A simple, slow, outpatient paracentesis was done by using an intravenous polyethylene catheter. I told her that I could not know, but it was my hope that, just as in the past, the fluid would not reaccumulate. I urged her to get back to her life, and so she returned to Florida. About 1 month later, by telephone, she said that she was tiring easily, but everyone was urging her to be more active. I also urged her on. One week later her fatigability had increased, and she complained of pain in her back, which she blamed on nervousness. I asked that she and her husband come to New York, even though the trip might be difficult. It is very important that the doctor does not urge a patient to function past his or her physical capacity because the patient often takes the blame for failure. Though it is true for all, this is especially important in terminal illness, where the primary resource that has been constructed, reinforced, and depended upon is the patient's sense of being in control. Led to believe that the only reason she was not being more active was "nerves," she might lose her confidence in the control that had served her well for 2 years. On May 18, 1977, the Gordons went from the airport to the emergency room, where I met them. She was obviously ill and jaundiced. Moderate ascites was present, but a tumor mass occupied much of the lower abdomen and liver. The back pain came from a pathologic fracture of the right fourth rib in the posterior axillary line, with a 10-cm tumor mass surrounding. It was only painful when pressed. I did not x-ray her or do other studies. The bone ends could be heard clicking on auscultation.

I explained that she was ill because of her disease, which had gotten worse. The lump on her back, I said, was from her disease. She was relieved that it was not her old back pain. She did not want to hear the word tumor. "Does that mean I'm on my way out?"

"Yes, it may mean that, but I cannot be sure that you won't start getting better again." As initially 2 years earlier she heard only the good news, now she heard only the bad. She wanted to know how long she would live. I explained that if she remained in control and "kept her cool," that she would probably die within 10 days or 2 weeks after she had finished saying goodbye to everyone. I told her that death is not the enemy, and that disease is not the enemy; the enemy is fear. Every symptom that she may have had could be controlled, except weakness. But if she did not get frightened and remained in control, she would have very little pain. I wrote prescriptions for meperidine, chlorpromazine, hydroxyzine, and propoxyphene, and explained in writing how they were to be used. Hydroxyzine is also effective in reducing the amount of analgesics necessary (25 mg or 50 mg four times daily), and usually does not produce as much sedation as chlorpromazine.

She and her husband were dismayed by what I said. Only a few weeks earlier, they said, I had told them everything was going to be fine. I pointed out that I had not said that, but did not press the point. Patients hear when and what they need to hear. Now they could hear bad news. Despite being shocked by the information, she remained calm. Before they left for their daughter's home, I cautioned again that her only real enemy was fear, and that she had done so remarkably well and handled everything so beautifully up until now that I was sure she would be able to do whatever was necessary.

Fear of Death

And fear *is* the enemy, but fear of what? It is generally assumed that dying patients are afraid of death. Some insight into the fear of death is necessary for physicians who care for the dying. How many of us are there who have not given thought to the fear of death? It fills the fantasies of children and adolescents, occupies countless midnight hours in the healthy, and infuses the contemplation of students of the human condition. People mark themselves for a lifetime on how well they have met that fear. Whole cultures and societies develop mechanisms to deny death and handle the fear of its omnipresence. Religions speak directly to the issue, and many people with a deep and abiding belief in God and the hereafter seem little afflicted by a fear of death. From all of this, we know that the fear of death is ubiquitous and that, considering the simple finality of its source, it should be understood easily. I think not, however, and some paradoxes point to its complexity. Generally speaking, the aged fear death less than the young. How odd it is that the closer one gets to death through the natural unfolding of years, the less frightening it becomes. Sir William Osler once wrote

that he could hardly remember a dying patient who was afraid of death. That too
has been my experience. What studies have been done show the same thing.
Avery Weisman concluded that the absence from his subjects of a fear of dying
was an artifact of observation and not a true indication of lack of concern.[23]
More recent work confirms those results, but shows that questions that elicit
below-awareness responses to death-related materials are handled differently by
the dying (but similarly in patients with heart disease and cancer) than they are by
healthy subjects. It is concluded that such responses indicate greater fear of
death.[24]

But concern and fear are very different, and it is an error to confuse the two.
We would be very surprised if the dying had no concern about their impending
death, if it did not occupy their thought.

The fear of death that most of us know is, I believe, quite different. It first
appears in children so young (age 4 or 5) and so devoid of life experience as to
cast doubt that the fear is of the unknown, future nonexistence, or the body's rotting in the grave. What then is the fear of death? In the child, it is the fear of
nothingness, the fear of separation and disappearance, the fear of loss of object
or separation from the object. All these fears have their basis in a very recent
reality for the child. In adults who have a fear of death, the same mechanism is
commonly the basis. We, the living, remote from our own deaths but standing at
the bedside of the dying, must not confuse our own fear of death with the patient's fear of dying. To do so would be to deny dying patients a means to remain
in control of their own deaths. Our fear is a luxury of the living, an abstraction of
our past. The sick deal with the concrete—pain, nausea, thirst, weakness, and the
fear that they will not be able to "take it," and so on. Those are the things that
form the basis of the fears of the dying, and with good reason. But those are
things for which we have excellent tools. Our enemies are not vague apparitions
like the fear of death, but instead are well-grounded apprehensions that are common to all the ill. Doctors have done battle with symptoms like pain and nausea
since the beginning of time, because those things rob patients of independence
and of their ability to rise above the ever-narrowing confines of the dying body.
To the extent that we work against the symptoms and teach patients how to
manage them so that they can maintain control over their own deaths, we are successful in treating the illness called dying.

You might believe that when Sally Gordon heard that death would come, she
would lose all hope and fall apart. But that did not happen. She remained calm
and tranquil. She had things to do. She must say goodbye to her family. She and
her husband were angry with me for a few days, but the anger passed. During one
conversation, she related how her sister suggested she take the current quack an-
ticancer drug, Laetrile. She said, "I told her that was just silly." Not the comment of someone who was hopeless and grasping at straws. We are always hearing that we must not take hope away from our patients by telling them of their
cancer or impending deaths. Yet these patients do not seem without hope or act
hopeless. Others have made the same observations.[25,26] Neither do old people
who know that death is near act hopeless. To know that one will die, therefore, is

not the same as having no hope. On the other hand, hope is a future word, and these patients would seem to have no future. They may not have a day after tomorrow, but they have a tomorrow and they know what it contains. It is not a tomorrow of awful uncertainty, but rather of concrete realities that they have learned to surmount. These are sick people, and the sick are rooted in the concrete present. The larger future abstractions of the healthy do not concern them. Once again, the physician must not confuse personal mentation or the thoughts and dreams of the healthy with the concerns of the sick. To do so may be to deny them what they require—the control of now.

After about 10 days in New York with her sisters, daughter, son-in-law, and grandchild, she went to Atlanta, where her other daughter and family lived. I transmitted the details of her case to the physician who would be caring for her there. During her last visit, I assured her that the doctor knew about her, but that he could call me if needed. She thanked me for everything, the way patients do.

I heard from her son-in-law that after a week or so in Atlanta she began to get quite weak and had to be helped back and forth to the bathroom, which distressed her, as did some rectal bleeding that occurred. She was grateful to be admitted to the hospital. After 2 days, on June 20, 1977, she died, 2 years and 9 months after the original surgery that had shown the metastatic disease. During those 33 months, her total illness disability time, including the surgery and subsequent hospitalizations, was perhaps 2 months, of which 1 month was the terminal illness—a rather typical career for a dying patient who has been treated as I have described.

HOSPITAL VERSUS HOME

It has been pointed out repeatedly that in this era more patients die in institutions and fewer at home. The modern hospital, devoted as it is to the aggressive care of acute illness, is said to be a very poor place to die. That need not be the case. On the other hand, families may be grateful for the opportunity to care for the patient's terminal illness at home. Often the family would like to keep the patient at home, but feels inadequate in the face of the responsibility and what appear to be overwhelming details. Economics may dictate the choice when the patient's insurance will cover hospitalization but not care at home. Even in the absence of insurance coverage, use of community resources and agencies, such as Cancer Care or The Muscular Dystrophy Association, may make home care of the terminal illness possible. Planning is required, and the physician may have to invest considerable time in providing the necessary instruction. Adequate medications to meet almost any contingency should be provided, along with detailed instructions about their use. In this era, many laypersons are capable of handling the most sophisticated drugs, and even injectables. However, if any major barrier, emotional, language, intelligence, or other, suggests that instructions cannot be given or followed, the patient should not be cared for at home. The decision should not be based on current ideology, but rather on what is most desirable and practical.[20]

There is no reason why a terminal illness cannot be handled extremely well in the hospital when the goals are understood. Only things that contribute to comfort should be done. As with Mrs. Gordon, the patient is often grateful to be hospitalized. Some things that are generally avoided, such as the Foley catheter, become objects of mercy, since they allow the patient who is in pain or is extremely weak to avoid moving. Where weakness is very distressing to the patient, it may respond to 15 or 20 mg of prednisone daily in divided doses. This is particularly true of terminal carcinoma of the lung,[20] where the weakness may be attributable to hypercalcemia. Discomfiting anorexia and mild nausea will often improve when the diet contains very little protein. In any case, patients should be reassured that eating is not necessary but that adequate fluid intake will make them more comfortable.

The Relief of Pain

There is absolutely no excuse for suffering caused by pain. Patients in pain require analgesia. The only important criterion for choosing dose and type of drug is whether adequate relief is obtained for an adequate period of time. When an agent appears ineffective it should be changed, the dose increased, and/or the interval between doses shortened. The patient's statement is sufficient evidence that pain has not been relieved. When pain is mild, simple drugs such as codeine given orally are preferable. But where pain is severe, particularly in a patient seen for the first time, give whatever is necessary to stop the pain. Remember that you are not only trying to relieve pain, but to demonstrate to the patient that control is possible and that you can be trusted to help. Although Sally Gordon was given meperidine because she was afraid of morphine, I prefer morphine because it can be given subcutaneously and seems to provide greater comfort. The intramuscular injection of meperidine is in itself painful, and after days of use produces buttocks that look like a purple pincushion. When you do not know whether the patient will become nauseated or vomit with an analgesic, give chlorpromazine or another phenothiazine at the same time. I do not like to substitute retching or vomiting for pain. After initial pain control has been achieved, you may, in working with the patient, try other regimens, in order to produce fewer side effects while maintaining comfort. Orders written ''as needed'' or ''p.r.n.'' have no place in the treatment of pain in fatal disease. I often write my orders this way:

    1   Morphine sulfate 10 mg subcutaneously every 3 hours, unless the patient is asleep or refuses.
    2   Codeine sulfate 30 mg p.o. every 3 hours, unless the patient is asleep or refuses.
    3   Patient may have morphine even if he (or she) has recently had codeine.
    4   The object is to achieve complete relief from pain.

Then I show the order to the nurses and also to the patient, so that both understand the goal. Considerable ingenuity is sometimes required to find the proper drug or combination and the proper timing, because pain patterns differ from patient to patient. Almost invariably when analgesics are given in this manner, the patient's need for medication will quickly diminish within 2 or 3 days. Patients may be avoiding the stronger agents because they do not like the grogginess or other side effects. Some pain may remain, but with fear gone the discomfort may be minimal. Whenever pain has been present for long periods, muscle spasm is almost invariably present, and thus hot or cold application or physical therapy may be useful. Other modalities, such as nerve block, may also be tried when necessary.[27] I have no experience with Brompton's mixture (oral narcotic, cocaine, and alcohol) used at St. Christopher's Hospice in London and elsewhere, [20,28] but I would not hesitate to use it. The basic principle is simple—do whatever is necessary to relieve pain. The success in the management of terminal illness achieved at St. Christopher's comes in part from the recognition that chronic pain is a combination of physical, psychological, and social factors for which analgesics are necessary but not sufficient. The patient must be cared for as a person whose needs, desires, opinions, and fears are respected and dealt with. The patient should never have the sense of being abandoned.

At this late stage in the illness, when death may be near, the family must be given prime consideration. People frequently want to be nearby when a loved one dies, and this should be accommodated when possible. It is misplaced kindness to spare them unhappiness by false optimism or by denying access to a deathbed. I am frequently asked whether a son or daughter should be called back from college, or whether a young child should be told. My answer is invariably yes. The preventive treatment of grief starts before death. In this and other aspects of the care of the dying, the Golden Rule is a good guide.

The physician who has been open, direct, and honest with the patient throughout a fatal illness has an important tool with which to deal with the terminal phase. His or her relationship with the patient will be good, and a strong bond based on performance will have been formed. The patient has seen that the doctors' prognostications have generally been accurate, and symptom relief and other promises have been fulfilled. It is within the power of the doctor-patient relationship for the physician to suggest to the patient that the time has come to die. We spend our lives fighting sickness, regression, disability, and death. Physicians spend their lives in the service of that fight, exhorting and abetting the will to live, the life-force. Call it what you will, measurable or not, we know that the life-force exists, and that it is potent. But there is a time to stop—not merely to stop the application of technology but to actively help the dying patient develop the will to die.

This can be done with the terminally ill in the most practical terms. It is possible to suggest to patients that the time has come to leave, but at the same time to reassure them that it is all right to leave and that it is not going to hurt. When this is explained to patients, you will discover that they become more peaceful; that pain, if present, becomes less severe and more bearable; and that within a relatively short time death follows. Since in the terminally ill what is being done is tantamount to telling the patient to die, one must have the technical and clinical evidence, as well as consultations where indicated, to support that judgment. The doctor must face the responsibility openly. He or she must be certain, in the light of medical science and of personal experience and judgment, that the time has indeed come for the patient to leave. The process is based on trust. The patient is being told that it is permissible, indeed necessary, to stop doing what has been done for a whole life—namely, battling for life—and that it will not hurt. To accept that assurance requires the deep and abiding trust of one human in another. It is not necessary to be blunt or direct, although some patients wish that. One can say "All right, you've done a good job, now just lie back and be peaceful," or "You don't have to struggle with your breathing anymore, just give way and let it happen—like sleep, it won't hurt." As the days go by, you must assure them of what a good job they are doing—and how well they have handled everything. We all deserve praise for things well done, even our dying. They have no standard for comparison, but you do, and you can point that out to the patient and the family. You may not actually ever use the word death or dying, although the word should not be avoided if the patient desires. Those last days are not the time to back away from medications. Morphine with or without chlorpromazine can reduce restlessness, and the patient's clouded consciousness is not a contraindication. Around-the-clock orders are preferable because they relieve the nurses of the burden of decision making. Predicting time of death is difficult, but the family will often want to be near so one does the best one can.[29] It is permissible to make it clear on the chart that the patient is not to be resuscitated, especially if that has been discussed with the family.[30]

The physician's ability to help the patient die comes not only from the patient's trust but from part of a doctor's function, the giving of permission. The social scientists, who have pointed out that physicians validate their patients' illnesses for society, fail to see the constant battle between self and body, between pain and will, that takes place in illness. The disease may be the cause and the social setting may be the stage, but the battle is in the person. It is the physician who gives permission for a person who becomes ill to stop and do battle for the body. And, once health has returned, it is the physician who gives permission to get on with life without fear of or for the body. In the care of the dying the physician can, based on trust and in the service of his or her patient, give permission for the person to stop the battle for life.[31]

Mr. Gordon came to see me early in September. He wanted to tell me about his wife's last days, and to thank me and to express his doubts about some things and clarify others. The visit only took about 20 minutes, but it was very important to him. In those situations I am always somewhat worried that the survivors will be angry with me, but that is not their purpose. They come to effect closure, and it is often several months before they are prepared to do it.

He described her last few days in detail and wondered, typically, whether it would have made any difference if he had brought her to the hospital sooner, when she did not want to go, and whether she should have gotten a blood transfusion a few hours earlier. One wants to dismiss those things as silly—death was inevitable—but should not. I listened until he was finished, and explained that those and the other details he mentioned would not have made a substantial difference. I think the survivors, who inevitably feel guilty no matter how well they have done, really want to ask whether all kinds of things, parts of the past and of the way lives were lived and relationships unfolded, made a difference. But survivors usually do not know or cannot say those things, so they ask about terminal details.

He thanked me for my help and for keeping her alive so long, and wanted me to thank the thoracic surgeon who had handled the chest tube so well. Out of modesty or embarrassment, one tends to brush away the thanks but should not. "Thank you" is the only meaningful gift the survivors have to offer, and it should be accepted gracefully.

He wanted to know more about her disease. I explained in complete detail how much disease and how much evidence of metastases there had been for so long. "I didn't know that," he said, "why didn't you tell me?" I replied that he had not asked, and I saw no purpose—would he have been able to do anything better or act differently if he had known? He agreed. Then he said he was not sure whether it had been correct to tell her, at the end, that she was dying. However, when they discussed it she had told him that she already knew. He left feeling much better.

The care of Mrs. Sally Gordon had ended.

REFERENCES

1 Gilmore, Anne J. J.: "The Care and Management of the Dying Patient in General Practice," *The General Practioner,* **213**:833–842, 1974.

2 Kahn, Sidmund, and Vincent Zarro: "The Management of the Dying," *Seminars in Drug Treatment,* **3**:37–44, 1973.

3 Dunphy, J. Englehert: "Annual Discourse—On Caring for the Patient with Cancer," *N.E.J.M.,* **295**:313–319, 1976.

4 Isaacs, Bernard: "Treatment of the 'Irremedicable' Elderly Patient," *Brit. Med. Jr.,* September 8, 1973, pp. 526–528.

5 Feigenberg, Loma: "Care and Understanding of the Dying: A Patient Centered Approach," *Omega,* **6**:81–93, 1975.

6 Krantz, Melvin J. et al.: "The Role of a Hospital-Based Psychosocial Unit in Terminal Cancer Illness and Bereavement," *J. Chron. Dis.,* **29**:115–127, 1976.

7 Davies, Robert K. et al.: "Organic Factors and Psychological Adjustment in Advanced Cancer Patients," *Psychosom. Med.,* **35**:464–471, 1973.

8 Kraus, Hans: *Clinical Treatment of Back and Neck Pain,* New York: McGraw-Hill, 1970, Chapter 5.

9 Friedman, Henry J.: "Physician Management of Dying Patients: An Exploration," *Psychiat. Med.,* **1**:295–305, 1970.

10 Erickson, Richard C., and Bobbie J. Hyerstay: "The Dying Patient and the Double-Bind Hypothesis," *Omega,* **5**:287–298, 1974.

11 Noyes, Russell, Jr., and Terry A. Travis: "The Care of Terminally Ill Patients," *Arch. Intern. Med.,* **132**:607–611, 1973.

12 Hinton, John: "The Influence of Previous Personality on Reactions to Having Cancer," *Omega,* **6**:95–111, 1975.

13 Pattison, E. Mansell: "Psychosocial Predictions of Death Prognosis," *Omega,* **5**:145–160, 1974.

14 Weisman, Avery D., and J. William Worden: "Psychosocial Analysis of Cancer Deaths," *Omega,* **6:**61-75, 1975.
15 Abrams, Ruth D.: "Denial and Depression in the Terminal Cancer Patient," *Psychiat. Quart.,* **45:**394-404, 1971.
16 Vispo, Raul H.: "Critique of 'Denial and Depression,'" *Psychiat. Quart.,* **45:**405-409, 1971.
17 Johnston, Barbara: "Relief of Mixed Anxiety-Depression in Terminal Cancer Patients," *N.Y.S. J. Med.,* **72:**2315-2317, 1972.
18 Levinson, Peritz: "Obstacles in the Treatment of Dying Patients," *Am. J. Psychiatry,* **132:**28-32, 1975.
19 Cramond, W. A.: "Psychotherapy of the Dying Patient," *Brit. Med. J.,* **3:**389-393, 1970.
20 Twycross, R. G.: "The Terminal Care of Patients with Lung Cancer," *Postgrad. Med. J.,* **49:**732-737, 1973.
21 Binger, C. M. et al.: "Childhood Leukemia: Emotional Impact on Patient and Family," *N.E.J.M.,* **280:**414-418, February 2, 1969.
22 Mount, Balfour M.: "The Problem of Caring for the Dying in a General Hospital: The Palliative Care Unit as a Possible Solution," *Can. Med. Assoc. J.,* **115:**119-121, 1976.
23 Weisman, Avery: *On Dying and Denying,* New York: Behavioral Publications, 1972.
24 Feifel, Herman et al.: "Death Fear in Dying Heart and Cancer Patients," *J. Psychosom. Res.,* **17:**161-166, 1973.
25 Imbus, Sharon H., and Bruce E. Zawacki: "Autonomy for Burn Patients When Survival is Unprecedented," *N.E.J.M.,* **297**(6), 1977.
26 Cassell, Eric J.: "Autonomy and Ethics in Action," *N.E.J.M.,* **297**(6), 1977.
27 Swerdlow, M.: "Relieving Pain in the Terminally Ill," *Geriatrics,* **28:**100-103, 1973.
28 Mount, B. M. et al.: "Use of the Brompton Mixture in Treating the Chronic Pain of Malignant Disease," *Can. Med. Assoc. J.,* **115:**122-124, 1976.
29 Parkes, C. Murray: "Accuracy of Predictions of Survival in Later Stages of Cancer," *Brit. Med. J.,* **2:**29-31, 1972.
30 Bergen, Richard P.: "Management of Terminal Illness: Medicolegal Rounds," *J.A.M.A.,* **229:**1352-1353, 1974.
31 Milton, G. W.: "Self-Willed Death or the Bone-Pointing Syndrome," *Lancet,* **817:**1435-1436, 1973.

BIBLIOGRAPHY

Brin, O. et al. (eds.): *The Dying Patient,* New York: Russell Sage Foundation, 1970.
Glaser, B. G., and A. L. Strauss: *Awareness of Dying,* Chicago: Aldine, 1965.
Grollman, Earl A.: *Concerning Death: A Practical Guide for the Living,* Boston: Beacon Press, 1974.
Kastenbaum, R., and R. Aisenberg: *The Psychology of Death,* New York: Springer, 1972.
Krant, Melvin J.: *Dying and Dignity,* Springfield: Charles C Thomas, 1974.
Weisman, Avery D.: *On Dying and Denying,* New York: Behavioral Publications, 1972.

Appendix

Generic and Trade Names of Some Drugs Commonly Used in Psychiatry

Generic names	Trade names	Generic names	Trade names
Amitriptyline	Amitril, Elavil, Endep	Meperidine	Demerol
Amphetamine	Benzedrine	Meprobamate	Equanil, Miltown
Amphetamine and dextroamphetamine	Biphetamine	Mesoridazine besylate	Serentil
		Methamphetamine	Desoxyn
Benztropin	Cogentin	Methaqualone	Quaalude
Biperiden	Akineton	Methylphenidate	Ritalin
Carphenazine	Proketazine	Methyprylon	Noludar
Chloral hydrate	Noctec	Molindone	Lidone, Moban
Chlordiazepoxide	Librium	Nortriptyline	Aventyl, Pamelor
Chlorpromazine	Thorazine	Nylidrin	Arlidin
Chlorprothixene	Taractan	Oxazepam	Serax
Clorazepate	Azene, Tranxene	Pemoline	Cylert
Deanol	Deaner	Perphenazine	Trilafon
Desipramine	Norpramin, Pertofrane	Phenelzine	Nardil
		Phenmetrazine	Preludin
Dextroamphetamine	Dexedrine	Phenytoin	Dilantin
Diazepam	Valium	Piperacetazine	Quide
Disulfiram	Antabuse	Prazepam	Verstran
Doxepin	Adapin, Sinequan	Prochlorperazine	Compazine
Ethchlorynol	Placidyl	Procyclidine	Kemadrin
Fluphenazine	Permitil, Prolixin	Promazine	Sparine
Flurazepam	Dalmane	Protriptyline	Vivactil
Glutethimide	Doriden	Rauwolfia Serpentina	Raudixin
Haloperidol	Haldol	Reserpine	Rau-sed, Sandril, Serpasil
Hydroxyzine	Atarax, Vistaril		
Imipramine	Imavate, Janimine, Presamine, SK-Pramine, Tofranil	Succinylcholine chloride	Anectine, Sucostrin
		Thioridazine	Mellaril
		Thiothixene	Navane
Isocarboxazid	Marplan	Tranylcypromine	Parnate
Lithium Carbonate	Eskalith, Lithane, Lithonate	Triclofos	Triclos
		Trifluoperazine	Stelazine
Lorazepam	Ativan	Triflupromazine	Vesprin
Loxapine	Daxolin, Loxitane	Trihexyphenidyl	Artane

Index